I0065972

Current Status and Future Perspectives of Gynecological Oncology

Current Status and Future Perspectives of Gynecological Oncology

Edited by Aurora Moran

hayle
medical

New York

Hayle Medical,
750 Third Avenue, 9th Floor,
New York, NY 10017, USA

Visit us on the World Wide Web at:
www.haylemedical.com

© Hayle Medical, 2019

This book contains information obtained from authentic and highly regarded sources. Copyright for all individual chapters remain with the respective authors as indicated. All chapters are published with permission under the Creative Commons Attribution License or equivalent. A wide variety of references are listed. Permission and sources are indicated; for detailed attributions, please refer to the permissions page and list of contributors. Reasonable efforts have been made to publish reliable data and information, but the authors, editors and publisher cannot assume any responsibility for the validity of all materials or the consequences of their use.

ISBN: 978-1-63241-694-0

Trademark Notice: Registered trademark of products or corporate names are used only for explanation and identification without intent to infringe.

Cataloging-in-Publication Data

Current status and future perspectives of gynecological oncology / edited by Aurora Moran.
p. cm.
Includes bibliographical references and index.
ISBN 978-1-63241-694-0
1. Generative organs, Female--Cancer. 2. Cancer in women. 3. Generative organs, Female--Tumors.
4. Gynecology. 5. Oncology. I. Moran, Aurora.
RC280.G5 C87 2019
616.994 65--dc23

Table of Contents

Preface

The purpose of the book is to provide a glimpse into the dynamics and to present opinions and studies of some of the scientists engaged in the development of new ideas in the field from very different standpoints. This book will prove useful to students and researchers owing to its high content quality.

Gynecological oncology is a specialization of gynecology that deals with cancers related to the female reproductive system. After breast cancer, cervical cancer is the second most common cause of female-specific cancer occurring globally. The greatest cause associated with cervical cancer is infection with HPV. Uterine cancer is the tenth most common cause of death due to cancer globally. Vaginal cancer can occur in women of all ages, even in infants. Children diagnosed with cancers can be treated with radiation therapy, surgery and chemotherapy. Vaginectomy is a surgical procedure involving the removal of the complete or part of the vagina. It is performed for the treatment of vaginal cancer. Depending on the severity of the cancer, it can be radical or partial. After a radical vaginectomy, vaginal reconstruction or vaginoplasty may be performed for preserving normalcy in terms of aesthetics. This book provides comprehensive insights into the field of gynecological oncology. From theories to research to clinical applications, case studies related to all contemporary topics of relevance to this field have been included in this book. It includes contributions of experts and scientists, which will provide innovative insights into the current status and future perspectives of this field.

At the end, I would like to appreciate all the efforts made by the authors in completing their chapters professionally. I express my deepest gratitude to all of them for contributing to this book by sharing their valuable works. A special thanks to my family and friends for their constant support in this journey.

Editor

Dasatinib (BMS-35482) potentiates the activity of gemcitabine and docetaxel in uterine leiomyosarcoma cell lines

Micael Lopez-Acevedo[1,5*], Lisa Grace[1], Deanna Teoh[2], Regina Whitaker[1], David J Adams[3], Jingquan Jia[4], Andrew B Nixon[3] and Angeles Alvarez Secord[1]

Abstract

Background: To explore the activity of dasatinib alone and in combination with gemcitabine and docetaxel in uterine leiomyosarcoma (uLMS) cell lines, and determine if dasatinib inhibits the SRC pathway.

Methods: SK-UT-1 and SK-UT-1B uLMS cells were treated with gemcitabine, docetaxel and dasatinib individually and in combination. SRC and paxcillin protein expression were determined pre- and post-dasatinib treatment using Meso Scale Discovery (MSD) multi-array immunogenicity assay. Dose-response curves were constructed and the coefficient of drug interaction (CDI) and combination index (CI) for drug interaction calculated.

Results: Activated phosphorylated levels of SRC and paxillin were decreased after treatment with dasatinib in both cell lines ($p < 0.001$). The addition of a minimally active concentration of dasatinib (IC_{25}) decreased the IC_{50} of each cytotoxic agent by 2-4 fold. The combination of gemcitabine-docetaxel yielded a synergistic effect in SK-UT-1 ($CI = 0.59$) and an antagonistic effect in SK-UT-1B ($CI = 1.36$). Dasatinib combined with gemcitabine or docetaxel revealed a synergistic anti-tumor effect ($CDI < 1$) in both cell lines. The triple drug combination and sequencing revealed conflicting results with a synergistic effect in SK-UT-1B and antagonistic in SK-UT-1.

Conclusion: Dasatinib inhibits the *SRC* pathway and yields a synergistic effect with the two-drug combination with either gemcitabine or docetaxel. The value of adding dasatinib to gemcitabine and docetaxel in a triple drug combination is uncertain, but may be beneficial in select uLMS cell lines. Based on our pre-clinical data and known activity of gemcitabine and docetaxel, further evaluation of dasatinib in combination with these agents for the treatment of uLMS is warranted.

Keywords: Dasatinib, Leiomyosarcoma, SRC pathway, Targeted agents, Uterine sarcoma

Background

Leiomyosarcomas (LMS) are a rare and aggressive type of uterine malignancy that has an extremely poor prognosis. Uterine sarcomas represent only 3-9% of all uterine malignancies and LMS account for 40% of all uterine sarcomas [1,2]. Even in the setting of early-stage disease 53 to 71% of women will develop recurrences that are often extra-pelvic and incurable. The prognosis is dismal with a historical progression-free survival rate at 2 years (PFS$_{2 yrs}$) of only 30% for patients treated with surgery alone [3].

Chemotherapy with a combination of gemcitabine and docetaxel has shown the most promise to date. The overall response rate has ranged from 42% to 53% with a median duration of response of greater than 7 months in women with unresectable LMS [4]. Most recently, adjuvant gemcitabine and docetaxel was evaluated in women with completely resected stage I to IV uterine LMS. The PFS$_{2 yrs}$ was 45% with a median PFS of 13 months and the median survival was not yet reached [3]. Despite these modest improvements, there is an urgent need for innovative therapeutic approaches.

* Correspondence: micael.lopez@duke.edu
[1]Division of Gynecologic Oncology, Duke Cancer Institute, Durham, NC 27710, USA
[5]DUMC 3079, Gynecologic Oncology, Duke University Medical Center, Durham, NC 27710, USA
Full list of author information is available at the end of the article

One novel and promising therapeutic agent is dasatinib (BMS-354825) (NSC 732517). Dasatinib is a potent, orally-bioavailable, small molecule inhibitor that has been shown to inhibit at least five protein tyrosine kinases/kinase families: SRC family kinases, BCR-ABL, c-KIT, EPHA2 and the PDGFβ receptor [5,6]. SRC kinase interacts with a variety of receptor tyrosine kinases such as EGFR, PDGFR, and c-KIT as well as other cellular factors such as focal adhesion kinase (FAK). These pathways are integral components of cellular function and regulate cellular migration, proliferation, survival, angiogenesis, and metastasis. The SRC pathway and its substrates (FAK) as well as c-KIT, EGFR and PDGF tyrosine kinase receptors have been found to be overexpressed in a wide variety of sarcomas including LMS [7-9]. Most recently, Shank et al. showed that EGFR, VEGF and c-KIT is expressed in uterine LMS specimens [9]. In particular, 57% of uterine LMS specimens express c-KIT.

Given the activity of gemcitabine and docetaxel as well as the pre-clinical data regarding the SRC pathway in LMS, we sought to explore the activity of dasatinib (a SRC inhibitor) in combination with these cytotoxic agents in uLMS.

Methods

Drugs
Gemcitabine and docetaxel were purchased from Sigma (St. Louis, MO). Dasatinib (BMS-354825) was provided by Bristol-Myers-Squibb (Princeton, NJ) via the National Cancer Institute (NCI). Dasatinib, gemcitabine and docetaxel were dissolved in dimethylsulfoxide (DMSO). Concentrated stock solutions of all drugs were stored at -25°C.

Cell culture
SK-UT-1 and SK-UT-1B cell lines were obtained from the American Type Culture Collection (Manassas, VA). SK-UT-1 and SK-UT-1B cell lines are uterine in origin. Cell lines were grown and maintained in monolayer culture in RPMI 1640 (Gibco) media supplemented with 10% fetal bovine serum (Hyclone, Logan UT), 1% sodium pyruvate, 100 units/ml penicillin, 100 ug/ml stremptomycin and 1% nonessential amino acids in a humidified chamber containing 5% CO_2.

Meso scale discovery (MSD) analysis
MSD analysis was performed for SRC and paxillin. Paxillin is a SRC pathway substrate that is phosphorylated by SRC and FAK upon integrin binding or growth factor stimulation. Cells were seeded at 3×10^6 cells per plate of each cell line, and allowed to reach confluence over 24 hours. Cells were incubated at 37°C for 24 hours with dasatinib at a escalating concentrations of 30, 100 and 500 nmol/L. Controls were treated with DMSO. Anti-total Src antibody (tSrc) (Cell Signaling Technology, Inc.,

Danvers, MA, Cat#2108), anti-pSrc pY418 antibody (Invitrogen, Carlsbad, CA, Cat# 44660G), anti-total paxillin antibody (Cell Signaling Technology, Inc., Danvers, MA, Cat#2542), or anti-phospho paxillin (Tyr118) antibody (Cell Signaling Technology, Inc., Danvers, MA, Cat#2541) were added at 1ug/ml to bare, goat anti-mouse plates (MSD, Gaithersburg MD), and incubated at room temperature (R.T.) for 1 hour. The plates were washed with TBS/ 0.05% Tween-20 three times and protein lysate from SK-UT-1 (20 ug total protein) or SK-UT-1B (20 ug total protein) cells were added and incubated for 2 hours at R.T. Sulfo-TAG (MSD, Cat#R91AN-1) labeled anti-Src antibody (R&D, Cat# AF3389) were then added to the plates and incubated for 1 hour at room temperature after plates were washed. The plates were imaged and analyzed using a MSD Sector Imager 2400 and associated software. The electroluminescence value was normalized to each control and plotted as a percent of control. Statistical analysis was performed using two-tailed unpaired t-test.

Cell proliferation assay
Tumor cells were seeded at a density of 2,500 cells/well in a 96-well plate, and allowed to reach 70% confluence over 24 hours. Cells were then incubated with each drug at 37°C for 72 hours with escalating doses: docetaxel (0.1 nmol/L-1000 nmol/L), gemcitabine (0.1 nmol/L-100 nmol/L) and dasatinib (10 nmol-4000 nmol/L). Control wells contained RPMI media only. All experiments were done using exponentially proliferating cells. After the 72 hours drug incubation period, 5 μl of ATP luminescence solution was added to each well and cell proliferation was measured by ATP content using the Luminescence ATP cell detection assay system according to manufacturer's recommendations. Experiments to determine the IC_{50} were performed in triplicate.

The percentage of growth inhibition was calculated using the following: survival ratio = # live cells$_{treated\ group}$ /#live cells$_{control\ group}$ × 100. The half maximal inhibitory concentration (IC_{50}) was defined as the drug concentration at which the 50% of the cell growth was inhibited and was analyzed using GraphPad Prism software (version 4.03 San Diego, CA). Single-agent dose response curves were constructed and the IC_{50} for gemcitabine and docetaxel was computed from the best fitting transition functions (determined by F-statistic). The average IC_{50} of all experiments performed was chosen as the final IC_{50}. Given the lack of significant activity of dasatinib as a single-agent, the IC_{25} was calculated from the dose response curve. The cells were subsequently treated with combinations of gemcitabine and docetaxel; dasatinib and gemcitabine; dasatinib and docetaxel; and the three-drug simultaneous and sequential combination of gemcitabine, docetaxel, and dasatinib. For gemcitabine and docetaxel, fixed-ratio molar concentrations ranging from 0.125 to 4 multiples of the single-drug IC_{50} was used. Dasatinib was added at a fixed 1:1 ratio using the IC_{25}.

Two-drug combination effect evaluation and statistical methodologies

The IC_{50} obtained for single-agent gemcitabine and docetaxel was compared to the IC_{50} calculated for each cytotoxic agent after adding dasatinib IC_{25}. To analyze the drug interaction between both cytotoxic agents and dasatinib combined with either agent, the coefficient of drug interaction (CDI) was calculated. CDI is defined by the following formula; $CDI = AB/(A \times B)$ [10,11]. According to the absorbance of the luminescence of each group, AB is the ratio of the two-drug combination group to the control group, and A or B is the ratio of the single drug group to the control group. $CDI < 1$ indicates synergism, $CDI < 0.7$ significant synergism, $CDI = 1$ additivity and $CD > 1$ antagonism [11]. Due to the lack of significant activity of dasatinib and the inability to obtain an IC_{50} for this agent, the CDI formula was utilized to evaluate the anti-proliferative effect between dasatinib and each cytotoxic agent. This formula permits calculation of drug-to-drug interaction without a requisite IC_{50}. All experiments were performed in duplicate.

Triple drug simultaneous and sequential combination effect evaluation and statistical methodologies

To evaluate the growth inhibition effect of dasatinib with gemcitabine and docetaxel in a triple-drug combination, we used the median effect method, which takes into account the potency of each drug combination and the shape of the dose-response curve [12,13]. Composite dose response curves were obtained from three independent experiments and the median effective dose, Dm (equivalent to the IC_{50}) was computed using CalcuSyn software (Biosoft, Cambridge, UK). Drug interaction was assessed by the combination index (CI) method of Chou and Talalay [12,13]:

$$CI = (D)A /(Dx)A + (D)B /(Dx)B + \alpha(D)A (D)B /(Dx)A(Dx)B$$

where D is the dose that yields x% growth inhibition and $\alpha = 0$ for mutually exclusive drugs (the drugs have similar sites of action). Combination index scale was defined as: CI <0.9 synergistic, CI = 0.9-1.1 additive, CI = 1.1-1.2 slight antagonism, CI = 1.2-1.45 moderate antagonism, CI = 1.45-3.3 antagonism, CI = 3.3-10 strong antagonism.

In contrast to the two-drug combination where the CDI formula was used, the median effect (CI formula) method was utilized to evaluate triple-drug interaction. This was possible because both gemcitabine and docetaxel reached an IC_{50} as single agents. For sequencing studies,

drug exposures were separated by 24 hours. The combination index between gemcitabine and docetaxel was computed with and without the addition of dasatinib IC_{25}. All experiments were performed in triplicate.

Results
Meso scale discovery (MSD) analysis
SRC protein expression

The level of SRC activation (pSRC) was determined using MSD analysis. In SK-UT-1, treatment with dasatinib resulted in a loss of SRC activation (pSRC/tSRC) at 30 nm (16%; p < 0.001), 100 nm (8%; p < 0.001) and 500 nm (2%; p < 0.001) (Figure 1). The pSRC signal from SK-UT-1 was at least 15-fold higher than the pSRC signal from the control cells (Additional file 1: Figure S1). In SK-UT-1, there was an increase in tSRC after treatment with single-agent dasatinib at 30 nm (148%, p < 0.001), 100 nm (181%, p < 0001) and 500 nm (172%, p < 0.001) compared to controls (Additional file 2: Figure S2). In contrast, pSRC levels were significantly decreased after treatment with dasatinib at 30 nm (24%, p < 0.001), 100 nm (14%, p < 0.001) and 500 nm (3%, p < 0.001) (Additional file 3: Figure S3).

In SK-UT-1B, there was a loss of SRC activation at 30 nm (11%, p < 0.001), 100 nm (11%, p < 0.001) and 500 nm (5%, p < 0.001) compared to controls (Figure 1). There was a decrease in pSRC levels after treatment with single-agent dasatinib at 30 nm (17%, p < 0.001), 100 nm (7%, p < 0.001) and 500 nm (4%, p < 0.001) and an increase in tSRC after treatment with single-agent dasatinib at 30 nm (152%, p < 0.001), but a decrease at 100 nm (64%, p < 0.001) and 500 nm (74%, p < 0.001) (Additional file 2: Figure S2 and Additional file 3: Figure S3).

Paxillin protein expression

In SK-UT-1, the ratio of p-paxillin/t-paxillin was unchanged after treatment with dasatinib at 30 nm (90%, p < 0.001) and 100 nm (110%, p < 0.001), but there was a significant reduction at 500 nm (16%, p < 0.001) (Figure 2). There was a significant loss of t-paxillin expression after treatment with dasatinib at 500 nm (73%, p = 0.01), but no change at 30 nm (113%, p = 0.06) and 100 nm (92%, p = 0.2) compared to controls (data not shown). Similar results were observed for p-paxillin levels, with a significant loss after treatment with dasatinib at 500 nm (11%, p < 0.001), but no change at 30 nm (100%) or 100 nm (100%) (data not shown).

In SK-UT-1B, activation of paxillin (p-paxillin/t-paxillin) was significantly inhibited by the presence of dasatinib at 30 nm (76%), 100 nm (1%) and 500 nm (3%) (Figure 2). There was an increase in t-paxillin expression after treatment with dasatinib at 100 nm (198%, p < 0.001), but no change at 30 nm (76%, p = 0.02) or 500 nm (93%, p = 0.2) (data not shown). The expression of p-paxillin was reduced by 42% after treatment with dasatinib at 30 nm (p < 0.001)

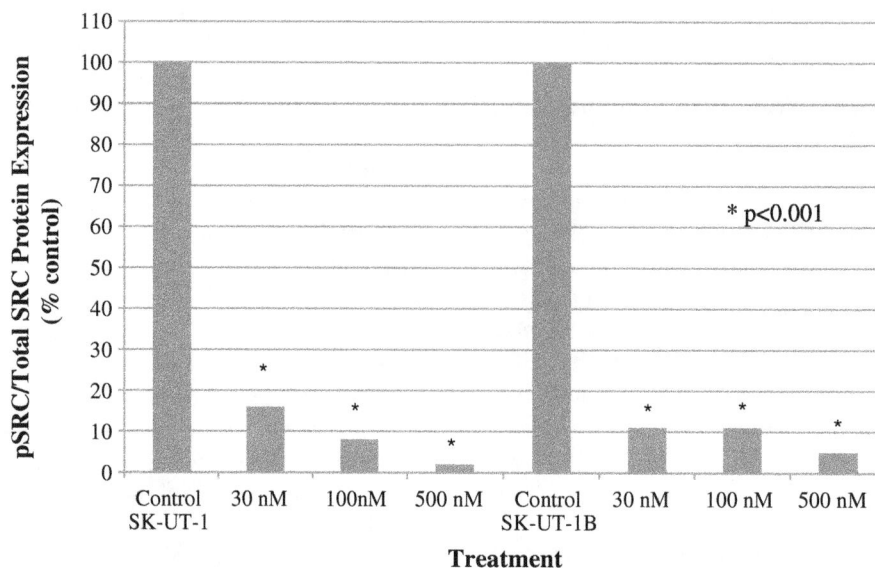

Figure 1 The pSRC/tSRC ratio after treatment with single-agent dasatinib. In SK-UT-1, activation of the SRC kinase (pSRC/tSRC) pathway was inhibited by dasatinib at 30 nm (84%), 100 nm (92%) and 500 nm (98%). In SK-UT-1B, the SRC kinase activity was reduced in the presence of dasatinib at 30 nm (91%), 100 nm (91%) and 500 nm (95%).

and by 97% (p < 0.001) at 100 and 500 nm (data not shown).

Anti-proliferative activity of single-agent gemcitabine, docetaxel and dasatinib

The IC_{50} for gemcitabine and docetaxel as single agents was calculated for each cell line (Table 1). Growth inhibition with dasatinib was first detected at 100 nmol for

SK-UT-1 (21.7% inhibition) and for SK-UT-1B (32.8%). Using increasing concentrations of dasatinib, the maximal growth inhibitory effect of dasatinib for SK-UT-1 was 42.8% (1000 nm) and 55.5% (4000 nm) for SK-UT-1B (Figure 3). The dasatinib IC_{50} for SK-UT-1B was 381 nmol/L. Higher concentrations did not achieve greater growth inhibition. In the SK-UT-1 cell line an IC_{50} was not reached. The IC_{25} (25% growth inhibition)

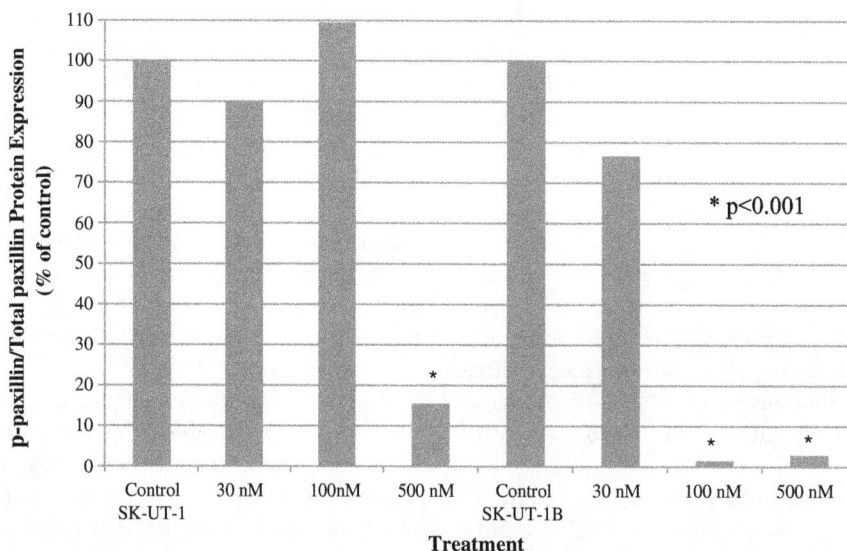

Figure 2 The p-paxillin/t-paxillin ratio after treatment with single-agent dasatinib. Activation of paxillin (p-paxillin/t-paxillin) was inhibited by the presence of dasatinib at 500 nm in SK-UT-1 (16%); and 30 nm (14%), 100 nm (1%) and 500 nm (3%) in SK-UT-1B.

Table 1 IC$_{50}$ of each cytotoxic agent alone and in combination with dasatinib (IC$_{25}$) and coefficient of drug interaction (CDI)

Cell Line	Drugs	IC$_{50}$	CDI
SK-UT-1			
	Gemcitabine	4.02 (SD ± 1.0)	
	Docetaxel	4.30 (SD ± 0.5)	
	Gemcitabine:Dasatinib IC$_{25}$	2.35 (SD ± 1.4)	0.72
	Docetaxel:Dasatinib IC$_{25}$	1.15 (SD ± 0.07)	0.80
SK-UT-1B			
	Gemcitabine	2.97 (SD ± 0.5)	
	Docetaxel	0.94 (SD ± 0.6)	
	Gemcitabine:Dasatinib IC$_{25}$	0.85 (SD ± 0.6)	0.83
	Docetaxel:Dasatinib IC$_{25}$	0.52 (SD ± 0.4)	0.93

SD = standard deviation.
IC$_{50}$ = 50% of maximal inhibitory concentration.
IC$_{25}$ = 25% of maximal inhibitory concentration.
CDI = Coefficient of drug interaction. Calculation utilize when one drug does not achieve an IC$_{50}$.
CDI scale = CDI < 1 indicates synergism between dasatinib and cytotoxic agents, whereas CDI < 0.7 indicates significant synergism.

was therefore calculated from dose response curves for each cell line. The IC$_{25}$ for dasatinib was 100 nm for both cell lines.

Drug interaction assessment for combination dasatinib and cytotoxic chemotherapy

The IC$_{25}$ of dasatinib calculated for each cell line was used in combination with different concentrations of gemcitabine (e.g. 10, 7.5, 5, 2.5, 1 nm) and docetaxel (e.g. 40, 20, 10, 5, 1 nm) mixed at a fixed ratio (1:1), respectively. The IC$_{50}$ obtained from the single agent response curves for both gemcitabine and docetaxel was then compared to the IC$_{50}$ calculated after adding dasatinib (IC$_{25}$). Results showed that the minimally active dose of

dasatinib reduced the IC$_{50}$ of both gemcitabine and docetaxel for each cell line ranging from 2:1 to 4:1 (2-4 fold inhibition) (Table 1) (Figure 4).

For SK-UT-1 and SK-UT-1B, the combination of gemcitabine-dasatinib at all concentrations analyzed demonstrated decreased cell viability (Figure 5A and E) and yielded a CDI <1 indicating synergistic effects (average CDI = 0.72 and 0.83 for SK-UT-1 and SK-UT-1B, respectively) (Figure 5B and F). Similarly, in both cell lines the combination of docetaxel-dasatinib demonstrated decreased cell viability (Figure 5C and G) and synergistic effects (average CDI = 0.80 and 0.93 for SK-UT-1 and SK-UT-1B, respectively) (Figure 5D and H).

The median effect analysis for combining gemcitabine and docetaxel revealed synergistic effect in SK-UT-1 (CI = 0.59) and moderate antagonism in SK-UT-1B (CI = 1.36) (Table 2). The results of the simultaneous and sequential drug experiments using dasatinib IC$_{25}$, gemcitabine and docetaxel in a triple-drug combination are shown in Table 2. The greatest anti-proliferative activity (synergistic) in SK-UT-1 was seen with the simultaneous triple-drug combination of dasatinib, gemcitabine and docetaxel (CI = 0.46). The remainder of the sequential triple-drug combinations revealed a moderate antagonistic effect (CI = 1.07-1.8) (Table 2). In SK-UT-1B, the simultaneous triple-drug combination of gemcitabine, docetaxel and dasatinib revealed moderate antagonistic effect (anti-proliferative effect (CI = 1.4)). Sequential dasatinib followed by combination gemcitabine and docetaxel as well as gemcitabine followed by combination docetaxel and dasatinib yielded synergistic effects (CI = 0.9 for both). In contrast, combination dasatinib and docetaxel followed by gemcitabine demonstrated an additive effect (CI = 1.0). The remaining sequential combinations produced an antagonistic effect (CI ranging from 1.21-1.5) (Table 2).

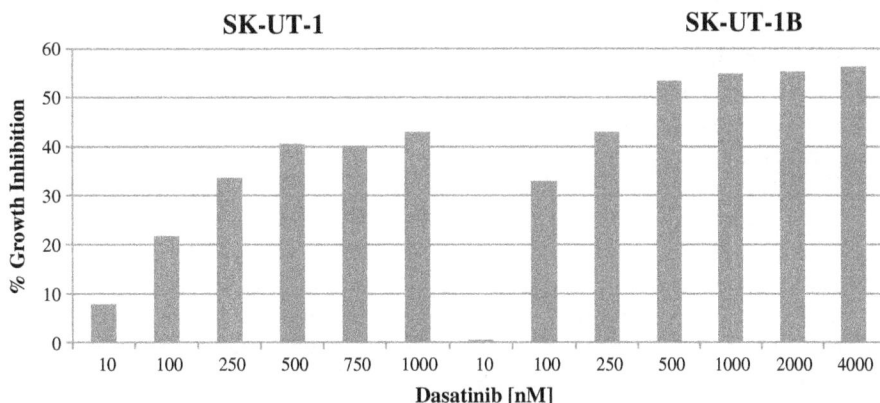

Figure 3 Growth inhibition assay. Dasatinib showed minimal to modest activity against leiomyosarcoma cell lines. Maximal growth inhibitory effect for SK-UT-1 and SK-UT-1B was 42.8% and 55% respectively.

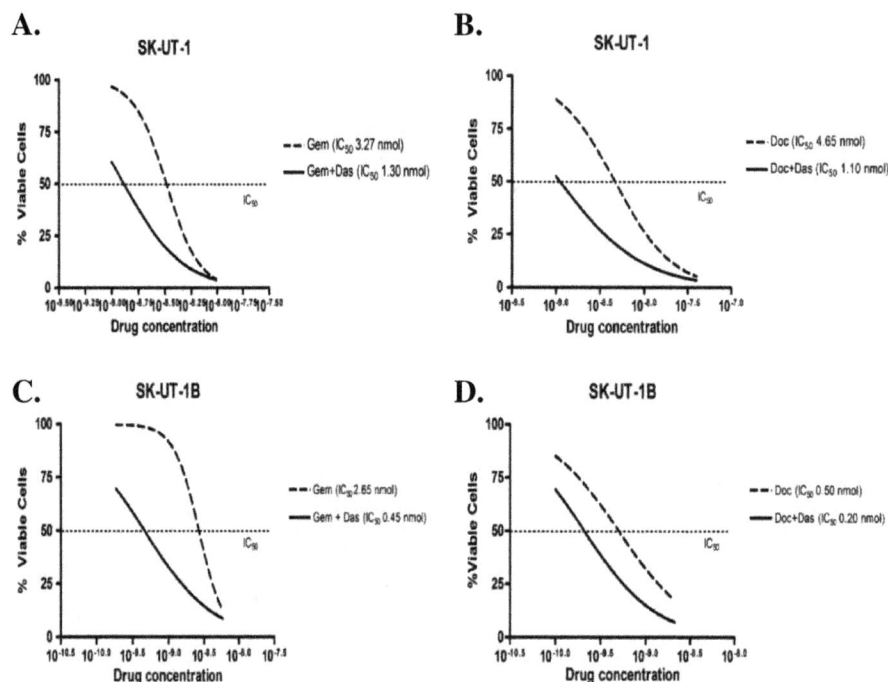

Figure 4 IC$_{50}$ obtained from single agent response curves for gemcitabine and docetaxel was compared to the IC$_{50}$ obtained after adding dasatinib at a minimally active concentration (IC$_{25}$). Graphics above represents the results of a single experiment for SK-UT-1 (**A & B**) and SK-UT-1B (**C & D**). (Gem = gemcitabine; Das = dasatinib; Doc = docetaxel).

Discussion and conclusion

Dasatinib has not been shown to be a potent agent when used alone in a variety of solid tumors [14]. Schrage *et al.* previously reported their findings of dasatinib in chondrosarcoma cell lines [15]. The maximum percent of growth inhibition in the chondrosarcoma cell lines was approximately 50%. They also explored dasatinib's effect on SRC phosphorylation and caspase-3- mediated apoptosis. Although dasatinib treatment of chondrosarcoma decreased SRC phosphorylation, indicating target inhibition, it did not result in an increase in apoptosis. Therefore, the inhibition of SRC and its family of kinases was not sufficient to promote cell death. In a large clinical trial of patients with incurable sarcoma, which included 47 participants with LMS, dasatinib did not have a significant anti-tumor activity as a single agent [16]. Based on pre-clinical and clinical data, it appears that single agent dasatinib does not have significant clinical activity in soft tissue sarcomas.

However, our pre-clinical study investigating the activity of dasatinib in combination with gemcitabine and docetaxel in uterine LMS demonstrates that dasatinib acts synergistically with gemcitabine or docetaxel in a two-drug combination and in select triplet combinations in the analyzed uterine LMS cell lines. Our findings in sequential and triple combination yielded conflicting results. Interestingly, the simultaneous triple-drug combination of dasatinib IC$_{25}$, gemcitabine and docetaxel in SK-UT-1 yielded a synergistic effect, although the magnitude of that effect is probably minimal (CI = 0.59 to 0.46). Conversely, the gemcitabine and docetaxel doublet demonstrated an antagonistic effect in SK-UT-1B cells and that effect was not reversed with the addition of dasabinib in the simultaneous triple-drug combination. However, in select sequencing experiments, dasatinib enhanced the anti-proliferative effect of gemcitabine and docetaxel; gemcitabine + docetaxel + dasatinib; dasatinib followed by docetaxel + gemcitabine; and gemcitabine followed by docetaxel + dasatinib. In the latter two experiments, this finding may be due to avoidance of the antagonistic interaction of the gemcitabine and docetaxel doublet in the SK-UT-1B cell line as well as partially attributed to the synergistic effect of the dasatinib doublet. The results with the sequential dasatinib followed by combination gemcitabine and docetaxel indicate a possible role for priming with dasatinib.

We hypothesize that our synergistic findings may in part be due to the inhibition of the SRC pathway. Our MSD analysis revealed that dasatinib inhibited the SRC pathway based on reduction of pSRC and p-paxillin protein expression and ratios pSRC/tSRC and p-paxcillin/t-paxillin. Even at very low doses of dasatinib (30 nM), the SRC pathway was inhibited in both uLMS cell lines. This suggests that an optimal biologic effect on SRC can occur with low doses of dasatinib. However, expression of paxillin was only inhibited at high doses. A possible

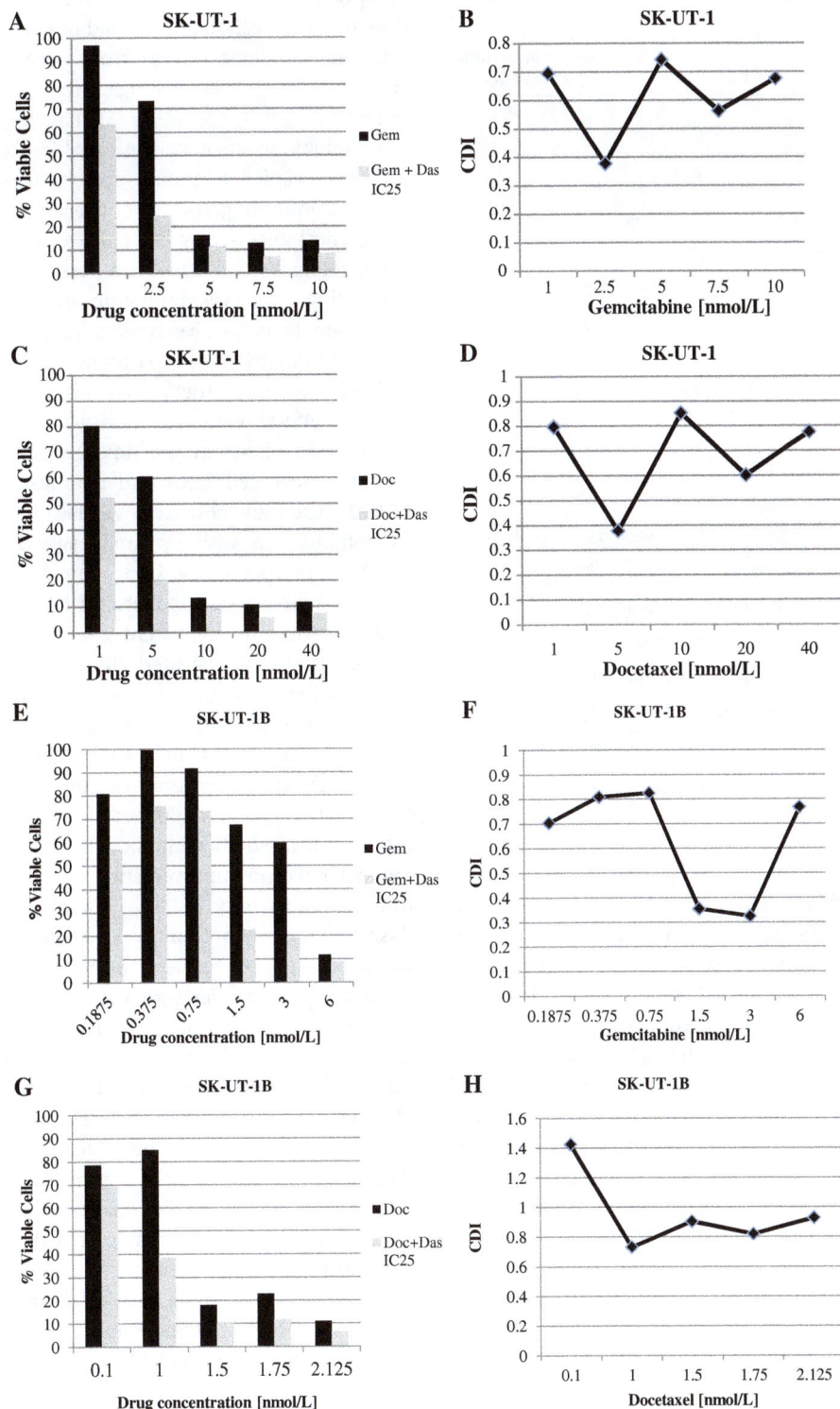

Figure 5 The inhibitory effect of gemcitabine and docetaxel at different concentrations combined with dasatinib IC$_{25}$ and the coefficient of drug interaction (CDI). CDI < 1 indicates synergism, CDI < 0.7 significant synergism, CDI = 1 additivity and CD > 1 antagonism. In SK-UT-1, the combination of gemcitabine-dasatinib, at all concentrations analyzed demonstrated decreased cell viability **(A)** and yielded a CDI <1 indicating synergistic effects (average CDI = 0.72) **(B)**; the combination of docetaxel-dasatinib demonstrated decreased cell viability **(C)** and synergistic effects (average CDI = 0.80) **(D)**. In SK-UT-1B the combination of gemcitabine-dasatinib, at all concentrations analyzed demonstrated decreased cell viability **(E)** and yielded a CDI <1 indicating synergistic effects (average CDI = 0.83) **(F)**; the combination of docetaxel-dasatinib demonstrated decreased cell viability **(G)** and synergistic effects (CDI = 0.93) **(H)**.

Table 2 The combination index (CI) in uterine LMS cell lines

Cell Line	Drugs	Combination index (CI) at the IC$_{50}$
SK-UT-1		
	Gemcitabine:Docetaxel	0.59
	Gemcitabine + Docetaxel + Dasatinib	0.46
	Dasatinib- > Gemcitabine + Docetaxel	1.77
	Gemcitabine + Docetaxel- > Dasatinib	1.14
	Dasatinib + Gemcitabine- > Docetaxel	1.32
	Dasatinib + Docetaxel- > Gemcitabine	1.07
	Gemcitabine- > Docetaxel + Dasatinib	1.8
	Docetaxel- > Gemcitabine + Dasatinib	N/D
SK-UT-1B		
	Gemcitabine:Docetaxel	1.36
	Gemcitabine + Docetaxel + Dasatinib	1.4
	Dasatinib- > Gemcitabine + Docetaxel	0.9
	Gemcitabine + Docetaxel- > Dasatinib	1.36
	Dasatinib + Gemcitabine- > Docetaxel	1.21
	Dasatinib + Docetaxel- > Gemcitabine	1.0
	Gemcitabine- > Docetaxel + Dasatinib	0.9
	Docetaxel- > Gemcitabine + Dasatinib	1.5

Combination index scale: CI <0.9 synergistic, CI = 0.9-1.1 additive, CI = 1.1-1.2 slight antagonism,
CI = 1.2-1.45 moderate antagonism, CI = 1.45-3.3 antagonism, CI = 3.3-10 strong antagonism.
N/D = not determined.

explanation for this is that downstream substrates of SRC pathway may be activated via different pathways. The SRC pathway is a complex pathway with convergent and divergent interactions. It is not clear that the anti-proliferative effect we noted in our study was a direct result of inhibition of the SRC pathway. Most recently, Shank et al. showed that EGFR, VEGF and especially c-KIT were expressed in uterine LMS specimens [9]. In particular, 57% of uterine LMS specimens expressed c-KIT. Therefore, dasatinib's anti-proliferative effect seen in our study may be via the inhibition of the c-KIT pathway in addition to or instead of inhibition of the SRC pathway.

Another important property of dasatinib not related to cytotoxicity, lies in its ability to inhibit migration and cell invasion. Dasatinib has been shown to inhibit cell migration in non-small cell lung cancer, head and neck squamous cell cancer, neuroblastoma, and multiple soft tissue and bone sarcoma cell lines [8,17,18]. Johnson and colleagues reported that the anti-migratory effects of dasatinib were present regardless of the effects seen on proliferation and survival [17]. In addition, Shor et al. showed that dasatinib significantly inhibited cellular invasion using matrigel invasion chambers. With the

exception of one rhabdomyosarcoma cell line, the IC$_{50}$ dose to inhibit cell migration and invasion in the soft tissue sarcoma cell lines ranged from 4-65 nmol/L and was similar to the IC$_{50}$ dose (range 3 nmol/L to 68 nmol/L) to inhibit SRC phosphorylation [8]. This finding suggests that SRC inhibition may be responsible for suppression of sarcoma cellular migration and invasion. The universal effects seen on migration and invasion suggest that beneficial clinical effects may be achieved without direct cancer cell cytotoxicity and provides a possible role of dasatinib in preventing metastasis. Inhibition of metastasis is especially important in aggressive tumors such as LMS which are known to rapidly spread to distant sites.

While we and others have reported synergistic and additive effects with dasatinib and a variety of chemotherapeutic agents in preclinical studies of ovarian and breast cancer cell lines and ovarian cancer xenografts [19-21], the clinical activity of dasatinib either alone or in combination with cytotoxic agents in solid tumors has been disappointing. In a phase I trial of dasatinib in combination with paclitaxel and carboplatin in patients with advanced or recurrent ovarian cancer, the triplet combination demonstrated clinical activity but was also associated with a higher than expected rate of hematologic toxicity. Pharmacokinetic analysis showed that concurrent administration of dasatinib with paclitaxel did not significantly alter either dasatinib or paclitaxel drug concentrations [14]. Two randomized studies of another SRC inhibitor, saracatinib, with chemotherapy in ovarian cancer demonstrated no improvement in response rate or survival, but higher toxicity [22,23]. Therefore, the addition of dasatinib to chemotherapy is unlikely to be beneficial in an unselected patient population and there is a need to identify biomarkers that can be used to direct therapy. Of note, these studies used the maximum tolerated dose (MTD). In our data, we observed an increased antiproliferative effect of dasatinib in combination with cytotoxic agents at a minimal active dose. Hence, combination effects may be beneficial at lower doses of dasatinib in the treatment of uterine leiomyosarcoma.

Up-regulation of the SRC pathway has been shown to be associated with resistance to cytotoxic therapy. In mucinous ovarian cancer cell lines, Matsuo et al. revealed that treatment with oxaliplatin induced phosphorylation of SRC kinase and this contributed to the chemoresistance observed in this tumor. This induced activity was subsequently inhibited by concurrent administration of dasatinib, which resulted in a synergistic anti-tumor effect [24].

To our knowledge, there are no clinical trials that have evaluated the toxicity of gemcitabine and docetaxel in combination with dasatinib. In a prospective trial of women with completely resected uterine leiomyosarcoma, treatment with gemcitabine plus docetaxel was generally well-tolerated.

Potential serious toxicities associated with gemcitabine plus docetaxel in the advanced disease setting included pulmonary toxicity and myelosuppression requiring administration of granulocyte-colony stimulating factor [3]. Based on our prior experience, we anticipate that the addition of dasatinib to gemcitabine and docetaxel would be associated with even greater hematologic toxicity. A phase I evaluation would be required to determine if biologically relevant doses could be delivered with the triplet combination. However, the disparate sequential combination results in our cell lines was not expected and requires further study. Alternatively, doublet therapy with dasatinib plus gemcitabine or docetaxel may be more effective than triplet therapy.

We acknowledge the limitations of our study, which include the use of only two LMS cell lines rather than primary tumor, and the use of *in vitro* models. Further investigation in *in vivo* models is warranted to confirm our *in vitro* results. Further study is also needed to determine if dasatinib exerts its function via inhibition of the SRC pathway or via other tyrosine kinases, such as BCR-ABL, c-KIT, EPHA2, EGFR and PDGF, or a combination. In summary, we are the first to report an anti-proliferative effect of dasatinib in combination with cytotoxic agents in uterine leiomyosarcoma.

Competing interest

The authors declare that they have no competing interests to be disclosed.

Authors' contributions

AAS, DT, DJA and MLA provided substantial contributions to conception and design, acquisition, interpretation of data, drafting the article and final approval of the version to be published. LG and RW were responsible for supervising proper laboratory techniques and assure compliance with established protocols. They actively participated in all laboratories task including: growth of cell cultures, mixing chemotherapy agents in investigation with cell lines and recording results. They provided substantial contributions to drafting the article and final approval of the version to be published. JJ and ABN performed all immunogenicity assays and provided substantial contributions to drafting the article and final approval of the version to be published. All authors agree to be accountable for all aspects of the work in ensuring that questions related to the accuracy or integrity of any part of the work are appropriately investigated and resolved.

Acknowledgments

We thank the Charles Hammond Research Fund and the Sandra H. Barbeau Foundation for granting financial assistance to conduct this project the National Cancer Institute for providing the cytotoxic agents.

Author details

[1]Division of Gynecologic Oncology, Duke Cancer Institute, Durham, NC 27710, USA. [2]Division of Gynecologic Oncology, University of Minnesota, Minneapolis, MN 55455, USA. [3]Department of Medicine, Duke University Medical Center, Durham, NC 27710, USA. [4]East Carolina University School of Medicine, Greenville, NC 27834, USA. [5]DUMC 3079, Gynecologic Oncology, Duke University Medical Center, Durham, NC 27710, USA.

References

1. Nordal RR, Thoresen SO: Uterine sarcomas in Norway 1956-1992: incidence, survival and mortality. *Eur J Cancer* 1997, **33**(6):907–11.

2. Lurain J, Piver M: Uterine sarcomas: clinical features and management. In *Gynecological Oncology*. Edited by Coppleson M. Edinburgh; London; Melbourne: Churchill Livingstone; 1992:827–42.

3. Hensley ML, Ishill N, Soslow R, Larkin J, Abu-Rustum N, Sabbatini P, Konner J, Tew W, Spriggs D, Aghajanian CA: Adjuvant gemcitabine plus docetaxel for completely resected stages I-IV high grade uterine leiomyosarcoma: Results of a prospective study. *Gynecol Oncol* 2009, **112**(3):563–7.

4. Hensley ML, Maki R, Venkatraman E, Geller G, Lovegren M, Aghajanian C, Sabbatini P, Tong W, Barakat R, Spriggs DR: Gemcitabine and docetaxel in patients with unresectable leiomyosarcoma: results of a phase II trial. *J Clin Oncol* 2002, **20**(12):2824–31.

5. Luo FR, Barrett YC, Yang Z, Camuso A, McGlinchey K, Wen ML, Smykla R, Fager K, Wild R, Palme H, Galbraith S, Blackwood-Chirchir A, Lee FY: Identification and validation of phospho-SRC, a novel and potential pharmacodynamic biomarker for dasatinib (SPRYCEL), a multi-targeted kinase inhibitor. *Cancer Chemother Pharmacol* 2008, **62**(6):1065–74.

6. Lombardo LJ, Lee FY, Chen P, Norris D, Barrish JC, Behnia K, Castaneda S, Cornelius LA, Das J, Doweyko AM, Fairchild C, Hunt JT, Inigo I, Johnston K, Kamath A, Kan D, Klei H, Marathe P, Pang S, Peterson R, Pitt S, Schieven GL, Schmidt RJ, Tokarski J, Wen ML, Wityak J, Borzilleri RM: Discovery of N-(2-chloro-6-methyl- phenyl)-2-(6-(4-(2-hydroxyethyl)-piperazin-1-yl)-2-methylpyrimidin-4- ylamino)thiazole-5-carboxamide (BMS-354825), a dual Src/Abl kinase inhibitor with potent antitumor activity in preclinical assays. *J Med Chem* 2004, **47**(27):6658–61.

7. Weiner TM, Liu ET, Craven RJ, Cance WG: Expression of growth factor receptors, the focal adhesion kinase, and other tyrosine kinases in human soft tissue tumors. *Ann Surg Oncol* 1994, **1**(1):18–27.

8. Shor AC, Keschman EA, Lee FY, Muro-Cacho C, Letson GD, Trent JC: Dasatinib inhibits migration and invasion in diverse human sarcoma cell lines and induces apoptosis in bone sarcoma cells dependent on SRC kinase for survival. *Cancer Res* 2007, **67**(6):2800–8.

9. Shank J, Frisch N, Rhode J, Liu J: Identification of Molecular Markers for Targeted Treatment of Uterine Sarcomas. *Gynecol Oncol* 2013, **131**(1):282.

10. Cao SS, Zhen YS: Potentiation of antimetabolite antitumor activity in vivo by dipyridamole and amphotericin B. *Cancer Chemother Pharmacol* 1989, **24**(3):181–6.

11. Xu SP, Sun GP, Shen YX, Peng WR, Wang H, Wei W: Synergistic effect of combining paeonol and cisplatin on apoptotic induction of human hepatoma cell lines. *Acta Pharmacol Sin* 2007, **28**(6):869–78.

12. Chou TC: Theoretical basis, experimental design, and computerized simulation of synergism and antagonism in drug combination studies. *Pharmacol Rev* 2006, **58**(3):621–81.

13. Chou TC, Talalay P: Quantitative analysis of dose-effect relationships: the combined effects of multiple drugs or enzyme inhibitors. *Adv Enzyme Regul* 1984, **22**:27–55.

14. Secord AA, Teoh DK, Barry WT, Yu M, Broadwater G, Havrilesky LJ, Lee PS, Berchuck A, Lancaster J, Wenham RM: A phase I trial of dasatinib, an SRC-family kinase inhibitor, in combination with paclitaxel and carboplatin in patients with advanced or recurrent ovarian cancer. *Clin Cancer Res* 2012, **18**(19):5489–98.

15. Schrage YM, Briaire-de Bruijn IH, de Miranda NF, van Oosterwijk J, Taminiau AH, van Wezel T, Hogendoorn PC, Bovée JV: Kinome profiling of chondrosarcoma reveals SRC-pathway activity and dasatinib as option for treatment. *Cancer Res* 2009, **69**(15):6216–22.

16. Schuetze S, Wathen K, Choy E, Samuels BL, Ganjoo KN, Staddon AP, von Mehren M, Chow WA, Trent JC, Baker LH: Results of a Sarcoma Alliance for Research through Collaboration (SARC) phase II trial of dasatinib in previously treated, high-grade, advanced sarcoma. *J Clin Oncol* 2010, **28**(suppl; abstr 10009):15s.

17. Johnson FM, Saigal B, Talpaz M, Donato NJ: Dasatinib (BMS-354825) tyrosine kinase inhibitor suppresses invasion and induces cell cycle arrest and apoptosis of head and neck squamous cell carcinoma and non-small cell lung cancer cells. *Clin Cancer Res* 2005, **11**(19 Pt 1):6924–32.

18. Timeus F, Crescenzio N, Fandi A, Doria A, Foglia L, Cordero di Montezemolo L: In vitro antiproliferative and antimigratory activity of dasatinib in neuroblastoma and Ewing sarcoma cell lines. *Oncol Rep* 2008, **19**(2):353–9.

19. Teoh D, Ayeni TA, Rubatt JM, Adams DJ, Grace L, Starr MD, Barry WT, Berchuck A, Murphy SK, Secord AA: **Dasatinib (BMS-35482) has synergistic activity with paclitaxel and carboplatin in ovarian cancer cells.** *Gynecol Oncol* 2011, **121**(1):187–92.

20. Chen T, Pengetnze Y, Taylor CC: **Src inhibition enhances paclitaxel cytotoxicity in ovarian cancer cells by caspase-9-independent activation of caspase-3.** *Mol Cancer Ther* 2005, **4**(2):217–24.

21. Company BMS: **Preclinical pharmacology of dasatinib, a SRC protein kinase inhibitor.** 2003, Control No. 930003300.

22. Poole C, Lisyanskaya A, Rodenhuis S, Kristensen G, Pujade-Lauraine E, Cantarini M, Emeribe U, Stuart M, Ray CI: **A randomized phase II clinical trial of the SRC inhibitor saracatinib (AZD0530) and carboplatin 1 paclitaxel (C1P) versus C1P in patients with advanced platinumsensitive epithelial ovarian cancer.** *Ann Oncol* 2010, **21**(Suppl 8):S313.

23. McNeish IA, Ledermann JA, Webber LC, James LE, Kaye SB, Rustin GJS, Hall G, Clamp A, Earl HM, Banerjee SN, Kristeleit RS, Raja F, Feeney A, Lawrence C, Dawson-Athey L, Persic M, Khan I: *A Randomized Placebo-Controlled Trial of Saracatinib (AZD0530) Plus Weekly Paclitaxel in Platinum-Resistant Ovarian, Fallopian-Tube, Or Primary Peritoneal Cancer (SaPPrOC).* Chicago, IL: American Society of Clinical Oncology annual meeting; 2013.

24. Matsuo K, Nishimura M, Bottsford-Miller JN, Huang J, Komurov K, Armaiz-Pena GN, Shahzad MM, Stone RL, Roh JW, Sanguino AM, Lu C, Im DD, Rosenshien NB, Sakakibara A, Nagano T, Yamasaki M, Enomoto T, Kimura T, Ram PT, Schmeler KM, Gallick GE, Wong KK, Frumovitz M, Sood AK: **Targeting SRC in mucinous ovarian carcinoma.** *Clin Cancer Res* 2011, **17**(16):5367–78.

2

Fifth annual workshop of cytoreductive surgery for advanced ovarian cancer and peritoneal surface malignancies

Krishnansu S. Tewari

Abstract

The Fifth Annual Advanced Course in Cytoreductive Surgery for Ovarian Cancer and Peritoneal Surface Malignances was held at and sponsored by the Division of Gynecologic Oncology at the the University of California, Irvine on Friday and Saturday, October 9-10, 2015. The workshop was comprised of didactic modules, historical treatise, an impassioned tribute, a cadaver laboratory, and heated intraperitoneal chemotherapy demonstration. This was a not-for-profit workshop, and registration fees were used to support course faculty travel to U.C. Irvine and to pay for the cadavers. The original 56 available spots were filled within three weeks of the initial announcement, prompting procurement of two additional cadavers to satisfy registration overflow and accommodate the six U.C. Irvine fellows-in-training. While international participation in the Workshops continues to rise, we have also noted more U.S.-trained Gynecologic Oncologists among the registrants.

Keywords: Ovarian cancer, Cytoreduction, Workshop

Introduction: ovarian cancer – the clinical problem

Cytoreductive surgery followed by adjuvant systemic platinum- and taxane-based combination chemotherapy continues to represent standard treatment of advanced ovarian cancer. Median 10-year survival rates, however, are still below 20 %, even as the optimal debulking paradigm has evolved from 1 cm^3 residual volume of disease to that of complete resection (ie, microscopic residual or R_0) [1]. Enthusiasm for initially promising advancements in therapeutic dosing, scheduling and route of delivery, including weekly dose-dense pacliltaxel [2, 3] and combined intraveneous/intraperitoneal chemotherapy [4, 5], has been curtailed in recent months [6–8]. Furthermore, despite eight positive, phase III, randomized trials involving five different anti-angiogenesis agents [9], vascular endothelial growth factor inhibition has only been able to significantly improve progression-free survival, not overall survival (OS). Although supporters of antivascular strategies continue to regard PFS as a valid endpoint because post-progression therapy cannot be controlled in

the clinical trial setting [10], recent translational work suggests that the genomic instability which underlies ovarian carcinoma produces a phenotype comprised of different subgroups (eg., immune, *pro-angiogenic*) that limit the reach of the presumably wide net cast by anti-angiogenesis therapy [11]. The concept of oncogene addiction does not apply to this disease as prevalent driver mutations have not yet been identified [12]. Current research aims to identify and exploit somatic and germline homologous recombination deficiency mutations (eg, *BRCA1, BRCA2, RAD51*, etc.) via the synthetic lethality conferred through poly-ADP-ribose polymerase I inhibition [13–20]. In addition, strategies to break immune tolerance using programmed cell death ligand 1 and programmed death 1 inhibitors are being investigated [21–23].

Due to the absence of validated predictive biomarkers, only clinical and prognostic biomarkers are available to inform discussions with patients. Age, FIGO stage, grade, histology, performance status, volume of residual disease following cytoreductive surgery, and possibly time to initiation of adjuvant chemotherapy and rapidity of response to systemic therapy based on serial biochemical and radiographic analyses represent powerful

Correspondence: ktewari@uci.edu
The Division of Gynecologic Oncology, University of California, Irvine Medical Center, The City Tower, 333 City Blvd W., Orange, CA 92868, USA

prognostic factors for this disease. While performance status can be modified through medical and nutritional intervention, the time to initiation of chemotherapy is dependent on multiple factors including access to care, insurance authorizations, and perioperative sequelae. Thus, the only prognostic factor which is under control of the oncologist is the volume of tumor residual following cytoreductive surgery.

Workshop planning

The Fifth Annual Cytoreductive Surgery Workshop for Advanced Ovarian Carcinoma and Peritoneal Surface Malignancies was held in Orange County, California. Didactics were delivered at the Surf & Sand Hotel in Laguna Beach and cadaver dissections with demonstration of cardinal advanced cytoreductive surgical strategy were performed at the University of California, Irvine

Main Campus in Irvine. The assembled faculty included course director Robert E Bristow, MD from the home institution (radical oophorectomy), Krishnansu S. Tewari, MD (also from UC Irvine; extrapelvic colon and bowel), Scott M Eisenkop from the Women's Cancer Center in Sherman Oaks, CA (retroperitoneum), David Imagawa from UC Irvine (liver), William A. Cliby from the Mayo Clinic in Rochester, MN (spleen, diaphragm), Cyril W. Helm from St. Louis University Hospital (HIPEC), and Dennis S. Chi from Memorial Sloan-Kettering Cancer Center in New York (VATS), Similar to previous years, there was representation from the nations of six continents. Interestingly, while the international attendance which started off relatively high in 2011, continues to grow, this year there were many more attendees from the United States (Fig. 1, Table 1).

Didactics were subdivided into three components: 1) a history of the evolution of cytoreductive surgery

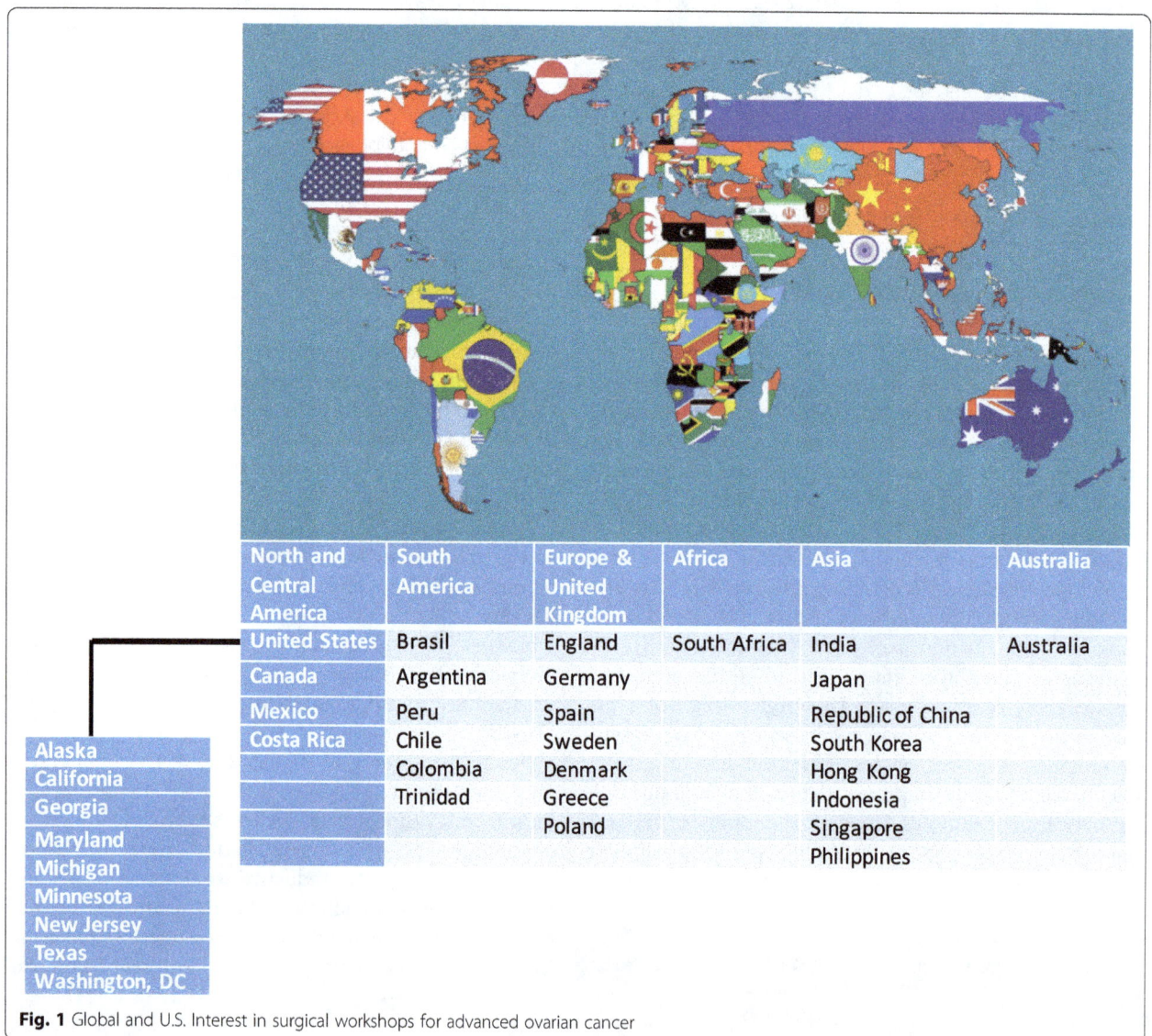

North and Central America	South America	Europe & United Kingdom	Africa	Asia	Australia
United States	Brasil	England	South Africa	India	Australia
Canada	Argentina	Germany		Japan	
Mexico	Peru	Spain		Republic of China	
Costa Rica	Chile	Sweden		South Korea	
	Colombia	Denmark		Hong Kong	
	Trinidad	Greece		Indonesia	
		Poland		Singapore	
				Philippines	

Alaska
California
Georgia
Maryland
Michigan
Minnesota
New Jersey
Texas
Washington, DC

Fig. 1 Global and U.S. Interest in surgical workshops for advanced ovarian cancer

Table 1 Six years of cytoreductive surgery workshops

Year	Course site	# Attendees	# Countries represented
2011	U.C. Irvine Medical Center, Orange, CA	25	12
2012[a]	St Louis University Medical Center		
2013	U.C. Irvine Main Campus (Irvine)[b]	36	18
2014[a]	Newcastle on Tyne, United Kingdom		
2015	U.C. Irvine Main Campus (Irvine)[b]	59	26
2016[c]	Newcastle on Tyne, United Kingdom		
	Philippine Society of Gynecologic Oncology, Manila, Philippines		
	U.C. Irvine Main Campus Fellows-in-Training Course		

[a]Satellite workshops
[b]Didactics given at the Surf & Sand Hotel in Laguna Beach, CA
[c]2016 workshops in Manila and in the UK have only recently been completed and therefore final registration data concerning number of participants and demographics is not yet available; the Fellows' Workshop is not scheduled to take place until November

including the advancement of a new thesis concerning the origins of cytoreduction for ovarian cancer (now regarded as the "2nd Law of Cytoreduction"); 2) lectures on surgical innovations and strategic planning in systematic anatomic manner based on intra-abdominal and extra-abdominal spread patterns of disease; 3) tribute to a pioneer in the field of surgery. At the 14 cadaver stations, faculty rotated among attendees to illustrate the principles of eight anatomic surgical procedures required to accomplish an R_0 designation at completion of cytoreduction.

Reiteration of the First Thesis

Introduced by faculty member, KS Tewari, at the 1st Workshop on November 4, 2011, the concept of cytoreduction for ovarian cancer evolved over three periods encompassing nearly 200 years [24]. Beginning with Ephraim McDowell's (1771-1830) first oophorectomy performed on 45-year old Jane Todd Crawford (1763-1842) on his kitchen table on Christmas Day, 1809, a surgical masterpiece was created for which McDowell was named the Father of Abdominal Surgery [25]. Attempts at oophorectomy or ovarian cystectomy preceding McDowell's time are not in short supply (including forays into antiquity and even Robert Houston's 1701 "puncture" of an ovarian cyst [26]), but McDowell was the first to safely remove an ovarian tumor and describe his technique in detail. The second period encompassed the idea that surgery could be performed even in the setting of metastatic disease, with proponents including Joe Vincent Meigs (1892-1963) of Boston Hospital [27],

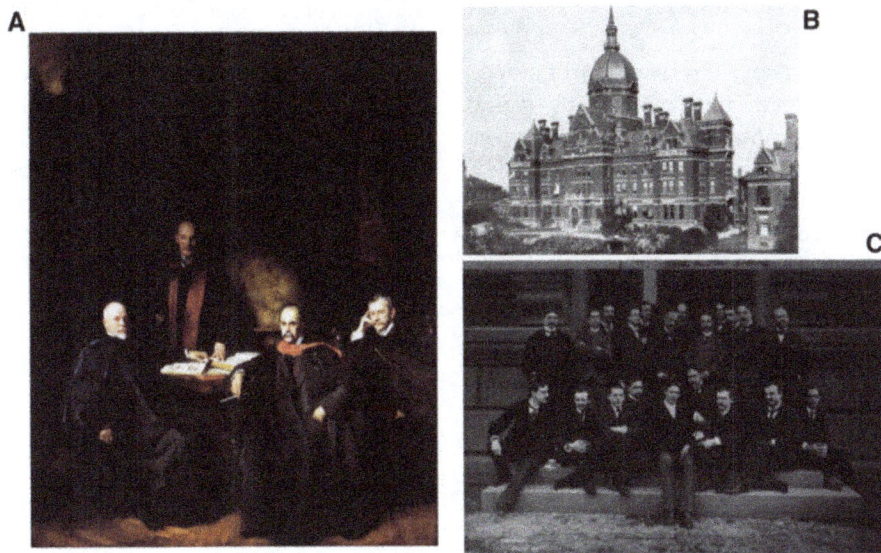

Fig. 2 Johns Hopkins University. **a** John Singer Sargent's The Four Doctors (1906) depicting the Founding Professors (left to right): Welch (pathologist & Dean), Osler (internist), Halstead (surgeon), and Kelly (gynecologist). **b** Early photograph of The Johns Hopkins Hospital. **c** Johns Hopkins Medical Class of 1892 with Dr(s) Kelly and Clark seated in the front row (third and second from the right, respectively). All images in the Public Domain

Hudson's radical oophorectomy for fixed cancers in the pelvis [28], and Hugh R. K. Barber (1918-2006) and Alexander Brunschwig (1901-1969) who used pelvic exenterative procedures (designed for women suffering from central, isolated recurrence of cervical cancer following radiotherapy) to treat 22 women with advanced and recurrent ovarian cancers [29]. The third and final period of the evolution of the concept of cytoreduction and inherent validity in advanced disease encompasses the 1973 report by McGrath on the survival advantage afforded patients with abdominal Burkitt's lymphoma who underwent extensive disease resections [30], the landmark study by Griffiths from 1974 in which the surgeon reported that among 102 consecutive cases of advanced ovarian cancer, those patients in whom residual disease greater than 1.5 cm in maximal diameter was left in the abdominal cavity were invariably dead within 2 years as compared to the 20 % 5-year survival rate conferred by tumor residuals under 1.5 cm [31], and finally, the watershed event by Bristow et al. in which a meta-analysis of 81 ovarian cancer cohorts (nearly 7,000 patients) treated with platinum-based chemotherapy demonstrated that the most important determinant of survival was maximal cytoreduction with each 10 % increase in tumor resection associated with a 5.5 % increase in median survival time [32]. This chronology appears in greater detail in our first Workshop Report [24]. The First Law of Cytoreduction is concerned with the temporal aspects and holds that the evolution traversed three distinct periods involving oophorectomy, surgery in the setting of metastatic disease, and validation of surgical effort to bring the residual disease volume to no visible tumor (ie, R_0).

The Road to Baltimore (New Thesis or 2nd Law)

The rationale for cytoreduction is supported by several hypotheses concerning intrinsic tumor drug resistance (which is independently described by both the Goldie Coldman hypothesis for acquisition of somatic mutations and Bayes Theorem) by which large areas of disease harboring chemoresistant clones are resected [24]. Increased tumor growth fraction (described according to Gompertzian cell kinetics) occurring after surgery shuttles resting phase G_0 cells into the cell cycle and thereby makes them more vulnerable to cycle-specific antineoplastic agents. Maximal cytoreduction also results in increased drug perfusion, a lower likelihood of developing acquired drug resistance, and enhanced host immunologic competence. To date the best outcomes among women with advanced ovarian cancer appear to be in the group of patients who can withstand cytoreductive surgery to optimal disease status (ie., low volume residual < 1 cm or R_0) and six cycles of combined intraperitoneal-intravenous chemotherapy.

Optimal cytoreduction and/or complete resection in the abdomen and pelvis is accomplished through radical pelvic surgery and in many cases upper abdominal procedures with complete parietal and visceral peritonectomy [33]. Interestingly, radical pelvic surgery was initially applied to cervical cancer. Although surgeons in Germany (A. K. Mackenrodt (1859-1925)) and in Austria (eg., Frederick Schauta (1849-1919), vaginal approach), Ernst Wertheim (1864-1920, abdominal approach) were developing the technique of radical hysterectomy for cervical cancer during the latter part of the 19th Century [34], it was in the United States, specifically in Baltimore, Maryland, that a formal treatise was prepared.

The Johns Hopkins University was founded in 1876 and named after its first benefactor the American entrepreneur, abolitionist, and philanthropist, Johns Hopkins. With the completion of Johns Hopkins Hospital in 1889 and the medical school in 1893, the university's research focus attracted faculty members with international reputations who would ultimately emerge as major figures in academic medicine. Among the "Big Four" founding professors of Johns Hopkins Hospital (Fig. 2a-b) was Sir William Osler, 1st Baronet (1849-1919), the internist who would bring medical students out of the lecture hall for bedside clinical training and become known as the "Father of Modern Medicine". William Henry Welch (1850-1934) was the pathologist (and bacteriologist) and served as the first Dean of the Johns Hopkins School of Medicine. William Stewart Halsted (1852-1922) was the surgeon who emphasized strict aseptic technique and developed the *en bloc* radical mastectomy for breast cancer [35]. Finally, Howard Atwood Kelly (1858-1943) was the gynecologist who had been trained by James Marion Sims (1813-1883), the "Father of Modern Gynecology" who developed the Sims speculum and the surgical technique for repair of vesicovaginal fistula due to obstructed childbirth. Kelly himself is credited for having established gynecology as a distinct specialty and developing new surgical instruments and surgical approaches to gynecologic diseases.

John Goodrich Clark (1867-1927) (Fig. 2c) had trained at the University of Pennsylvania and interned at a local Philadelphia hospital before coming to Johns Hopkins. He had originally been granted a residency position with Osler, but upon arrival he was told that that position had been committed to another physician. Fortunately, Kelly had an opening, and so through a quirk of fate, Clark changed career paths abruptly from internal medicine to gynecology [34]. Kelly assigned Clark the task of developing a more radical approach to the treatment of cervical cancer. At pathologic examination, Clark noted that in 15 of 20 cases, the disease had extended beyond the margins of resection. Having become influenced by the surgical doctrines of Halstead (Fig. 3a), Clark began

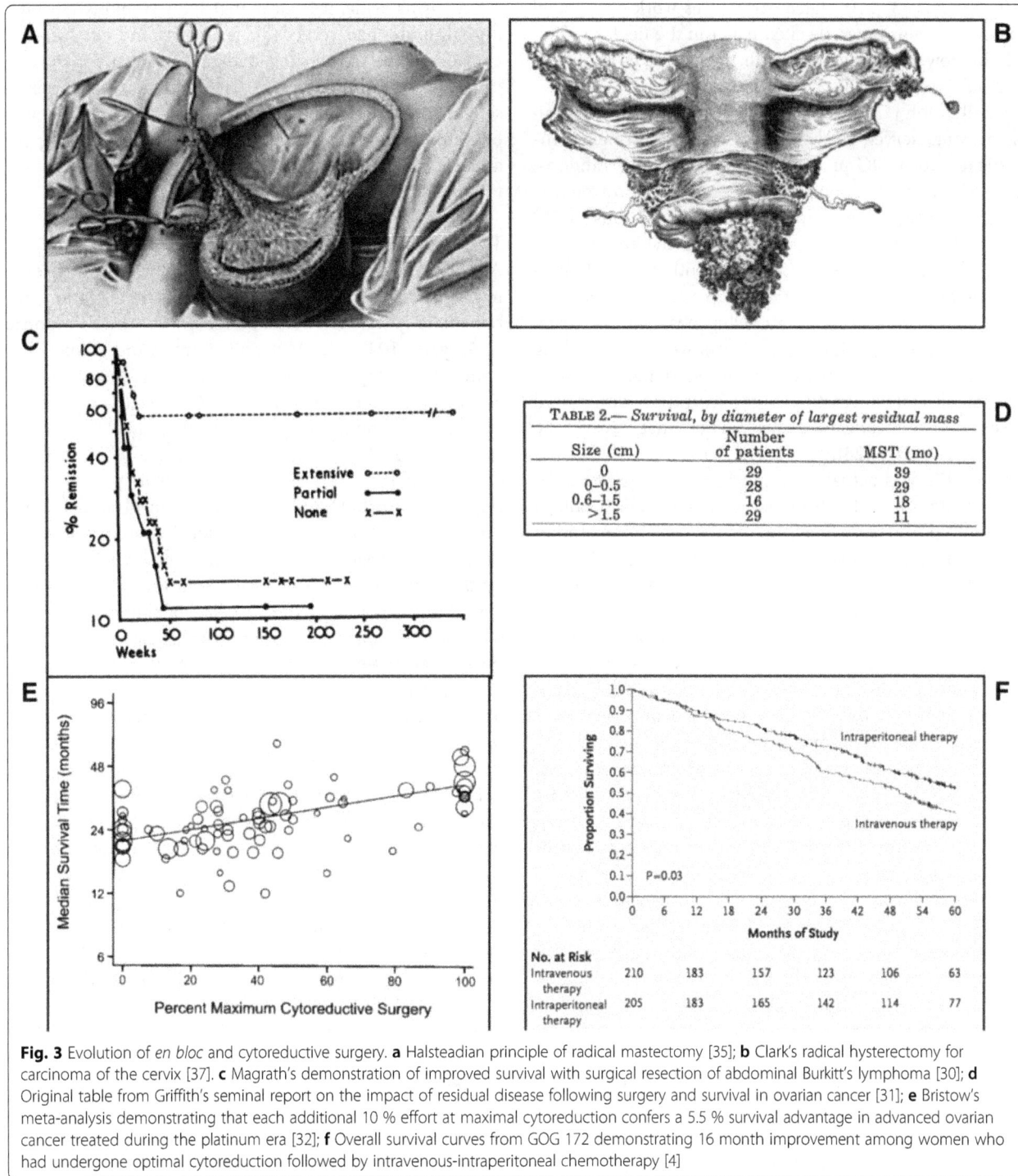

Fig. 3 Evolution of *en bloc* and cytoreductive surgery. **a** Halsteadian principle of radical mastectomy [35]; **b** Clark's radical hysterectomy for carcinoma of the cervix [37]. **c** Magrath's demonstration of improved survival with surgical resection of abdominal Burkitt's lymphoma [30]; **d** Original table from Griffith's seminal report on the impact of residual disease following surgery and survival in ovarian cancer [31]; **e** Bristow's meta-analysis demonstrating that each additional 10 % effort at maximal cytoreduction confers a 5.5 % survival advantage in advanced ovarian cancer treated during the platinum era [32]; **f** Overall survival curves from GOG 172 demonstrating 16 month improvement among women who had undergone optimal cytoreduction followed by intravenous-intraperitoneal chemotherapy [4]

considering the application of Halsteadian principles to *en bloc* radical hystererctomy for cervical cancer [34] (Fig. 3b). The difference between Clark and his more senior European contemporaries (eg., Mackenrodt, Schauta, Wertheim), was in rationale, thesis, and methodology [36].

John Hopkins Hospital is where Robert E Bristow (currently Chairman of Obstetrics & Gynecology at UC Irvine Medical Center in Orange, California) began collecting data on not only the performance of radical hysterectomy with radical oophorectomy (which encompassed in most cases a low anterior resection) for advanced ovarian cancer, but the performance of numerous other upper abdominal operations required to bring the residual disease burden down to zero (eg., splenectomy, full-thickness diaphragm resection, porta hepatis surgery, supra-renal lymphadenectomy, video-assisted thorascopic surgery

(VATS), etc.) [37]. As stated earlier, this work culminated in what remains a heavily cited paper in the field, specifically Bristow's meta-analysis performed while in Baltimore and published in 2002 [32] (Fig. 3d).

Finally, John Hopkins medical oncologist, Deborah Armstrong, served as the Study Chair and Principal Investigator for GOG protocol 172, the phase III randomized trial of intravenous chemotherapy vs intravenous-intraperitoneal chemotherapy which demonstrated a 16-month OS advantage in the combined therapy arm [4] (Fig. 3f). Regional therapy exploits both the prolonged confinement of disease within the peritoneal cavity and the steep dose-response relationship observed for many cytotoxic agents, allowing for a slower rate of drug clearance from the peritoneal to systemic compartments, ultimately creating a concentration differential across the peritoneal-plasma barrier that favors the peritoneal cavity [24].

GOG 172 was actually the third phase III randomized trial by the GOG to demonstrate a survival advantage with intraperitoneal chemotherapy, but all three studies had been subject to reasonable scrutiny, with GOG 104 (published in 1996 [38], the same year that GOG 111 was published and demonstrated the superiority of combining paclitaxel with cisplatin over cyclophosphamide plus cisplatin [39]) not including taxanes, and with GOG 114 (published in 2001) [40] being criticized for intravenous platinum dose escalation in the intraperitoneal arm (ie., prior to intraperitoneal therapy patients received 2 cycles of intravenous carboplatin at AUC 9). Not only was GOG 172 marred by significant toxicity which only permitted 40 % of patients on the combined intravenous-intraperitoneal arm to receive all six cycles of adjuvant therapy, but the schedule of paclitaxel on the intravenous-intraperitoneal arm (24 h intravenous paclitaxel (135 mg/m^2 BSA) on day 1 followed by intraperitoneal paclitaxel (60 mg/m^2 BSA) on day 8) suggested that weekly dose-dense taxane therapy could have accounted for the superior results. Despite these criticisms, a follow-up combined analysis of GOG 114 and GOG 172 by Tewari et al., does attest to the long-term survival (ie, 9 years) benefit of combined intravenous-intraperitoneal therapy [5]. Recent presentations at the 2016 Annual Meeting of the Society of Gynecologic Oncology (ie., GOG 252), have been disappointing with respect to intraperitoneal chemotherapy, with GOG 252 not having a proper control arm making the entire trial essentially uninterpretable [7]. Nevertheless, given the long-standing shortcomings of the three previous IV-IP vs IV phase III randomized trials described above, the negative results of GOG 252 have added to the growing disenchantment with IP therapy that has gained traction with many oncologists who treat women with advanced disease.

Criticisms aside, it is clear that John Hopkins Hospital in Baltimore has served as fertile ground for what is considered the treatment paradigm for advanced ovarian cancer. The Second Law of Cytoreduction concerns itself with geospatial constraints and holds that the development of radical pelvic surgery, together with upper abdominal procedures and adjuvant regional therapy took place at *ground zero* in Baltimore.

Tribute to Dr. Francis D. Moore (1913-2001)

At the 2015 Cytoreductive Surgery Workshop a tribute to Dr Francis Moore was made during the didactic component (Fig. 4a). His classic books, Metabolic Response to Surgery (1949) and Metabolic Care of the Surgical Patient (1959) (Fig. 4b), are regarded as masterpieces that according to Judah Folkman (1933-2008), the pioneer of angiogenesis and anti-angiogenesis therapy [41], changed the thinking of surgeons throughout the world and reduced suffering and mortality of their patients [42] (Fig. 4c). Before Moore, surgeons concentrated on improving their craft to effect the local anatomic changes necessary to treat disease, but they remained perplexed by the body's physiologic response to the trauma of surgery. Surgeons during the first half of the 20th Century did not understand how to optimize the physiologic status of their patients before surgery. A perfect anatomical operation could be followed by disastrous complications or death from a low level of circulating sodium chloride or magnesium, or a high level of potassium chloride, or an undetected loss of plasma water [43]. Dr Moore was among the first translational scientists and his studies carried out between the physiology laboratory and the patient's bedside culminated in his classic books which were regarded as the "Bible" of surgery for five generations of surgeons. The book was so well-written that in his lifetime, no updated/expanded edition needed to be written. At the 2015 Workshop, the purpose of the tribute was to recognize Moore's trailblazing work as that fundamental body of knowledge which has provided gynecologic oncologists with the knowledge base and confidence to pursue advanced surgical resections in women with ovarian cancer (Fig. 4b).

Surgery for Ovarian Cancer – A Surgical Atlas

The 2015 Workshop was held to coincide with publication of the 3rd edition of Surgery for Ovarian Cancer, which continues to be edited by Bristow RE, Karlan BY, and Chi DS. The 3rd edition is noteworthy for allowing access to the entire text as a VitalSource® ebook and contains instructions for creating a VitalSource Bookshelf upon redemption of the code contained on the scratch-off panel on the inside front cover. Internet links to high definition video illustrating many of the surgical procedures presented at the Workshop are also

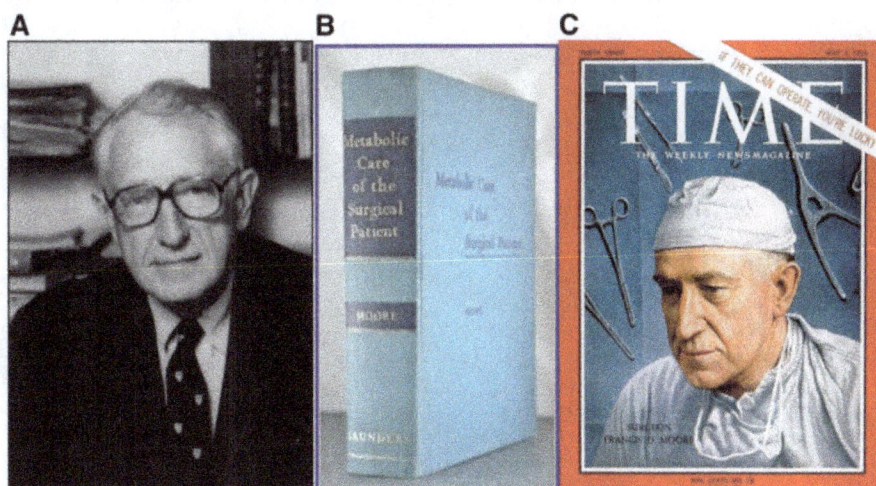

Fig. 4 Understanding the physiologic responses to surgery has allowed surgeons to safely perform the multiple surgical procedures required at times to completely cytoreduce women with advanced ovarian cancer. **a** Dr. Francis D. Moore (1913-2001); **b**: Metabolic Care of the Surgical Patient by Moore; **b** Dr. Moore on the cover of Time Magazine, May 1963

distributed throughout the text. All Workshop participants were provided a copy of this text book.

Cadaver stations

Coincident with the adaptation of surgical technique within the confines of this disease along with incorporation of procedures from other disciplines, cadaver dissections continue to evolve. For example, the attendees at the 2011 workshop were notably interested in the performance of low anterior resection with end-to-end anastomosis, splenectomy, and peritoneal stripping from the diaphragm. In 2015, cadaveric stations catering to the performance of the following were most popular:

A. Radical oophorectomy (key points):
a. The *en bloc* specimen includes the uterus, adnexae, anterior pelvic peritoneal tumor, cul-de-sac tumor, and rectosigmoid colon, all contained within the *peritoneal bag* to leave the pelvis macroscopically tumor-free (Fig. 5a).
b. The integrity of the rear admiral's circular end-to-end anastomosis is demonstrated by the production of two symmetrical, intact donuts and a negative bubble test.

B. Splenectomy with distal pancreatectomy (key points):
a. Identification of the left gastric vessels and the inferior mesenteric vein (IMV) (Fig. 5b).
b. Umbilical tape placed to the left of the IMV
c. Individual ligation of the splenic artery and vein

d. *En bloc* resection of distal pancreas with spleen by dividing the tail distal to ligated splenic vessels
e. Distal pancreas closed with running stitch of delayed absorbable suture followed by reinforcing layer of 2-0 silk mattress stitches.

C. Liver mobilization to allow full-thickness resection of the right diaphragm (key points):
a. Following division of the round ligament, the falciform ligament is divided towards its apex where it bifurcates into the coronary ligament
b. Incision of the coronary ligament exposes the right hepatic vein and inferior vena cava and the dissection is maintained superficial to these vessels (Fig. 5c)
c. The liver is drawn inferiorly and medially by releasing the ligamentous attachments of the left lobe
d. In sequence, the left triangular ligament, the anterior and posterior layers of the left coronary ligament, the hepatogastric ligament, the anterior layer of the right coronary ligament, and the right triangular ligament are divided, exposing the right paracolic gutter and Morison's pouch.
e. The incision for diaphragm resection should include a 0.5-1.0 cm margin and run parallel to the path of the branching phrenic nerve.

In addition to the stations listed above, the 2015 Workshop included cadaver dissections to demonstrate suprarenal aortic lymphadenectomy, resection of porta hepatis disease, and the Pringle maneuver in which the

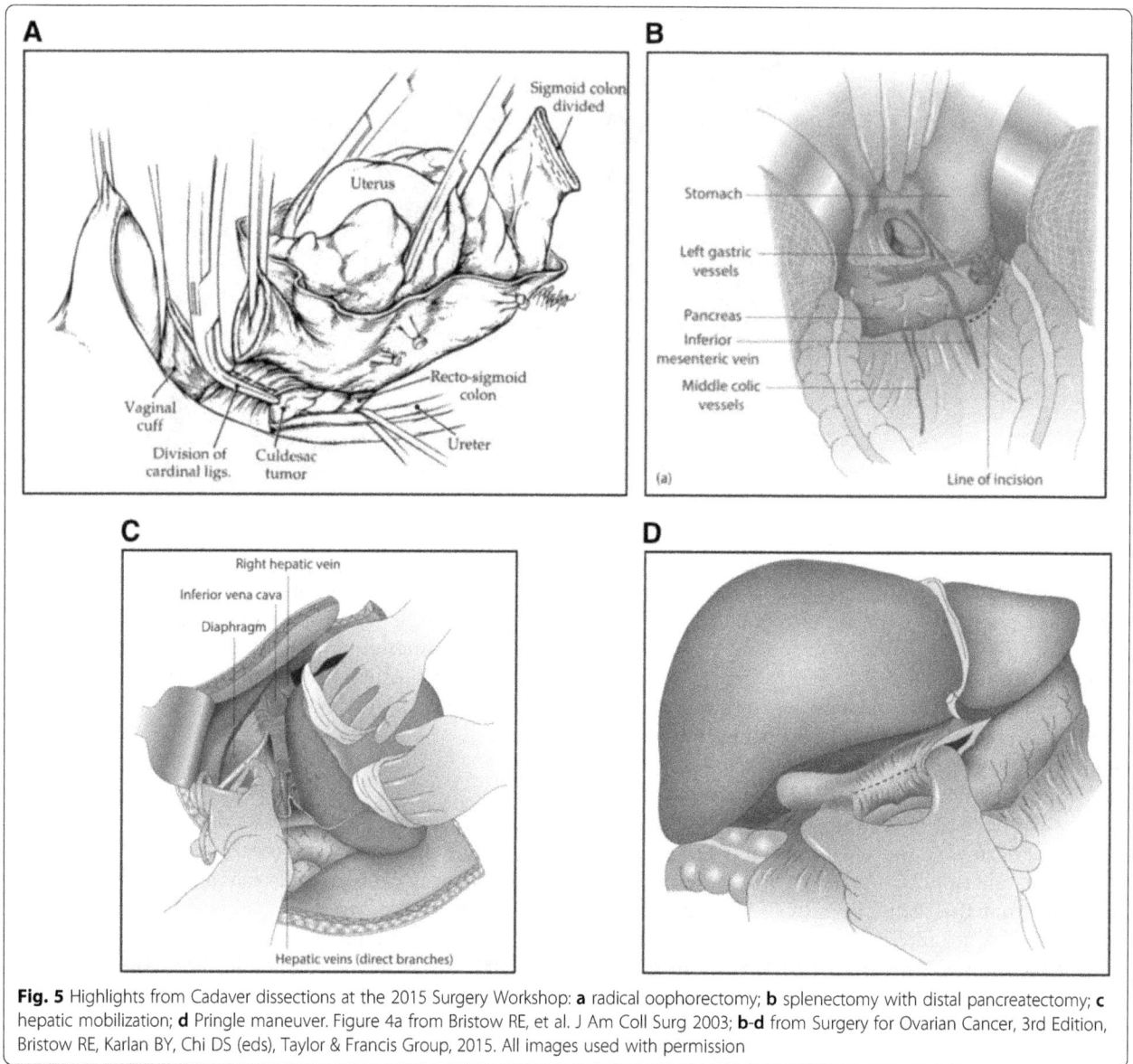

Fig. 5 Highlights from Cadaver dissections at the 2015 Surgery Workshop: **a** radical oophorectomy; **b** splenectomy with distal pancreatectomy; **c** hepatic mobilization; **d** Pringle maneuver. Figure 4a from Bristow RE, et al. J Am Coll Surg 2003; **b-d** from Surgery for Ovarian Cancer, 3rd Edition, Bristow RE, Karlan BY, Chi DS (eds), Taylor & Francis Group, 2015. All images used with permission

index finger is inserted through the foramen of Winslow and the thumb through a defect in the gastrohepatic ligament to access the porta hepatis, allowing for total inflow occlusion via an atraumatic clamp or silastic vessel loop to prevent unnecessary blood loss during wedge and/or hepatic resections (Fig. 5d). Both heated intraperitoneal chemotherapy (HIPEC) and video-assisted thoracoscopic surgery (VATS) were also featured in the cadaver laboratory, with the latter representing a new addition to the 2015 Workshop.

Discussion

The discipline of surgery requires life-long learning. In the subspecialty of Gynecologic Oncology, this principle has been best exemplified by the introduction of minimally invasive surgery into the management of clinical stage I endometrial cancer, FIGO stage I cervical cancer (including lesions amenable to fertility-preserving radical trachelectomy), and select adnexal masses. Some practicing Gynecologic Oncologists had little or no laparoscopic training during fellowship, and many had no robotics training. Minimally invasive workshops held by the American Association of Gynecologic Laparoscopists and by the Society of Gynecologic Oncology in collaboration with industry partners (eg., Intuitive Surgical, Ethicon, Covidien, etc.) have helped disseminate the knowledge of minimally invasive surgery throughout the subspecialty and brought many surgeons up to speed with this essential treatment modality.

While the principles of cytoreductive surgery are taught in Gynecologic Oncology fellowship training programs throughout the world, the demonstration of

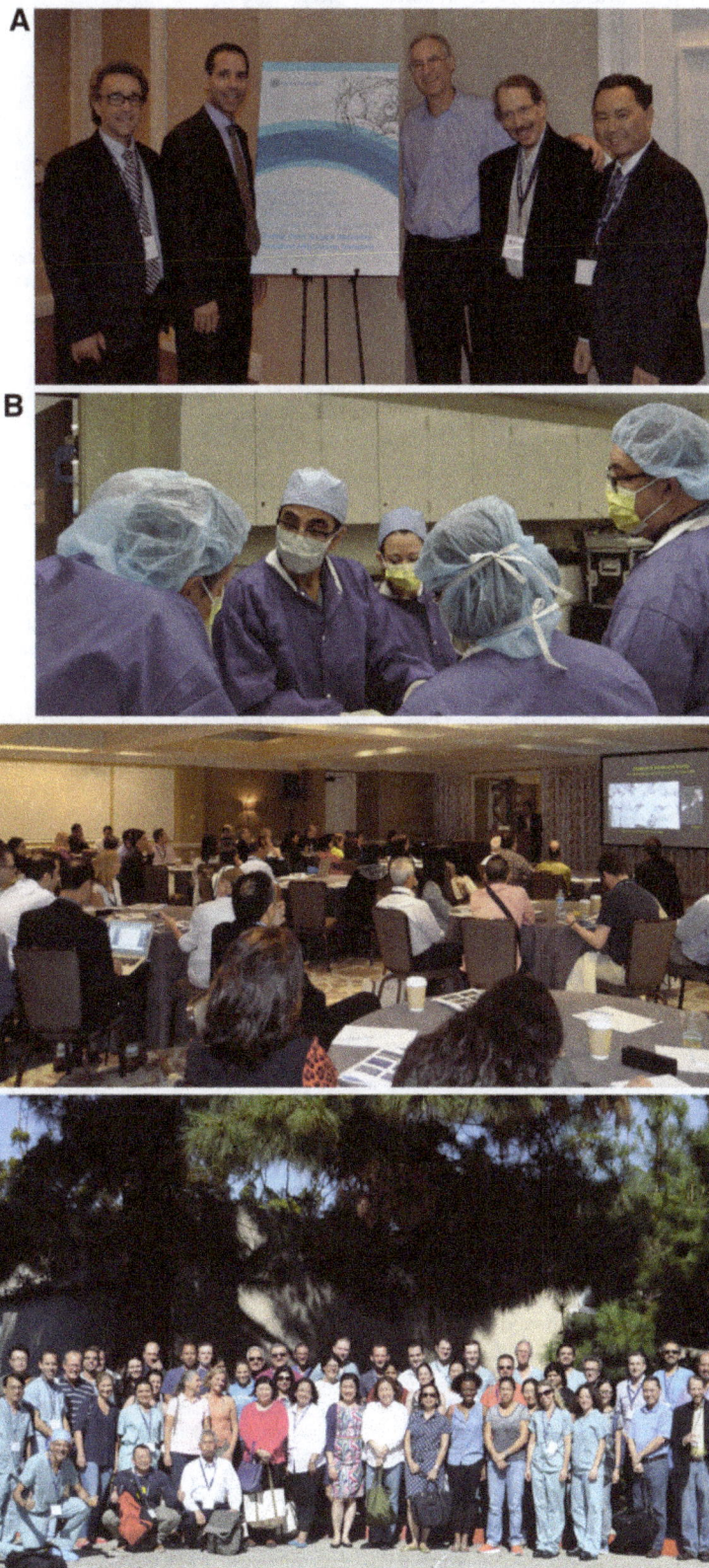

Fig. 6 The Fifth Annual Cytoreductive Surgery Workshop (2015). **a** Workshop faculty (from left to right): Dr(s) Cliby, Bristow, Helm, Eisenkop, and Chi; **b** An astonished Ramirez Escobar attempts to dissect a cadaver in the laboratory; **c** Dr. Tewari presents his thesis, *The Road to Baltimore*, during didactics; **d** Participants (attendees, faculty, and UCI fellows) seen outside of the cadaver dissection laboratory

technique and how to safely push the envelope to accomplish optimal debulking status or even an R_0 resection appears to vary to some degree. In the EORTC randomized trial of primary surgery vs neoadjvuant chemotherapy, Vergote et al. reported that the hazard ratio (HR) for death in the group assigned to neoadjvuant chemotherapy followed by interval debulking surgery, (as compared with the group assigned to primary debulking surgery followed by chemotherapy), was 0.98 (90 % CI, 0.84-1.13; p-0.01 for non-inferiority) and the HR for PFS was 1.01 (90 % CI, 0.89-1.15) [44]. Although postoperative rates of adverse effects and mortality tended to be higher after primary debulking than after interval cytoreduction, this study raised a number of controversies, particularly regarding the quality of debulking surgery. While complete resection of all macroscopic disease (at primary or interval surgery) was the strongest independent variable in predicting OS, only 41.6 % of patients were rendered optimally debulked to 1 cm or less of residual tumor following primary cytoreduction, as compared to 80.6 % of patients after interval cytoreduction. Similarly, in the MRC CHORUS Trial which also demonstrated significant non-inferiority between primary and interval cytoreduction arms, only 25 % of patients in the primary surgery cohort were left with $\leq$ 1 cm residual disease [45]. These results for optimal cytoreduction rates are much lower than what is reported by many U.S. centers. For these reasons it was not surprising that beginning with the First Annual Cytoreductive Surgery Workshop in 2011 that attendees were registering from around the world, with each succeeding Workshop receiving even more participation from our global partners.

Interestingly, each succeeding workshop has also been met with increased registration from graduates of American Board of Obstetrics & Gynecology certified training programs. The high numbers of U.S. participants in the 2015 workshop (Fig. 6) may be the result of the aftermath following plenary presentation of GOG data at the 2015 SGO Annual Meeting in which notable discrepancies were reported between surgeon's assessment of cytoreduction status and pre-treatment imaging on a U.S.-led phase III randomized clinical trial of anti-angiogenesis therapy for newly diagnosed advanced ovarian carcinoma [46]. Enthusiasm for these types of activities has led directly to our first Cytoreductive Surgery Workshop designed specifically for fellows-in-training. All 24 spots for this 2016 Fellows Cytoreductive Surgery Workshop were filled within two hours of its announcement.

Acknowledgements
None.

Funding
Registration fees paid for the cadavers and travel for out of state faculty.

Author contributions
I wrote the entire manuscript (KST).

Author's information
On Title Page of manuscript.

Competing interests
The author (KST) declares that he has no competing interest. None; this workshop is not for profit.

References

1. Tewari KS, Monk BJ. The 21st Century Handbook of Clinical Ovarian Cancer. Adis; 2015.
2. Katsumata N, Yasuda M, Takahashi F, Isonishi S, Jobo T, Aoki D, et al. Dose-dense paclitaxel once a week in combination with carboplatin every 3 weeks for advanced ovarian cancer: a phase 3, open-label, randomized controlled trial. Lancet. 2009;374:1331–8.
3. Pignata S, Scambia G, Katsaros D, Gallo C, Pujade-Lauraine E, De Placido S, et al. Carboplatin plus paclitaxel once a week versus every 3 weeks in patients with advanced ovarian cancer (MITO-7): a randomized, multicenter, open-label, phase 3 trial. Lancet Oncol. 2014;15:396–405.
4. Armstrong DK, Bundy B, Wenzel L, Huang HQ, Baergen R, Lele S, et al. Intraperitoneal cisplatin and paclitaxel in ovarian cancer. N Engl J Med. 2006;354:34–43.
5. Tewari D, Java JJ, Salani R, Armstrong DK, Markman M, Herzog T, et al. Long-term survival advantage and prognostic factors associated with intraperitoneal chemotherapy treatment in advanced ovarian cancer: A Gynecologic Oncology Group study. J Clin Oncol. 2015;33:1460–6.
6. Chan JK, Brady MF, Penson RT, Huang H, Birrer MJ, Walker JL, et al. Weekly vs every-3-week paclitaxel and carboplatin for ovarian cancer. N Engl J Med. 2016;374:738–48.
7. Walker JL, Brady MF, DiSilvestro PA, Fujiwara K, Alberts D, Zheng W, et al. A phase III clinical trial of bevacizumab with IV versus IP chemotherapy in ovarian, fallopian tube, and primary peritoneal carcinoma: An NRG Oncology Study. Gynecol Oncol. 2016;141 Suppl 1:208(LBA6).
8. Wenzel L, Huang HQ, Walker JL, Brady MF, DiSilvestro PA, Fujiwara K, et al. Patient-reported outcomes of a phase III clinical trial of bevacizumab with IV versus IP chemotherapy in ovarian, fallopian tube, and primary peritoneal carcinoma: a Gynecologic Oncology Group/NRG Oncology tria. Gynecol Oncol. 2016;141(Suppl1):208(LBA7).
9. Eskander RN, Tewari KS. Incorporation of anti-angiogenesis therapy in the management of advanced ovarian carcinoma – Mechanistics, review of phase III randomized clinical trials, and regulatory implications. Gynecol Oncol. 2014;132:496–505.
10. Herzog TJ, Armstrong DK, Brady MF, Coleman RL, Einstein MH, Monk BJ, et al. Ovarian cancer clinical trial endpoints: Society of Gynecologic Oncology white paper. Gynecol Oncol. 2014;132:8–17.
11. Gourley C, McCavigan A, Perren T, Paul J, Michie CO, Churchman M, et al. Molecular subgroup of high-grade serous ovarian cancer (HGSOC) as a predictor of outcome following bevacizumab. J Clin Oncol. 2014;32:5s (suppl; abstr 5502).
12. Hodeib M, Serna-Gallegos T, Tewari KS. A review of HER2-targeted therapy in breast and ovarian cancer: Lessons from antiquity – CLEOPATRA and PENELOPE. Future. 2015;11:3113–31.
13. Ledermann J, Harter P, Gourley C, Friedlander M, Vergote I, Rustin G, et al. Olaparib maintenance therapy in platinum-sensitive relapsed ovarian cancer. N Engl J Med. 2012;366:1382–92.
14. Eskander RN, Tewari KS. PARP inhibition and synthetic lethality in ovarian cancer. Expert Rev Clin Pharmacol. 2014;7:613–22.
15. Kaufman B, Shapira-Frommer R, Schmutzler RK, Audeh MW, Friedlander M, Balmana J, et al. Olaparib monotherapy in patients with advanced cancer and a germline BRCA 1/2 mutation. J Clin Oncol. 2015;33:244–50.
16. Tewari KS, Eskander RN, Monk BJ. Development of olaparib for BRCA-deficient recurrent epithelial ovarian cancer. Clin Cancer Res. 2015;21:3829–35.
17. McNeish IA, Oza AM, Coleman RL, Scott CL, Konecny GE, Tinker A, et al.

Results of ARIEL2: A Phase 2 trial to prospectively identify ovarian cancer patietns likely to respond to rucaparib using tumor genetic analysis. J Clin Oncol. 2015;33:suppl; abstr 5508.

18. Liu FW, Tewari KS. New targeted agents in gynecologic cancers: Synthetic lethality, homologous recombination deficiency, and PARP inhibitors. Curr Treat Options Oncol. 2016;17:12–26.

19. LaFargue CJ, Forde G, Tewari KS. Recent patents for homologous recombination deficiency assays among women with ovarian cancer. Recent Pat Biotechnol. 2016;9:86–101.

20. Tesaro's niraparib significantly improved progression-free survival for patients with ovarian cancer in both cohorts of the phase 3 NOVA trial. Press Release, 29 June 2016, 0700 ET. http://www.ir.tesarobio.com/releasedetail.cfm?ReleaseID=977524.

21. Topalian SSL, HOdi FS, Brahmer JR, Gettinger SN, Smith DC, McDermott DF, et al. Safety, activity, and immune correlates of anti-PD-1 antibody in cancer. N Engl J Med. 2012;366:2443–54.

22. Brahmer JR, Tykodi SS, Chow LQ, Hwu WJ, Topalian SL, Hwu P, et al. Safety and activity of anti-PD-L1 antibody in patietns with advanced cancer. N Engl J Med. 2012;366:2455–65.

23. Hamanishi J, Mandai M, Ikeda T, Minami M, Kawaguchi A, Murayama T, et al. Safety and antitumor activity of anti-PD-1 antibody, niolumab, in patients with platinum-resistant ovarian cancer. J Clin Oncol. 2015;33:4015–22.

24. Tewari KS. Advanced Cytoreductive Surgery Workshop report. Int J Gynecol Cancer. 2012;22:1604–10.

25. McDowell E. Three cases of extirpation of diseased ovaria. Eclectic Repertory Anal Rev. 1817;7:242–44.

26. Houston R. An account of a dropsy in the left ovary of a woman, aged 58, cured by a large incision made in the side of the abdomen. Trans R Soc. 1724;33:2–4.

27. Meigs JV. The surgical treatment of cancer of the ovary. Clin Obstet Gynecol. 1961;4:846–54.

28. Hudson CN. A radical operation for fixed ovarian tumours. J Obstet Gynaecol Br Commonw. 1968;75:1155–60.

29. Barber HR, Brunschwig A. Pelvic exenteration for locally advanced and recurrent ovarian cancer. Review of 22 cases. Surgery. 1965;58:935–7.

30. Magrath IT, Lwanga S, Carswell W, Harrison N. Surgical reduction of tumour bulk in management of abdominal Burkitt's lymphoma. Br Med J. 1974;2:308–12.

31. Griffiths CT. Surgical resection of tumor bulk in the primary treatment of ovarian carcinoma. Natl Cancer Inst Monogr. 1975;42:101–4.

32. Bristow RE, Tomacruz RS, Armstrong DK, Trimble EL, Montz FJ. Survival effect of maximal cytoreductive surgery for advanced ovarian carcinoma during the platinum era: A Meta-analysis. J Clin Oncol. 2002;20:1248–59.

33. Sugarbaker PH. Complete parietal and visceral peritonectomy of the pelvis for advanced primary and recurrent ovarian cancer. Cancer Treat Res. 1996; 81:75–87.

34. Tewari KS. History of radical and reconstructive surgery for gynecologic cancer. In: Radical and Reconstructive Gynecologic Cancer Surgery. Bristow RE, Chi DS (eds). New York, USA: McGraw-Hill Education; 2015.

35. Halstead WS. The results of operations for the cure of cancer of the breast performed at the Johns Hopkins Hospital from June 1889 to January 1894. Johns Hopkins Hosp Rep 1894-1895;4:297

36. Clark JG. A more radical method for performing hysterectomy for cancer of the uterus. Maryland: Johns Hopkins Bulletin; July and August 1895.

37. Tewari KS. Historical development of cytoreductive surgery for ovarian cancer. In: Surgery for Ovarian Cancer: Principles and Practice. 3rd ed. Bristow RE, Karlan BY, Chi DS (eds). Zug: Informa Healthcare; 2010.

38. Alberts DS, Liu PY, Hannigan EV, O'Toole R, Williams SD, Young JA, et al. Intraperitoneal cisplatin plus intravenous cyclophosphamide versus intravenous cisplatin plus intravenous cyclophosphamide for stage III ovarian cancer. N Engl J Med. 1996;335:1950–5.

39. McGuire WP, Hoskins WJ, Brady MF, Kucera PR, Partridge EE, Look KY, et al. Cyclophosphamide and cisplatin compared with paclitaxel and cisplatij in patients with stage III and stage IV ovarian cancer. N Engl J Med. 1996;334:1–6.

40. Markman M, Bundy BN, Alberts DS, Fowler JM, Clark-Pearson DL, Carson LF, An Intergroup Study of the Gynecolgoic Oncologoy Group, Southwestern Oncology Group, and Eastern Cooperative Oncology Group, et al. Phase III trial of standard-dose intravenous cisplatin plus paclitaxel versus moderately high-dose carboplatin followed by intravenous paclitaxel and intraperitoneal cisplatin in small-volume stage III ovarian carcinoma. J Clin Oncol. 2001;19: 1001–7.

41. Folkman J. Tumor angiogenesis: therapeutic implications. N Engl J Med. 1971;285:1182–6.

42. Folkman J. Francis Daniels Moore. In: Biographical Memoirs: Volume 88. Washington, DC: The National Academies Press; 2006.

43. Brennan MF, Francis D. Moore, MD 1913-2001. Ann Surg. 2002;235:600–1.

44. Vergote I, Trope CG, Amant F, Kristensen GB, Ehlen T, Johnson N, et al. Neoadjuvant chemotherapy or primary surgery in stage IIIC or IV ovarian cancer. N Engl J Med. 2010;363:943–53.

45. Kehoe S, Hook J, Nankivell M, Jayson GC, Kitchener HC, Lopes T, et al. Chemotherapy or upfront surgery for newly diagnosed advanced ovarian cancer: Results of the MRC CHORUS trial. J Clin Oncol. 2013;31: suppl; abstr 5500.

46. Eskander RN, Kauderer J, Tewari KS, Bristow RE, Burger RA. Correlation between surgeon's assessment of residual disease and findings on postoperative pre-treatment computed tomography scan in women with advanced stage ovarian cancer reported to have undergone optimal cytoreduction: An NRG Oncology/GOG study. Gynecol Oncol. 2015;137: Suppl 1:4 (abstr 5).

3

Willingness and acceptability of cervical cancer screening among women living with HIV/AIDS in Addis Ababa, Ethiopia: a cross sectional study

Netsanet Belete[1], Yosief Tsige[2] and Habtamu Mellie[3*]

Abstract

Background: In Ethiopia, cervical cancer (CC) ranks the 2nd most frequent cancer and the country had 27.19 million women at risk of developing the disease though only 0.6 % women age 18-69 years was screened every 3 years. Nearly a quarter (22.1 %) of southern Ethiopia HIV (Human Immunodeficiency Virus) infected Women were positive for precancerous cervical cancer. Doing regular screening can prevent the disease by around half (45 %) of the cases in age of 30s and three quarter (75 %) cases in 50s and 60s.In the presence of high risk for acquiring cervical cancer among HIV patients, willingness and acceptance of the screening is low in Addis Ababa, Ethiopia thus the current study was aimed to assess willingness and acceptability of cervical cancer screening and its determinants among women living with HIV/AIDS in Addis Ababa, Ethiopia.

Method: A facility based cross sectional study was conducted among HIV positive women attending HIV treatment centers in Addis Ababa. The respondents were identified using systematic random sampling method. Data was collected using pretested questionnaire and were entered in to Epi-info version 3.5.1 software and exported in to SPSS version 20 statistical package for analysis. The criterias for entering independent variables into multivariate analysis were having p-value 0.05 or less at bivariate analysis and not co-linear.

Result: One third (34.2 %) of participants knew cervical cancer and two third (62.7 %) were willing for the test though only a quarter (24.8 %) were accepted the test. The independent variables significantly associated with acceptance of screening were educational level, source of information, awareness for the test and preventability of the disease.

Conclusion: In current study willingness and acceptance of CC (cervical cancer) were low thus organizations working on cancer and HIV/AIDS should establish cervical cancer screening program and further enhance awareness creation.

Keywords: Cervical cancer, HIV/AIDS, Screening, Willingness, Acceptability, Ethiopia

Background

In women, cervical cancer is the fourth most common cancer accounting about 20.4 % of all cancers globally, with an estimated 528,000 new cases in 2012 [1, 2]. Majority (85 %) of the global burden occurs in the less developed regions, where it accounts for almost 12 % of all female cancers. In sub-Saharan Africa, 34.8 new cases of cervical cancer are diagnosed per 100, 000

women annually and it happens in about 60 % women living with HIV infection [3–5].

There were an estimated 266,000 global deaths from cervical cancer in 2012, accounting for 7.5 % of all female cancer deaths. Almost nine out of ten (87 %) CC deaths occur in less developed regions. In sub-Saharan Africa, the mortality is 22.5 per 100,000 though it is less than 2 per 100,000 in Western Asia, Western Europe and Australia/New Zealand [1, 2].

In 2014, the expected diagnosis and death from invasive cervical cancer in America was 12,360 and 4,020 respectively [6].

* Correspondence: habtamumellie@yahoo.com
[3]Debre Markos University, College of Medicine and Health Science, Department of Public Health, Debre Markos, Ethiopia
Full list of author information is available at the end of the article

More than one fifth of all new cervical cancer cases globally are diagnosed in India. In the country, the disease ranked 2nd cause of female cancer. According to 2012 estimate, the country annual diagnosed cases and deaths from the disease was 122,844 and 67,477 respectively [2, 7]. In Taiwan the incidence rate of the disease among HIV infected women was 712.08/100,000 person-years [8].

In 2012, Ethiopia has a population of 27.19 million women aged 15 years and older who are at risk of developing cervical cancer. Current estimates indicate that every year 7095 women are diagnosed with cervical cancer and 4732 die from the disease. The disease ranks 2nd most frequent cancer among women. The disease has crude incidence rate of 16.3 per 100,000 populations per year in the country. Only 0.6 % women age 18–69 years was screened every 3 years [9].

As evidences showed HIV infected women are at risk for CC [10–13]. Cervical cancer is about 7.9 times more common in HIV infected women than none infected ones [10]. Cervical squamous intraepithelial lesion was about 7.04 times higher in HIV positive compared HIV negative women [12]. Nearly a quarter (22.1 %) of Southern Ethiopia HIV-Infected Women were positive for precancerous cervical cancer [13].

Cervical cancer which is caused by persistent infection with human papillomavirus [1, 7, 12, 14–17] is preventable disease, yet the number of cases globally is expected to almost double by the year 2025 [18]. Doing regular screening (no more than once every three to five years) can prevent the disease by around 45 of the cases in age of 30s and 75 % cases in 50s and 60s [19, 20]. Screening can be done using Pap smear [20], human papillomavirus testing [21] and visual inspection with acetic acid [22].

In the presence of high risk for acquiring cervical cancer among HIV patients, awareness and acceptance of the screening is low. In Boston, of eligible women for screening about 53.0 % had not undergone screening [23]. In Kenya teaching and referral hospital the self-reported screening uptake was 17.5 % [24]. About half (56.2 %) of HIV positive Nigerian women were aware of cervical cancer. In same country, only one every ten (9.4 %) of HIV positive women were screened for cervical cancer [25].

In Addis Ababa, Ethiopian women had very low awareness of cervical cancer and the etiology of cervical cancer was thought to be due to breaching social taboos or undertaking unacceptable behaviors. As a result, the perceived benefits of modern treatment were very low [26].

Although cervical cancer is a leading cause of cancer related morbidity and mortality among women in Ethiopia, its screening coverage as part of HIV care was low, only covers less than 1 % due to have no national screening program [18, 27, 28]. Hence the current study used to assess the willingness and acceptability of cervical cancer screening and its determinants among HIV positive women. The obtained information will be used for decision makers and organizations working on cancer and HIV/AIDS to consider and integrate cervical cancer screening as part of HIV/AIDS diagnosis and treatment guideline since there is no prior local evidence up to our knowledge.

Methods and materials
Study design and setting
A cross-sectional study design using both quantitative and qualitative research method was conducted on HIV treatment centers in Addis Ababa which is the capital city of Ethiopia. In the town, there are 45 hospitals, 72 health centers, and 43 health posts owned by ministry of health [29, 30]. These service sites were providing HIV diagnosis and treatment and its related supportive services. There are about 210,306 people living with HIV/AIDS in Addis Ababa of which 124,609 are women [31].

All HIV infected women above age of 17 years and coming for chronic HIV care in public health institutions of Addis Ababa during study period were the study populations.

Sample size determination and sampling strategy
The sample size for quantitative part was determined by a single population proportion formula using 95 % confidence interval (a = 0.05), 5 % margin of error (d) and the proportion (p) of cervical cancer screening in women living with HIV/AIDS from prior studies, which was 27.0 % [32].

$$n = \left(Z_{a/2}\right)^2 (p(1-p))/d^2$$

The final sample size after adding 10 % contingency was 333.

For qualitative part two women from each referral hospital and one woman from each health centers was selected for in-depth interview.

Among Addis Ababa regional health bureau owned public health institutions, three referral hospitals and eight health centers providing ART service were selected for study by lottery method. To calculate the sampling interval for quantitative study, the HIV patient flow for the past six consecutive months before data collection period was taken from each selected health institutions and added for approximation of future sampling frame. Selection of participants was done using systematic random sampling method based on arrival order of HIV infected women to the health institution for medical care. The staring participant was selected by lottery method from sample interval. The interviewed participant's corresponding medical record was reviewed for assessing laboratory measurements like CD4 count and clinical stages of HIV/AIDS.

For qualitative data, purposive sampling method was used to select women for the in-depth interview in selected health institutions. Women who were not selected for interview in quantitative study were included for qualitative part.

Data collection procedure and data quality management

For quantitative study, a structured questionnaire which was developed by reviewing different literatures was used for data collection. The questionnaire was translated in to local language (Amharic) and back translated to check consistency. The data collection tool was pretested among 16 patients and identified errors were corrected accordingly. The outcome variable of the study was cervical cancer screening acceptability. For the qualitative aspect a semi-structured interview guide was prepared in English and translated to local language of Amharic version. The in-depth interview was tape recorded and note was taken during interview.

To maintain quality of data; standardized and pretasted data collection tools were used for both quantitative and qualitative studies. Appropriate training was given for data collectors and supervisors. Daily supervision was carried out by supervisors and principal investigators to check completeness of the questionnaire. The quantitative data was entered twice by trained data clerk to check correct data entry. In addition at the end of data entry data cleaning were done using frequencies, cross tabulations, sorting and listing to check missed values and outliers. Errors identified during data collection were corrected accordingly at the field and those errors occurred during/after data entry were corrected by revising the original questionnaire.

Operational definitions

- Willingness to be screened for cervical cancer - if a women willing for testing but not decided to be screened in the near future [25].
- Acceptance to be screened for cervical cancer- if a women willing for testing and decided to be screened in the near future" [25].
- Knowledgeable about cervical cancer- if participant answers 7 questions out of 13 Knowledge assessment questions.

Data analysis

For quantitative data, code was given and entered in to Epi-info version 3.5.1 software and exported in to SPSS version 20 statistical package for analysis. Multi-colinearity was checked using Pearson correlation, tolerance or variance inflation factor and there were not multi-co-

linearity. Independent Variables associated with outcome variable with p-value 0.05 or less at bivariate analysis and not co-linear were entered into multivariate analysis via binomial logistic regression to get adjusted predictors. Descriptive statics of continuous variables were presented using mean, median and discrete variables were presented using percentage, and tables. P-value <0.05 was used as cut off point of statistical significance for analytical analysis.

The qualitative in-depth interview was translated to English version by arranging the points according to forwarded questions. Then framework analysis method was employed to grasp the detail information.

Ethical issue

The study proposal was approved by the institutional review board of Addis Ababa University. Letter from the Research Ethics Committee was submitted to Addis Ababa regional health bureau to get permission for conducting the study. To protect anonymity and confidentiality of the participants, both data collectors and supervisors were working in ART clinics in addition personal identifier data was not collected. Informed written consent was obtained from respondents after explaining the purpose of the study.

Results

A total of 322 study participants were included with a response rate of 96.7 % and about 14 in depth interviews were conducted based on saturation of information.

Characteristics of the study participants

The dominant ethnicity and religion were Amhara (53.7 %) and orthodox Christianity (71.7 %) respectively. Mean age of the study participants was 35.65 (SD ±10.17). Most of them were educated (78.3 %) and about half of them were have no regular source of income (51.2 %), had experience of pregnancy 1–2 times (47.5 %), diagnosed as having HIV before 6–10 Years ago (49.1 %). Most of (91.9 %) the participants were initiated ART and were WHO clinical stage 2 (34 %) HIV patients.

On card review, CD4 count of 211 (65.5 %) participants were less than or equal to 500 cells/ul, and the remaining 111(34.5 %) were CD4 count greater than 500 cells/ul. Most of the participants in the qualitative were attended secondary education, married and were between the age of 29 and 35.

Cervical cancer awareness, knowledge and test acceptance

Of the whole participants 110 (34.2 %) know about cervical cancer. And their major sources were health professionals during contact on routine HIV chronic care 59

(53.6 %), media 64 (58.2 %), reading books 13 (11.8 %), and friends 11(10.0 %) and the least was from family 3 (2.7 %). Regarding knowledge assessment only 81 (25.1 %) was found to be knowledgeable.

Even though they didn't have detail knowledge regarding the disease, most of the in-depth participants were aware of cervical cancer. Some of the participants agree as it is the cancer of the female reproductive tract. Medias are mentioned as a source of knowledge about the disease for most of the participants and some of them also experience the disease in their family members and neighbors.

Majority of participants 97 (88.2 %) believe as the disease is a preventable. Similarly from the qualitative part, most of the participants believed as cervical cancer is a preventable disease. A young respondent mention that *"one can get prevented from cervical cancer by having the screening test regularly"*.

About one third 31.4 % (101) participants knowing the availability of the screening procedures for the disease and about one third (62.7 %) were willing to screened for cervical cancer and a quarter (24.8 %) of them were decided to screened in the near future.

Most of the participants repudiate to take the screening test due to assuming, the test is time consuming 43 (35.8 %) (Table 1). The mentioned reasons in in depth interview were high cost of the test and timing consuming, fear of result of the test (being diagnosed as having cervical cancer), and a recently HIV diagnosed woman noted that *"the word you have a cancer diagnosis is really irritating beside my HIV, I think I will get hopeless, if I am diagnosed as having cervical cancer"*.

Only 37 (11.5 %) of the study participants were ever tested for cervical cancer in their life time. The time of screening was before HIV/AIDS diagnosis (29.7 %), within one year of HIV/AIDS diagnosis (32.5 %) and after one year of HIV/AIDS diagnosis (37.8 %). Of those

who get the screening test, about 11(29.7 %) were positive for the test.

In multiple logistic regression, after adjustment for potential cofounders, the factors that enhance accepting of screening were being in age group of 40–49, 50–59 and >60 years compared <29; having above 12 grade educational level compared to read and write; having regular source of income; getting information about cervical cancer from health professionals, having awareness of the test and needing the screening to take early measure. Respondents not knowing cervical cancer as preventable were less likely to accept the screening (Table 2).

Discussion

In this study one third (34.2 %) participants knew the availability of screening test for CC and this finding was similar with HIV positive women in Lagos, Nigeria (34.5 %) [25] and it was higher than two studies in Nigeria (15.5 %) [33], (6.5 %.) [34]. The possible reasons for discrepancy of the result might be variation in study populations i.e. all women [33, 34] vs HIV infected women in current study, regional state or country specific promotion policy variations, variations in involvement of the CC education in media and its exposure and differences in socio-cultural condition.

In current study majority of participants mentioned as health professionals were their main source of information for CC and the finding is in agreement with prior studies [33, 35–37].

The current finding of two third participants (62.7 %) willing to be screened for cervical cancer were lower than a study done in Nigeria (96.5 %) [38] and Mozambique (84 %) [39] and the difference might be attributed by variations in health policy on promotion of CC, variations on awareness creation using mass-media and socio-economic variations.

The current study revealed as one every ten (11.5 %) participants were ever tested for CC in their life time and this is in line with a study in rural Mozambique (11 %) [39], Sokoto, Nigeria, (10 %) [40], two studies in Kenya (12.3 %) [41] and (17.5 %) [25] and HIV positive women in Lagos, Nigerian (9.4 %) [25]. The finding was higher than two studies in Ogun State, Nigeria (4.8 %) [34] and (9.5) [42] and it was lower than a study among HIV-positive women Ottawa, Ont (58 %) [23]. The reason of being higher than Ogun State, Nigeria [34, 42] might be attributed by variations of study populations i.e. all women in [35] since HIV infected women may frequently visit health institutions and can get health professionals which are the main source of information for screening [33, 35–37].

The current finding of most of the participants not willing to take the test due to assuming that the test is time consuming (35.8 %), fear of being positive for the

Table 1 Reason for not having screening test among study participants in Addis Ababa, 2014

Reason for not having the screening test	Variable	Frequency	Percentage (%)
	High cost of the test	36	30.0
	Religious denial	12	10.0
	Partner acceptance	12	10.0
	Time consuming	43	35.8
	Recently delivered/ Pregnant	16	13.3
	Fear of test result	37	30.8
	Lack of female screeners	16	13.3
	No reason	25	20.8
	Others	9	10.8

Table 2 The association of variables with accepting of cervical cancer screening among study participants, 2014

Variable	(AOR, 95 % CI)
Socio-demographic characteristics	
Age in completed years	
<29 Years	1
30-39 Years	0.96 (0.372, 1.671)
40-49 Years	3.8 (1.212, 12.290)*
50-59 Years	4.2 (1.505, 17.482)*
>60 Years	8.2 (1.104, 61.543)*
Level of education	
Read and write	1
Primary Education (1–8)	1.2 (0.417, 3.846)
secondary Education (9–12)	1.6 (0.479, 5.600)
Higher education above 12	1.2 (1.313, 5.269)*
Regular source of income	
Yes	3.2 (1.346, 8.005)*
No	1
First most cause of cervical cancer	
Viral	1.8 (0.011, 3.895)
I don't know	0.619 (0.001, 2.233)
Others	1
Health professional source	
Yes	6.0 (1.440, 83.933)*
No	1
Is cervical cancer preventable	
Yes	1
No	0.07 (0.001, 0.249)*
Aware of the test used	
Yes	3.6 (1.395, 33.76)*
No	1
Reason of testing to take early measure	
Yes	9.9 (1.423, 309.316)*
No	1
High cost of the test	
Yes	1.001 (0.811, 29.268)
No	1
WHO Clinical staging	
WHO stage 1	1
WHO stage 2	0.68 (0.079, 5.870)
WHO stage 3	0.67 (0.042, 10.675)
WHO stage 4	0.011 (0.463, 3.282)

AOR adjusted odds ratio, *WHO* world health organization
* = statistically significant

test (30.8 %) and high cost of the test (30.0 %) was in agreement with the a similar study in HIV positive women in Lagos, Nigerian [25] and Kenya [41].

In this study, participants having above 12th grade educational level compared to read and write, and having awareness about CC were 1.2 and 3.6 times respectively more likely accepting the screening and the finding was in parallel with a study among HIV positive women in Lagos, Nigerian in which having a tertiary education were enhancing screening by 1.4 times (OR = 1.4; 95 % CI: 1.03-1.84) and those aware of cervical cancer were 1.5 times (OR: 1.5; 95 % CI: 1.2-2.0) more likely accepting the screening [25].

In current study, participants who were getting information about cervical cancer from health professionals were 6 times more likely accepting the screening and this finding was supported by prior studies [33, 40].

Conclusion and recommendation

One third (34.2 %) participants knew cervical cancer and two third (62.7 %) were willing for the test though only a quarter (24.8 %) were accepted the test. After adjustment in multivariate analysis, the factors that enhance accepting of screening were being in age group of 40–49, 50–59 and >60 years compared <29; having above 12th grade educational level compared to read and write; having regular source of income; getting information about cervical cancer from health professionals, having awareness of the test, needing screening to take early measure and knowing cervical cancer as preventable disease. Thus organizations working on cancer and HIV/AIDS should further work to enhance awareness, and acceptability of the test. Ethiopian ministry of health should establish CC screening program since two third participants were willing for screening. Screening refusals as a result of assuming time consuming of the test, fear of the test result and anticipated high cost need to be addressed through advocacy and public mobilization. A further study with a large sample size is recommended to validate the current finding.

Abbreviations
AIDS: Acquired immunodeficiency syndrome; ART: Antiretroviral treatment; CC: Cervical cancer; HIV: Human Immunodeficiency Virus.

Competing interests
The authors declare that they have no competing interests.

Authors' contributions
NB has brought the research idea, develops the proposal, coordinated the data collection and performed the statistical analysis. YT has participated in development of the proposal, coordinated the data collection and performed the statistical analysis. HM was participated in development of the proposal, coordinated the data collection and performed the statistical analysis and prepares the manuscript. All authors read and approved the final manuscript.

Acknowledgment
We would like to thank Addis Ababa University for its financial support. The authors thank the counselors at each institution and health providers working in each HIV treatment unit and study participants for their cooperation in the success of this work.

Author details

[1]Ethiopian Public Health Institute, Health System Research Directorate, Addis Ababa, Ethiopian. [2]Addis Ababa University, Allied School of Health Science, Addis Ababa, Ethiopian. [3]Debre Markos University, College of Medicine and Health Science, Department of Public Health, Debre Markos, Ethiopia.

References

1. Integrated Africa Cancer Factsheet. Focusing on Cervical Cancer, Girls & Women Health, Sexual & Reproductive Health, HIV & Maternal Health. 2014.
2. WHO. International agency for research on cancer. Latest world cancer statistics. 2013.
3. Sam MM, Kishor B, Clement A, Annie JS. HIV and cancer in Africa: mutual collaboration between HIV and cancer programs may provide timely research and public health data. Infect Agents Cancer. 2011;6:16. http://www.infectagentscancer.com/content/6/1/16.
4. UNAIDS. AIDS epidemic update Geneva, Switzerland. November 2009. www.unaids.org.
5. Global report UNAIDS report on the global aids epidemic. 2010. http://www.unaids.org/documents/2010.
6. American Cancer Society. Cancer Facts & Figures. Atlanta: American Cancer Society; 2014.
7. Human Papillomavirus and Related Diseases Report INDIA. August 22nd, 2014. www.hpvcentre.net.
8. Chen M, Jen I, Chen YH, Lin MW, Bhatia K, Sharp GB, et al. Cancer incidence in a Nationwide HIV/AIDS patient cohort in Taiwan in 1998–2009. J Acquir Immune Defic Syndr. 2014;65(4):463–72. doi:10.1097/QAI.0000000000000065.
9. Bruni L, Barrionuevo-Rosas L, Albero G, Aldea M, Serrano B, Valencia S, et al. ICO Information Centre on HPV and Cancer (HPV Information Centre). Human Papillomavirus and Related Diseases in Ethiopia. Summary Report 2014; 12: 18. www.hpvcentre.net.
10. Tanon A, Jaquet A, Ekouevi DK, Akakpo J, Adoubi I, et al. The pectrum of Cancers in West Africa: Associations with Human Immunodeficiency Virus. PLoS One. 2012;7(10), e48108. doi:10.1371/journal.pone.0048108.
11. Moscicki AB, Ellenberg JH, Vermund SH, Holland CA, Darragh T, Crowley-Nowick PA, et al. Prevalence of and risks for cervical human papillomavirus infection and squamous intraepithelial lesions in adolescent girls: impact of infection with human immunodeficiency virus. Arch Pediatr Adolesc Med. 2000;154(2):127–34.
12. Meijer CJ, Rozendaal L, Voorhorst FJ, Verheijen R, Helmerhorst TJ, Walboomers JM. Human papillomavirus and screening for cervical cancer: state of art and prospects. Ned Tijdschr Geneeskd. 2000;144(35):1675–9.
13. Gedefaw A, Astatkie A, Tessema GA. The Prevalence of Precancerous Cervical Cancer Lesion among HIV-Infected Women in Southern Ethiopia: A Cross-Sectional Study. PLoS One. 2013;8(12), e84519. doi:10.1371/journal.pone.0084519.
14. Smith JS, Lindsay L, Hoots B, Keys J, Franceschi S, et al. Human papillomavirus type distribution in invasive cervical cancer and high-grade cervical lesions: a meta-analysis update. Int J Cancer. 2007;121(3):621–32.
15. Walboomers JM, Jacobs MV, Manos MM, Bosch FX, Kummer JA, Shah KV, et al. Human papillomavirus is a necessary cause of invasive cervical cancer worldwide. J Pathol. 1999;189:12–9.
16. Schiffman M, Castle PE, Jeronimo J, Rodriguez AC, Wacholder S. Human papillomavirus and cervical cancer. Lancet. 2007;370:890–907.
17. Agaba PA, Thacher TD, Ekwempu CC, Idoko JA. Cervical dysplasia in Nigerian women infected with HIV. Int J Gynaecol Obstet. 2009;107(2):99–102. doi:10.1016/j.ijgo.2009.06.006. Epub 2009 Jul 19.
18. WHO/ICO Information Centre on HPV and Cervical Cancer (HPV Information Centre). Human Papillomavirus and Related Cancers in World. Summary Report 2010. [Date accessed]. www.who.int/hpvcentre.
19. Cancer Research UK Registered charity in England and Wales (1089464), Scotland (SC041666) and the Isle of Man (1103). 2014. cruk.org/cancerstats.
20. Minjee L, Eun-Cheol P, Hoo-Sun C, Jeoung AK, Ki Bong Y, et al. Socioeconomic disparity in cervical cancer screening among Korean women: 1998–2010. MC Public Health. 2013;13:553. doi:10.1186/1471-2458-13-553.
21. Mutyaba T, Mirembe F, Sandin S, Weiderpass E. Evaluation of 'see-see and treat' strategy and role of HIV on cervical cancer prevention in Uganda. Reprod Health. 2010;7:4.
22. Gravitt PE, Belinson JL, Salmeron J, Shah VK. Looking ahead: a case for human papillomavirus testing of self-sampled vaginal specimens as a cervical cancer screening strategy. Int J Cancer. 2011;129:517–27.
23. Pamela L, Claire K, Claire T, Kevin P, Jonathan BA, James J. Cervical cancer screening among HIV-positive women Retrospective cohort study from a tertiary care HIV clinic. Can Fam Physician. 2010;56:e425–31.
24. Everlyne NM, Harrysone EA, Rosebella OO, Joyce HO, Collins O. Determinants of Cervical screening services uptake among 18–49 year old women seeking services at the Jaramogi Oginga Odinga Teaching and Referral Hospital, Kisumu, Kenya. BMC Health Serv Res. 2014;14:335. http://www.biomedcentral.com/1472-6963/14/335.
25. Oliver CE, Chidinma VGO, Per OO, Karen OP. Willingness and acceptability of cervical cancer screening among HIV positive Nigerian women. BMC Public Health. 2013;13:46. http://www.biomedcentral.com/1471-2458/13/46.
26. Zewdie B, Alemseged A, Tefera B, Amare D, Hailemariam S, Vivien T, et al. Health seeking behavior for cervical cancer in Ethiopia: a qualitative study. Int J Equity Health. 2012;11:83. http://www.equityhealthj.com/content/11/1/83.
27. Meredith SS, Ruth MPH, Irene H, Jianmin L, James JG, et al. Proportions of Kaposi Sarcoma, Selected Non-Hodgkin Lymphomas, and Cervical Cancer in the United States Occurring in Persons with AIDS, 1980–2007. JAMA. 2011;305(14):1450–9. doi:10.1001/jama.2011.396.
28. Joint United Nations Program on HIV/AIDS. (UNAIDS) report on the global AIDS epidemic. 2010.
29. Profile on General Hospital, the number of registered and number of Health Facilities in Addis Ababa City by Types of ownership. 2004/ 2005. www.ethiopianembassy.org/About.Ethiopia.
30. Profile on referral Hospital, the number of registered and number of Health Facilities in Addis Ababa city by types of ownership. 2004/ 2005. www.ethiopianembassy.org/About.Ethiopia
31. Central statistical agency, Addis Ababa, Ethiopia. 2007.
32. Peter M, Wangeci M, Grace K, Solomon A, Francesca O. Prevalence and Risk Factors Associated with Precancerous Cervical Cancer Lesions among HIV-Infected Women in Resource-Limited Settings. AIDS Research and Treatment. 2012. doi:10.1155/2012/953743.
33. Nwankwo KC, Aniebue UU, Aguwa EN, Anarado AN, Agunwah E. Knowledge attitudes and practices of cervical cancer screening among urban and rural Nigerian women: a call for education and mass screening. European J Cancer Care. 2011;20:362–7.
34. Abiodun OA, Fatungase OK, Olu-Abiodun OO, Idowu-Ajiboye BA, Awosile JO. An assessment of women's awareness and knowledge about cervical cancer and screening and the barriers to cervical screening in Ogun State, Nigeria. IOSR. J Dental Med Sci. 2013;10(3):52–8. www.iosrjournals.org.
35. Maree JE, Moitse KA. Exploration of knowledge of cervical cancer and cervical cancer screening amongst HIV-positive women. Curationis. 2014;37(1):1209. http://dx.doi.org/10.4102/curationis.v37i1.1209.
36. Gichangi P, Estambale B, Bwayo J, Rogo K, Ojwang S, Opiyo A, et al. Knowledge and practice about cervical cancer and pap smear testing among patients at Kenyatta National Hospital, Nairobi, Kenya. Int J Gynaecol Cancer. 2003;3:827–33.
37. Gharoro EP, Ikeanyi EN. An appraisal of the level of awareness and utilization of the Pap smear as a cervical cancer screening test among female health workers in a tertiary health institution. Int J Gynaecol Cancer. 2006;16:1063–8.
38. Solomon O, Kwasi T, Hadiza K, Edward O, Oluwasanmi A, Otto C, et al. Integrating cervical cancer screening with HIV care in a district hospital in Abuja, Nigeria. Niger. Med J. 2013;54(3):176–84. doi:10.4103/0300-1652.114590. doi:10.4103%2F0300-1652.114590#pmc_ext.
39. Carolyn M. Audet, Carla Silva Matos, Meridith Blevins, Aventina Cardoso and Troy D. Moon. Acceptability of cervical cancer screening in rural Mozambique. Health Education Research February 3, 2012. doi:10.1093/her/cys008.
40. Oche MO, Kaoje AU, Gana G, Ango JT. Cancer of the cervix and cervical screening: Current knowledge, attitude and practices of female health workers in Sokoto, Nigeria. Int J Med Med Sci. 2013;5(4):184–90. doi:10.5897/IJMMS2013.0886. http://www.academicjournals.org/IJMMS.
41. Were E, Nyaberi Z, Buziba N. Perceptions of risk and barriers to cervical cancer screening at Moi Teaching and Referral Hospital (MTRH), Eldoret. Kenya African Health Sci. 2011;11(1):58–64.
42. Sylvia C M, Carolyn MS, and Timothy RBJ. Knowledge, Attitudes, and Demographic Factors Influencing Cervical Cancer Screening Behavior of Zimbabwean Women. Journal Of Women's Health 2011; 20(6). doi:10.1089/jwh.2010.2062.

4

Surgical safety and personal costs in morbidly obese, multimorbid patients diagnosed with early-stage endometrial cancer having a hysterectomy

Andreas Obermair[1,2,8*], Donal J. Brennan[3], Eva Baxter[4], Jane E. Armes[5], Val Gebski[6] and Monika Janda[7]

Abstract

Background: Many women who develop endometrial cancer (EC) or endometrial hyperplasia with atypia are obese and therefore at high risk of surgical complications. Recently clinical trials have been initiated offering non-surgical treatment to these women, but not all may agree to participate in such trials. This paper aims to describe the patient characteristics, and surgical outcomes of women with suspected early stage endometrial cancer and body mass index (BMI) of 30 or greater, who declined enrolment in the feMMe trial, which offers non-surgical hormonal treatment, hormonal plus metformin or hormonal plus weight loss as primary treatment.

Methods: Consecutive case series from a tertiary gynaecological oncology unit. Over the course of the first 2 years of the feMMe trial, 27 patients met the initial eligibility screening, but declined enrolment in the feMMe trial and opted for upfront surgery. The main surgical outcome measures were type of surgical approach, need for conversion from laparoscopic to open approach, length of stay in hospital and adverse events.

Results: Patients' median age was 63 years (range 40 to 86); median BMI was 37.3 kg/m2 (range 30.7 to 54.7); median medical co-morbidities were six (range 3–10). Of the 26/27 surgeries planned to be undertaken laparoscopically, 2/26 patients had to be converted (7 %). Overall, the average hospital stay was 4.5 days, and 11/27 (41 %) of the patients developed one or more adverse events grade 2+ rated according to the Common Toxicity Criteria Version 3.

Conclusions: Adverse surgical outcomes are common in multi-morbid, obese or morbidly obese patients diagnosed with early stage EC or endometrial hyperplasia with atypia and who have a hysterectomy.

Keywords: Endometrial cancer, Endometrial hyperplasia with atypia, Obesity, Surgery, Adverse event

Background

Obesity is a massive health issue in many countries around the world and is also the major risk factor for Endometrial Cancer (EC) [1–4]. It has previously been reported that obesity causes at least 39 % of cases of EC [5]. Obesity is also associated with increased risk of medical co-morbidities (e.g., diabetes, cardiovascular) [6–8]; the need for intense preoperative assessments;

perioperative complications [9]; conversion from laparoscopic to open surgery [10]; intensive postoperative care [11, 12]; treatment costs [11, 13]; and reduced recurrence-free survival [9, 14, 15].

While surgical treatment of EC is generally effective, it does not address the specific needs of the steadily growing group of morbidly obese and multi-morbid patients as well as young obese patients still desiring fertility [16, 17]. For these growing groups of patients treatment often comes at a high personal cost (long hospital stay, protracted recovery from surgery, high incidence of postoperative complications) and subsequent high healthcare cost. We previously estimated hospital costs of $12,872 vs

* Correspondence: obermair@powerup.com.au
[1]Queensland Centre for Gynaecological Cancer, The University of Queensland, Brisbane, QLD, Australia
[2]Greenslopes Private Hospital, Brisbane, QLD, Australia
Full list of author information is available at the end of the article

$25,652 for patients without or with a surgical complication, respectively [11].

The challenges of pre- and postoperative care for multi-morbid and morbidly obese EC patients impact on a variety of resources. Thus, as highlighted by the Royal College of Obstetricians and Gynaecologists, treatment for EC needs to be reassessed in this complex and increasingly common situation [18]. The search for treatment alternatives that are safe, effective and less harmful than surgery is warranted.

Recently, the Gynecologic Cancer InterGroup identified conservative treatment for fertility sparing purposes and to treat morbidly obese women as a most pressing research priority at their EC Clinical Trials Planning Meeting in the Netherlands [19].

To address this need the feMMe trial was initiated in 2013 [20]. It is an open-label, randomised clinical trial exploring conservative, non-surgical treatment options to achieve a pathological complete response in patients diagnosed with early-stage EC (ANZGOG #1301, NCT01686126).

The aim of the present study was to describe the safety and clinical outcomes of consecutive patients who would have fulfilled the eligibility criteria for the feMMe trial and who were offered participation in the feMMe trial, but declined enrolment and opted for hysterectomy at two institutions instead.

Methods

Approval for this study was received from the Royal Brisbane & Women's Hospital Human Research Ethics Committee (HREC/15/QRBW/113). All patients reported here have been identified through gynaecological oncology services at Royal Brisbane and Women's Hospital and Greenslopes Private Hospital. These patients would have been considered potentially eligible to be enrolled in the feMMe trial.

The feMMe trial is an open label, randomised phase II trial with three treatment arms and is recruiting patients at present [20]. The three arms consist of Intrauterine Progestin (IUP) placed into the uterine cavity (45 patients); IUP plus Metformin 1000 mg daily (75 patients); or IUP plus weight loss through Weight Watchers (45 patients). Weight Watchers is a standardised, evidence-based and formally tested weight loss intervention including diet, physical activity, social networking and support via a network of lifestyle centres, one-on-one support and an online program [21, 22]. It has been shown to be the most cost-effective among a range of currently available weight loss programs [22].

In this phase II trial randomisation aims to eliminate selection bias rather than allow a formal comparison of groups. Trial methodology, in-/exclusion criteria, randomisation /stratification and study assessments were published recently [20]. Human Research and Ethics Committee and site-specific approvals are underway in various Australian States but only sites in the state of Queensland are fully approved and enrolling at present. All patients are followed for 6 months and a central pathology review will be conducted once all patients are enrolled.

Eligibility criteria: Only patients with histologically confirmed innocuous EC or endometrial hyperplasia with atypia, Body Mass Index (BMI) >30 kg/m2 who wish to retain fertility or who suffer from medical impairments and are considered suboptimal candidates for hysterectomy are eligible [20].

Patients are excluded from enrolment if they had a histological type other than endometrioid adenocarcinoma of the endometrium, clinically advanced disease, involvement of the uterine cervix or enlarged retroperitoneal lymph nodes.

To be eligible for this study, patients had to have a CT scan of the abdomen and pelvis as well as imaging (CT or X-Ray to the chest) suggesting the absence of extra-uterine disease. Patients are also only considered eligible if their baseline serum CA-125 reading was 30 U/ml or less.

Patients who agree to proceed with enrolment into the feMMe trial receive a pelvic MRI to ensure that the depth of invasion is not greater than 50 % of myometrium and to re-confirm the absence of extrauterine dissemination. Patients who decline participation in feMMe (including the patients reported herein) however do not receive an MRI as it is not part of the standard imaging workup in our institutions.

In addition to the established criteria for low-risk disease (CT and MRI scan showing the absence of extrauterine disease, FIGO grade = 1) we offer enrolment only to patients with serum CA125 of 30 U/ml or less [23]. Considering the strict criteria above, we expect that the risk of enrolling patients with advanced or aggressive disease is minimal.

All patients reported here did not qualify for feMMe because they preferred hysterectomy and as a consequence declined enrolment into the feMMe trial. Hence, following standard protocols, a pelvic MRI was not offered (as has been explained above).

In all 27 patients, pre-existing medical co-morbidities were recorded as well as any intra- or post-operative Adverse Events (AEs) up to 30 days post-operatively. We coded AEs according to the post-operative Common Toxicity Criteria (CTC) Version 3 and report any AEs grade 2+ (moderate to severe AEs). Analyses were restricted to women who completed 30 days of follow-up after surgery.

Results

The clinical outcomes of 27 patients who fulfilled the eligibility criteria but declined participation in the feMMe trial and have chosen primary surgical treatment instead are reported here.

Patients' median age was 63 years (range 40 to 86 years) and the median BMI was 37.3 kg/m2 (range 30.7 to 54.7 kg/m2), median ASA was 3 (range 2–3). At baseline a total of 167 medical co-morbidities were recorded among the 27 patients including hypertension, hyperlipidemia, hypercholesterolemia, diabetes, obstructive sleep apnoea, fatty liver and many other lifestyle-related ailments.

Twenty-six patients had a total laparoscopic procedure of which two patients (7 %) had to be converted to a laparotomy. One patient required an abdominal hysterectomy through a midline incision (Table 1).

The reasons for conversion to open surgery in two patients included an inadvertent gastrotomy through a trocar at primary port entry, which required primary surgical closure. The second patient sustained an enterotomy to the small bowel during adhesiolysis. The

Table 1 Patient characteristics

Patient #	Age (years)	D&C histology	BMI	Surgical approach	Node dissection	LOS	Stage	FIGO grade	Depth of invasion (%)	Intra-, Postoperative complications
1	40	EHA	31.0	TLH	0	2	1a	1	15	
2	56	G1 EAC	49.2	TLH	0	1	1a	1	0	Post-operative bleeding
3	62	G1 EAC	35.1	TLH	0	2	1a	2	11	
4	69	G1 EAC	54.7	TLH	0	2	1a	2	38	Vault haematoma, abdominal cramping, urinary frequency
5	75	G1 EAC	39.6	TLH	0	2	1a	1	0	
6	65	G1 EAC	40.9	TLH	0	2	1b	2	60	
7	56	G1 EAC	42.7	TLH	0	5	1a	1	0	
8	74	G1 EAC	46.8	TLH	0	1	1b	2	52	
9	73	G1 EAC	44.8	TLH	0	8	2	2	18	Post-operative bleeding, anaemia, retroperitoneal haematoma, rise in Troponin
10	68	EHA	35.4	TLH	1	2	1b	2	60	
11	75	G1 EAC	38.9	TLH converted to TAH	0	14	1b	2	57	Unplanned gastrostomy, unplanned stay in ICU
12	69	EHA	45.5	TLH	0	2	1a		0	
13	67	G1 EAC	32.5	TLH	0	3	1a	2	8	Vault haematoma, hypokalaemia, sinus tachycardia
14	57	G1 EAC	30.7	TLH	0	2	1a	1	50	Vault haematoma, pain
15	73	G1 EAC	34.3	TLH	0	5	1a	1	10	
16	69	EHA	29.4	TLH	0	2	1a	1	0	Vault haematoma, hypotension, hypokalaemia
17	68	G1 EAC	43.9	TLH	0	2	1a	2	45	
18	78	G1 EAC	32.0	TLH	0	2	1a	1	45	
19	63	EHA	33.5	TLH	0	2	0		0	Hypertension
20	66	EHA	40.6	TLH	0	2	1a	1	1	Atrial fibrillation
21	60	EHA	37.1	TLH	0	7	1a	1	37	
22	70	EHA	43.1	TLH	0	5	1b	2	75	Chest infection, wound dehiscence, vault haematoma, pain
23	72	G1 EAC	42.7	TLH	1	3	3b	1	100	
24	50	EHA	35.6	TLH	0	9	1a	1	39	Fluid overload, pulmonary oedema
25	55	G1 EAC	33.3	TAH	0	4	2	1	7	
26	73	G1 EAC	47.0	TLH	0	2	1a1	1	0	
27	86	G1 EAC	43.6	TLH converted to TAH	1	28	1a	1	31	Unplanned enterotomy, wound infection, Atrial fibrillation, renal failure

Abbreviations: BMI body mass index, *EAC* endometriod adencocarcinoma, *EHA* endometrial hyperplasia with atypia, *TLH* total laparoscopic hysterectomy, *TAH* total abdominal hysterectomy, *LOS* length of stay, *FIGO* the international federation of gynecology and obstetrics

adhesions could not be dissected from the anterior abdominal wall laparoscopically. The enterotomy was recognised at surgery and the operation was completed through open surgery. The median percentage of invasion into the endometrium was 31 % (range 0–100 %).

The average postoperative hospital stay was 4.5 days (median 2 days), ranging from 1 to 28 days. The patient with a 28-day hospital stay was a patient with a body mass index of 43.6 kg/m2 who required conversion from laparoscopic to open surgery. She developed a wound infection (limited to the subcutaneous adipose tissue), atrial fibrillation resulting in a stay at the Cardiac Care Unit followed by acute renal failure. The patient was discharged into rehab on day 28 post surgery.

Within 30 days from surgery, 12 patients developed at total of 30 AEs. One of 27 patients developed an AE CTC grade 1 and 11/12 patients developed one or more AEs CTC grade 2+ (41 %). All but 5 AEs were surgery related (Table 1).

Nine patients were enrolled to treat endometrial hyperplasia with atypia based on a pre-hysterectomy endometrial biopsy or curette and 18 of 27 patients had surgery for histologically proven endometrioid endometrial adenocarcinoma on endometrial biopsy or curette.

Of those nine patients who were treated for endometrial hyperplasia with atypia, seven patients were found to have endometrial adenocarcinoma in the final histopathology specimen of the uterus.

In patients with the final histopathological outcomes confirming endometrial adenocarcinoma, all patients were diagnosed with endometrioid cell type. In those patients FIGO grade was grade 1 in 14/25 patients and grade 2 in 10/25 patients. In one patient there was no residual disease at hysterectomy. The depth of invasion was limited to inner half in all but five patients.

Two patients had extension of disease into the endocervix (stage 2) and one patient had full thickness myomterial invasion of a grade 1 adenocarcinoma and focal involvement of a fallopian tube (FIGO stage 3b).

Discussion
Main findings
Adverse surgical outcomes are common in multi-morbid and morbidly obese patients diagnosed with early stage EC who have a hysterectomy. Obesity is an independent risk factor for AEs, regardless of the surgical approach [12]. Obese women will have a higher risk of conversion to open surgery [10] and their risk of surgical AEs is higher [24].

For comparison we quote data from the prospective randomised and multi-institutional LACE trial below [12, 25]. The LACE trial compared open with laparoscopic surgery for early stage EC or endometrial hyperplasia with atypia. It was an international trial but the vast majority of patients were treated in Australian institutions.

In the case series reported here, all but one operations were planned to be performed laparoscopically; two of the 27 patients required a conversion from laparoscopy to laparotomy (7 %) and one patient required a primary laparotomy, implying that 10 % of patients required a laparotomy to accomplish the surgical task of a hysterectomy. By contrast, the conversion rate from laparoscopic to open in the prospective randomised and multi-institutional LACE trial was only 3.8 %, most likely due to omitting the requirements for a comprehensive pelvic and aortic retroperitoneal node dissection in these patients and a smaller proportion of patients with a BMI of 30 or greater.

By contrast, pelvic and aortic lymph node dissection was mandatory in the LAP-2 trial corresponding to a 25.8 % conversion rate. Patients with a high BMI had an up to 60 % risk of conversion to open surgery [24].

In the context of morbidly obese and multi-morbid patients we typically aim to minimise the risk of conversion, which may attract further intraoperative and postoperative morbidity. In those instances patients' adjuvant treatment may be guided by their general medical health and histopathological features available from the primary tumour. At present only low-level evidence is available on the feasibility and safety of robotic surgery in morbidly obese patients requiring a retroperitoneal node dissection. Deaths due to complications of robotic surgery have also been reported [26].

In this sample, the mean length of hospital stay (LOS) was 4.5 days. Length of stay was largely associated with the development of postoperative complications. However, in some patients an uneventful postoperative recovery still required a longer than expected LOS due to slow recovery. In the LACE trial, reflecting the Australian health care situation the LOS was 2.4 days for patients assigned to have a laparoscopic hysterectomy and 5 days for patients who were randomised to have a laparotomy.

In this series of patients the per-patient incidence of surgical AE's CTC grade 2+ was high at 41 %.

Strength and limitations
Innovatively this case series details the outcomes of patients who were offered enrolment in a non-surgical clinical trial, but preferred surgery. These results again highlight the increased risk of obese patients to develop complications as previously shown in other international series. This group of morbidly obese and multi-morbid patients carries a high risk of conversion to laparotomy, a longer hospital stay and a three to four times higher risk of surgical AEs compared to previous series with a wider range of BMI. LOS and AEs are significant contributors to health care costs and funders of health care services

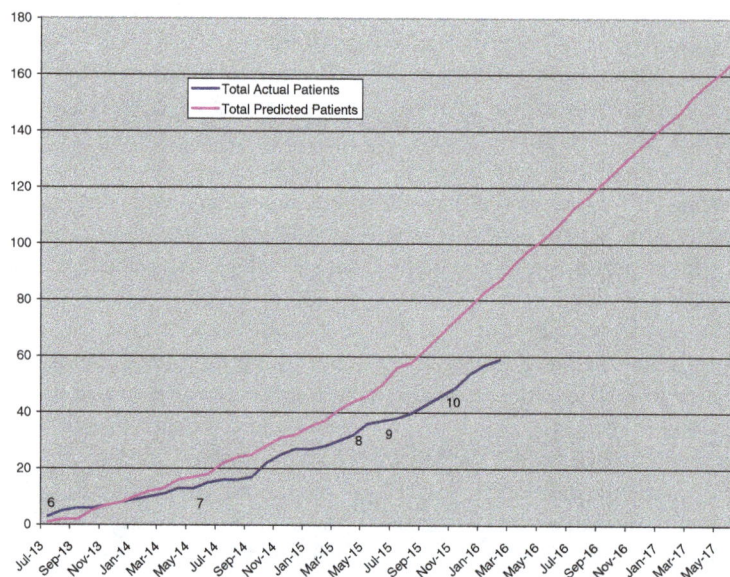

Fig. 1 Recruitment chart for the FeMMe trial

must therefore expect high costs among obese patients treated surgically for EC [13]. Limitations of this study include the non-random assignment to surgery, which was based on patients' preference, as well as the relatively small number of patients available for data collection.

Conclusions

While hysterectomy for EC offers excellent survival outcomes, it also comes at a price: slow recovery from surgery, surgical AEs, loss of fertility, financial and societal treatment costs [27, 28].

Importantly these results indicate that current risk estimations do not take populations at high surgical risk (e.g. obese and multi-morbid patients) into sufficiently account. Thus, the efficacy of treatment alternatives need to be assessed in the complex and increasingly common situation of obesity and EC or endometrial hyperplasia with atypia [18]. We envisage that for obese and multimorbid patients less invasive treatments will achieve equivalent survival outcomes at a lower personal and financial cost to patients and society [13].

Historically intracavitary brachytherapy has been used to treat patients at advanced age and severe medical illnesses and with the advent of IMRT [29], radiotherapy may be well positioned to be evaluated in clinical trials as an alternative to major surgery.

By contrast, others units currently investigate the effectiveness of a levonorgestrel containing intrauterine device for the treatment of endometrial cancer. The feMMe trial (ANZGOG #1301, NCT01686126) is an international, phase II, 3-arm randomised clinical trial exploring conservative, non-surgical treatment options to achieve a pathological complete response in early-stage endometrial cancer patients who are suboptimal candidates for hysterectomy [20].

In addition to the eligibility criteria for this case series, patients have to have an MRI of the pelvis to determine the depth of myometrial invasion. In the context of the results reported here this is well warranted, and the pelvic MRI will also be critical to exclude involvement of the cervix and/or adnexae.

The trial is recruiting at present (Fig. 1 shows the recruitment chart) and also includes a molecular component investigating the mechanisms of change associated with response or non-response to feMMe intervention (tumour polymorphisms; molecular phenotype of tumours; circulating cytokines, such as adipokines, hormones and growth factors). Phase II results are expected for 2017, and early discussion about the optimal Phase III trial design to follow have been initiated in 2015.

Ethics approval

Royal Brisbane & Women's Hospital Human Research Ethics Committee (HREC/15/QRBW/113).

Competing interests

AO acts as a consultant for Covidien and receives research support from Ethicon, a Johnson and Johnson company. AO has received travel support from Gate healthcare. AO is the founder and director of SurgicalPerformance.com, an online audit software. All other authors have declared no conflicts of interest.

Authors' contributions

The authors conceived and designed the feMMe trial and contributed to the conception of the present analyses of patients who preferred surgical treatment. All authors contributed to the writing of this article or revised it critically. All authors gave final approval of the version to be published and will be accountable for all aspects of the work.

Acknowledgments

The authors thank the feMMe study staff Anne Hughes, Vanessa Taylor, Trudi Cattley, Vanessa Behan, Kerry Millgate, as well as Karen Sanday. Interested clinicians could enquire with the corresponding author about enrolment of suitable patients into the feMMe trial.

Funding

The feMMe trial is funded by Cancer Australia #1044900 and #1078121, UQ academic Title Holders Grant, Royal Brisbane and Women's Hospital Foundation, Lord Mayor's community fund, Cherish Women's Cancer Foundation and Australian and New Zealand Gynaecologic Oncology Group. MJ is funded by NHMRC Career Development Fellowship #1045247.

Author details

[1]Queensland Centre for Gynaecological Cancer, The University of Queensland, Brisbane, QLD, Australia. [2]Greenslopes Private Hospital, Brisbane, QLD, Australia. [3]Rotunda Hospital, Dublin, Ireland. [4]QIMR Berghofer Medical Research Institute, Brisbane, QLD, Australia. [5]Anatomical Pathology Mater Health Services, Mater Adult Hospital, and Mater Research Institute-University of Queensland, Brisbane, QLD, Australia. [6]University of Sydney NHMRC Clinical Trials Centre, Sydney, NSW, Australia. [7]School of Public Health, Institute for Health and Biomedical Innovation, Queensland University of Technology, Brisbane, QLD, Australia. [8]Queensland Centre for Gynaecological Cancer, c/o Royal Brisbane and Women's Hospital, Butterfield Street, Herston, Brisbane, QLD 4029, Australia.

References

1. Renehan AG, Tyson M, Egger M, Heller RF, Zwahlen M. Body-mass index and incidence of cancer: a systematic review and meta-analysis of prospective observational studies. Lancet. 2008;371(9612):569–78.
2. Kaaks R, Lukanova A, Kurzer MS. Obesity, endogenous hormones, and endometrial cancer risk: a synthetic review. Cancer Epidemiol Biomarkers Prev. 2002;11(12):1531–43.
3. Nagle CM, Marquart L, Bain CJ, O'Brien S, Lahmann PH, Quinn M, et al. Impact of weight change and weight cycling on risk of different subtypes of endometrial cancer. Eur J Cancer. 2013;49(12):2717–26.
4. Park SL, Goodman MT, Zhang ZF, Kolonel LN, Henderson BE, Setiawan VW. Body size, adult BMI gain and endometrial cancer risk: the multiethnic cohort. Int J Cancer. 2010;126(2):490–9.
5. Bergstrom A, Pisani P, Tenet V, Wolk A, Adami HO. Overweight as an avoidable cause of cancer in Europe. Int J Cancer. 2001;91(3):421–30.
6. Bhaskaran K, Douglas I, Forbes H, dos-Santos-Silva I, Leon DA, Smeeth L. Body-mass index and risk of 22 specific cancers: a population-based cohort study of 5.24 million UK adults. Lancet. 2014;384(9945):755–65.
7. Calle EE, Kaaks R. Overweight, obesity and cancer: epidemiological evidence and proposed mechanisms. Nat Rev Cancer. 2004;4(8):579–91.
8. Lucenteforte E, Bosetti C, Talamini R, Montella M, Zucchetto A, Pelucchi C, et al. Diabetes and endometrial cancer: effect modification by body weight, physical activity and hypertension. Br J Cancer. 2007;97(7):995–8.
9. Gunderson CC, Java J, Moore KN, Walker JL. The impact of obesity on surgical staging, complications, and survival with uterine cancer: a Gynecologic Oncology Group LAP2 ancillary data study. Gynecol Oncol. 2014;133(1):23–7.
10. Mourits MJ, Bijen CB, Arts HJ, ter Brugge HG, van der Sijde R, Paulsen L, et al. Safety of laparoscopy versus laparotomy in early-stage endometrial cancer: a randomised trial. Lancet Oncol. 2010;11(8):763–71.
11. Kondalsamy-Chennakesavan S, Gordon LG, Sanday K, Bouman C, De Jong S, Nicklin J, et al. Hospital costs associated with adverse events in gynecological oncology. Gynecol Oncol. 2011;121(1):70–5.
12. Kondalsamy-Chennakesavan S, Janda M, Gebski V, Baker J, Brand A, Hogg R, et al. Risk factors to predict the incidence of surgical adverse events following open or laparoscopic surgery for apparent early stage endometrial cancer: results from a randomised controlled trial. Eur J Cancer. 2012;48(14):2155–62.
13. Graves N, Janda M, Merollini K, Gebski V, Obermair A, committee Lt. The cost-effectiveness of total laparoscopic hysterectomy compared to total abdominal hysterectomy for the treatment of early stage endometrial cancer. BMJ Open. 2013; 3(4): e001884. doi:10.1136/bmjopen-2012-001884.
14. Canlorbe G, Bendifallah S, Raimond E, Graesslin O, Hudry D, Coutant C, et al. Severe Obesity Impacts Recurrence-Free Survival of Women with High-Risk Endometrial Cancer: Results of a French Multicenter Study. Ann Surg Oncol. 2014;22:2714–21.
15. McTiernan A, Irwin M, Vongruenigen V. Weight, physical activity, diet, and prognosis in breast and gynecologic cancers. J Clin Oncol. 2010;28(26):4074–80.
16. Linkov F, Elishaev E, Gloyeske N, Edwards R, Althouse AD, Geller MA, et al. Bariatric surgery-induced weight loss changes immune markers in the endometrium of morbidly obese women. Surg Obes Relat Dis. 2014;10(5):921–6.
17. Nevadunsky NS, Van Arsdale A, Strickler HD, Moadel A, Kaur G, Levitt J, et al. Obesity and age at diagnosis of endometrial cancer. Obstet Gynecol. 2014;124(2 Pt 1):300–6.
18. Endometrial Cancer in Obese Women. Scientific Impact Paper No. 32. London, United Kingdom: Royal College of Obstetricians and Gynaecologists; 2012.
19. Creutzberg CL, Kitchener HC, Birrer MJ, Landoni F, Lu KH, Powell M, et al. Gynecologic Cancer InterGroup (GCIG) endometrial cancer clinical trials planning meeting: taking endometrial cancer trials into the translational era. Int J Gynecol Cancer. 2013;23(8):1528–34.
20. Hawkes AL, Quinn M, Gebski V, Armes J, Brennan D, Janda M, et al. Improving treatment for obese women with early stage cancer of the uterus: rationale and design of the levonorgestrel intrauterine device +/– metformin +/– weight loss in endometrial cancer (feMME) trial. Contemp Clin Trials. 2014;39(1):14–21.
21. Jebb SA, Ahern AL, Olson AD, Aston LM, Holzapfel C, Stoll J, et al. Primary care referral to a commercial provider for weight loss treatment versus standard care: a randomised controlled trial. Lancet. 2011;378(9801):1485–92.
22. Finkelstein EA, Kruger E. Meta- and cost-effectiveness analysis of commercial weight loss strategies. Obesity (Silver Spring). 2014;22(9):1942–51.
23. Nicklin J, Janda M, Gebski V, Jobling T, Land R, Manolitsas T, et al. The utility of serum CA-125 in predicting extra-uterine disease in apparent early-stage endometrial cancer. Int J Cancer. 2012;131(4):885–90.
24. Walker JL, Piedmonte MR, Spirtos NM, Eisenkop SM, Schlaerth JB, Mannel RS, et al. Laparoscopy compared with laparotomy for comprehensive surgical staging of uterine cancer: Gynecologic Oncology Group Study LAP2. J Clin Oncol. 2009;27(32):5331–6.
25. Obermair A, Janda M, Baker J, Kondalsamy-Chennakesavan S, Brand A, Hogg R, et al. Improved surgical safety after laparoscopic compared to open surgery for apparent early stage endometrial cancer: results from a randomised controlled trial. Eur J Cancer. 2012;48(8):1147–53.
26. Shields K, Minion L, Willmott L, Sumner D, Monk B. Ten-Year Food and Drug Administration Reporting on Robotic Complications in Gynecologic Surgery. J Gynecol Surg. 2015;31(6):331–5.
27. Tangjitgamol S, Anderson BO, See HT, Lertbutsayanukul C, Sirisabya N, Manchana T, et al. Management of endometrial cancer in Asia: consensus statement from the Asian Oncology Summit 2009. Lancet Oncol. 2009;10(11):1119–27.
28. Zullo F, Falbo A, Palomba S. Safety of laparoscopy vs laparotomy in the surgical staging of endometrial cancer: a systematic review and metaanalysis of randomized controlled trials. Am J Obstet Gynecol. 2012;207(2):94–100.
29. Paganetti H. Changes in tumor cell response due to prolonged dose delivery times in fractionated radiation therapy. Int J Radiat Oncol Biol Phys. 2005;63(3):892–900.

Surgical management of lung, liver and brain metastases from gynecological cancers

Neville F. Hacker[1,2*] and Archana Rao[1,2]

Abstract

Background: The management of patients with recurrent gynecological malignancy is complex, and often contentious. While historically, patients with metastases in the lungs, liver or brain have been treated with palliative intent, surgery is proving to have an increasing role in the management of such patients.

Methods: In this review article, the surgical management of lung, liver and brain metastases from gynecological cancers is examined. A search of the English language literature over the last 25 years was conducted using the Medline and PubMed databases.

Results: The results for management of metastases from the endometrium, ovary and cervix to the lung, brain and liver show that surprisingly good long-term survival results can be achieved for resection of metastases from all three organs. Patient selection is critical, and surgery is often used in conjunction with other treatment modalities.

Conclusions: From this review, it is apparent that surgery should play an increasing role in the management of patients with parenchymal metastases from gynecological cancers. The surgery should ideally be performed in high volume, tertiary centers where there is a committed multi-disciplinary team with the necessary infrastructure to achieve the best possible outcomes in terms of both survival and morbidity.

Keywords: Gynecological malignancy, Cervix, Endometrium, Ovary, Metastasis, Brain, Lung, Liver, Survival

Background

The primary management of patients with a gynecological malignancy is usually protocol driven, and is seldom controversial, but the management of patients with recurrent disease is often contentious. It requires a multidisciplinary team discussion, and complex decisions around the possible roles of surgery, chemotherapy, radiation therapy or hormonal therapy. Often, a combination of therapies will be required.

Historically, patients with metastases in the lungs, liver or brain have been treated with palliative intent. Surgery is proving to have an increasing role in the management of such patients, and survivals are surprisingly good in many cases.

We undertook a search of the English literature over the past 25 years to seek references to the surgical management of lung, liver or brain metastases from cancers of the endometrium, ovary or cervix. The MEDLINE/PubMed database was searched, using the keywords metastases, lungs, liver, brain, endometrium, ovary and cervix.

Surgical management of lung metastases

The first successful lobectomy for lung metastases in the 20th century was reported by Barney and Churchill in 1939 [1]. The patient was a 55-year old woman with a metastatic renal cell carcinoma, and she survived disease-free for 23 years Subsequently, there have been a number of reports of pulmonary metastasectomy for a variety of tumors [2–8], and the commonest primary epithelial tumour sites have been the colon, rectum, kidney and breast [9].

* Correspondence: n.hacker@unsw.edu.au
[1]Gynaecological Cancer Centre, Royal Hospital for Women, Randwick, NSW 2031, Australia
[2]School of Women's and Children's Health, University of New South Wales, Kensington, NSW 2052, Australia

Endometrial cancer is the commonest gynecological cancer in Western countries, and the majority of patients are diagnosed with disease confined to the corpus [10]. The lungs are the commonest site of hematogenous spread for patients with advanced endometrial cancer [11, 12], but lung metastasis may occasionally occur with very early stage disease [13].

The commonest gynaecological cancer in developing countries is cervical cancer [14]. A review of the records of 2075 Sri Lankan women treated for cervical cancer from 1989 to 1993 reported that 38 patients (1.8 %) developed lung metastases, with a median interval from diagnosis of 9 months [15].

Diagnosis
Most recurrences in the lungs are diagnosed by the investigation of symptoms, or of rising CA125 titers in the case of ovarian cancer. Barter et al. reported that there was no indication for routine chest x-ray in the follow-up of patients with cervical cancer, as there was no significant survival difference between symptomatic and asymptomatic patients [16].

Imaging
Thoracic metastases from gynecologic malignancies exhibit various imaging patterns [17]. Metastases from endometrial cancer typically manifest as pulmonary nodules and lymphadenopathy, whereas ovarian cancer often manifests with small pleural effusions and subtle pleural nodules. Most squamous cervical carcinomas manifest as solid pulmonary nodules, but cavitation occurs reasonably frequently. A "halo sign" is sometimes seen in hemorrhagic metastatic choriocarcinoma. Metastases from common gynecologic malignancies may be subtle and mimic benign condition such as intrapulmonary lymph nodes or granulomatous disease [17]. If a solitary lung lesion is found, it is always important to consider the possibility of primary lung cancer.

The spiral computed tomographic (CT) scan has revolutionized the identification of small lung metastases. Before the advent of spiral CT technology, bimanual palpation of the lung through an open thoracotomy or sternotomy was considered necessary to avoid missing small lesions [9]. The spiral CT scan has allowed better characterisation of both location and resectability of pulmonary nodules, so minimally invasive surgery has become a more attractive option [18].

A preoperative PET/CT is desirable to exclude disease beyond the lungs, which would make pulmonary resection inadvisable in most cases.

Indications for pulmonary metastasectomy
Specific criteria vary considerably in the literature. Clearly, there needs to be an adequate pulmonary reserve, and a limited number of lung metastases. A solitary metastasis is ideal, and 2 papers have reported a 100 % 5-year survival for a total of 21 patients with a solitary endometrial lung metastasis treated with wedge resection and adjuvant hormonal therapy [11, 19]. The estrogen and progesterone receptor (ER/PR) status should be obtained at the time of metastacectomy for endometrial cancer [20].

Except for patients with ovarian cancer, whose tumors are often quite sensitive to chemotherapy or targeted therapy, it is preferable to have no spread beyond the thorax. A disease-free interval of at least 12, but preferably 24 months, is an important prognostic factor [9, 19, 21–23].

Surgical technique
The operative procedure of choice is a wedge resection. Seki et al. stated that this should be performed with a disease-free margin of at least 2 cm for patients with metastatic lesions smaller than 3 cm diameter. Lobectomy was recommended for lesions larger than 3 cm, because of the greater risk of microscopic satellite lesions [24].

Although most reports are of open thoracotomies, video-assisted thoracic surgery (VATS) has recently become an accepted and often preferred modality in patients with a limited number of metastases, either unilateral or bilateral [18]. It is usually associated with a shorter hospital stay, and preserves the ability of the patient to undergo repeated resections, which may be necessary to achieve cure [9].

Mediastinal lymphadenectomy was recommended by Seki et al. for metastatic squamous cell carcinomas 3 cm or more in diameter [24]. In the paper from the Mayo clinic, there was no association between lymphadenectomy and survival, but the number of positive nodes was small [23]. On the evidence available, resection of at least bulky nodes only would seem to be a reasonable option.

Reported series
The findings of reported series with 5 or more patients are summarised in Table 1. Although small series had been reported earlier [2, 25, 26], the first major report of resection of pulmonary metastases from a gynecological cancer came from Memorial Sloan Kettering Cancer Center in 1992 [27]. The study involved 45 patients whose pulmonary metastases from uterine sarcomas were resected between 1960 and 1989. All patients had a prior hysterectomy for uterine sarcoma, no extrathoracic tumor, and disease that was thought to be resectable. The mean age of the patients was 50 years, and the mean interval from hysterectomy to thoracotomy was 44 months (range 1 to 193 months).

Table 1 Major series reporting surgical management of pulmonary metastases from gynaecological malignancies

First Author Year of Publication	Number of Cases	Primary Tumour	Pattern of Metastasis	Surgery	Survival/Recurrence Outcomes	Prognostic Factors
Adachi [29] 2015	23	Epithelial gynecologic cancers Major series reporting suCervical – 60.9 % Endometrial – 17.4 % Ovarian – 21.7 %	1 nodule – 69.6 % 2–3 nodules – 30.4 %	VATS – 56.5 % Conventional thoracotomy – 43.5 %	5 year OS: Cervical – 61 % Endometrial – 100 % Ovarian – 100 % Recurrence – 43.4 %	Univariate analysis – positive prognostic factors for survival: Endometrioid vs mucinous adenoca DFI >2 years
Gonzalez Casaurran [19] 2011	27	Uterine and cervical cancer	1 metastasis – 66.7 % 2 metastases – 18.5 % ≥2 metastases – 14.8 %	Surgical approach: - thoracotomy – 81.5 % - sequential bilateral – 7.4 % - unilateral VATS – 3.7 % - sequential bilateral VATS – 3.7 % - VATS + thoracotomy – 3.7 % Lung resection: - Wedge resection – 81.5 % - Lobectomy – 11.1 % - Other – 7.4 % Second surgery for metastases – 18.5 %	Median survival from diagnosis of metastases – 94 months 5-year OS after diagnosis of metastases – 84.1 % Overall relapse rate 44 %	Positive prognostic factors Primary site – endometrial vs cervical ($P = 0.023$) DFI >24 months ($p = 0.054$)
Burt [22] 2011	82	Sarcoma Included male and female patients Leiomyosarcoma – 31 cases (38 %) – 24 pts (77 %) of these were female In female pts, uterus most common primary site	Solitary metastases – 16 pts (52 %) Bilateral disease – 19 %	- Wedge resection – 71 % - Lobectomy – 23 % - Segmentectomy – 6 % - VATS – 58 %	5 year survival: - Leiomyosarcoma – 52 % - other sarcoma – 32 % 2nd pulmonary metastasectomy – 58.5 % Second pulmonary recurrence – 30.5 %	Multivariate analysis – DFI >12 months from time of primary tumour resection
Lim [90] 2010	21	Primary and recurrent cervical cancer	Not reported	23 resections in 21 patients - thoracotomies – 43.5 % - VATS – 52.2 % - VATS following thoracotomies – 4.3 % Procedures – 49 - wedge resections – 51.1 % - lobectomies – 18.4 % - mediastinal LN dissections – 24.5 % - segmentectomy – 2.0 % - diaphragmatic resection – 2.0 % - pleurectomy – 2.0 %	Note – only 14 patients had recurrent cervical cancer, and 1 patient had primary lung cancer and mediastinal LN metastasis from cervical cancer Median f/up 16 months (range 2–67) - 2 pts died of disease - 3 pts alive with disease - 16 pts alive without disease	Not reported
Clavero [23] 2006	70	Uterine corpus – 52.9 % Endometrium – 32.9 % Cervix – 10.0 % Ovaries – 2.9 % Vagina – 1.3 % Histopathology: Leiomyosarcoma – 41.4 % Adenocarcinoma – 32.9 %	Median number of lung metastases – 2 (range 1–19)	Wedge excision – 63 % Lobectomy – 20 % Bilobectomy – 3 % Pneumonectomy – 2.5 % Combination – 12.5 %	5-year OS 46.8 % (95 % CI 34.2–63.0 %) 10 year OS – 34.3 % (95 % CI 19.7–52.5 %)	Factors that adversely affected survival: DFI between 1st gynecologic procedure and pulmonary resection <24 months ($p = 0.004$) Primary site in cervix ($p < 0.001$)

Table 1 Major series reporting surgical management of pulmonary metastases from gynaecological malignancies (*Continued*)

Study	Number	Histology	Solitary vs multiple	Surgery	Survival	Prognostic factors
		Other sarcoma – 15.7 % SCC – 7.1 % Other – 2.9 %				
Yamomoto [28] 2004	29 (out of 7748 = 0.37 %)	Cervical cancer (Stage Ib or II treated with curative intent surgery or radiotherapy)	Solitary metastasis – 58.6 % Multiple metastases – 43.4 %	Wedge resection – 27.6 % Segmentectomy – 6.9 % Lobectomy – 65.5 % Hilar or mediastinal lymph node dissection – 55.2 %	5 year DFS after pulmonary metastasectomy – 32.9 %	For DFS: - ≤2 metastases - SCC
Anraku [21] 2004	133	Uterine malignancies (cervix and endometrium) Histopathology: SCC – 43.6 % Cervical adenocarcinoma – 9.8 % Endometrial adenocarcinoma – 17.3 % Choriocarcinoma – 12.0 % Leiomyosarcoma – 4.7 %	Solitary metastasis –58 % 2–3 mets – 23 % ≥4 mets – 17 %	Wedge resection – 50 % Lobectomy – 45 % Bilobectomy – 2.5 % Pneumonectomy – 2.5 %	Overall survival after surgical resection: 5-year – 54.6 % 10-year – 44.9 % 5-year survival by histpathological type: SCC – 46.8 % Cervical adenoca – 40.3 % Endometrial adenoca – 75.7 % Choriocarcinoma – 86.5 % Leiomyosarcoma – 37.9 %	Univariate analysis – negative prognostic factors: Primary tumour in cervix DFI <12 months Resection ≥ 4 mets Large tumour size (≥3 cm) Multivariate analysis: DFI < 12 months
Anderson [20] 2001	82 eligible pts 25 underwent pulmonary resection	Eligible patients: Uterine – 73.2 % Cervical – 26.8 % Patients undergoing resection: Uterine – 76.0 % Cervical – 24.0 %	Solitary – 28 % Multiple – 72 %	Uterine: - Wedge – 63.1 % - Lobectomy – 10.5 % - Lobectomy/wedge – 15.8 % - Bilobectomy – 5.3 % - Segmentectomy – 5.3 % Cervix: - Wedge – 66.7 % - Lobectomy – 33.3 %	Uterine cancer - median survival 26 months - Leiomyosarcoma –25 months - Adenocarcinoma – 46 months Cervix cancer - median survival 36 months	Uterine cancer – favourable prognostic factors: Leiomyosarcoma vs adenocarcinoma (p = 0.02)
Levenback [27] 1992	45	Uterine sarcomas: - Leiomyosarcoma – 84 % - Endometrial stromal sarcoma – 9 % - Mesodermal mixed tumours – 7 %	Unilateral lesions – 71 % 1 lesion – 51 % Nodules >2 cm – 70 %	Staged thoracotomies – 100 % Median sternotomy and bilateral resections – 4.4 % Incomplete resection – 36 %	From time of pulmonary resection: - 5 year survival – 43 % - 10 year survival – 35 % Median follow-up – 89 months Disease recurrence – 42 %	Significant predictors: - unilateral vs bilateral disease Not significant: - metastasis size - number of metastases - disease free interval - patient age

VATS video-assisted thoracoscopic surgery, *OS* overall survival, *DFI* disease free interval

All gross disease could be resected in 29 patients (64 %), the vast majority by wedge resection. The postoperative mortality was 2 % (one patient). The 5- and 10-year survival from the time of the pulmonary resection was 43 % and 35 % respectively, with a mean follow-up of 25 months. The mean survival for patients with bilateral disease was 27 months, while it was 39 months for patients with unilateral disease ($p = 0.02$).

A more recent paper looked at 82 male and female patients who underwent pulmonary resection for metastatic sarcoma with curative intent at the Brigham and Women's Hospital from 1989 to 2004 [22]. Leiomyosarcomas accounted for 31 cases (38 %), and 77 % of leiomyosarcomas were in females. Patients with leiomyosarcomas had a better overall survival than patients with other sarcoma subtypes (70 versus 24 months; $p = 0.049$). Disease-free survival of greater than 12 months from time of primary tumor resection was the only significant prognostic factor in multivariate analysis. Systemic chemotherapy had no significant effect on long term survival.

In 2004, the Metastatic Lung Tumor Study Group of Japan reported the results of the largest series of patients having pulmonary metastasectomy for uterine malignancies. They reported on 133 patients undergoing surgery between March 1984 and February 2002 [21]. The postoperative mortality was 0.8 % (1 case). The only significant prognostic factor in multivariate analysis was a disease-free interval of less than 12 months [21].

Another Japanese study published in 2004 evaluated the role of resection of pulmonary metastases from patients with stage Ib or II cervical cancer who underwent curative initial treatment [28]. The 5-year disease-free survival was 42 % for patients with one or two metastases, compared to 0 % for patients with three or four ($p = 0.0003$). Patients with squamous cancers had a 5-year disease-free survival of 47.4 %, compared to 0 % for patients with glandular cancers ($p = 0.014$)

A large series of surgical resections for lung metastases from gynaecological malignancies was reported from the Mayo Clinic in 2006 [23]. They reported 70 patients with metastatic disease limited to the lungs who were treated between 1985 and 2001. Synchronous lung metastases were present in 9 patients (13 %). Post-operative morbidity occurred in 18 patients (26 %), and there was one postoperative death (1.4 %) [23]. The overall survival for the group was 47 % at 5 years and 34 % at 10 years.

The most recent report was from Nagoya University Hospital in 2015 [29]. They reviewed 37 patients with isolated lung metastases (<3 nodules). They compared 23 patients who underwent surgical resection (cervical (14), endometrial (4) or ovarian (5) carcinomas), with 10 patients who underwent chemotherapy only. Among 6 patients who recurred in the lung a second time, 5

underwent a second pulmonary metastasectomy and all 5 patients were alive and well at the time of reporting. There was no significant difference in overall survival between patients having surgery or chemotherapy, but the numbers were small and the trend favoured surgery (81.7 % versus 49.5 %; $p = 0.072$). There was a significant survival advantage for patients with a disease-free survival of > 24 months ($p = 0.006$).

Surgical management of brain metastases

Brain metastases are common with breast, lung, and renal carcinomas, and malignant melanoma [30, 31], but are rare with gynaecological cancers, with the exception of choriocarcinoma [32, 33]. They are usually associated with widely disseminated disease.

Diagnosis

Symptoms of brain metastases may be subtle initially, and may include headaches, nausea, vomiting, confusion, dizziness, decreased mental status, general or extremity weakness, urinary incontinence, gait disturbance, ataxia, visual disturbance including diplopia, photophobia, speech impairment, syncope or seizures [32–36]. Increased intracranial pressure caused by associated brain edema leads to the development of papilledema in the fundus of the eye, which is a classical sign of a brain tumor [37].

Imaging

Most brain metastases are diagnosed with a computed tomographic (CT) scan of the brain, which has been performed to investigate suspicious symptoms. The metastasis appears as a heterogeneous, contrast enhancing lesion [35] (Fig. 1). Metastatic ovarian cancers can occasionally be calcified [38]. Contrast-enhanced magnetic resonance imaging (MRI) is the most accurate modality to image the brain [39].

Surgical Technique

Traditionally, patients with solitary metastases have undergone metastasectomy and whole brain radiotherapy (WBRT) [37, 39]. The latter is associated with a number of late complications, including brain atrophy, necrosis, dementia, and endocrine dysfunction [40].

More recently, stereotactic radiosurgery using a "gamma-knife" (GKRT) has become available [37, 41, 42]. This is a technique that enables the precise delivery of a high-dose of gamma radiation to a small intracranial target, while sparing the surrounding normal brain. If there is a solitary lesion, surgical resection followed by GKRT to the tumor bed is ideal. GKRT offers an advantage if the lesion is inaccessible. Lesions larger than 3 cm are less likely to be controlled by GKRT [41].

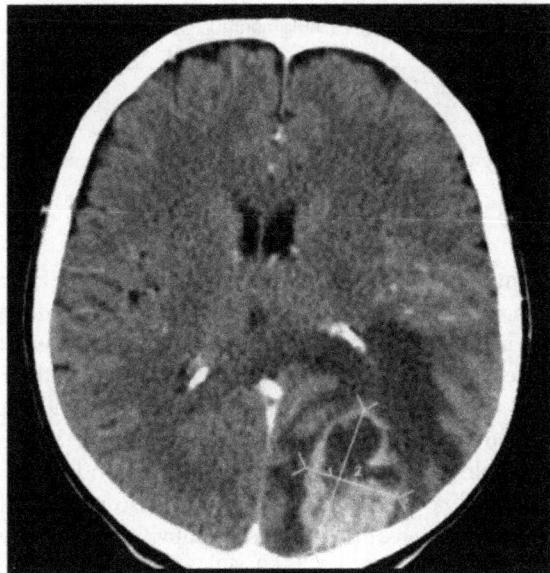

Fig. 1 CT scan of the brain showing a solitary metastasis, 5x4 cm, in the right occipital lobe, with some extension to the parietal lobe. Note the heterogeneic appearance of the metastasis and the surrounding brain edema

Indications for surgical resection

Ideally, suitable patients for brain metastasectomy would have a solitary lesion and no evidence of extracranial disease [35, 43–45]. Such patients are uncommon, as the majority of patients have multiple brain metastases [39, 46–49]. A well controlled primary tumor [42, 50] and a disease-free interval of at least 12 months is desirable, but Petru et al. reported a patient who had a solitary brain metastasis diagnosed prior to the diagnosis of endometrial cancer. She had stereotactic radiosurgery to the brain lesion, followed by aggressive cytoreductive surgery and doxorubin-based chemotherapy for the primary tumor, and remained alive and free of disease at 171 months [51].

Brain metastases by primary site

There have been comprehensive reviews by Piura and Piura regarding brain metastases from gynaecological cancers [32, 33, 37]. The incidence, pattern of brain metastasis, and survival by primary site are summarised in Tables 2 and 3.

Ovarian cancer

Of the gynaecological cancers, ovarian cancer is associated with the highest incidence of brain metastases, and there have been two comprehensive reviews in the past 5 years. In 2011, Piura and Piura reported 521 cases between 1978 and 2011 [32], while in 2014, Pakneshan et al. reported 591 cases between 1978 and 2013 [45]. Piura and Piura determined the incidence of brain metastases from ovarian cancer to be 1.2 % [32], which was twice the incidence associated with cervical [37] or endometrial cancer [33]. Pakneshan et al. reported that the incidence among the various studies ranged from 0.49 to 11.4 %, with an average of 2.55 % [45]. A review of the literature reveals several case reports and small series, the largest being 72 patients [47].

Since the advent of chemotherapy over 50 years ago, the incidence of brain metastases from ovarian cancer has increased, presumably because these patients are living longer, and because the chemotherapy has difficulty crossing the blood–brain barrier [31]. A review of 3,690 patients with epithelial ovarian cancer treated at the Royal Marsden Hospital from 1980 to 2000 reported that the incidence of brain metastases increased from 0.2 % in 1980–84 to 1.3 % in 1995–99 ($p < 0.001$) [34].

Most patients have advanced stage, high-grade serous cancers at initial presentation [35, 45, 47, 48, 52–54], and the brain metastasis often follows a negative second-look laparotomy [54–56]. CA125 titers are not absolutely reliable in the screening for brain metastases [57], although they are elevated in the majority of patients [45, 46].

In the review by Piura and Piura, the median interval from diagnosis to brain metastasis in 31 series was 24.3 months (range 11 to 46 months) [32], although there was a case report of a patient who developed a brain metastasis 11 years after diagnosis of the primary cancer [58]. The disease was confined to the central nervous system in 236 of 504 patients (46.8 %) [32]. The brain parenchyma, most commonly the cerebrum, was the site of metastasis in 489 patients (97 %) and the leptomeninges in 15 cases (3 %). Most brain metastases were multiple (269 of 474; 56.8 %) [32].

Prognosis

Survival by treatment type in patients with brain metastases from ovarian cancer is summarised in Table 4. Surgical resection significantly improved the survival

Table 2 Summary of incidence, disease-free survival, and pattern of brain metastasis [32, 33, 37]

Primary Site	Incidence	Median Disease-Free Interval	Only site of metastatic disease	Solitary metastasis
Ovarian (n = 521)	1.19 % (413/34 728)	24.3 months (11–46)	46.8 % (236/504)	41.9 % (205/489)
Endometrial (n = 115)	0.59 % (61/10 199)	17 months (2–108)	49 % (48/98)	56.8 % (50/88)
Cervical (n = 100)	0.57 % (n = 65/11 249)	18 months (0.25-105 months)	46.8 % (37/79)	50.6 % (40/79)

Table 3 Summary of survival outcomes after diagnosis of brain metastases [32, 33, 37]

Primary Site	Median survival (months)	Surgery alone (months)	WBRT (months)	Surgery + WBRT (months)	Multimodal Surgery + RT +/− Chemo (months)
Ovarian	6.4 (1–28)	6.7	4.5	17	20
Endometrial	5 (0.1-171)	2.25 (1–18)	2 (0.25-17)	Not available	22 (2.1-84)
Cervical	4 (0.1-72)	4 (1–7)	3 (0.1-22.6) (+/− chemo)	7.1 (1–72) (+/− chemo)	SRS + other modality13.7 (5–22.5)

WBRT whole brain radiotherapy, *RT* radiotherapy, *SRS* stereotactic radiosurgery

compared to other methods of treatment [35, 43, 45, 47, 48, 52, 54, 59, 60]. Solitary metastases generally have a better prognosis [35, 43, 45]. Cormio et al. reported 22 patients who had resection of a solitary metastasis [44]. They reported that extracranial disease and the time interval between diagnosis of ovarian cancer and central nervous system involvement were the only factors significantly affecting survival. There were no operative deaths, and low morbidity. The majority of patients had complete resolution of their neurological symptoms [44].

Aggressive management of multiple metastases is justified [39, 46–49], particularly if the patient meets the criteria for Class I of the Radiation Therapy Oncology Group's recursive partitioning analysis system, ie., age < 65 years, Karnofsky score > 70, controlled primary disease and no extracranial metastases [43]. Kawana et al. described a patient who was initially diagnosed with stage IVB ovarian cancer, and developed 3 brain metastases after a disease-free interval of 27 months [41]. She underwent surgical resection of the two accessible lesions, and then gamma-knife radiotherapy for a third inaccessible lesion after 30Gy external beam local radiation to the bed of the resected tumors and the inoperable tumor. She remained disease-free at 5 years, with good quality of life [41].

In their recent literature review, Piura and Piura reported that the median survival for patients having whole brain radiation was 4.5 months, compared to

Table 4 Ovarian cancer with brain metastases – survival by treatment modality after diagnosis of brain metastases [32]

Treatment modality	Median survival (months)	% of patients (n) Total = 538
WBRT* only	4.5	35 % (182)
Surgery + WBRT	17	15.2 % (79)
WBRT + chemo	9.1	13.5 % (70)
Surgery + WBRT + chemo	20	13.3 % (69)
Surgery only	6.7	5 % (26)
SRS* or GKRS*	18	3.8 % (20)
Chemo only	7.5	1.9 % (10)
Surgery + chemo	Not available	1.3 % (7)
No treatment (steroids only)	1.4	11 % (57)

*WBRT whole brain radiationtherapy, SRS stereotactic radiosurgery, GKRS gamma knife radiosurgery

17 months for patients having surgical resection plus radiation, and 20 months for the addition of chemotherapy [32]. The outcomes for patients with brain metastases by treatment modality are summarised in Table 4. In the review by Pakneshan et al., combination surgery, radiation and chemotherapy was associated with longer survival than whole brain radiation alone (20.5 months versus 9.1 months; $p = 0.04$) [45]. Others have also stressed the need for aggressive multimodal therapy, including adjuvant chemotherapy [47, 52, 59–62], as the patients usually succumb to extracranial disease [63].

Long term survival is possible. Micha el al reported a patient with a stage IIIC high-grade serous carcinoma who recurred in the cerebellum 27 months after diagnosis, and following primary cytoreductive surgery and platinum-based chemotherapy [64]. She had surgery and whole brain radiation and was still alive and well 7 years post treatment for her brain metastasis. McMeekin also described a 7-year survivor [60].

Cervical cancer

The most common site of distant metastases from cervical cancer is the lung [65, 66]. Brain metastases are rare. In a literature review in 2012, Piura and Piura reported only 96 cases, with an incidence of 0.57 % [37]. The majority of patients had early stage disease at diagnosis – 42.2 % had stage IB and 36.6 % stage II – although 80 % of patients had poorly differentiated (grade 3) tumors. Histologic types basically reflected those expected in the general population, although there were 3 (3.6 %) small cell neuroendocrine carcinomas [37].

The interval between primary diagnosis and brain metastasis ranged from 1 week to 105 months, with a median of 18 months. The brain metastasis was part of a disseminated recurrence in 53.2 % of patients, was solitary in 50.6 %, and was located only in the cerebrum in 73 % of patients. Some authors have noted that brain metastases from cervical cancer were rarely accompanied by systemic disease, but they were commonly accompanied by uncontrolled local-regional disease [42, 50].

Prognosis

Based on limited data in the literature, Piura and Piura determined that the median survival for no treatment was 0.6 months, for whole brain radiation (WBRT)

4 months, while for surgical resection followed by WBRT it was 7.1 months. The best median survival (13.7 months) was achieved with stereotactic radiation, either alone or combined with another modality [37].

Robinson and Morris reported a patient with a brain metastasis from a squamous cell carcinoma of the cervix who remained disease free 6 years following surgical resection and whole brain radiation [67]. Chura et al. reported 12 patients with brain metastases from cervical cancer, 8 of whom received WBRT, but their median survival was only 2.3 months [68].

Endometrial Cancer

Brain metastases from endometrial cancer are rare, with Piura and Piura documenting only 115 cases from 35 published papers, with an incidence of 0.59 % [33]. The brain metastasis was diagnosed after a median interval of 17 months (range 2 to 108 months). In 4 patients (4.2 %), the primary and metastatic diagnoses were made simultaneously, and in 9 patients (9.5 %), the brain metastases were detected before the primary.

In the review by Piura and Piura, 63 % of patients (50 of 79) had advanced disease at initial diagnosis, and 78.1 % (57 of 73) had poorly differentiated tumors [33]. Almost half the patients had metastases confined to the brain (48 of 98 patients; 49 %), and 56.8 % of patients (50 of 88) had a solitary metastasis. Site of metastasis was available for 66 patients, of whom 48 (72.7 %) had disease confined to the cerebellum [33]. Of the 20 patients reported by Chura et al., 8 (40 %) had a single metastasis, 4 (20 %) had two, 7 (35 %) had 3 or more, and 1 patient (5 %) had leptomeningeal disease [69].

Prognosis

In the review by Piura and Piura, the overall median survival after diagnosis of brain metastasis was 5 months (0.1 to 171 months). Patients having WBRT alone had a median survival of 2 months (0.25-17 months) while patients having surgical resection followed by WBRT had a median survival of 22 months (2.1-84 months) [33]. Orrru et al. reported 2 patients treated by surgical resection followed by WBRT who were alive and well at 16 and 64 months respectively [70].

Surgical management of liver metastases

The literature on liver resection for metastatic gynecological cancer is limited. It has been estimated that up to 50 % of patients who die of cervical, endometrial or ovarian cancer will have liver metastases at autopsy [71, 72], but probably only 1 - 10 % would be suitable for liver resection [73]. Gynecologic cancers that metastasize to the liver usually do so in the setting of obvious regional or systemic dissemination [71, 74].

Surgical technique

Hepatic resection has evolved, with improved surgical techniques, instrumentation, anesthesia and perioperative care, and now carries a very low morbidity and mortality [73, 75, 76].

Hepatic resection usually involves non-anatomical wedge resection (Fig. 2), but anatomical resection of one or more liver segments may also be performed [77]. Resection of as much as 70 % of the liver can be performed, with a mortality rate of less than 5 % in major hepatobiliary centers [77, 78]. Over the past 15 years, radiofrequency ablation, usually in conjunction with surgical resection, has extended the cohort of patients with surgically treatable disease, and helped achieve better locoregional control [79, 80].

Indications

Liver surgery should only be considered when all other metastatic disease is well controlled, when disease in the liver can be completely resected, or when liver resection is part of the achievement of optimal cytoreduction for patients with ovarian cancer [81, 82].

Results

The findings of reported series with 5 or more patients are summarised in Table 5.

The first study by Brunchwig in 1963 [83] reported 24 cases of hepatic lobectomy for metastatic carcinoma, 4 of whom were from the cervix or endometrium. Three of the four died in the perioperative period, and the fourth died of disease at 18 months..

In most large series of patients having partial hepatectomy for metastatic malignancy, gynaecological cancers represent less than 10 % of cases [73, 76, 84–86]. A large, multi-centre French study reported that during the 1980's, the median number of partial hepatectomies

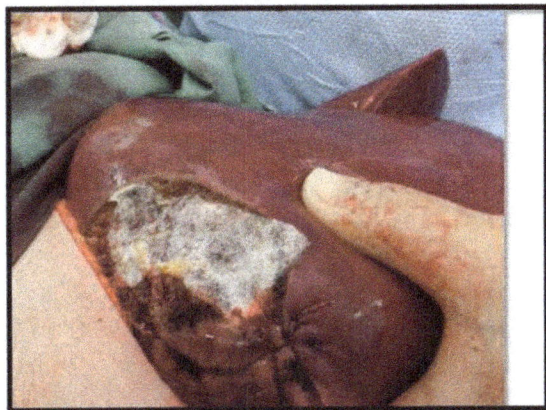

Fig. 2 Non-anatomical liver resection for a patient with ovarian cancer with involvement of the liver capsule and underlying parenchyma

Table 5 Major series reporting surgical management of hepatic metastases from gynaecological malignancies

First Author Year of Publication	Number of patients	Primary vs Recurrent Disease	Primary Site	Median overall survival (from time of liver resection unless otherwise stated)	Factors associated with longest survival
Kolev [91] 2014	27	Recurrent	Ovary	12 months (2–190)	Interval from primary surgery of >24 months (P = 0.044) Secondary cytoreduction to <1 cm (P = 0.014)
Neumann [82] 2012	41	Primary	Ovary	R0 – 42 months R1 – 4 months R2 – 6 months	Post operative residual tumour mass
Roh [77] 2011	18	Recurrent	Ovary	38 months (3–78)	Less abdominal than pelvic disease (38 vs 11 months, P = 0.032) Optimal cytoreduction (40 vs 9 months, P = 0.0004) Negative margin status of hepatic resection (40 vs (months, P = 0.0196
Kamel [92] 2011	52	Primary	Ovary	53 months 5-year survival 41 %	Not reported
Knowles [93] 2010	5	Recurrent	Endometrioid (Ovarian or Endometrial)	Median OS not reported DFS range 8–66 months	Not reported
Lim [75] 2009	14	Primary	Ovary	5-year PFS by Stage: - IIIC – 25 % - IV – 23 % 5-year OS by Stage: - IIIC – 55 % - IV – 51 %	Not reported
Loizzi [94] 2005	29	Primary (Group 1) – 8 1st Recurrence (Group 2) – 10 2nd recurrence (Group 3) – 11	Ovary	Median survival from time of liver metastasis diagnosis: Group 1 – 19 months Group 2 – 24 months Group 3 – 10 months	Cell type Performance status Number of hepatic lesions Presence of other sites of disease at time of diagnosis of hepatic metastasis Platinum based chemotherapy
Weitz [76] 2005	19	Recurrent	Ovary – 63.2 % Endometrium – 21.1 % Cervix – 10.5 % Fallopian tube – 5.2 %	Reproductive tract tumours (note – included testicular cancer pts, but no difference between ovary and testicular survival) Median cancer specific survival reproductive tract primary – 115 months Ovary - 3 year recurrence free survival 58 %	Primary tumour type Length of disease free interval from primary tumour
Yoon [95] 2003	24	Recurrent	Ovary Fallopian tube	62 months (6–94)	No significant prognostic factors for OS identified on univariate analysis
Merideth [89] 2003	26	Recurrent	Ovary	Overall median disease-related survival 26.3 months	>12 months since original diagnosis (27.3 vs 5.7 months, P = 0.004) ≤1 cm residual disease (27.3 vs 8.6 months, P = 0.031)
Fan [96] 2001	18		Ovary – immature teratoma	3-year survival – 77.8 % 5-year survival – 55.6 % 10-year survival – 38.9 %	Not reported
Naik [97] 2000	37	Primary	Ovary	11 months 2-year survival 23 % 5-year survival 9 %	Optimal surgery with residual <2 cm (P = 0.0029) or <1 cm (P = 0.0086)

Table 5 Major series reporting surgical management of hepatic metastases from gynaecological malignancies *(Continued)*

Bristow [81] 1999	37	Primary	Ovary	Optimal extrahepatic and hepatic resection – 50.1 months Optimal extrahepatic resection with residual hepatic tumour – 27.0 months Suboptimal with residual extrahepatic and heaptic tumour – 7.6 months	Optimal extrahepatic resection ($P = 0.0001$)
Elias [84] 1998	6	Not stated	Gynecologic	5-year survival – 45 %	Not reported
Chi [71] 1997	12	Recurrent	Ovary – 58 % Cervix – 17 % Endometrium – 17 % Fallopian tube – 1 8 %	27 months (Median f/up 25 months, range 8–94 months)	Not reported

OS overall survival, *DFS* disease-free survival, *PFS* progression-free survival

for non-colorectal, non-endocrine metastases per annum did not exceed 17, whereas it rose to 70 during the 1990's and 115 during the 2000's [73].

In patients with colorectal and gut-associated endocrine tumors, the most likely mode of spread is via the portal venous system. The majority of the patient's tumor burden is thus confined to the abdomen [73], and 5-year survivals of 45-50 % are routinely reported [87, 88]. By contrast, liver metastases from gynaecological cancers reach the liver via the systemic circulation, so other extra-abdominal sites are likely to be involved, which has fostered caution. Liver surgery should only be considered when the metastatic disease is well controlled or responding to systemic therapy, or when liver resection is part of the achievement of optimal cytoreduction for ovarian cancer [81, 82].

Lim et al. reported 16 patients who had parenchymal liver metastases at the time of diagnosis with advanced ovarian cancer [75]. Two patients (12.5 %) had hematogenous metastases which were unresectable, while 14 (87.5 %) had parenchymal invasion from peritoneal seeding, and were able to undergo complete resection. These patients, who were officially FIGO stage IV, had the same survival as patients with Stage IIIC disease.

A series of 26 patients undergoing hepatic resection for metachronous metastases from ovarian cancer was reported from the Mayo Clinic in 2003 [89]. The median age of the patients was 62 years and a solitary liver lesion was present in 17 patients (63.4 %). All patients had pelvic and abdominal disease in addition to the liver metastases and 42 % had a simultaneous bowel resection. Optimal cytoreduction (<1 cm) was achieved in 21 patients (80.7 %). Segmentectomy was required in 18 patients (69.2 %) and right hepatectomy in 4 (15.4 %). There was no serious morbidity or mortality from the surgery. There was a significant survival advantage for patients whose disease-free interval was >12 months (27.3 versus 5.7 months; $p < 0.004$)), and for those having optimal cytoreduction (27.3 versus 8.6 months; $p < 0.031$)

In 2006, a multicentre French study reported the largest series (1452) of patients who underwent hepatic resection for non-colorectal, non-endocrine liver metastases [73]. Gynecologic cancer represented 126 cases (8.7 %), and although the patients were highly selected, the results were very satisfactory. Overall, the 5-year survival was 48 %. It was 50 % for patients with ovarian cancer and 35 % for patients with a uterine primary [73]. For the 1452 patients the 60-day operative mortality was 2.3 %.

Conclusions

From a review of the current literature, it is apparent that surgery should play an increasing role in the management of patients with parenchymal metastases from gynecological cancers to the lungs, brain or liver. Appropriate patient selection is critical, but surprisingly good long-term survival results can be achieved for resection of metastases from all three organs, in conjunction usually with the use of adjuvant radiation, chemotherapy or hormonal therapy.

This requires the development of a committed, multidisciplinary team, working in a high volume tertiary center, where the necessary infrastructure for postoperative management is available. In these circumstances, postoperative morbidity and mortality are low.

Ideally, patients should have metastatic disease confined to the lungs, brain or liver, except in the case of a patient with a chemosensitive ovarian cancer, where resection of pulmonary or liver metastases may form part of the initial cytoreductive surgical effort. A solitary metastasis is ideal, but good results may be obtained with multiple metastases, as long as all macroscopic disease can be resected. A disease-free interval of at least 12 months, and preferably 24 months is desirable, together with a satisfactory performance status, and adequate functional reserve in the organ being partially resected.

Authors contributions

NFH wrote the manuscript, based on a lecture he had given to the ESGO meeting in 2015. AR did the tables and checked all references. Both read and approved the final manuscript.

Competing interests

The authors declare that they have no competing interests.

References

1. Barney JD, Churchill CE. Adenocarcinoma of the kidney with metastasis to the lung. J Urol. 1939;42:269–76.

2. Mountain CF, McMurtrey MJ, Hermes KE. Surgery for pulmonary metastasis: a 20-year experience. Ann Thorac Surg. 1984;38:323–30.

3. Casson AG, Putnam JB, Natarajan G, Johnston DA, Mountain C, McMurtrey M, Roth JA. Five-year survival after pulmonary metastasectomy for adult soft tissue sarcoma. Cancer. 1992;69:662–8.

4. Headrick JR, Miller DL, Nagorney DM, Allen MS, Deschamps C, Trastek VF, Pairolero PC. Surgical treatment of hepatic and pulmonary metastases from colon cancer. Ann Thorac Surg. 2001;71:975–9. discussion 979–980.

5. Martini N, McCormack PM. Evolution of the surgical management of pulmonary metastases. Chest Surg Clin N Am. 1998;8:13–27.

6. Monteiro A, Arce N, Bernardo J, Eugenio L, Antunes MJ. Surgical resection of lung metastases from epithelial tumors. Ann Thorac Surg. 2004;77:431–7.

7. Murthy SC, Kim K, Rice TW, Rajeswaran J, Bukowski R, DeCamp MM, Blackstone EH. Can we predict long-term survival after pulmonary metastasectomy for renal cell carcinoma? Ann Thorac Surg. 2005;79: 996–1003.

8. Piltz S, Meimarakis G, Wichmann MW, Hatz R, Schildberg FW, Fuerst H. Long-term results after pulmonary resection of renal cell carcinoma metastases. Ann Thorac Surg. 2002;73:1082–7.

9. Pastorino U, Buyse M, Friedel G, Ginsberg RJ, Girard P, Goldstraw P, Johnston M, McCormack P, Pass H, Putnam JB Jr, International Registry of Lung M. Long-term results of lung metastasectomy: prognostic analyses based on 5206 cases. J Thoracic & Cardiovasc Surg. 1997;113:37–49.

10. Creasman WT, Odicino F, Maisonneuve P, Quinn MA, Beller U, Benedet JL, Heintz AP, Ngan HY, Pecorelli S. Carcinoma of the corpus uteri. FIGO 26th Annual Report on the Results of Treatment in Gynecological Cancer. Int J Gynaecology & Obstetrics. 2006;95 Suppl 1:S105–43.

11. Blecharz P, Urbanski K, Mucha-Malecka A, Malecki K, Reinfuss M, Jakubowicz J, Skotnicki P. Hematogenous metastases in patients with Stage I or II endometrial carcinoma. Strahlenther Onkol. 2011;187:806–11.

12. Bouros D, Papadakis K, Siafakas N, Fuller Jr AF. Patterns of pulmonary metastasis from uterine cancer. Oncology. 1996;53:360–3.

13. Labi FL, Evangelista S, Di Miscia A, Stentella P. FIGO Stage I endometrial carcinoma: evaluation of lung metastases and follow-up. Eur J Gynaecol Oncol. 2008;29:65–6.

14. Torre LA, Bray F, Siegel RL, Ferlay J, Lortet-Tieulent J, Jemal A. Global cancer statistics, 2012. CA Cancer J Clin. 2015;65:87–108.

15. Gunasekera PC. Emergency contraception. Ceylon Med J. 1999;44:60–2.

16. Barter JF, Soong SJ, Hatch KD, Orr JW, Shingleton HM. Diagnosis and treatment of pulmonary metastases from cervical carcinoma. Gynecol Oncol. 1990;38:347–51.

17. Martinez-Jimenez S, Rosado-de-Christenson ML, Walker CM, Kunin JR, Betancourt SL, Shoup BL, Pettavel PP. Imaging features of thoracic metastases from gynecologic neoplasms. Radiographics. 2014;34:1742–54.

18. Paramanathan A, Wright G. Pulmonary metastasectomy for sarcoma of gynaecologic origin. Heart Lung Circ. 2013;22:270–5.

19. Gonzalez Casaurran G, Simon Adiego C, Penalver Pascual R, Moreno Mata N, Lozano Barriuso MA, Gonzalez Aragoneses F. Surgery of female genital tract tumour lung metastases. Arch Bronconeumol. 2011;47:134–7.

20. Anderson TM, McMahon JJ, Nwogu CE, Pombo MW, Urschel JD, Driscoll DL, Lele SB. Pulmonary resection in metastatic uterine and cervical malignancies. Gynecol Oncol. 2001;83:472–6.

21. Anraku M, Yokoi K, Nakagawa K, Fujisawa T, Nakajima J, Akiyama H, Nishimura Y, Kobayashi K, Metastatic Lung Tumor Study Group of J. Pulmonary metastases from uterine malignancies: results of surgical resection in 133 patients. J Thoracic & Cardiovasc Surg. 2004;127:1107–12.

22. Burt BM, Ocejo S, Mery CM, Dasilva M, Bueno R, Sugarbaker DJ, Jaklitsch MT. Repeated and aggressive pulmonary resections for leiomyosarcoma metastases extends survival. Ann Thorac Surg. 2011;92:1202–7.

23. Clavero JM, Deschamps C, Cassivi SD, Allen MS, Nichols 3rd FC, Barrette BA, Larson DR, Pairolero PC. Gynecologic cancers: factors affecting survival after pulmonary metastasectomy. Ann Thorac Surg. 2006;81:2004–7.

24. Seki M, Nakagawa K, Tsuchiya S, Matsubara T, Kinoshita I, Weng SY, Tsuchiya E. Surgical treatment of pulmonary metastases from uterine cervical cancer. Operation method by lung tumor size. J Thorac Cardiovasc Surg. 1992;104:876–81.

25. Fuller Jr AF, Scannell JG, Wilkins Jr EW. Pulmonary resection for metastases from gynecologic cancers: Massachusetts General Hospital experience, 1943–1982. Gynecol Oncol. 1985;22:174–80.

26. McCormack PM, Martini N. The changing role of surgery for pulmonary metastases. Ann Thorac Surg. 1979;28:139–45.

27. Levenback C, Rubin SC, McCormack PM, Hoskins WJ, Atkinson EN, Lewis Jr JL. Resection of pulmonary metastases from uterine sarcomas. Gynecol Oncol. 1992;45:202–5.

28. Yamamoto K, Yoshikawa H, Shiromizu K, Saito T, Kuzuya K, Tsunematsu R, Kamura T. Pulmonary metastasectomy for uterine cervical cancer: a multivariate analysis. Ann Thorac Surg. 2004;77:1179–82.

29. Adachi M, Mizuno M, Mitsui H, Kajiyama H, Suzuki S, Sekiya R, Utsumi F, Shibata K, Taniguchi T, Kawaguchi K, et al. The prognostic impact of pulmonary metastasectomy in recurrent gynecologic cancers: a retrospective single-institution study. Nagoya J Med Sci. 2015;77:363–72.

30. Schouten LJ, Rutten J, Huveneers HA, Twijnstra A. Incidence of brain metastases in a cohort of patients with carcinoma of the breast, colon, kidney, and lung and melanoma. Cancer. 2002;94:2698–705.

31. Tosoni A, Ermani M, Brandes AA. The pathogenesis and treatment of brain metastases: a comprehensive review. Crit Rev Oncol Hematol. 2004;52:199–215.

32. Piura E, Piura B. Brain metastases from ovarian carcinoma. ISRN Oncol. 2011; 2011:527453.

33. Piura E, Piura B. Brain metastases from endometrial carcinoma. ISRN Oncol. 2012;2012:581749.

34. Kolomainen DF, Larkin JM, Badran M, A'Hern RP, King DM, Fisher C, Bridges JE, Blake PR, Barton DP, Shepherd JH, et al. Epithelial ovarian cancer metastasizing to the brain: a late manifestation of the disease with an increasing incidence. J Clin Oncol. 2002;20:982–6.

35. LeRoux PD, Berger MS, Elliott JP, Tamimi HK. Cerebral metastases from ovarian carcinoma. Cancer. 1991;67:2194–9.

36. Plaxe SC, Dottino PR, Lipsztein R, Dalton J, Cohen CJ. Clinical features and treatment outcome of patients with epithelial carcinoma of the ovary metastatic to the central nervous system. Obstet Gynecol. 1990;75:278–81.

37. Piura E, Piura B. Brain metastases from cervical carcinoma: overview of pertinent literature. Eur J Gynaecol Oncol. 2012;33:567–73.

38. Kawamura D, Tanaka T, Fuga M, Yanagisawa T, Tochigi S, Irie K, Hasegawa Y, Abe T. Slow progression of calcified cerebellar metastasis from ovarian cancer: a case report and review of the literature. Neurol Med Chir. 2013;53:722–6.

39. Kim TJ, Song S, Kim CK, Kim WY, Choi CH, Lee JH, Lee JW, Bae DS, Kim BG. Prognostic factors associated with brain metastases from epithelial ovarian carcinoma. Int J Gynecol Cancer. 2007;17:1252–7.

40. Schultheiss TE, Kun LE, Ang KK, Stephens LC. Radiation response of the central nervous system. Int J Radiat Oncol Biol Phys. 1995;31:1093–112.

41. Kawana K, Yoshikawa H, Yokota H, Onda T, Nakagawa K, Tsutsumi O, Taketani Y. Successful treatment of brain metastases from ovarian cancer using gamma-knife radiosurgery. Gynecol Oncol. 1997;65:357–9.

42. Mahmoud-Ahmed AS, Suh JH, Barnett GH, Webster KD, Kennedy AW. Tumor distribution and survival in six patients with brain metastases from cervical carcinoma. Gynecol Oncol. 2001;81:196–200.

43. Chen PG, Lee SY, Barnett GH, Vogelbaum MA, Saxton JP, Fleming PA, Suh JH. Use of the Radiation Therapy Oncology Group recursive partitioning analysis classification system and predictors of survival in 19 women with brain metastases from ovarian carcinoma. Cancer. 2005;104:2174–80.

44. Cormio G, Maneo A, Colamaria A, Loverro G, Lissoni A, Selvaggi L. Surgical resection of solitary brain metastasis from ovarian carcinoma: an analysis of 22 cases. Gynecol Oncol. 2003;89:116–9.

45. Pakneshan S, Safarpour D, Tavassoli F, Jabbari B. Brain metastasis from ovarian cancer: a systematic review. J Neurooncol. 2014;119:1–6.

46. Anupol N, Ghamande S, Odunsi K, Driscoll D, Lele S. Evaluation of prognostic factors and treatment modalities in ovarian cancer patients with brain metastases. Gynecol Oncol. 2002;85:487–92.

47. Cohen ZR, Suki D, Weinberg JS, Marmor E, Lang FF, Gershenson DM, Sawaya R. Brain metastases in patients with ovarian carcinoma: prognostic factors and outcome. J Neurooncol. 2004;66:313–25.

48. Geisler JP, Geisler HE. Brain metastases in epithelial ovarian carcinoma. Gynecol Oncol. 1995;57:246–9.

49. Ratner ES, Toy E, O'Malley DM, McAlpine J, Rutherford TJ, Azodi M, Higgins SA, Schwartz PE. Brain metastases in epithelial ovarian and primary peritoneal carcinoma. Int J Gynecol Cancer. 2009;19:856–9.

50. Cormio G, Colamaria A, Loverro G, Pierangeli E, Di Vagno G, De Tommasi A, Selvaggi L. Surgical resection of a cerebral metastasis from cervical cancer: case report and review of the literature. Tumori. 1999;85:65–7.

51. Petru E, Lax S, Kurschel S, Gucer F, Sutter B. Long-term survival in a patient with brain metastases preceding the diagnosis of endometrial cancer. Report of two cases and review of the literature. J Neurosurg. 2001;94:846–8.

52. Kaminsky-Forrett MC, Weber B, Conroy T, Spaeth D. Brain metastases from epithelial ovarian carcinoma. Int J Gynecol Cancer. 2000;10:366–71.

53. Pectasides D, Pectasides M, Economopoulos T. Brain metastases from epithelial ovarian cancer: a review of the literature. Oncologist. 2006;11:252–60.

54. Pothuri B, Chi DS, Reid T, Aghajanian C, Venkatraman E, Alektiar K, Bilsky M, Barakat RR. Craniotomy for central nervous system metastases in epithelial ovarian carcinoma. Gynecol Oncol. 2002;87:133–7.

55. Akhan SE, Isikoglu M, Salihoglu Y, Bengisu E, Berkman S. Brain metastasis of ovarian cancer after negative second-look laparotomy. Eur J Gynaecol Oncol. 2002;23:330–2.

56. Deutsch M, Beck D, Manor D, Brandes J. Metastatic brain tumor following negative second-look operation for ovarian carcinoma. Gynecol Oncol. 1987;27:116–20.

57. Tay SK, Rajesh H. Brain metastases from epithelial ovarian cancer. Int J Gynecol Cancer. 2005;15:824–9.

58. Longo R, Platini C, Eid N, Elias-Matta C, Buda T, Nguyen D, Quetin P. A late, solitary brain metastasis of epithelial ovarian carcinoma. BMC Cancer. 2014;14:543.

59. Cormio G, Loizzi V, Falagario M, Lissoni AA, Resta L, Selvaggi LE. Changes in the management and outcome of central nervous system involvement from ovarian cancer since 1994. International Journal of Gynaecology & Obstetrics. 2011;114:133–6.

60. McMeekin DS, Kamelle SA, Vasilev SA, Tillmanns TD, Gould NS, Scribner DR, Gold MA, Guruswamy S, Mannel RS. Ovarian cancer metastatic to the brain: what is the optimal management? J Surg Oncol. 2001;78:194–200. discussion 200–191.

61. D'Andrea G, Roperto R, Dinia L, Caroli E, Salvati M, Ferrante L. Solitary cerebral metastases from ovarian epithelial carcinoma: 11 cases. Neurosurg Rev. 2005;28:120–3.

62. Rodriguez GC, Soper JT, Berchuck A, Oleson J, Dodge R, Montana G, Clarke-Pearson DL. Improved palliation of cerebral metastases in epithelial ovarian cancer using a combined modality approach including radiation therapy, chemotherapy, and surgery. J Clin Oncol. 1992;10:1553–60.

63. Kastritis E, Efstathiou E, Gika D, Bozas G, Koutsoukou V, Papadimitriou C, Pissakas G, Dimopoulos MA, Bamias A. Brain metastases as isolated site of relapse in patients with epithelial ovarian cancer previously treated with platinum and paclitaxel-based chemotherapy. Int J Gynecol Cancer. 2006;16:994–9.

64. Micha JP, Goldstein BH, Hunter JV, Rettenmaier MA, Brown JV. Long-term survival in an ovarian cancer patient with brain metastases. Gynecol Oncol. 2004;92:978–80.

65. Bodurka-Bevers D, Morris M, Eifel PJ, Levenback C, Bevers MW, Lucas KR, Wharton JT. Posttherapy surveillance of women with cervical cancer: an outcomes analysis. Gynecol Oncol. 2000;78:187–93.

66. Elit L, Fyles AW, Devries MC, Oliver TK, Fung-Kee-Fung M, Gynecology Cancer Disease Site G. Follow-up for women after treatment for cervical cancer: a systematic review. Gynecol Oncol. 2009;114:528–35.

67. Robinson JB, Morris M. Cervical carcinoma metastatic to the brain. Gynecol Oncol. 1997;66:324–6.

68. Chura JC, Shukla K, Argenta PA. Brain metastasis from cervical carcinoma. Int J Gynecol Cancer. 2007;17:141–6.

69. Chura JC, Marushin R, Boyd A, Ghebre R, Geller MA, Argenta PA. Multimodal therapy improves survival in patients with CNS metastasis from uterine cancer: a retrospective analysis and literature review. Gynecol Oncol. 2007; 107:79–85.

70. Orrru S, Lay G, Dessi M, Murtas R, Deidda MA, Amichetti M. Brain metastases from endometrial carcinoma: report of three cases and review of the literature. Tumori. 2007;93:112–7.

71. Chi DS, Fong Y, Venkatraman ES, Barakat RR. Hepatic resection for metastatic gynecologic carcinomas. Gynecol Oncol. 1997;66:45–51.

72. Rose PG, Piver MS, Tsukada Y, Lau TS. Metastatic patterns in histologic variants of ovarian cancer. An autopsy study. Cancer. 1989;64:1508–13.

73. Adam R, Chiche L, Aloia T, Elias D, Salmon R, Rivoire M, Jaeck D, Saric J, Le Treut YP, Belghiti J, et al. Hepatic resection for noncolorectal nonendocrine liver metastases: analysis of 1,452 patients and development of a prognostic model. Ann Surg. 2006;244:524–35.

74. Kim GE, Lee SW, Suh CO, Park TK, Kim JW, Park JT, Shim JU. Hepatic metastases from carcinoma of the uterine cervix. Gynecol Oncol. 1998; 70:56–60.

75. Lim MC, Kang S, Lee KS, Han SS, Park SJ, Seo SS, Park SY. The clinical significance of hepatic parenchymal metastasis in patients with primary epithelial ovarian cancer. Gynecol Oncol. 2009;112:28–34.

76. Weitz J, Blumgart LH, Fong Y, Jarnagin WR, D'Angelica M, Harrison LE, DeMatteo RP. Partial hepatectomy for metastases from noncolorectal, nonneuroendocrine carcinoma. Ann Surg. 2005;241:269–76.

77. Roh HJ, Kim DY, Joo WD, Yoo HJ, Kim JH, Kim YM, Kim YT, Nam JH. Hepatic resection as part of secondary cytoreductive surgery for recurrent ovarian cancer involving the liver. Archives of Gynecology & Obstetrics. 2011;284:1223–9.

78. Chang YC. Low mortality major hepatectomy. Hepatogastroenterology. 2004;51:1766–70.

79. Goering JD, Mahvi DM, Niederhuber JE, Chicks D, Rikkers LF. Cryoablation and liver resection for noncolorectal liver metastases. Am J Surg. 2002; 183:384–9.

80. Mateo R, Singh G, Jabbour N, Palmer S, Genyk Y, Roman L. Optimal cytoreduction after combined resection and radiofrequency ablation of hepatic metastases from recurrent malignant ovarian tumors. Gynecol Oncol. 2005;97:266–70.

81. Bristow RE, Montz FJ, Lagasse LD, Leuchter RS, Karlan BY. Survival impact of surgical cytoreduction in stage IV epithelial ovarian cancer. Gynecol Oncol. 1999;72:278–87.

82. Neumann UP, Fotopoulou C, Schmeding M, Thelen A, Papanikolaou G, Braicu EI, Neuhaus P, Sehouli J. Clinical outcome of patients with advanced ovarian cancer after resection of liver metastases. Anticancer Res. 2012;32:4517–21.

83. Brunschwig A. Hepatic lobectomy for metastatic cancer. Cancer. 1963; 16:277–82.

84. Elias D, Cavalcanti de Albuquerque A, Eggenspieler P, Plaud B, Ducreux M, Spielmann M, Theodore C, Bonvalot S, Lasser P. Resection of liver metastases from a noncolorectal primary: indications and results based on 147 monocentric patients. J Am Coll Surg. 1998;187:487–93.

85. Ercolani G, Grazi GL, Ravaioli M, Ramacciato G, Cescon M, Varotti G, Del Gaudio M, Vetrone G, Pinna AD. The role of liver resections for noncolorectal, nonneuroendocrine metastases: experience with 142 observed cases. Ann Surg Oncol. 2005;12:459–66.

86. O'Rourke TR, Tekkis P, Yeung S, Fawcett J, Lynch S, Strong R, Wall D, John TG, Welsh F, Rees M. Long-term results of liver resection for non-colorectal, non-neuroendocrine metastases. Ann Surg Oncol. 2008;15:207–18.

87. Adam R, Pascal G, Azoulay D, Tanaka K, Castaing D, Bismuth H. Liver resection for colorectal metastases: the third hepatectomy. Ann Surg. 2003; 238:871–83. discussion 883–874.

88. Jaeck D, Bachellier P, Guiguet M, Boudjema K, Vaillant JC, Balladur P, Nordlinger B. Long-term survival following resection of colorectal hepatic metastases. Association Francaise de Chirurgie. Br J Surg. 1997;84:977–80.

89. Merideth MA, Cliby WA, Keeney GL, Lesnick TG, Nagorney DM, Podratz KC. Hepatic resection for metachronous metastases from ovarian carcinoma. Gynecol Oncol. 2003;89:16–21.

90. Lim MC, Lee HS, Seo SS, Kim MS, Kim JY, Zo JI, Park SY. Pathologic diagnosis and resection of suspicious thoracic metastases in patients with cervical cancer through thoracotomy or video-assisted thoracic surgery. Gynecol Oncol. 2010;116:478–82.

91. Kolev V, Pereira EB, Schwartz M, Sarpel U, Roayaie S, Labow D, Momeni M, Chuang L, Dottino P, Rahaman J, Zakashansky K. The role of liver resection at the time of secondary cytoreduction in patients with recurrent ovarian cancer. Int J Gynecol Cancer. 2014;24:70–4.

92. Kamel SI, de Jong MC, Schulick RD, Diaz-Montes TP, Wolfgang CL, Hirose K, Edil BH, Choti MA, Anders RA, Pawlik TM. The role of liver-directed surgery in patients with hepatic metastasis from a gynecologic primary carcinoma. World J Surg. 2011;35:1345–54.

93. Knowles B, Bellamy CO, Oniscu A, Wigmore SJ. Hepatic resection for metastatic endometrioid carcinoma. HPB. 2010;12:412–7.

94. Loizzi V, Rossi C, Cormio G, Cazzolla A, Altomare D, Selvaggi L. Clinical features of hepatic metastasis in patients with ovarian cancer. Int J Gynecol Cancer. 2005;15:26–31.

6

Protein profiling of ovarian cancers by immunohistochemistry to identify potential target pathways

Cassandra D Foss[1,2], Heather J Dalton[3], Bradley J Monk[1,2], Dana M Chase[1,2] and John H Farley[1*]

Abstract

Background: To determine the protein expression profile (PEP) of primary and recurrent ovarian cancer patients in order to predict therapeutic targets for chemotherapy.

Methods: Tissue samples were submitted for PEP in two formats, including formalin-fixed paraffin-embedded tissue for immunohistochemistry (IHC) and fresh frozen tissue for oligonucleotide microarray (MA) gene expression assays. Specimens were analyzed for 18 protein markers and 88 MA genes. A series of Generalized Linear Models (GLM) was used to predict the proportion of positive results by histology for each biomarker.

Results: Four hundred and twenty-eight specimens were analyzed for IHC and 67 specimens for MA analysis. The majority of specimens, 82%, were serous histology and 35.3% of specimens were poorly differentiated. Sixty percent of specimens were advanced stage, 62% were from a primary diagnosis, and 53% were obtained from a metastatic site. BCRP, ER, MGMT, and RRM1 proteins were overexpressed in 85%, 47%, 93%, and 47% of serous carcinomas, respectively. The MGMT and RRM1 biomarkers were significantly overexpressed in serous ($p < .001$) and endometrioid ($p = .01$) histologies when compared to clear cell histology. MGMT was significantly elevated in 93% of serous and endometrioid samples, compared to 62% of samples with clear cell histology. Those proteins most often underexpressed included Her2/neu, SPARC, and c-kit, seen in less than 1%, 4%, and 5% of specimens, respectively.

Conclusions: PEP is a reliable and effective way of analyzing ovarian cancer specimens. PEP target identification does not appear to vary significantly with site evaluated, ovarian or other abdominal pelvic tissue, or primary versus recurrent disease. Variability in the expression of drug targets, including BCRP, ER, MGMT, and RRM1 could impact decision making pertaining to which therapeutic strategies carry the best chances for controlling disease.

Keywords: Protein profiling, Ovarian cancer, Immunohistochemistry

Background

Ovarian cancer is the fifth-leading cause of cancer death among women in the United States [1]. The current standard initial treatment of epithelial ovarian cancer includes surgical staging with optimal tumor debulking, followed by the administration of six cycles of intravenous chemotherapy with carboplatin and placlitaxel [2]. Although more than 80% of patients benefit from first-line therapy, tumor recurrence develops in nearly all patients, at a median of 15 months from completion of treatment

[2]. Moreover, platinum resistance occurs in 25% of patients within 6 months from the last administration of platinum-agent [3], and the overall five-year survival rate of advanced stage disease is 37% [1]. For this reason, ovarian cancer is considered a systemic disease, and systemic therapies are being increasingly relied upon for treatment.

In the recurrent setting, tumor molecular profiling has been an area of recent investigation in an attempt to improve patient outcomes by employing targeted chemotherapeutic agents. In a pilot study, Von Hoff et al. [4] performed molecular profiling (MP) in 86 patients with refractory metastatic cancers. Of the 27% of patients who received targeted chemotherapy, the MP approach resulted in a longer progression-free survival than the

* Correspondence: john.farley@chw.edu
[1]Division of Gynecologic Oncology, Department of Obstetrics and Gynecology, University of Arizona Cancer Center, 500 W. Thomas Road, Suite 600, Phoenix, AZ 85013, USA
Full list of author information is available at the end of the article

regimen on which the patient had just experienced progression.

In another study, The Cancer Genome Atlas (TCGA) researchers reported DNA gene mutations on tumor samples in patients with high-grade serous ovarian carcinomas (HGS-OvCa) [3]. Their findings were significant for TP53 mutations being identified in nearly all tumors (96%), while BRCA1 and BRCA2 mutations were identified in 22% of tumors. Their results indicated that the mutational spectrum of HGS-OvCa is distinct from other histological subtypes of ovarian cancer. Further study would therefore warrant the investigation of targeted therapies based on the specific molecular alterations identified in a specific histology of ovarian cancer.

To date, there is modest data regarding MP of ovarian cancer specimens. Of the 86 patients in the Von Hoff study, only 5 had ovarian cancer [4]. Furthermore, the TCGA data was limited to specimens with high-grade serous histology. The objective of the current study, therefore, is to determine the protein expression profile of primary and recurrent ovarian cancer patients of all histological types in order to predict potential therapeutic targets for chemotherapy.

Methods

The Target Now® (Caris Life Sciences®) database was accessed to obtain MP results for ovarian cancer tissue samples. De-identified results of Target Now®, as well as available histopathologic and clinical data from the Caris Life Sciences'® database were obtained after Institutional Review Board (IRB) approval. Because the research involved data collected previously for clinical utility (non-research purposes), this study qualified and was approved for expedited review by the IRB at St. Joseph's Hospital and Medical Center. Data was transferred from Caris Life Sciences® to the investigators in the form of a limited data set in compliance with a Data Transfer Agreement.

Immunohistochemistry

The database was used to analyze formalin fixed tissue samples for protein expression profile (PEP) by immunohistochemistry (IHC), which were obtained from women with primary and recurrent ovarian carcinoma, 62% and 37% respectively. Specimens were collected between January 2010 and December 2010. A total of 428 specimens were analyzed for 18 protein markers specific to the Target Now® PEP: Androgen Receptor, BCRP, c-kit, ER/PR, ERCC1, Her2/Neu, MGMT, MRP1, PDGFR, PGP, PTEN, RRM1, SPARC, TOP2A, TOPO1, TS, cMET, TUBB3. Analyses were performed by Caris Life Sciences® (Irving, Tx). The tests performed by Caris Life Sciences® were part of the Target Now® MP service. Staining protocols employed the Ventana Medical Systems, Inc. (Tucson, AZ) automated staining systems. Following heat-induced epitope retrieval,

antibody incubation was for 20–40 minutes (antibody-specific), and visualization procedure was based on the staining system. Appropriate positive and negative control specimens and slides were included for all of the proteins tested. Slides were evaluated semi-quantitatively for staining intensity on a scale of 0 (no staining) to 3 and by the percentage of the tumor cells showing the reactivity. For IHC scoring appropriate positive and negative thresholds were defined and considered in the subsequent statistical analyses with intermediate and unknown results considered not evaluable. Comparison of IHC results with clinical variables was performed with Fisher's exact test.

Oligonucleotide microarray (MA) gene expression

A total of 67(25%) of the 264 primary specimens were analyzed for MA. Normal tissue from the abdominal pelvic cavity was used as a control organ. No specific site was ever designated as a control, the only requirement being that it was uninvolved with cancer. The arrays contain probes for 88 genes for which there is a therapeutic agent that could potentially interact with that gene. Those 88 genes are listed in Additional file 1: Table S1. The frozen tumor fragments for MA were placed in a glass tube on 0.5 mL of frozen 0.5 M guanidine isothiocyanate solution, thawed, and homogenized with a Covaris S2 (Covari, Woburn, MA). RNA was bound and then eluted. RNA was tested for integrity by assessing the ratio of 28S to 18S ribosomal RNA on an Agilent BioAnalyzer (Agilent, Santa Clara, CA). Tumor RNA (2 to 5 µg) and control RNA from a sample of a normal tissue representative of the tumor's tissue of origin (2 to 5 µg) were converted to cDNA and labeled during T7 polymerase amplification with contrasting fluor tagged (Cy3, Cy5) cytidine triphosphate. The labeled tumor and its tissue of origin reference were hybridized to an Agilent H1Av2 60-mer oligo array chip with 17,085 unique probes. The chips were then scanned on an Agilent Microarray Scanner (Agilent, Santa Clara, CA). Fluorescence intensity data were extracted, normalized, and analyzed using Agilent Feature Extraction Software. The MA was considered positive for a target if the difference in expression for a gene between tumor and control organ tissue was at a significance level of $P \leq .001$. Cut points were chosen for gene expression of the cancer based on stringent P values ($P < .001$) compared with the normal mRNA expression levels. It was decided that using the mRNA level from the tissue of the organ of tumor origin would be the most informative comparison. To provide stringent quality control, these MA studies were performed in a Clinical Laboratory Improvement Amendments–certified environment.

Statistical analysis

Generalized Linear Models (GLM) were used with binomial distribution and link logit specified to predict the dichotomous outcome variable overexpression from the categorical predictor histology. Histologies classified as other was set as the reference group for the computation of parameter estimate odds ratios. One GLM model per biomarker was conducted resulting in eighteen models. The False Discovery Rate [SITE] correction used to adjust for multiple comparisons for significant GLM models. SPSS version 20 was used for statistical analyses.

Results

Specimens were obtained from 428 females with a median age of 62 years (Table 1). The majority of specimens analyzed by IHC were of serous and carcinoma histology (82%, Table 2). Thirty-five percent of specimens were poorly differentiated, while 27% were of unknown histological grade. Of the primary specimens, 62% were from adnexa, while 53% were obtained from a metastatic site and not the adnexa. Of the 67 specimens analyzed by MA, 55 (82%) were serous histology, 4 (6%) endometrioid, 2 (3%) clear cell, and 6 (9%) other. An advanced-stage diagnosis was represented in 60% of specimens. Five of the eighteen binomial GLM models predicting protein overexpression were significant. Significant models were for BCRP, ER, MGMT, RRM1, and PTEN at the trend level (Table 3). Twelve pairwise post hoc comparisons were performed for each significant model resulting in sixty post hoc contrasts (Table 4).

ER protein was significantly overexpressed in 47% of serous and 50% of endometrioid samples, while only elevated in only 14% of clear cell samples. Post-hoc testing demonstrated the ER protein was significantly overexpressed in serous (p < .001) and endometrioid (p = .003) histologies when compared to clear cell histology (Table 2). The MGMT and RRM1 biomarkers were also significantly overexpressed in serous (p < .001) and endometrioid (p = .01) histologies when compared to clear cell histology. MGMT was significantly elevated in 93% of serous and endometrioid samples, compared to 62% of samples with clear cell histology. Only 14% of clear cell samples were found to have overexpression of RRM1, compared to 47% of serous and 25% of endometrioid samples. Those proteins most often underexpressed included Her2/neu, SPARC, and c-kit, seen in less than 1%, 4%, and 5% of specimens, respectively. None of the post hoc comparisons for histology were significant for biomarkers BCRP and PTEN with the FDR correction applied.

There were 88 genes evaluated by MA gene expression and included in statistical analysis for association with histology. Those genes most overexpressed, defined as a difference in expression of mRNA between tumor and control organ tissue at a significance level of $P \leq .001$, in serous histology included TOP2A, MSH2, OGFR, RRM2, GART, and PARP1. A description of proportion of positive expression is shown in Figure 1. There were fourteen genes that were never expressed in serous histology and are not shown in Figure 1: ABCG2, AR, CES2, KIT, MS4A1, PDGFRA, PDGFRB, POLA1, RXRB, SPARC, SSTR1, SSTR2, SSTR4, and TOP1. There was no difference in protein or gene overexpression identified when analyzed by age, FIGO stage, grade, primary or recurrent tumor, and ovary or other biopsy site.

Discussion

TCGA project has analyzed post-transcriptional messenger RNA expression, microRNA expression, promoter methylation, and DNA copy number in 489 high-grade serous ovarian adenocarcinomas [3]. They reported that high-grade serous ovarian cancer is characterized by TP53 mutations in almost all tumors (96%); and a low prevalence but statistically significant recurrent somatic mutations in nine further genes including NF1, BRCA1, BRCA2, RB1, and CDK12. Pathway analyses suggested that homologous recombination was a potentially important pathway and was defective in about half of the high grade serous cancers analyzed. NOTCH and FOXM1 signaling were involved in serous ovarian cancer pathophysiology.

Molecular PEP is a powerful approach to identify clinical markers for diagnosis and prognosis as in epithelial ovarian

Table 1 Patient characteristics at diagnosis

	(N)	Percent%
TOTAL	428	
Median age (years)	61.7	
Tumor histology		
Serous	351	82
Clear cell	21	5
Endometrioid	28	7
Other	28	6
Tumor stage		
I	36	8
II	24	6
III	224	52
IV	34	8
Missing	110	26
Tumor grade		
Well differentiated	117	27
Moderately differentiated	43	10
Poorly differentiated	151	35
Unknown	117	28
Timing		
Primary	264	62
Recurrent	157	37
Unknown	7	1

Table 2 Counts and proportions of overexpression for biomarkers by histology

Biomarker	Serous mean (sd)	Clear cell mean (sd)	Endometrioid mean (sd)	Other mean (sd)
1 Androgen receptor	.27(.44)	.10(.31)	.27(.45)	.12(.33)
2 BCRP*	.85(.36)	.85(.37)	.65(.49)	.72(.46)
3 c-kit	.05(.22)	.00(.00)	.00(.00)	.00(.00)
4 ER*	.47(.50)	.14(.36)	.50(.51)	.39(.50)
5 ERCC1	.24(.43)	.33(.48)	.04(.19)	.25(.44)
6 Her2/Neu	.01(.09)	.00(.00)	.00(.00)	.00(.00)
7 MGMT***	.93(.25)	.62(.50)	.93(.26)	.89(.32)
8 MRP1	.89(.32)	.85(.37)	.92(.27)	.92(.27)
9 PDGFR	.18(.38)	.15(.37)	.23(.43)	.16(.37)
10 PGP	.19(.39)	.24(.47)	.21(.42)	.14(.36)
11 PR	.39(.49)	.19(.40)	.50(.51)	.36(.49)
12 PTEN	.65(.48)	.48(.51)	.43(.50)	.61(.50)
13 RRM1**	.47(.50)	.14(.36)	.24(.44)	.57(.50)
14 SPARC MONO	.11(.32)	.24(.47)	.10(.30)	.16(.37)
15 SPARC POLY	.04(.20)	.00(.00)	.00(.00)	.00(.00)
16 TOP2A	.39(.49)	.20(.41)	.23(.43)	.40(.50)
17 TOPO1	.89(.32)	.86(.36)	.89(.32)	.93(.26)
18 TS	.15(.35)	.05(.22)	.08(.27)	.16(.37)

*P < .05, **P < .01, ***P < .001.

cancer. In a previous smaller study, a tissue array composed of 244 serous tumors of different grades (0–3) and stages (I–IV) was evaluated by comprehensive IHC for proteins not necessarily associated with response to selective chemotherapeutic agents [5]. Ccne1, Ran, Cdc20, and Cks1 showed significant differences of expression in association with the clinical stage of disease. The application of these biomarkers in both the initial diagnosis and prognostic attributes of patients with epithelial ovarian tumors could prove to be useful in patient management.

The main objective of this study was to characterize and identify the characteristics of epithelial ovarian cancers through PEP of ovarian tumors in order to predict targeted therapies. The current study is one of the largest PEP

Table 3 Parameter estimates predicting overexpression from histology

		OR	95% CI	P	Wald chi-square
BCRP	Carcinoma and serous	2.21	.88-5.58	0.09	8.39, p = .039
	Clear cell	2.2	.49-9.94	0.3	
	Endometriod	0.735	.22-2.41	0.61	
ER	Carcinoma and serous	1.39	.63-3.05	0.42	7.76, p = .051
	Clear Cell	0.26	.06-1.09	0.07	
	Endometriod	1.55	.54-4.46	0.42	
MGMT	Carcinoma and serous	1.64	.46-5.81	0.48	18.57, p < .001
	Clear cell	0.2	.04-.86	0.03	
	Endometriod	1.56	.24-10.14	0.64	
PTEN	Carcinoma and serous	1.19	.54-2.61	0.67	7.01, p = .071
	Clear cell	0.59	.19-1.85	0.36	
	Endometriod	0.49	.17-1.41	0.18	
RRM1	Carcinoma and serous	0.67	.31-1.46	0.32	13.06, p = .005
	Clear cell	0.13	.03-.52	0.004	
	Endometriod	0.25	.08-.78	0.017	

Table 4 Post hoc comparisons for significant glm models predicting overexpression

		BCRP					ER				
		Mean diff	SE	95% LCL	95% UCL	p	Mean diff	SE	95% LCL	95% UCL	p
Carcinoma and serous	Clear cell	0	0.08	-0.16	0.16	.993	0.33	0.08	0.17	0.49	.000*
Carcinoma and serous	Endometriod	0.2	0.10	0.01	0.38	.039	-0.03	0.10	-0.22	0.17	.783
Carcinoma and serous	Other	0.13	0.09	-0.05	0.31	.155	0.08	0.10	-0.11	0.27	.405
Clear cell	Endometriod	0.2	0.12	-0.04	0.44	.110	-0.36	0.12	-0.60	-0.12	.003*
Clear cell	Other	0.13	0.12	-0.11	0.37	.279	-0.25	0.12	-0.48	-0.02	.037
Endometriod	Other	-0.07	0.13	-0.32	0.19	.609	0.11	0.13	-0.15	0.37	.417

		MGMT					RRM1				
		Mean diff	SE	95% LCL	95% UCL	p	Mean diff	SE	95% LCL	95% UCL	p
Carcinoma and serous	Clear cell	0.31	0.11	0.10	0.52	0.00*	0.33	.081	.17	.49	.000*
Carcinoma and serous	Endometriod	0.00	0.05	-0.10	0.10	0.95	0.22	.086	.05	.39	.010*
Carcinoma and serous	Other	0.04	0.06	-0.08	0.16	0.52	-.10	.097	-.29	.09	.311
Clear cell	Endometriod	-0.31	0.12	-0.54	-0.08	0.00*	-.11	.112	-.33	.11	.338
Clear cell	Other	-0.27	0.12	-0.51	-0.04	0.02	-0.43	.121	-.67	-.19	.000*
Endometriod	Other	0.04	0.08	-0.11	0.18	0.95	-0.32	.124	-.56	-.08	.010*

		PTEN				
		Mean diff	SE	95% LCL	95% UCL	p
Carcinoma and serous	Clear cell	.17	.112	-.05	.39	.128
Carcinoma and serous	Endometriod	0.22	.097	.03	.41	.024
Carcinoma and serous	Other	.04	.096	-.15	.23	.679
Clear cell	Endometriod	.05	.144	-.23	.33	.740
Clear cell	Other	-.13	.143	-.41	.15	.359
Endometriod	Other	-.18	.131	-.44	.08	.174

*P < 0.05.

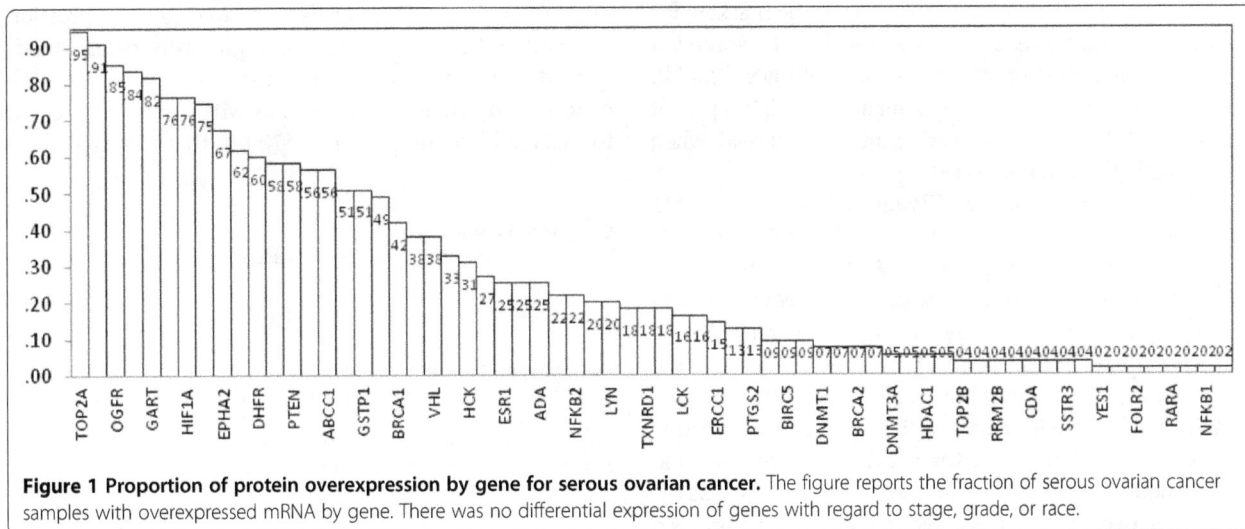

Figure 1 Proportion of protein overexpression by gene for serous ovarian cancer. The figure reports the fraction of serous ovarian cancer samples with overexpressed mRNA by gene. There was no differential expression of genes with regard to stage, grade, or race.

analyses of epithelial ovarian cancers in the literature. This study demonstrates that PEP is a reliable and effective way of analyzing ovarian cancer specimens. In this study, protein expression target identification did not appear to vary significantly with the site evaluated, ovarian or other abdominal pelvic tissue, or with primary versus recurrent disease.

Several markers have been identified which may predict a specific tumor's response to chemotherapy (Table 3). Breast cancer resistance protein (BCRP), an atypical drug efflux pump, mediates multidrug resistance in breast cancer, as well as other cancer types, by reducing the intracellular concentration of cytotoxic drugs [6]. BCRP has been described in breast, colon, gastric cancer, and fibrosarcoma cell lines but has also had documented overexpression in ovarian cancer cell lines [7]. Studies in topotecan-resistant ovarian cancer cell lines have demonstrated a substantial overexpression of BCRP. Moreover, these cell lines demonstrated resistance to other topoisomerase I inhibitors, SN-38 (the active metabolite of irinotecan, and 9-aminocamptothecin, as well as the topoisomerase II inhibitor, mitoxantrone [6,7]). Topotecan, etoposide, mitoxantrone, 5-FU, anthracyclines such as doxorubicin and pirarubicin, as well as methotrexate have all been identified as substrates of BCRP [8,9], and therefore would be less effective in tumors that overexpress this protein. However, paclitaxel, vincristine, vindesine, mitomycin c, and cisplatin are not mediated by BCRP [9] and would likely be more successful in treating patients with tumors that overexpress BCRP.

Tumors which overexpress estrogen receptor (ER) may have an enhanced response to anti-estrogens such as megestrol, tamoxifen, and aromatase inhibitors. These therapies have been used extensively in the treatment of ER-positive breast cancer. However, there is sparse data

on ER-positivity in ovarian tumors. In the 'MALOVA' Ovarian Cancer Study, the investigators identified that ER was expressed in 36% of epithelial ovarian tumors [10]. The authors suggested ER is a prognostic indicator of improved survival in ovarian cancer patients, though no targeted therapy was used in this study. Data on the use of anti-estrogens in the treatment of ovarian cancer is limited to phase II trials with results indicating these therapies, if successful, are predominantly able to achieve disease stabilization, with only marginal rates of partial or complete treatment responses [11-15].

MGMT, or O6-methylguanine-DNA methyltransferase, is an enzyme that repairs methylated DNA and plays a crucial role in the protection against alkylating agents [16,17]. MGMT expression in cancer cells can inhibit the success of chemotherapy treatment with alkylating agents, which work by triggering DNA methylation [18]. If MGMT is overexpressed in the tumor, alkylating agents such as temozolomide may be less effective. Low expression of MGMT has been associated with successful response to treatment with temozolomide [19]. Furthermore, inhibition of MGMT activity has been shown to increase the toxicity of alkylating agents [17,18].

RRM1 is a subunit of Ribonucleotide reductase (RR), an enzyme that acts as the rate-limiting step in DNA synthesis, as it is the only known enzyme to convert ribonucleotides to deoxyribonucleotides for DNA polymerization and repair. It functions with the p53-regulated RRM2 homologue p53R2 and is important in DNA repair secondary to genotoxic stress [20]. Gemcitabine is an analog of deoxycytidine and is converted intracellularly into active diphosphate and triphosphate nucleosides, which become incorporated into the DNA chain, leading to termination of chain elongation and inhibition of DNA synthesis [21]. In preclinical studies, increased RRM1 expression and activity have been shown to be markers for gemcitabine resistance, suggesting that RRM1 expression is a negative predictor of gemcitabine efficacy [20-24]. However, patients with low as compared to high levels of tumoral RRM1 expression had improved survival when treated with gemcitabine-based therapy [25].

In this particular study, BCRP, ER, MGMT, and RRM1 proteins were overexpressed in 85%, 47%, 93%, and 47% of serous carcinomas, respectively. As these proteins have been shown to be associated with various resistances to specific chemotherapeutic agents, targeted therapy may be helpful in identifying successful treatments. Because of the increased expression of BCRP, MGMT, and RRM1 identified in serous carcinomas, in theory chemotherapeutic agents such as etoposide, adriamycin, temozolomide, and gemcitabine may be avoided in the treatment of serous tumors that overexpress these biomarkers and considered only for other histologies of ovarian cancer.

On the other hand, for a segment of the ovarian cancer population, drugs that have not been developed in ovarian cancer, such as temozolomide, could be useful for patients with the right biomarker profile, such as low MGMT expression, perhaps even in preference to giving a standard drug like topotecan to a patient with suboptimal biomarker expression, such as low TOPO1. In this way, PEP offers a laboratory-based approach to drug selection, rather than the empiric method of selecting drugs blindly. Accordingly, PEP could impact medical decision-making by prioritizing which standard agents are most likely and least likely to offer benefit to the individual patient, as well as identifying drugs outside the standard armamentarium with previously unrecognized potential to control disease. Admittedly, future studies measuring outcomes in patients undergoing PEP are sorely needed before PEP becomes a standard of care.

This study is limited by its retrospective design and descriptive nature, and the absence of clinical information such as response rates, disease status, which might allow correlation with response at this time. Another limitation of the current study pertains to the absent inclusion of a variety of molecular markers that appear to play a significant role in driving malignant behavior or in producing drug resistance. These include P53 and PIK3CA mutation, cMET, NOTCH, and FOXM1. To the extent that pathways that cause chemotherapeutic resistance were not assayed, the report of optimal protein expression for a given patient could overestimate the chance for benefit from the associated agent.

Conclusion

We observed that a majority of patients with serous histology demonstrated protein expression associated with resistance to one or more chemotherapeutic agents. Furthermore, the resistance pattern in each individual cancer was unpredictable. Future studies could include clinical benefit analysis of MP in ovarian cancer patients

in prospective trials or analysis of MA gene expression in ovarian tumors. Given the high proportion of advanced stage at diagnosis and the proclivity of ovarian cancer recurrence, efforts such as MP have the potential to make a large impact on survival of this disease.

Competing interests

The authors disclose that they have no financial relationships and/or competing interests.

Authors' contributions

CF drafted manuscript, HD assisted id data acquisition and manuscript drafting, BM reviewed manuscript, manuscript concept, DC data acquisition manuscript review, JF manuscript concept, manuscript draft and editing. All authors read and approved the final manuscript.

Acknowledgement

The authors wish to recognize Caris Life Sciences® staff Nancy Doll, RN, CTR and Diane Stapleton, CTR, for data extraction and quality control as well as Sheri Sanders, RN, BSN, MBA for administrative and operational oversight. The authors also wish to thank Daniele A. Sumner, BA, and Angela Barber for their assistance in editing this manuscript. The authors are solely responsible for the content of this manuscript.

Author details

[1]Division of Gynecologic Oncology, Department of Obstetrics and Gynecology, University of Arizona Cancer Center, 500 W. Thomas Road, Suite 600, Phoenix, AZ 85013, USA. [2]Creighton University School of Medicine at Dignity Health St. Joseph's Hospital and Medical Center, 500 W. Thomas Road, Suite 600, Phoenix, AZ 85013, USA. [3]Department of Gynecologic Oncology and Reproductive Medicine, The University of Texas MD Anderson Cancer Center, Houston, TX, USA.

References

1. Siegel R, Naishadham D, Jemal A: **Cancer Statistics 2013.** *CA Cancer J Clin* 2013, **63:**11–30.
2. Hennessy BT, Coleman RL, Markman M: **Ovarian Cancer.** *Lancet* 2009, **374:**1371–1382.
3. The Cancer Genome Atlas Research Network: **Integrated genomic analyses of ovarian carcinoma.** *Nature* 2011, **474:**609–614.
4. Von Hoff DD, Stephenson JJ, Rosen P, Loesch DM, Borad MJ, Anthony S, Jameson G, Brown S, Cantafio N, Richards DA, Fitch TR, Wasserman E, Fernandez C, Green S, Sutherland W, Bittner M, Alarcon A, Mallery D, Penny R: **Pilot study using molecular profiling of patient's tumors to find potential targets and select treatments for their refractory cancers.** *J Clin Onc* 2010, **28:**4877–4883.
5. Ouellet V, Guyot MC, Le Page C, Filali-Mouhim A, Lussier C, Tonin PN, Provencher DM, Mes-Masson AM: **Tissue array analysis of expression microarray candidates identifies markers associated with tumor grade and outcome in serous epithelial ovarian cancer.** *Int J Cancer* 2006, **119:**599–607.
6. Jia P, Wu X, Li F, Xu Q, Wu M, Chen G, Liao G, Wang S, Zhou J, Lu Y, MA D: **Breast cancer resistance protein-mediated topotecan resistance in ovarian cancer cells.** *Int J Gynecol Cancer* 2005, **15:**1042–1048.
7. Maliepaard M, van Gastelen MA, de Jong LA, Pluim D, van Waardenburg RC, Ruevekamp-Helmers MC, Floot BG, Schellens JH: **Overexpression of the BCRP/MXR/ABCP gene in a topotecan-selected ovarian tumor cell line.** *Cancer Res* 1999, **59:**4559–4563.
8. Mao Q, Unadkat JD: **Role of the breast cancer resistance protein (ABCG2) in drug transport.** *AAPS J* 2005, **7:**E118–E133.
9. Yuan J, Lv H, Peng B, Wang C, Yu Y, He Z: **Role of BCRP as a biomarker for predicting resistance to 5-fluorouracil in breast cancer.** *Cancer Chemother Pharmacol* 2009, **63:**1103–1110.

10. Hogdall EV, Christensen L, Hogdall CK, Blaakaer J, Gayther S, Jacobs IJ, Christensen IJ, Kjaer SK: **Prognostic value of estrogen receptor and progesterone receptor tumor expression in Danish ovarian cancer patients: from the 'MALOVA' Ovarian Cancer Study.** *Oncol Rep* 2007, **18:**1051–1059.

11. Pan Y, Kao MS: **Endometrioid ovarian carcinoma benefits from aromatase inhibitors: case report and literature review.** *Current Oncol* 2010, **17:**82–85.

12. Bowman A, Gabra H, Langdon SP, Lessells A, Stewart M, Young A, Smyth JF: **CA125 response is associated with estrogen receptor expression in a phase II trial of letrozole in ovarian cancer: identification of an endocrine-sensitive subgroup.** *Clin Cancer Res* 2002, **8:**2233–2239.

13. del Carmen MG, Fuller AF, Matulonis U, Horick NK, Goodman A, Duska LR, Penson R, Campos S, Roche M, Seiden MV: **Phase II trial of anastrozole in women with asymptomatic Mullerian cancer.** *Gynecol Oncol* 2003, **91:**596–602.

14. Papadimitriou CA, Markaki S, Siapkaras J, Viachos G, Efstathiou E, Grimani I, Hamilos G, Zorzou M, Dimopoulos MA: **Hormonal therapy with letrozole for relapsed epithelial ovarian cancer. Long-term results of a phase II study.** *Oncology* 2004, **66:**112–117.

15. Smyth JF, Gourley C, Walker G, MacKean MJ, Stevenson A, Williams AR, Nafussi AA, Rye T, Rye R, Stewart M, McCurdy J, Mano M, Reed N, McMahon T, Vasey P, Gabra H, Landon SP: **Antiestrogen therapy is active in selected ovarian cancer cases: the use of letrozole in estrogen-receptor positive patients.** *Clin Cancer Res* 2007, **13:**3617–3622.

16. Kaina B, Christmann M, Naumann S, Roos WP: **MGMT: key node in the battle against genotoxicity, carcinogenicity and apoptosis induced by alkylating agents.** *DNA Repair (Amst)* 2007, **6:**1079–1099.

17. Casorelli I, Russo MT, Bignami M: **Role of mismatch repair and MGMT in response to anticancer therapies.** *Anticancer Agents Med Chem* 2008, **8:**368–380.

18. Gerson SL: **Clinical relevance of MGMT in the treatment of cancer.** *J Clin Oncol* 2002, **20:**2388–2399.

19. McCormack AI, McDonald KL, Gill AJ, Clark SJ, Burt MG, Campbell KA, Braund WJ, Little NS, Cook RJ, Grossman AB, Robinson BG, Clifton-Bligh RJ: **Low O-6-methylgaunine-DNA methyltransferase (MGMT) expression and response to temozolomide in aggressive pituitary tumours.** *Clin Endocrinol (Oxf)* 2009, **71:**226–233.

20. Davidson JD, Ma L, Flagella M, Geeganage S, Gelbert LM, Slapak CA: **An increase in the expression of ribonucleotide reductase large subunit 1 is associated with gemcitabine resistance in non–small cell lung cancer cell lines.** *Cancer Res* 2004, **64:**3761–3766.

21. Zhao LP, Xue C, Zhang JW, Hu ZH, Zhao YY, Zhang J, Huang Y, Zhao HY, Zhang L: **Expression of RRM1 and its correlation with sensitivity to gemcitabine-based chemotherapy in advanced nasorpharyngeal carcinoma.** *Chin J Cancer* 2012, **31:**476–483.

22. Bergman AM, Eijk PP, van Haperen VW R, Smid K, Veerman G, Hubeek I, van den Ijssel P, Ylstra B, Peters GJ: *In vivo* **induction of resistance to gemcitabine results in increased expression of ribonucleotide reductase subunit M1 as the major determinant.** *Cancer Res* 2005, **65:**9510–9516.

23. Bepler G, Kusmartseva I, Sharma S, Gautam A, Cantor A, Sharma A, Simon G: **RRM1 modulated in vitro and in vivo efficacy of gemcitabine and platinum in non–small-cell lung cancer.** *J Clin Oncol* 2006, **24:**4731–4737.

24. Nakahira S, Nakamori S, Tsujie M, Takahashi Y, Okami J, Yoshioka S, Yamasaki M, Marubashi S, Takemasa I, Miyamoto A, Takeda Y, Nagano H, Dono K, Umeshita K, Sakon M, Monden M: **Involvement of ribonucleotide reductase M1 subunit overexpression in gemcitabine resistance of human pancreatic cancer.** *Int J Cancer* 2007, **120:**1355–1363.

25. Rosell R, Danenberg KD, Alberola V, Bepler G, Sanchez JJ, Camps C, Provencio M, Isla D, Taron M, Diz P, Artal A, Spanish Lung Cancer Group: **Ribonucleotide reductase mRNA expression and survival in gemcitabine/ cisplatin-treated advanced non-small-cell lung cancer patients.** *Clin Cancer Res* 2004, **10:**1318–1325.

7

Disparities in the surgical staging of high-grade endometrial cancer in the United States

Jonathan R. Foote[1*], Stephanie Gaillard[1], Gloria Broadwater[2], Julie A. Sosa[3,4], Brittany Davidson[1], Mohamed A. Adam[3], Angeles Alvarez Secord[1], Monica B. Jones[1], Junzo Chino[5] and Laura J. Havrilesky[1]

Abstract

Background: The National Comprehensive Cancer Network (NCCN) and the Society of Gynecologic Oncology (SGO) recommend lymph node sampling (LNS) as a key component in the surgical staging of high-grade endometrial cancer. Our goal was to examine surgical staging patterns for high-grade endometrial cancer in the United States.

Methods: The National Cancer Data Base (NCDB) was searched for patients who underwent surgery for serous, clear cell, or grade 3 endometrioid endometrial cancer. Outcomes were receipt of LNS and overall survival (OS). Multivariate logistic regression was used to examine receipt of LNS in Stage I–III disease based on race (White vs. Black), income, surgical volume, and distance traveled to care. Multivariate Cox proportional hazards regression modeling was used to assess OS based on stage, race, income, LNS, surgical volume, and distance traveled.

Results: Forty-two thousand nine hundred seventy-three patients were identified: 76% White, 53% insured by Medicare/Medicaid, 24% traveled >30 miles, and 33% stage III disease. LNS was similar among White and Black women (81% vs 82%). LNS was more common among >30 miles traveled (84% vs 81%, $p < 0.001$), higher surgical volume (83% vs 80%, $p < 0.001$), and academic centers (84% vs 80%, $p < 0.001$). In multivariate analysis, higher income, higher surgical volume, Charlson-Deyo score, and distance traveled were predictors of LNS. Stage III disease (HR 3.39, 95% CI 3.28–3.50), age (10-year increase; HR 1.63, 95% CI 1.61–1.66), lack of LNS (HR 1.64, 95% CI 1.56–1.69), and low income (HR 1.20, 95% CI 1.14–1.27) were predictors of lower survival.

Conclusions: Surgical care for high-grade endometrial cancer in the United States is not uniform. Improved access to high quality care at high volume centers is needed to improve rates of recommended LNS.

Keywords: Endometrial cancer, Disparity, High-grade, Staging, NCDB, Surgical volume

Background

Endometrial cancer is the most common form of gynecologic cancer in the United States, with more than 60,000 new cases and 10,470 deaths estimated to occur in 2016 [1]. The majority of endometrial cancers are Type I, grade 1–2 endometrioid adenocarcinoma and have an excellent prognosis, most often presenting as low-grade and at an early stage. Conversely, Type II cancers, including uterine papillary serous carcinoma (UPSC), clear cell carcinoma (CC), and grade 3 endometrioid adenocarcinoma, often have a much worse prognosis, presenting with extra-uterine disease [2–5]. UPSC, CC, and grade 3 endometrioid adenocarcinoma represent 10–27% of incident endometrial cancer cases, but account for over 70% of endometrial cancer deaths [6].

The National Comprehensive Cancer Network (NCCN) and the Society of Gynecologic Oncology (SGO) support pelvic and para-aortic lymphadenectomy for patients with high-grade endometrial cancer, including UPSC, CC, and grade 3 endometrioid adenocarcinoma [7–9]. Although the surgical guidelines are clear, there is a demonstrated racial disparity between Whites and Blacks in de facto surgical management [10]. Black women are less likely to undergo surgery for endometrial cancer [11–13]. While

* Correspondence: jonathan.foote@dm.duke.edu
[1]Division of Gynecologic Oncology, Duke University Medical Center, 2301 Erwin Rd, Durham, NC 27710, USA
Full list of author information is available at the end of the article

many authors have examined associations between race and the epidemiology, treatment, and outcomes of endometrial cancer, no author has explored the relationship between race and the type of surgery performed. Disparities also exist for the distance traveled to receive care for endometrial cancer, although the available data are limited. In 2011, Benjamin et al. performed a statewide analysis of endometrial cancer care in Arizona and found that minorities travel farther than Whites to receive care, while patients with government-funded insurance travel farther than patients with other types of insurance [14]. There are no other regional or national studies examining the relationship between receipt of care for endometrial cancer and travel distance. Based on the NCCN and the SGO recommendations of lymph node sampling during the surgical staging of high-grade endometrial cancer, we explored surgical practice patterns and disparities in the treatment of UPSC, CC, and grade 3 endometrioid adenocarcinoma in the United States.

Methods

Data source

The National Cancer Data Base (NCDB) is a national oncology outcomes database in the United States, founded in 1989 by the American College of Surgeons (ACS) and its Commission on Cancer (CoC) Program. One of the largest cancer registries in the world, the NCDB collects data on 70% of all new cancer diagnoses in the U.S. from over 1,500 reporting hospitals [15]. The NCDB data coding process is standardized according to the CoC Registry Operations and Data Standards Manual, the American Joint Committee for Cancer (AJCC) Manual for Staging of Cancer, and the International Classification of Disease for Oncology, Third Edition (ICD-O3). For the current study, all data were extracted from medical records by trained and certified tumor registrars. Our Institutional Review Board granted this study an exemption status due to the de-identified nature of the dataset.

Case selection

The NCDB Participant User File was searched for all patients who underwent surgery for UPSC, CC, or grade 3 endometrioid adenocarcinoma. Data were available from the years 1998 to 2012. Demographic and socioeconomic information was recorded for each patient, including age, race, income, education and insurance status. Clinical and pathologic data collected included International Federation of Gynecology and Obstetrics (FIGO) staging, Charlson-Deyo comorbidity score, number of regional lymph nodes examined, number of para-aortic lymph nodes examined, peritoneal cytology status,

and performance of omentectomy. While FIGO staging criteria were updated in 2009, we did not reclassify patients for our analysis. The FIGO 2009 staging criteria changes to Stage I would not alter our Stage I designation; and changes to Stage II and Stage III designation could not be fully addressed from data available in the NCDB. Patients were further categorized based on treatment center type (academic research center, community cancer program/other, comprehensive community cancer program), hospital endometrial cancer surgical volume, and distance travelled to receive care ($\leq$ or $>$ 30 miles). Surgical volume was defined based on strategies previously utilized in NCDB-related publications [16]. Hospital surgical volume was annualized based on the total number of endometrial cancer patients and the total number of years of reported data. Surgical volume groups were then categorized by quartile rank: 75th percentile = very-high volume ($>$31.7 cases/year); 51st–75th percentile = moderately-high volume (13.3–31.6 cases/year); 25th–50th percentile = intermediate volume (6.7–13.2 cases/year); and $<25^{th}$ percentile = low volume ($<$6.7 cases/year). While distance to care was recorded continuously in the NCDB, we stratified distance in two groups, $\leq$ 30 miles and $>$ 30 miles, based on the overall mean distance traveled (mean = 30).

Statistical analysis

The main outcomes examined were the rates of lymph node sampling and overall survival (OS). Multivariate logistic regression was used to explore differences in receipt of lymph node sampling (LNS). Stage IV patients were excluded as LNS may not always be necessary or indicated in this patient population. Given that there is not a standard number of sampled lymph nodes to constitute 'adequate' staging, we performed a sensitivity analysis using replicate logistic models considering various cut points for the number of lymph nodes sampled: (1) 0 vs. 1 +; (2) 0–1 vs. 2+; (3) 0–4 vs. 5+; (4) 0–9 vs. 10+; (5) 0–14 vs. 15+; (6) 0–19 vs. 20+. In addition, logistic regression modeling was used to explore a subset of patients with available data on para-aortic LNS. The following variables were assessed for possible associations with receipt of LNS (as categorized by the NCDB): race (White, Black, other), median-household income (defined based on a specific patient's zip code at the time of diagnosis compared against 2012 American Community Survey data: <$38,000; $38,000 to $47,999; $48,000 to $62,999; or > $63,000), education (defined as the percentage of the population with a high school diploma as the highest degree obtained in a specific patient's zip code: $\geq$21%, 13–20%, 7–12.9%, or <7%), insurance status (not insured, private insurance, Medicaid, Medicare, or other), Charlson-Deyo comorbidity score (Charlson score of 0, 1, or $\geq$2), type of treatment center (comprehensive

Table 1 Patient characteristics of patients with UPSC, CC, or grade 3 endometrioid carcinoma

	Overall n (%)	Black n (%)	White n (%)	Other n (%)	p-values
Total	42,973 (100)[a]	5,285 (12.2)	35,694 (76.1)	1,417 (3.3)	
Age at diagnosis					
Mean (SD)	66.0 (11.5)	65.7 (11.7)	66.2 (11.7)	61.5 (11.6)	<0.001
Income					
< $38,000	7,708 (17.9)	2,352 (44.5)	5,119 (14.3)	167 (11.8)	<0.001
$38,000–$47,999	9,814 (22.9)	1,175 (22.2)	8,304 (23.3)	216 (15.2)	
$48,000–$62,999	11,218 (26.1)	921 (17.4)	9,747 (27.3)	375 (26.5)	
≥ $63,000	13,192 (30.7)	707 (13.4)	11,668 (32.7)	627 (44.2)	
Unknown	1,041 (2.4)				
Insurance status					
Uninsured	1,418 (3.3)	256 (4.8)	1,060 (3.0)	81 (5.7)	<0.001
Private Insurance	17,582 (40.9)	1,807 (34.2)	14,845 (40.6)	683 (48.2)	
Medicaid and Medicare	22,750 (52.9)	3,081 (58.3)	18,823 (52.7)	578 (40.8)	
Other	282 (0.7)	30 (0.6)	218 (0.6)	33 (2.3)	
Unknown	941 (2.2)				
Education[b]					
≥ 21%	7,196 (16.7)	1,928 (36.5)	4,881 (13.7)	318 (22.4)	<0.001
13–20%	10,792 (25.1)	1,923 (36.4)	8,393 (23.5)	344 (24.3)	
7.0–12.9%	13,867 (32.3)	933 (17.7)	12,314 (34.5)	413 (29.1)	
< 7.0%	10,107 (23.5)	373 (7.1)	9,277 (26.0)	310 (21.9)	
Unknown	1,011 (2.4)				
Charlson-Deyo Score					
0	24,653 (57.4)	2,858 (54.1)	20,540 (57.5)	890 (62.8)	<0.001
≥ 1	8,128 (18.9)	1,307 (24.7)	6,465 (18.1)	258 (18.2)	
Unknown	10,192 (23.7)				
Histology					
Uterine papillary Serous	8,238 (19.1)	1,506 (28.5)	6,413 (18.0)	211 (14.9)	<0.001
Clear cell	3,631 (8.5)	576 (10.9)	2,873 (8.0)	134 (9.5)	
Grade 3 endometrioid	31,104 (72.4)	3,203 (60.6)	26,408 (74.0)	1,072 (75.6)	
FIGO Stage					
I	24,052 (55.9)	2,622 (49.6)	20,348 (57.0)	756 (53.4)	<0.001
II	4,888 (11.4)	764 (14.5)	3,911 (11.0)	152 (10.7)	
III	14,033 (32.7)	1,899 (35.9)	11,435 (32.0)	509 (35.9)	
Lymph node sampling[c]					
Yes	35,158 (81.8)	4,265 (80.7)	29,211 (81.8)	1,214 (85.7)	<0.001
No	7,815 (18.2)	1,020 (19.3)	6,483 (18.2)	203 (14.3)	
Treatment center type					
Community Cancer Program	2,647 (6.2)	269 (5.1)	2,258 (6.3)	108 (7.6)	<0.001
Comprehensive Community Cancer Program	22,272 (51.8)	2,225 (42.1)	19,191 (53.8)	621 (43.8)	
Academic/ Research Program	18,054 (42.0)	2,791 (52.8)	14,245 (39.9)	688 (48.6)	
Hospital surgical volume[d]					
Very–high	30,518 (71.0)	3,880 (73.4)	25,146 (70.5)	1,006 (71.0)	<0.001

Table 1 Patient characteristics of patients with UPSC, CC, or grade 3 endometrioid carcinoma *(Continued)*

Moderately–high	7,998 (18.6)	926 (17.5)	6,709 (18.8)	296 (20.9)	
Intermediate	3,272 (7.6)	379 (7.2)	2,796 (7.8)	83 (5.9)	
Low	1,185 (2.8)	100 (1.9)	1,043 (2.9)	32 (2.2)	
Distance to care					
≤ 30 miles	31,645 (73.6)	4,246 (80.3)	25,884 (72.5)	1,152 (81.3)	<0.001
> 30 miles	10,366 (24.1)	913 (17.3)	9,025 (25.3)	234 (16.5)	
Unknown	962 (2.3)				

[a]Race data is available for 42,396 patients
[b]Defined as the percentage of the population with a high school diploma in a specific patient's area code
[c]Defined based on the number of regional lymph nodes sampled during surgery. Yes = 1+; No = 0
[d]Surgical volume groups were identified based on quartile rank of the total number of endometrial cancer patients undergoing surgery and the total number of years of reported data: 75th percentile = very-high volume (>31.7cases/year); 51st–75th percentile = moderately-high volume (13.3–31.6 cases/year); 25th–50th percentile = intermediate volume (6.7–13.2 cases/year); and <25th percentile = low volume (<6.7 cases/year)

community cancer program, community cancer program/other, or academic research center), hospital endometrial cancer surgical volume, and distance traveled to receive care. Receipt of peritoneal cytology and omentectomy were inconsistently reported, and therefore excluded from our assessment. Given limited numbers regarding minorities other than Blacks, we grouped additional minorities as 'other' for model parsimony. Table 1 lists patient and clinical characteristics based on race for patients with Stage I–III disease. Categorical variables were compared using chi-square tests. Multivariate Cox proportional hazards regression modeling and Kaplan Meier curves were used to assess associations between clinical variables and OS. OS models were explored utilizing distance to care as both continuous and dichotomous (≤30 miles and >30 miles). Statistical significance was considered a priori at a two-sided p-value of <0.05. We defined a clinically significant difference between categorical groups to exist if a p-value of <0.05 was associated with a ≥5% difference. Statistical analyses were conducted using SAS v. 9.3 software (SAS Institute, Inc., Cary, NC) and survival plots were created using Spotfire S+ v. 8.1 (TIBCO, Palo Alto, CA).

Results

Patient and cancer characteristics

A total of 53,841 patients were identified who underwent surgery and had available lymph node status data between 1998 and 2012 for high-grade endometrial cancer, including UPSC, CC, and grade 3 endometrioid adenocarcinoma. Patients were excluded from our analysis if lymph node status was not available. After excluding Stage IV patients, 42,973 patients were available for analysis. Table 1 lists demographic, socioeconomic, and clinical characteristics. Grade 3 endometrioid adenocarcinoma accounted for 31,104 cases (72%), while UPSC accounted for 8,238 cases (19%), and CC accounted for 3,631 cases (9%). Sixty–seven percent ($n = 28,940$) had Stage I/II disease,

while 33% ($n = 14,033$) had Stage III disease. Seventy–six percent of patients were White ($n = 35,694$), while 12% were Black ($n = 5,285$). The majority of patients were insured via Medicaid and Medicare (53%) or private insurance (41%). Most patients underwent surgery at a comprehensive community cancer program (52%) or at an academic/research center (42%). Seventy–one percent of patients received surgery at very-high volume centers (>31.7 cases/year). The mean distance traveled to care was 30 miles.

Receipt of surgical staging

In our cohort of 42,973 patients, 35,158 (82%) underwent regional LNS. In univariate analysis, receipt of care at an academic center (84% vs 70%, $p < 0.001$) and at a hospital with higher endometrial cancer surgical volume (>75th percentile, 83% vs 71% (all others), $p < 0.001$) were both associated with receipt of LNS (data not shown).

In multivariate analysis, income, distance traveled to care, Charlson-Deyo comorbidity score, and hospital surgical volume were all significant predictors of receipt of LNS. The sensitivity of these results were examined using replicate logistic models considering various cut points for the number of lymph nodes removed, which produced identical predictors of more complete staging to those reported above for all replicate models (0 vs. 1 +; 0–1 vs. 2+; 0–4 vs. 5+; 0–9 vs. 10+; 0–14 vs. 15+; 0–19 vs. 20+). Surgical volume and type of cancer center were strongly associated with each other, and thus were not considered concomitantly in multivariate analysis: Surgical volume was incorporated into the multivariate model. Receipt of LNS was less likely in patients with a Charleson-Deyo comorbidity score of ≥1 (OR 0.73, 95% CI 0.68 to 0.78) (Table 2), or with an annual income ≤ $38,000 (38 k-$47,999: OR 1.08, 95% CI 0.98 to 1.18; $48 k-$62,999: OR 1.20, 95% CI 1.10 to 1.32; >$63 k: OR 1.33, CI 1.21 to 1.46). Compared to very-high volume hospitals (>31.7 cases/year), receipt of LNS was also less

Table 2 Multivariate predictors of receipt of lymph node sampling in UPSC, CC, and grade 3 endometrioid carcinoma

Predictors	Odds Ratio (Reference =1)	95% CI	p-value
Race			
White	Reference		0.21
Black	0.97	0.88–1.06	
Other	1.15	0.96–1.36	
Income			
< $38,000	Reference		<0.001
$38,000–$47,999	1.08	0.98–1.18	
$48,000–$62,999	1.20	1.10–1.32	
≥ $63,000	1.33	1.21–1.46	
Surgical Volume[a]			
Very high	Reference		<0.001
Moderately high	0.65	0.61–0.71	
Intermediate	0.51	0.45–0.56	
Low	0.39	0.33–0.45	
Charlson-Deyo score			
0	Reference		<0.001
1	0.73	0.68–0.78	
Distance to care			
≤ 30 miles	Reference		0.0025
> 30 miles	1.12	1.04–1.21	

[a]Surgical volume groups were identified based on quartile rank: 75th percentile = very-high volume (>31.7cases/year); 51st–75th percentile = moderately-high volume (13.3–31.6 cases/year); 25th–50th percentile = intermediate volume (6.7–13.2 cases/year); and <25th percentile = low volume (<6.7 cases/year)

Table 3 Multivariate predictors of receipt of para-aortic lymph node sampling in UPSC, CC, and grade 3 endometrioid carcinoma

Predictors	Odds Ratio (Reference =1)	95% CI	p-value
Race			
White	Reference		0.79
Black	1.03	0.92–1.16	
Other	1.05	0.86–1.28	
Income			
< $38,000	Reference		
$38,000–$47,999	1.12	0.99–1.26	<0.001
$48,000–$62,999	1.23	1.09–1.38	
≥ $63,000	1.34	1.18–1.50	
Surgical Volume[a]			
Very high	Reference		<0.001
Moderately high	0.79	0.72–0.88	
Intermediate	0.72	0.61–0.85	
Low	0.57	0.46–0.72	
Charlson-Deyo score			
0	Reference		<0.001
1	0.69	0.63–0.76	
Distance to care			
≤ 30 miles	Reference		0.069
> 30 miles	1.09	0.99–1.19	

[a]Surgical volume groups were identified based on quartile rank: 75th percentile = very-high volume (>31.7cases/year); 51st–75th percentile = moderately-high volume (13.3–31.6 cases/year); 25th–50th percentile = intermediate volume (6.7–13.2 cases/year); and <25th percentile = low volume (<6.7 cases/year)

likely in patients receiving surgical care at moderately-high volume hospitals (OR 0.65, 95% CI 0.61 to 0.71), intermediate volume (OR 0.51, 95% CI 0.45 to 0.56), or low volume (OR 0.39, 95% CI 0.33 to 0.45). Receipt of LNS was more likely in patients who traveled >30 miles to receive their care (OR 1.12, 95% CI 1.04 to 1.21).

In our subset analysis of receipt of para-aortic LNS, there were 11,068 evaluable patients with para-aortic lymph node sampling status recorded. A total of 5,554 (50%) patients underwent para-aortic LNS. Significant predictors of receipt of para-aortic LNS were similar to our main model, including Black race not being associated with a difference in receipt of para-aortic LNS (OR 1.03, 95% CI 0.92 to 1.16) (Table 3).

Overall survival

Multivariate Cox proportional hazards analysis was performed to identify predictors of overall survival while controlling for patient age, race, income, receipt of lymph node staging, stage of disease, adjuvant chemotherapy or radiation, hospital surgical volume, and distance to care (Table 4). A total of 31,647 patients had

sufficiently matured data available for survival analysis. Compared to Stage I/II disease, Stage III disease was associated with lower overall survival (HR 3.39, 95% CI 3.28 to 3.50) (Fig. 1a). Patients who received LNS had improved overall survival (HR 0.61, 95% CI 0.59 to 0.64) (Fig. 1b). Although LNS was more common at higher volume surgical centers, surgical volume was not a statistically significant predictor of overall survival (Table 4). Black women compared to White women had a poorer overall survival (HR 1.36, 95% CI 1.29 to 1.42) (Fig. 1c). While patients who traveled >30 miles were more likely to receive LNS, distance to care was not associated with overall survival (HR 1.00, 95% CI 0.99 to 1.00, $p = 0.758$) (Fig. 1d).

In our multivariate subset analysis of para-aortic LNS, significant predictors of OS were similar to our main model, including Black race (HR 1.27, 95% CI 1.10 to 1.46). Other significant predictors included Stage III/disease (HR 3.14, 95% CI 2.80 to 3.52) and receipt of para-aortic LNS (HR 0.65, 95% CI 0.59 to 0.73). Similar to our main cohort, surgical volume and distance to care were not associated with OS.

Table 4 Multivariate predictors of overall survival in UPSC, CC, and grade 3 endometrioid carcinoma

Predictors	Hazard Ratio (Reference = 1)	95% CI	p-value
Stage			
I/II	Reference		
III	3.39	3.28–3.50	<0.001
Age			
10-year increase	1.63	1.61–1.66	<0.001
Race			
White	Reference		<0.001
Black	1.36	1.29–1.42	
Other	0.92	0.83–1.02	
Income			
< $38,000	Reference		<0.001
$38,000–$47,999	0.96	0.91–1.01	
$48,000–$62,999	0.92	0.88–0.97	
≥ $63,000	0.83	0.79–0.87	
Lymph node sampling			
No	Reference		<0.001
Yes[a]	0.61	0.59–0.64	
Surgical Volume			
Highest (4th) Quartile	Reference		0.59
Third Quartile	0.97	0.94–1.02	
Second Quartile	1.02	0.96–1.08	
Lowest (1st) Quartile	1.01	0.91–1.11	
Distance to care[b]			
10-mile increase	1.00	0.99–1.00	0.48

[a]Defined based on the number of regional lymph nodes sampled during surgery. Yes = 1+; No = 0
[b]"Great circle" distance: defined as the distance between the reporting hospital and the patient's zip code centroid. Defined here continuously. Results were similar when distance was defined as ≤30 miles versus >30 miles

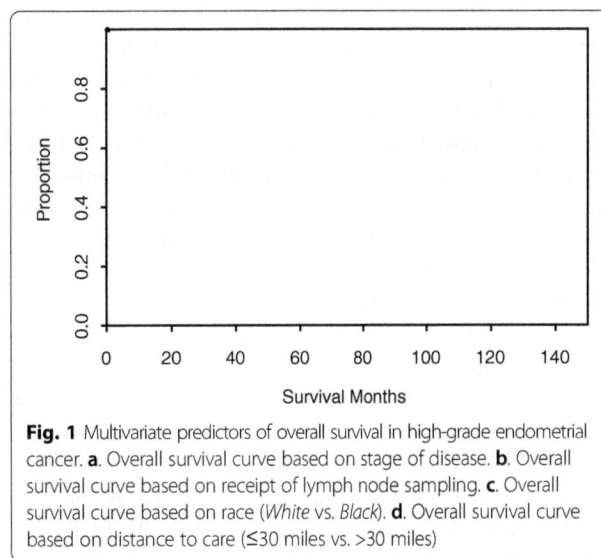

Fig. 1 Multivariate predictors of overall survival in high-grade endometrial cancer. **a.** Overall survival curve based on stage of disease. **b.** Overall survival curve based on receipt of lymph node sampling. **c.** Overall survival curve based on race (*White* vs. *Black*). **d.** Overall survival curve based on distance to care (≤30 miles vs. >30 miles)

Discussion

The management of high-grade endometrial cancer relies on the cornerstone of surgical staging. The NCCN recommends that surgical staging for high-grade endometrial cancer, including UPSC, CC, and grade 3 endometrioid adenocarcinoma, consist of pelvic and para-aortic lymphadenectomy [7]. This removal of lymph nodes also affords the opportunity to appropriately tailor adjuvant therapy. In this cohort of high-grade endometrial cancer patients, our data, after controlling for the receipt of adjuvant therapy, demonstrate that receipt of regional LNS is associated with improved survival (HR 0.61, 95% CI 0.59 to 0.64). A number of observational studies have also shown that women who undergo lymph node staging have improved clinical outcomes [17–20]. While the interpretation of such observational studies is heavily limited by selection bias,

and no randomized trials specific to a high-risk histology cohort have been performed, the removal of lymph nodes not only follows NCCN recommendations for women with UPSC, CC, and grade 3 endometrioid adenocarcinoma, but also guides the use of appropriate adjuvant therapy [7]. Therefore, the lower rates of NCCN-recommended staging of high-grade endometrial cancer at lower surgical volume centers and among lower income women is a point of concern.

Epidemiological studies have demonstrated that Black women, as compared to White women, are disproportionately affected by high-risk histologic types of endometrial cancer and are less likely to undergo surgical management [11–13, 21–24]. Our study is the first to examine factors associated with the receipt of LNS as part of surgical management, and demonstrates that receipt of LNS for high-grade endometrial cancer is similar among Blacks and Whites (81% vs 80%, respectively). While disparities in the surgical management of high-risk endometrial cancer have improved, Black women, compared to White women, have worse overall survival (Table 4) (OR 1.36, 95% CI 1.29 to 1.42).

Prior studies have also demonstrated that women with endometrial cancer are more likely to undergo lymph node dissection at high-volume hospitals compared to low-volume hospitals (66% vs 35%, p < 0.001) [25]. However, treatment at high-volume centers has not been shown to improve overall survival [25–27]. Our data support these prior findings with the highest surgical volume centers significantly associated with receipt of LNS, but not resulting in an improved survival. However, lymph node staging remains a key component of surgical staging for endometrial cancer; and allows for tailoring of adjuvant therapies. Adherence to similar treatment guidelines in ovarian cancer has been associated with proximity to care, although similar reports are not available for endometrial cancer [28]. In our analysis, women with high-grade endometrial cancer who traveled farther for their surgical care were more likely to receive LNS (OR 1.12, 95% CI 1.04 to 1.21). Interestingly, 84% of women who traveled >30 miles for care received care at the highest volume centers. Our findings suggest that patients may have traveled farther initially to seek the surgical expertise of higher volume centers, thereby explaining the higher rates of LNS observed among those who traveled farther.

Several limitations to our study are inherent in the use of large clinical and administrative databases. While the Charlson-Deyo score accounts for comorbidities, the NCDB does not record data on body mass index (BMI), which can influence surgical decision making. Additionally, there was inadequate reporting of omentectomy and peritoneal cytology to include in our analysis. Another limitation is interpretation of the number of lymph nodes examined. The NCDB reports the number of lymph nodes examined by a pathologist; however, information distinguishing between pelvic and para-aortic nodal basins is largely incomplete. As sentinel lymph node mapping is being utilized more often in endometrial cancer, the number of lymph nodes needed for adequate surgical staging is likely to decrease while lymph node status becomes even more vital to the management and prognosis of endometrial cancer. In order to broadly examine the surgical staging issue without focusing on nodal counts, we chose to examine lymph node staging as a dichotomous variable.

Conclusions

Lymph node staging for high-grade endometrial cancer, whether comprehensive lymphadenectomy or sentinel lymph node mapping, is not only recommended by the NCCN and the SGO, but can also assist in the tailoring of adjuvant therapies. While medical comorbidities (as captured here in the Charlson-Deyo score) may provide inherent difficulties to completing surgical staging, the receipt of guideline-based care should not be limited. High-volume centers are best equipped to provide guideline-based care to these high-risk women.

Abbreviations
ACS: American College of surgeons; AJCC: American joint committee on cancer; BMI: Body mass index; CC: Clear cell; CoC: Commission on cancer; FIGO: International federation of gynecology and obstetrics; LNS: Lymph node sampling; NCCN: National comprehensive cancer network; NCDB: National cancer data base; OS: Overall survival; SGO: Society of gynecologic oncology; UPSC: Uterine papillary serous carcinoma

Acknowledgments
Not applicable.

Funding
No funding.

Authors' contributions
All authors contributed to the planning (conceptualization and methodology) of this research. JF, LH, and GB conducted the main investigation, while GB provided formal analysis of the data. All authors contributed to the writing and revision of this manuscript. While all authors have agreed to be accountable for this research, JF and LH are both guarantors of the overall content of this research. All authors read and approved the final manuscript.

Competing interests
The authors declare that they have no competing interests.

Required statement by the national cancer data base
The National Cancer Data Base (NCDB) is a joint project of the Commission on Cancer of the American College of Surgeons and the American Cancer Society. The data used in the study are derived from a de-identified NCDB file. The American College of Surgeons and the Commission on Cancer have not verified and are not responsible for the analytic or statistical methodology employed, or the conclusions drawn from these data by the investigator.

Author details
[1]Division of Gynecologic Oncology, Duke University Medical Center, 2301 Erwin Rd, Durham, NC 27710, USA. [2]Biostatistics, Duke Cancer Institute, Duke University, 2301 Erwin Rd, Durham, NC 27710, USA. [3]Department of Surgery, Duke University Medical Center, 2301 Erwin Rd, Durham, NC 27710, USA. [4]Duke Clinical Research Institute, Durham, USA. [5]Division of Radiation Oncology, Duke University Medical Center, 2301 Erwin Rd, Durham, NC 27710, USA.

References
1. Siegel RL, Miller KD, Jemal A. Cancer Statistics, 2016. CA Cancer J Clin. 2016;66:7–30.
2. Alektiar KM, McKee A, Lin O, et al. Is there a difference in outcome between stage I–II endometrial cancer of papillary serous/clear cell and endometrioid FIGO Grade 3 cancer? Int J Radiation Oncology Biol Phys. 2002;54:79–85.
3. Goff BA, Kato D, Schmidt RA, et al. Uterine papillary serous carcinoma: Patterns of metastatic spread. Gynecol Oncol. 1994;54:264–8.
4. Abeler VM, Vergote IB, Kjorstad KE, Trope CG. Clear cell carcinoma of the endometrium: Prognosis and metastatic pattern. Cancer. 1996;78:1740–7.
5. Cirisano FD, Robboy SJ, Dodge RK, et al. The outcome of stage I–II clinically and surgically staged papillary serous and clear cell endometrial cancers when compared with endometrioid carcinoma. Gynecol Oncol. 2000;77:55–65.
6. Hamilton CA, Cheung MK, Osann K, et al. Uterine papillary serous and clear cell carcinomas predict for poorer survival compared to grade 3 endometrioid corpus cancers. BJOC. 2006;94:642–6.
7. National Comprehensive Cancer Network. Uterine Neoplasms (Version 2. 2015). http://www.nccn.org/professionals/physician_gls/pdf/uterine.pdf. Accessed 6 Sept 2015
8. Boruta DM, Gehrig PA, Fader AN, Olawaiye AB. Management of women with uterine papillary serous cancer: A Society of Gynecologic Oncology (SGO) review. Gynecol Oncol. 2009;115:142–53.
9. Olawaiye AB, Boruta DM. Management of women with clear cell endometrial cancer: A Society of Gynecologic Oncology (SGO) review. Gynecol Oncol. 2009;113:277–83.
10. Madison T, Schottenfield D, James SA, Schwartz AG, Gruber SB. Endometrial cancer: Socioeconomic status and racial/ethnic differences in stage at diagnosis, treatment, and survival. Am J Public Health. 2004;94:2104–11.
11. Hicks ML, Phillips JL, Parham G, et al. The National Cancer Data Base report on endometrial carcinoma in African-American women. Cancer. 1998;83:2629–37.
12. Randall TC, Armstrong K. Differences in treatment and outcome between African-American and White women with endometrial cancer. J Clin Oncol. 2003;21:4200–6.
13. Rauh-Hain JA, Buskwofie A, Clemmer J, Boruta DM, Schorge JO, Del Carmen

MG. Racial disparities in treatment of high-grade endometrial cancer in the Medicare population. Obstet Gynecol. 2015;125:843–51.

14. Benjamin I, Dalton H, Qiu Y, Cayco L, Johnson WG, Balducci J. Endometrial cancer surgery in Arizona: A statewide analysis of access to care. Gynecol Oncol. 2011;121:83–6.

15. Mohanty S, Bilimoria KY. Comparing national cancer registries: The National Cancer Data Base (NCDB) and the Surveillance, Epidemiology, and End Results (SEER) program. J Surg Oncol. 2014;109:629–30.

16. Bristow RE, Palis BE, Chi DS, Cliby WA. The National Cancer Database report on advanced-stage epithelial ovarian cancer: Impact of hospital surgical case volume on overall survival and surgical treatment paradigm. Gynecol Oncol. 2010;118:262–7.

17. Mariani A, Webb MJ, Galli L, Podratz KC. Potential therapeutic role of para-aortic lymphadenectomy in node-positive endometrial cancer. Gynecol Oncol. 2000;76:348–56.

18. Kilgore LC, Partridge EE, Alvarez RD, et al. Adenocarcinoma of the endometrium: Survival comparisons of patients with and without pelvic node sampling. Gynecol Oncol. 1995;56:29–33.

19. Havrilesky LJ, Cragun JM, Calingaert B, et al. Resection of lymph node metastases influences survival in Stage IIIC endometrial cancer. Gynecol Oncol. 2005;99:689–95.

20. Todo Y, Kato H, Kaneuchi M, Watari H, Tokeda M, Sakuragi N. Survival effect of para-aortic lymphadenectomy in endometrial cancer (SEPAL) study: a retrospective cohort analysis. Lancet. 2010;375:1165–72.

21. Long B, Liu FW, Bristow RE. Disparities in uterine cancer epidemiology, treatment, and survival among African Americans in the United States. Gynecol Oncol. 2013;130:652–9.

22. Matthews RP, Hutchinson-Colas J, Maiman N, et al. Papillary serous and clear cell type lead to poor prognosis of endometrial carcinoma in Black women. Gynecol Oncol. 1997;65:206–12.

23. Barrett 2nd RJ, Harlan LC, Wesley MN, et al. Endometrial cancer: stage at diagnosis and associated factors in Black and White patients. Am J Obstet Gynecol. 1995;173:414–23.

24. Connell PP, Rotmensch J, Waggoner SE, Mundt AJ. Race and clinical outcome in endometrial carcinoma. Obstet Gynecol. 1999;94:713–20.

25. Wright JD, Hershman DL, Burke WM, et al. Influence of surgical volume on outcome for laparoscopic hysterectomy for endometrial cancer. Ann Surg Oncol. 2012;19:948–58.

26. Becker JH, Ezendam NPM, Boll D, van der Aa M, Pigenborg JMA. Effects of surgical volumes on the survival of endometrial cancer. Gynecol Oncol. 2015;139:306–11.

27. Wright JD, Lewin SN, Deutsch I, Burke WM, Sun X, Herzog TJ. Effect of surgical volume on morbidity and mortality of abdominal hysterectomy for endometrial cancer. Obstet Gynecol. 2011;117:1051–9.

28. Bristow RE, Chang J, Ziogas A, Anton-Culver H, Vieira VM. Spatial analysis of adherence to treatment guidelines for advanced-stage ovarian cancer and the impact of race and socioeconomic status. Gynecol Oncol. 2014;134:60–7.

8

New treatment option for ovarian cancer: PARP inhibitors

Robert S. Meehan and Alice P. Chen[*]

Abstract

Poly(ADP-ribose) polymerase (PARP), which was first described over 50 years ago by Mandel, are a family of protein enzymes involved in DNA damage response and works by recognizing the single-strand DNA break (ssDNA) and then effecting DNA repair. A double-strand DNA (dsDNA) break can be repaired by one of two different pathways: homologous recombination (HR) or non-homologous end joining (NHEJ). Homologous recombination occurs in the G2 or M phase of the cell cycle when a sister chromatid is available to use as a template for repair. Because a template is available, HR is a high fidelity, error-free form of DNA repair. With NHEJ there is not a template and the DNA is trimmed and ligated which is a very error-prone process of repair which can lead to genetic instability. Exploiting these mechanism led to development of PARP inhibitors with the idea of utilizing synthetic lethality, where two deficiencies each having no effect on the cellular outcome become lethal when combined, as single agent in BRCA deficient patients or as chemotherapy/radiotherapy combinations to inhibit ssDNA repair. The recent approval of olaparib in BRCA deficient ovarian cancer patients in US and Europe has opened up a whole new treatment option for ovarian cancer patients. This review will discuss the different PARP inhibitors in development and the potential use of this class of agents in the future.

Keywords: PARP inhibitor, Synthetic lethality, BRCA, Homologous recombinant pathway, Base excisional repair pathway

Background

Ovarian cancer is the leading cause of death from gynecological malignancies in the United States with an incidence rate of approximately 22,000 and 14,000 deaths per year. Despite all of the headway made in cancer overall, with a risk of dying from cancer decreasing by 20 % since 1991, the relative 5-years survival rates of ovarian cancer has remained poor 36 % in 1970's and still only 44 % in 2000's and much worse in late stage disease [1].

Cellular replication is a complex process which is the way living organisms are able to grow and propagate. Replication is a very controlled process with many points of error detection and redundancy to ensure that a high fidelity functioning copy of genetic material is maintained. Essential to this process is the unwinding of the DNA from histone complexes and followed by the active replication processes during S-phase, during this time period DNA is very susceptible to environmental damage or even errors in the replicative process itself [2]. There are a host of detection and repair mechanisms in place which try to minimize errors, which lead to mutations. The BRCA genes are a family of tumor suppressor genes responsible for helping to protect the genome, and the most widely known and studied with current clinical importance are BRCA1 and BRCA2 [3]. BRCA1 is located on chromosome 17 and has many cellular functions such as DNA repair, transcriptional regulation and chromatin remodeling and BRCA2 is located on chromosome 13 and is responsible for DNA recombination and repair primarily by chaperoning RAD51, the enzyme responsible for facilitating recombination [4]. These two genes were described in 1994 and 1995 and the repair pathways which they work have become clinical targets for molecular therapies [5, 6]. Deficiencies in these genes have been historically associated with hereditary breast and ovarian cancer but they also increase risk for uterine, cervical, colon, male breast, prostate, pancreatic cancers, and melanoma [7].

* Correspondence: chenali@mail.nih.gov
Early Clinical Trials Development Program Division of Cancer Treatment and Diagnosis (DCTD), National Institutes of Health (NIH) National Cancer Institute (NCI), 10 Center Drive, Bldg 31, 3A44, Bethesda MD 20892, USA

Poly(ADP-ribose) polymerase (PARP), which was first described over 50 years ago by Mandel [8], works by recognizing the single-strand DNA break (ssDNA) and then effecting DNA repair [9] through the base excisional pathway (BER). The proteins consist of two ribose moieties and two phosphates (Fig. 1), and DNA strand breaks are responsible for activating the protein [10].

The PARP catalytic domain binds NAD+ via a unique protein fold, PARP-1 has a combination of zinc fingers and PARP-2 and PARP-3 have different N-terminal domains with very specific regulatory functions in mitotic segregation as well as basal metabolism [11, 12]. PARP is also involved in methylation and transcription of genes coding for cell cycle and stress response, including *p53*. PARP

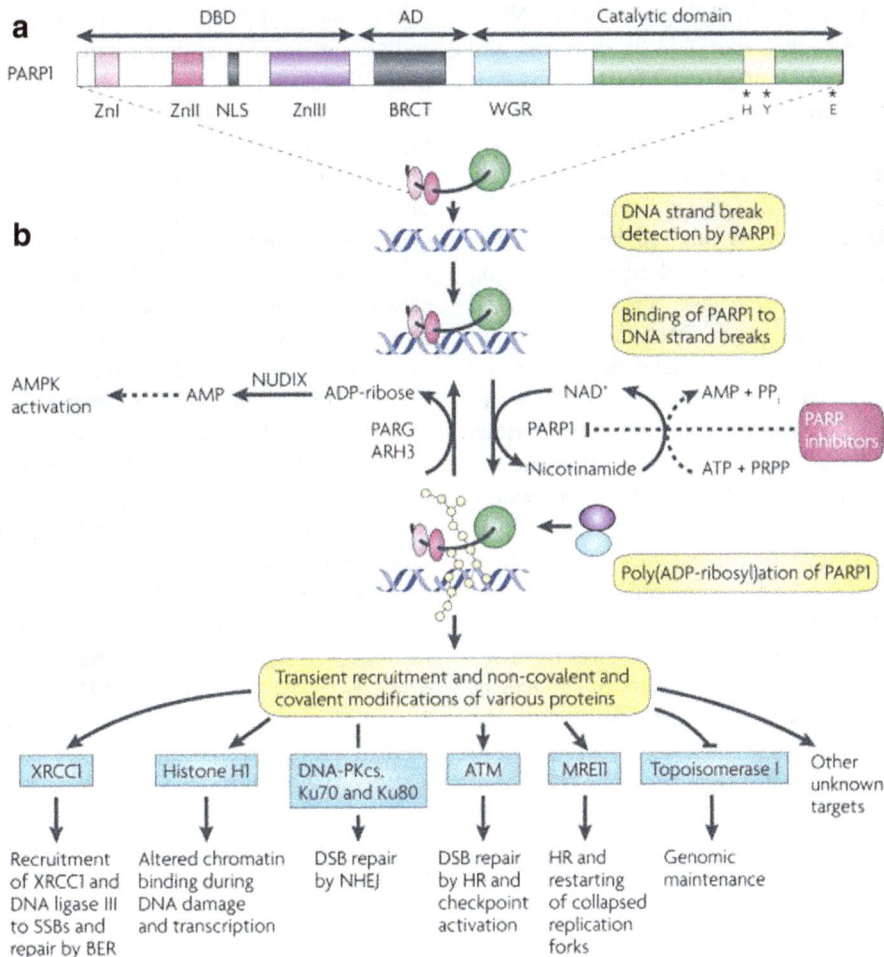

Fig. 1 Mechanism of PARP. **a** Poly(ADP-ribose) polymerase 1 (PARP1) is shown with its DNA-binding (DBD), automodification (AD) and catalytic domains. The PARP signature sequence (*yellow box* within the catalytic domain) comprises the sequence most conserved among PARPs. Crucial residues for nicotinamide adenine dinucleotide (NAD$^+$) binding (histidine; H and tyrosine; Y) and for polymerase activity (glutamic acid; E) are indicated. **b** | Consequences of PARP1 activation by DNA damage. Although not shown to simplify the scheme, PARP1 is active in a homodimeric form. PARP1 detects DNA damage through its DBD. This activates PARP1 to synthesize poly(ADP) ribose (pADPr; *yellow beads*) on acceptor proteins, including histones and PARP1. Owing to the dense negative charge of pADPr, PARP1 loses affinity for DNA, allowing the recruitment of repair proteins by pADPr to the damaged DNA (*blue* and *purple circles*). Poly(ADP-ribose) glycohydrolase (PARG) and possibly ADP-ribose hydrolase 3 (ARH3) hydrolyse pADPr into ADP-ribose molecules and free pADPr. ADP-ribose is further metabolized by the pyrophosphohydrolase NUDIX enzymes into AMP, raising AMP:ATP ratios, which in turn activate the metabolic sensor AMP-activated protein kinase (AMPK). NAD$^+$ is replenished by the enzymatic conversion of nicotinamide into NAD$^+$ at the expense of phosphoribosylpyrophosphate (PRPP) and ATP. Examples of proteins non-covalently (pADPr-binding proteins) or covalently poly(ADP-ribosyl)ated are shown with the functional consequences of modification. It is important to note that many potential protein acceptors of pADPr remain to be identified owing to the difficulty of purifying pADPr-binding proteins in vivo. PARP inhibitors prevent the synthesis of pADPr and hinder subsequent downstream repair processes, lengthening the lifetime of DNA lesions. ATM, ataxia telangiectasia-mutated; BER, base excision repair; BRCT, BRCA1 carboxy-terminal repeat motif; DNA-PKcs, DNA-protein kinase catalytic subunit; DSB, double-strand break; HR, homologous recombination; NHEJ, non-homologous end joining; NLS, nuclear localization signal; PP$_i$, inorganic pyrophosphate; SSB, single-strand break; Zn, zinc finger. Reprinted by permission from Macmillan Publishers Ltd: Nat Rev Cancer, 2010,10(4):293–301, copyright (2010) [10]

attaches DNA polymerase β to the DNA break site to re-place the missing bases [10].

A double-strand DNA (dsDNA) break can be repaired by one of two different pathways: homologous recombination (HR) or non-homologous end joining (NHEJ). Homologous recombination occurs in the G2 or M phase of the cell cycle when a sister chromatid is available to use as a template for repair [13]. Because a template is available, HR is a high fidelity, error-free form of DNA repair. With NHEJ there is not a template and the DNA is trimmed and ligated which is a very error-prone process of repair which can lead to genetic instability [14]. In patients that have BRCA deficient HR pathway the BER rescues the cell and leads to a viable cell [15]. When PARP is inhibited in a HR deficient cell, e.g. BRCA mutation, the ssDNA break is not repaired by either the BER or HR pathway. [16]. Solid tumors carrying various DNA repair defects have shown increased sensitivity to PARP inhibitors or DNA-damaging chemotherapies [17]. PARP inhibitors have shown activity as monotherapy in cells deficient for the repair of dsDNA breaks by HR as in case of BRCA deleterious mutation cells showcasing the principle of synthetic lethality. The concept of synthetic lethality is where two deficiencies each having no effect on the cellular outcome become lethal when combined. Cells which are BRCA deficient and then undergo PARP inhibition, leads to cell death [4].

PARP trapping is another recently described mechanism by which PARP inhibitors are able to kill cancer cells. PARP inhibitors trapped PARP1 and PARP2 to the sites of DNA damage and then the PARP enzyme-inhibitor complex locks onto the damaged DNA and stops DNA repair, transcription, and replication which then leads to cellular death [18]. Trapped PARP–DNA complexes were more cytotoxic than unrepaired single strand breaks (SSBs) caused by PARP inactivation, Murai et al. suggested that PARP inhibitors act in part as poisons that irreversibly trap PARP enzyme on DNA [19]. The potency in trapping PARP differed markedly among the PARP inhibitors in clinical development in a pattern not correlated with the catalytic inhibitory properties [20]. Thirty genetically altered avian DT40 cell lines with pre-established deletions in specific DNA repair genes were analyzed to reveal that, in addition to homologous recombination, post replication repair, the Fanconi anemia pathway, polymerase β, and FEN1 are critical for repairing trapped PARP–DNA complexes [18, 19]. This suggest that other defects in the HR pathway, including PTEN defects, Fanconi's anemia protein defects, ATM abnormalities, RAD51 dysfunction, and EMSY defects, may be sensitive to single agent PARP inhibitors [20].

PARP inhibitors
Olaparib (Astra Zeneca)

The idea of synthetic lethality has led to the use of single agent PARP inhibitors in BRCA deficient cancers. Olaparib (AZD 2281) is an oral PARP inhibitor that has shown activity in ovarian and breast tumors with known BRCA mutations and was the first FDA approved drug in this class [21]. The first hint of clinical activity in BRCA mutation patients was seen in a phase I single agent trial with 50 ovarian cancer patients with BRCA mutations. Twenty patients had CR or PR by response evaluation criteria in solid tumors (RECIST) and three patients had been SD for longer than 4 months, resulting in a clinical benefit rate of 46 % (23/50). The median duration of response was 28 months. The most common drug related toxicities were fatigue and mild gastrointestinal (GI) symptoms. A post analysis showed a statistically significant difference in response among platinum sensitive, resistant, and refractory populations (61, 42, and 15 %, respectively), though no differences were noted in the duration of response or time to progression between the three platinum response groups [22]. The FDA approval of olaparib in advanced ovarian cancer associated with defective BRCA genes was partially based on an international multicenter single-arm trail with 317 patients whom 193 had measurable germline BRCA mutation ovarian cancer with a mean of 4.3 prior lines of therapy and considered platinum resistant. They were given 400 mg oral olaparib twice a day until progression or toxicity. They showed an overall response rate of rate of 31 % (95 % CI, 24.6 to 38.1), and stable disease (at 8 weeks) of 40 % (95 % CI, 33.4 to 47.7) along with a median OS of 16.6 months [23].

PARP-1/2 inhibitors have been demonstrated to be effective in preclinical models in combination with platinum, alkylating and methylation agents, topoisomerase I inhibitors and radiation therapy [16]. In a phase I/Ib trial of olaparib with carboplatin in germline BRCA mutation breast/ovarian cancer patients with an expansion cohort treated with 400 mg twice a day D 1–7 along with carboplatin AUC 5 days one every 21 days followed by maintenance of olaparib 400 mg twice a day until progression showed an ORR of 52.4 %. Responses included one complete response (one breast cancer; 23 months) and 21 partial responses (50.0 %; 15 ovarian cancer; six breast cancer; median = 16 [4 to >45] in ovarian cancer and 10 [6 to >40] months in breast cancer) [24]. Olaparib was also combined with carboplatin and paclitaxel in a study aimed to determine the safety of olaparib in one of four dosing regimens: continuously with carboplatin, continuously with paclitaxel, continuously with both carboplatin and paclitaxel or intermittently with the chemotherapy combination. Eighty seven patients were enrolled, 12 of whom had known germline

BRCA one or two mutations. AEs were primarily myelotoxicity (neutropenia and thrombocytopenia of any grade occurring in 54 and 26 %, respectively). The dosing schedules deemed tolerable were olaparib with weekly paclitaxel (100 mg BD continuously and 80 mg/m2, respectively) and intermittent olaparib with 3-weekly doses of carboplatin and paclitaxel (200 mg BD d1-10 and AUC4 with 175 mg/m2, respectively). Sixteen percent of patients had an objective response and 28 % had stable disease that persisted for at least 4 months. Greater efficacy was evident in patients with *BRCA* mutations (two complete and four partial responses) [25]. Oza conducted a randomized phase II study, comparing six cycles of carboplatin and paclitaxel with olaparib (olaparib 200 mg/m2 BID d1-10 & carboplatin AUC 4 D1 & paclitaxel 175 mg/m2 D1, over a 21 day cycle) followed by maintenance olaparib (400 mg BID) until progression to six cycles of carboplatin and paclitaxel alone (AUC 6 and 175 mg/m2 respectively both D1, over a 21 days cycle), in patients with advanced serous ovarian cancer. The primary outcome, progression free survival, significantly favored those patients receiving olaparib in addition to chemotherapy (HR = 0.51, 95 % $P = 0.0012$) increasing median survival from 9.6 to 12.2 months [26].

Olaparib with cisplatin and gemcitabine was evaluated as a phase I trial by Rajan in advanced solid tumors. They saw high rates of myelosuppression even at early dose levels (DL1 olaparib 100 mg orally BID D1-4, gemcitabine 500 mg/m2 D3 & 10, and cisplatin 60 mg/m2 D3) which prompted dose reductions. Of the 21 patients which they evaluated two had PR. MTD was determined to be olaparib 100 mg orally once daily on D1, gemcitabine 500 mg/m2 on D1 & 8, and cisplatin 60 mg/m2 on D1. They were also able to demonstrate the olaparib inhibited PARP in PBMC and tumor tissue although they said that PARP levels were less efficiently inhibited when it was used for a short duration based on their observations that maximum inhibition of PAR was seen between 6 and 24 h after the first dose of administration and that PAR levels had started approaching baseline values within 36 h of the last dose of olaparib and exceeded baseline values in 80 % of cases before the next cycle of treatment [27]. There are a number of ongoing Phase I and II trials which various combinations currently underway and should have some promising results based on early phase trials.

After a number of early trials help to solidify the mechanism of action, the idea of maintenance therapy was explored. A randomized, double-blind, placebo-controlled study evaluated maintenance treatment with olaparib in patients with platinum-sensitive, relapsed, high-grade serous ovarian cancer who had received two or more platinum-based regimens and had had a partial or complete response to their most recent platinum-

based regimen. Two hundred sixty-five patients were randomized 1:1 to 400 mg bid of olaparib vs placebo. Their primary end point was progression-free survival. Progression-free survival was significantly longer with olaparib than with placebo (median, 8.4 months vs. 4.8 months from randomization at time of completion of chemotherapy; hazard ratio for progression or death, 0.35; 95 % confidence interval [CI], 0.25 to 0.49; $P < 0.001$) Subgroup analyses of progression-free survival showed that, regardless of subgroup, patients in the olaparib group had a lower risk of progression. The first interim analysis of overall survival (38 % maturity) showed no significant difference between groups (hazard ratio with olaparib, 0.94; 95 % CI, 0.63 to 1.39; $P = 0.75$) [28]. At the second interim analysis, subgroup analysis was included. *BRCA* status was known for 131 (96 %) patients in the olaparib group versus 123 (95 %) in the placebo group, of whom 74 (56 %) versus 62 (50 %) had a deleterious or suspected deleterious germline or tumor *BRCA* mutation. Of patients with a *BRCA* mutation, median PFS was significantly longer in the olaparib group than in the placebo group (11.2 months [95 % CI 8.3-not calculable] vs 4.3 months [3.0–5.4]; HR 0.18 [0.10–0.31]; $p < 0.0001$); similar findings were noted for patients with wild-type *BRCA*, although the difference between treated and placebo groups was lower (7.4 months [5.5–10.3] vs 5.5 months [3.7–5.6]; HR 0.54 [0.34–0.85]; $p = 0.0075$). OS did not significantly differ between the groups (HR 0.88 [95 % CI 0.64–1.21]; $p = 0.44$); similar findings were noted for patients with mutated *BRCA* (HR 0.73 [0.45–1.17]; $p = 0.19$) and wild-type *BRCA* (HR 0.99 [0.63–1.55]; $p = 0.96$). The investigators concluded that these results support the hypothesis that patients with platinum-sensitive recurrent serous ovarian cancer with a *BRCA* mutation have the greatest likelihood of benefiting from olaparib maintenance therapy [29]. Moore presented two AstraZeneca-sponsored Phase III trials of olaparib maintenance monotherapy in ovarian cancer patients with a *BRCA* mutation: SOLO1 & SOLO2 at the 2014 ASCO meeting. Both are double-blind multicenter studies in which pts are being randomized (2:1) to receive olaparib (300 mg [2 × 150 mg tablets] bid) or placebo SOLO1 is for newly diagnosed patients and SOLO2 is for pretreated patients who have failed therapy. They have a planned analysis at ≈ 60 % maturity which is not available at time of writing.

Angiogenesis inhibitors have been shown to be active in recurrent ovarian cancer [30], and in vivo have been tested with PARP inhibitors. In PARP-1 knockout mice [31] the combination showed additive effects. Olaparib was looked at with cediranib in a phase I trial and appeared to improve PFS in women with recurrent platinum-sensitive high-grade serous or endometrioid ovarian cancer with hematologic DLT's [32]. Sui looked at the combination of erlotinib and olaparib in EGFR-overexpressing ovarian tumor xenografts. They were able to show that erlotinib could slightly inhibit growth of A2780 tumor xenografts but the combination treatment had a markedly enhanced antitumor effect over either agent alone. They showed that the antitumor activity in BRCA-mutated xenograft models was 41 % compared with 24 % in BRCA wild-type. Western blot analysis revealed that treatment with erlotinib could significantly reduce the phosphorylation level of ERK1/2 and AKT in A2780 tumor tissue. It was shown that the autophagic effects were substantially enhanced when the agents were combined, which they postulated may be due to downregulation of apoptosis by decreasing p–p53 levels. Further investigations are underway to better understand these processes [33].

Veliparib (abbvie)

Veliparib (ABT 888), in preclinical studies, was demonstrated to be a strong inhibitor of PARP 1 and 2 and was found to potentiate the effects of temozolomide, platinum agents, cyclophosphamide, and radiation in syngeneic and xenograft tumor models. It was reported to have good bioavailability and able to cross the blood–brain barrier [34]. Based on these broad spectrums of chemopotentiation and radiopotentiation further clinical evaluation was undertaken.

Veliparib was combined with oral cyclophosphamide in a phase II trial where adult patients with pretreated *BRCA*-mutant ovarian cancer or primary peritoneal, fallopian tube, or high-grade serous ovarian cancers (HGSOC). The patients were randomized to receive cyclophosphamide alone (50 mg orally once daily) or with veliparib (60 mg orally once daily) in 21-day cycles, crossover was allowed at disease progression. There were 75 patients enrolled with 72 evaluable, 38 cyclophosphamide alone and 37 on the combination arm. Of the 70 patients with responses one in each arm had a CR. PR was seen in six patients in the cyclophosphamide-only arm [7/36 (19.4 %) responses overall; 95 % confidence interval (CI), 8.2–36.0 %] and three patients in the combination arm [4/34 (11.8 %) responses overall; 95 % CI, 3.3–27.5 %], and one patient who crossed over to the combination arm after progressing on the cyclophosphamide-only arm. Overall the addition of veliparib to cyclophosphamide did not improve the response rate or the PFS over cyclophosphamide alone [35].

A phase II trial of veliparib was reported by Coleman et al., looking at the clinical activity with use as a single agent in ovarian cancer patients with a gBRCA1 or gBRCA2 mutation. The eligibility criteria included patients with three or fewer lines of therapy none of which would have been a PARPi. Veliparib was given at

400 mg orally twice a day for 28 day cycles. They reported response of 26 % (90 % CI: 16–38 %, CR: 2, PR: 11); for platinum-resistant and platinum-sensitive patients the proportion responding was 20 and 35 %, respectively. Overall 62 % were taken off study for progression, 29 patients were alive at the end of study; two with SD remained on veliparib and the median PFS reported was 8.18 months [36].

Recently Veliparib has also been evaluated with whole brain XRT for brain metastasis [37], combination with temozolomide in metastatic melanoma [38], small cell lung cancer with cisplatin and etoposide [39], as well as whole abdominal radiation for peritoneal carcinomatosis [40] all with promising results.

Rucaparib (Clovis)

Rucaparib (AG014699) was initially studied as a first in class intravenous PARP inhibitor on an escalating dose design with temozolomide. There were 33 patients enrolled with PARP inhibition seen in PBMC at all doses through PK/PD studies with 74–97 % inhibition. The combination was well tolerated and there were encouraging responses in patients including one complete response and one partial response in melanoma, a partial response in a desmoid tumor, seven patients with prolonged disease stabilization (~6 months) [41]. The ongoing ARIEL 2/3 trails were presented at ASCO 2014 and consisted of two parts: ARIEL2 (NCT01891344), which is a Phase 2 trial of rucaparib trying to identify a molecular HRD signature which would predict response and Phase 3 ARIEL3 (NCT01968213), would then apply this signature prospectively to the analysis of a similar population. In ARIEL2, eligible patients (*n* = 180) who have relapsed, platinum-sensitive HGOC and measurable disease will have a pre-dose biopsy and provide archival tumor tissue. The design is then develop an initial HRD algorithm by using in vitro/in vivo and TCGA (and similar) bioinformatics data from Foundation Medicine's NGS platform and Univ. of Washington's BROCA-HR panel. The algorithm will be designed to correlate with tumor HRR status and PFS and response (RECIST v1.1, GCIG CA-125). Then prospectively in ARIEL3 (*n* = 540), optimized algorithm will then be tested an ongoing, randomized (2:1), placebo-controlled maintenance trial in platinum-sensitive HGSOC in remission after platinum-based therapy. The primary endpoint of ARIEL3 is PFS in HRD subgroups determined by NGS analysis of archival tumor tissue using the ARIEL2 optimized algorithm[42], these studies at time of manuscript writing are currently ongoing

Niraparib (tesaro)

Niraparib (MK4827) is another oral inhibitor of PARP1 and PARP2. It was tested in phase I trial as a single agent in advanced solid tumors, ovarian tumors, and prostate tumors, and as combination therapy with carboplatin, with or without paclitaxel, and carboplatin with liposomal doxorubicin in patients with advanced solid tumors [43]. In a phase I trial of single agent niraparib enriched with patients having *BRCA*1 or *BRCA*2 mutations, six patients, including five with *BRCA* mutation, achieved PR [44]. Niraparib has also been shown to be an effective radiosensatizer especially in lung and breast cancer cells [44, 45]. Additionally Tesaro is currently sponsoring the Phase 2 QUADRA trial for patients with heavily pretreated disease [46] as well as the NOVA trial looking at maintenance in platinum sensitive disease [47].

Talazoparib

Talazoparib (BMN 673) was designed as a potent novel inhibitor of PARP1 and PARP 2. Preclinical studies revealed selective antitumor cytotoxicity and causes expression of DNA repair biomarkers at much lower concentrations than that of earlier generations of PARP1/2 inhibitors [48]. Shen report that in vitro selectively targeted tumor cells with *BRCA*1, *BRCA*2, or PTEN gene defects with 20–to more than 200–fold greater potency than existing PARP1/2 inhibitors. BMN 673 is readily orally bioavailable and in vivo xenografted tumors that carry defects in *BRCA* or PTEN were profoundly sensitive to oral BMN 673 treatment. Synergistic or additive antitumor effects were also found when BMN 673 was combined with temozolomide, SN38, or platinum drugs in xenograft models. When evaluated in chicken DT40 cell lines, PALB2 mutation predicts exceptional in vivo response to BMN 673 [49]. Further studies showed that the nanomolar cytotoxicity is greater than that of rucaparib or olaparib and were believed to be related to the trapping of PARP-DNA complexes based on knockout mice models. All three drugs appeared to be equally effective at inhibiting PARP catalytic activity [50]. There are ongoing phase II trials in ovarian and phase III in breast cancer (EMBRACA) [51].

Radiotherapy

PARP inhibitors enhance the effects of ionizing radiation by means of inhibiting base excision repair and non-homologous end joining as well as altered regulation of cellular metabolism. [52] Both pre-clinical and clinical data has shown an improvement in tumor response to irradiation in the presence of PARP inhibitors. It had been unclear if this benefit was due to changes in the repair process or vasoactive effects contributing to tumor re-oxygenation. The two questions that were asked was if in S-phase the PARP inhibition increased the radiosensitivity of tumors and if at the tissue level it would affect the microvasculature [53]. Hirai, et al., looked at combination treatment with PARP inhibitors and single

fraction gamma-irradiation and showed that treatment with a PARP inhibitor enhanced the cytotoxic effect of gamma-irradiation. PARP inhibitor treatment induced S phase arrest and enhanced subsequent G2/M arrest after irradiation. These results suggest that the induction of S phase arrest through an enhanced DNA Damage Response (DDR) and a local delay in dsDNA break processing by PARP inhibition caused sensitization to irradiation [54].

Mechanisms of resistance

Multiple mechanisms of resistance to PARP inhibitors therapy have been identified. Intrinsic resistance to olaparib was show by increased up regulation of P-glycoprotein pumps in metaplastic breast carcinoma. This is a common pharmacological effect that reduces the efficacy of a number of drugs including PARP inhibitors by effluxing the drugs out of the cell and thus reducing the intracellular concentration of the drug available for the therapy [55]. Because PARP inhibitors can stabilize the cytotoxic PARP–DNA complexes, a loss-of-function of PARP1 can potentially lead to 100 fold resistance due to binding of PARP–DNA complexes and impaired catalytic inhibition of the PARP protein [56]. A mouse model resistant to olaparib showed up-regulation of a P-glycoprotein efflux pump caused by upregulating of ABCb1 a/b gene. The resistance can be reversed by inhibiting the pump with a P-glycoprotein inhibitor tariquidar [55]. Loss of 53BP1 leads to aberrant joining of complex chromosome rearrangements in Brca1-deficient cells by a process dependent on the non-homologous end-joining factors 53BP1 and DNA ligase 4. Loss of 53BP1 alleviates hypersensitivity of *BRCA*1 mutant cells to PARP inhibition and restores error-free repair by homologous recombination. 53BP1 deletion promotes ATM-dependent processing of broken DNA ends to produce recombinant single-stranded DNA competent for homologous recombination [57]. Another resistance mechanism to PARP inhibitor therapy that has been noted is via restoration of the homologous repair pathway in BRCA targeted tumors. BRCA2 mutant patients have shown resistance to PARP inhibitors by way of a secondary mutation in the BRCA2 gene that restores the open reading frame (ORF) which results in translation of a functional BRCA2 protein [58]. PARP inhibitor-resistant cells that up-regulation of NF-kappaB signaling is was suggested as a key mechanism underlying acquired resistance to PARP inhibition, and that NF-kappaB inhibition, or bortezomib are potentially effective anti-cancer agents after the acquisition of resistance to PARP inhibitors [59]. These are some of the mechanistic resistances to PARP inhibitors and more are being described as this class of drug continues to be studied.

Immunotherapy

Advances in immunotherapy have been at the forefront of cancer development over the past few years with exciting developments showing significant benefits to patients. Combining DNA repair mechanisms with immune based therapy offer new frontiers in clinical advancements. Preclinical data exists for combining various PARPi with anti-CTLA-4, anti-PD1, as well as anti-PDL1 but there is little clinical data at this time. Higuchi looked at CTLA-4 blockade with PARPi ABT-888(Veliparib) in BRCA1-deficient murine ovarian cancer models and showed that combination CTLA-4/PARPi was able to provide therapeutic benefit in these experiments supporting further clinical investigations [60]. Trial NCT02571725 which is about to open will be looking at combining olaparib with tremelimumab in BRCA1/2 positive patients with recurrent ovarian cancer [61]. Trial NCT02484404 at the NCI is enrolling to look at novel anti-PDL1 (Durvalumab) in a Phase 1/2 in combination either with olaparib or cediranib initially in recurrent solid tumor but then in recurrent ovarian, with no data reported at this time [62]. At time of writing there is recent announcement of a trial about to open looking at combing niraparib and pembrolizumab in BRCA-positive breast and ovarian patients. Immune based therapies are breakthrough advancements in cancer care and combinations are appearing to offer promising results.

Future directions

The approval of olaparib in the maintenance setting in Europe and metastatic setting in the US for patients with deleterious BRCA mutations in ovarian cancer is just the tip of the iceberg for the utilization for this class of agents. There are trials in progress to address the additional populations that may have deficiencies in the HR pathway that will benefit from PARP inhibitors. Additionally, combination trials with chemotherapy, radiation and TKIs are expanding the exploration of usage. Suggested by the cediranib and olaparib combination, combining PARP inhibitors with anther agent may not require additional DNA impairment for efficacy. Trials are also underway investigating agents that impair the DNA damage repair pathway, like veliparib and dinaciclib creating synthetic lethality without additional patient selection [63]. With greater understanding of resistance mechanisms, further trials utilizing combinations or sequential therapy to overcome the resistance to achieve greater efficacy. The duration of administration especially in the maintenance setting will also need to be considered to minimize resistance development. The current ongoing immune based combinations trials may bring additional synergistic efficacy and clinical benefit. This is a new class of agent that has endless possibilities for development and PARP inhibitors will be an important tool in the fight against cancer.

Conclusions

PARP inhibitors is a new class of agents that have shown activity in ovarian cancer. Activity in non BRCA mutation related tumors are being explored both in ovarian as well as outside of ovarian cancer. New combinations with other targeted agents and immunotherapy will be areas of great interest in the next few years.

Competing interest

The authors declare that they have no competing interests.

Authors' contributions

1) have made substantial contributions to conception and design, or acquisition of data, or analysis and interpretation of data (RM, AC); 2) have been involved in drafting the manuscript or revising it critically for important intellectual content (RM, AC) 3) have given final approval of the version to be published (AC); and 4) agree to be accountable for all aspects of the work in ensuring that questions related to the accuracy or integrity of any part of the work are appropriately investigated and resolved (AC). All authors read and approved the final manuscript.

References

1. Siegel R, et al. Cancer statistics, 2014. CA Cancer J Clin. 2014;64(1):9–29.
2. Boeger H, et al. Structural basis of eukaryotic gene transcription. FEBS Lett. 2005;579(4):899–903.
3. Gilks CB, Prat J. Ovarian carcinoma pathology and genetics: recent advances. Hum Pathol. 2009;40(9):1213–23.
4. Venkitaraman AR. Functions of BRCA1 and BRCA2 in the biological response to DNA damage. J Cell Sci. 2001;114(Pt 20):3591–8.
5. Wooster R, et al. Identification of the breast-cancer susceptibility gene Brca2. Nature. 1995;378(6559):789–92.
6. Miki Y, et al. A strong candidate for the breast and ovarian-cancer susceptibility gene Brca1. Science. 1994;266(5182):66–71.
7. Mersch J, et al. Cancers associated with BRCA1 and BRCA2 mutations other than breast and ovarian. Cancer. 2015;121(2):269–75.
8. Chambon P, Weill JD, Mandel P. Nicotinamide mononucleotide activation of new DNA-dependent polyadenylic acid synthesizing nuclear enzyme. Biochem Biophys Res Commun. 1963;11:39–43.
9. D'Amours D, et al. Poly(ADP-ribosyl)ation reactions in the regulation of nuclear functions. Biochem J. 1999;342(Pt 2):249–68.
10. Rouleau M, et al. PARP inhibition: PARP1 and beyond. Nat Rev Cancer. 2010;10(4):293–301.
11. Kim MY, Zhang T, Kraus WL. Poly(ADP-ribosyl)ation by PARP-1: 'PAR-laying' NAD(+) into a nuclear signal. Genes Dev. 2005;19(17):1951–67.
12. Schreiber V, et al. The human poly(ADP-ribose) polymerase nuclear localization signal is a bipartite element functionally separate from DNA binding and catalytic activity. EMBO J. 1992;11(9):3263–9.
13. Valerie K, Povirk LF. Regulation and mechanisms of mammalian double-strand break repair. Oncogene. 2003;22(37):5792–812.
14. Stecklein SR, et al. BRCA1 and HSP90 cooperate in homologous and non-homologous DNA double-strand-break repair and G2/M checkpoint activation. Proc Natl Acad Sci U S A. 2012;109(34):13650–5.
15. Ghosal G, Chen J. DNA damage tolerance: a double-edged sword guarding the genome. Transl Cancer Res. 2013;2(3):107–29.
16. Zaremba T, Curtin NJ. PARP inhibitor development for systemic cancer targeting. Anticancer Agents Med Chem. 2007;7(5):515–23.
17. Diavova II, Dianov GL. Poly(ADP-ribose) polymerase in base excision repair: always engaged, but not essential for DNA damage processing. Acta Biochim Pol, 2003. 50 (1): p. 169–79.
18. Pommier Y. Drugging topoisomerases: lessons and challenges. ACS Chem Biol. 2013;8(1):82–95.

19. Murai J, et al. Trapping of PARP1 and PARP2 by clinical PARP inhibitors. Cancer Res. 2012;72(21):5588–99.

20. Hopkins TA, et al. Mechanistic dissection of PARP1 trapping and the impact on in vivo tolerability and efficacy of PARP inhibitors. Mol Cancer Res. 2015; 13:1465–77.

21. Kim G, et al. FDA approval summary: olaparib Monotherapy in patients with deleterious germline BRCA-mutated advanced ovarian cancer treated with three or more lines of chemotherapy. Clin Cancer Res. 2015;21(19):4257–61.

22. Fong PC, et al. Poly(ADP)-ribose polymerase inhibition: frequent durable responses in BRCA carrier ovarian cancer correlating with platinum-free interval. J Clin Oncol. 2010;28(15):2512–9.

23. Kaufman B, et al. Olaparib Monotherapy in patients with advanced cancer and a germline BRCA1/2 mutation. J Clin Oncol. 2015;33(3):244–50.

24. Lee JM, et al. Phase I/Ib study of olaparib and carboplatin in BRCA1 or BRCA2 mutation-associated breast or ovarian cancer with biomarker analyses. J Natl Cancer Inst. 2014;106(6):dju089.

25. Oza AM, et al. Iaparib plus paclitaxel plus carboplatin (P/C) followed by olaparib maintenance treatment in patients (pts) with platinum-sensitive recurrent serous ovarian cancer (PSR SOC): A randomized, open-label phase II study. Journal of Clinical Oncology. 2012;30(15):Suppl 5001.

26. Oza AM, et al. Olaparib combined with chemotherapy for recurrent platinum-sensitive ovarian cancer: a randomised phase 2 trial. Lancet Oncol. 2015;16(1):87–97.

27. Rajan A, et al. A phase I combination study of olaparib with cisplatin and gemcitabine in adults with solid tumors. Clin Cancer Res. 2012;18(8):2344–51.

28. Ledermann J, et al. Olaparib maintenance therapy in platinum-sensitive relapsed ovarian cancer. N Engl J Med. 2012;366(15):1382–92.

29. Ledermann J, et al. Olaparib maintenance therapy in patients with platinum-sensitive relapsed serous ovarian cancer: a preplanned retrospective analysis of outcomes by BRCA status in a randomised phase 2 trial. Lancet Oncol. 2014;15(8):852–61.

30. Burger RA, et al. Phase II trial of Bevacizumab in persistent or recurrent epithelial ovarian cancer or primary peritoneal cancer: a gynecologic oncology group study. J Clin Oncol. 2007;25(33):5165–71.

31. Tentori L, et al. Poly(ADP-ribose) polymerase (PARP) inhibition or PARP-1 gene deletion reduces angiogenesis. Eur J Cancer. 2007;43(14):2124–33.

32. Liu JF, et al. Combination cediranib and olaparib versus olaparib alone for women with recurrent platinum-sensitive ovarian cancer: a randomised phase 2 study. Lancet Oncol. 2014;15(11):1207–14.

33. Sui H, et al. Combination of Erlotinib and a PARP inhibitor inhibits growth of A2780 tumor xenografts due to increased autophagy. Drug Des Devel Ther. 2015;9:3183–90.

34. Donawho CK, et al. ABT-888, an orallyactive poly(ADP-ribose) polymerase inhibitor that potentiates DNA-damaging agents in preclinical tumor models. Clin Cancer Res. 2007;13(9):2728–37.

35. Kummar S, et al. Randomized trial of oral cyclophosphamide and veliparib in high-grade serous ovarian, primary peritoneal, or fallopian tube cancers, or BRCA-mutant ovarian cancer. Clin Cancer Res. 2015;21(7):1574–82.

36. Coleman RL, et al. A phase II evaluation of the potent, highly selective PARP inhibitor veliparib in the treatment of persistent or recurrent epithelial ovarian, fallopian tube, or primary peritoneal cancer in patients who carry a germline BRCA1 or BRCA2 mutation—an NRG oncology/gynecologic oncology group study. Gynecol Oncol. 2015;137(3):386–91.

37. Mehta MP, et al. Veliparib in combination with whole brain radiation therapy in patients with brain metastases: results of a phase 1 study. J Neurooncol. 2015;122(2):409–17.

38. Middleton MR, et al. Randomized Phase 2 Study Evaluating Veliparib (ABT-888) With Temozolomide in Patients With Metastatic Melanoma. Ann Oncol, 2015. 26 (10). DOI: 10.1093/annonc/mdv308.

39. Owonikoko TK et al. A phase 1 safety study of veliparib combined with cisplatin and etoposide in extensive stage small cell lung cancer: a trial of the ECOG-ACRIN cancer research group (E2511). Lung Cancer. 2015;89(1):66–70.

40. Reiss KA, et al. A phase I study of veliparib (ABT-888) in combination with low-dose fractionated whole abdominal radiation therapy in patients with advanced solid malignancies and peritoneal carcinomatosis. Clin Cancer Res. 2015;21(1):68–76.

41. Plummer R, et al. Phase I study of the poly(ADP-ribose) polymerase inhibitor, AG014699, in combination with temozolomide in patients with advanced solid tumors. Clin Cancer Res. 2008;14(23):7917–23.

42. Swisher EM. ARIEL 2/3: an integrated clinical trial program to assess activity of rucaparib in ovarian cancer and to identify tumor molecular characteristics predictive of response. J Clin Oncol. 2014;32(5 supplement):TPS5619.

43. Jones P, et al. Niraparib: a poly(ADP-ribose) polymerase (PARP) inhibitor for the treatment of tumors with defective homologous recombination. J Med Chem. 2015;58(8):3302–14.

44. Wang L, et al. MK-4827, a PARP-1/-2 inhibitor, strongly enhances response of human lung and breast cancer xenografts to radiation. Invest New Drugs. 2012;30(6):2113–20.

45. Sandhu SK, et al. The poly(ADP-ribose) polymerase inhibitor niraparib (MK4827) in BRCA mutation carriers and patients with sporadic cancer: a phase 1 dose-escalation trial. Lancet Oncol. 2013;14(9):882–92.

46. A Study of Niraparib in Patients With Ovarian Cancer Who Have Received at Least Three Previous Chemotherapy Regimens. https://clinicaltrials.gov/ct2/show/NCT02354586.

47. A Maintenance Study With Niraparib Versus Placebo in Patients With Platinum Sensitive Ovarian Cancer. Available from: https://clinicaltrials.gov/ct2/show/NCT01847274.

48. Shen Y, et al. BMN 673, a novel and highly potent PARP1/2 inhibitor for the treatment of human cancers with DNA repair deficiency. Clin Cancer Res. 2013;19(18):5003–15.

49. Smith MA, et al. Initial testing (stage 1) of the PARP inhibitor BMN 673 by the pediatric preclinical testing program: PALB2 mutation predicts exceptional in vivo response to BMN 673. Pediatr Blood Cancer. 2015;62(1):91–8.

50. Murai J, et al. Stereospecific PARP trapping by BMN 673 and comparison with olaparib and rucaparib. Mol Cancer Ther. 2014;13(2):433–43.

51. Litton JK, et al. A phase 3, open-label, randomized, parallel, 2-arm international study of the oral PARP inhibitor talazoparib (BMN 673) in BRCA mutation subjects with locally advanced and/or metastatic breast cancer (EMBRACA). Journal of Clinical Oncology. 2015;33(15):Suppl 5001.

52. Calabrese CR, et al. Anticancer chemosensitization and radiosensitization by the novel poly(ADP-ribose) polymerase-1 inhibitor AG14361. J Natl Cancer Inst. 2004;96(1):56–67.

53. Pernin V, et al. PARP inhibitors and radiotherapy: rational and prospects for a clinical use. Cancer Radiother. 2014;18(8):790–8. quiz 799–802.

54. Hirai T, et al. Radiosensitization effect of poly(ADP-ribose) polymerase inhibition in cells exposed to low and high liner energy transfer radiation. Cancer Sci. 2012;103(6):1045–50.

55. Rottenberg S, et al. High sensitivity of BRCA1-deficient mammary tumors to the PARP inhibitor AZD2281 alone and in combination with platinum drugs. Proc Natl Acad Sci U S A. 2008;105(44):17079–84.

56. Henneman L, et al. Selective resistance to the PARP inhibitor olaparib in a mouse model for BRCA1-deficient metaplastic breast cancer. Proc Natl Acad Sci U S A. 2015;112(27):8409–14.

57. Bunting SF, et al. 53BP1 inhibits homologous recombination in Brca1-deficient cells by blocking resection of DNA breaks. Cell. 2010;141(2):243–54.

58. Lord CJ, Ashworth A. Mechanisms of resistance to therapies targeting BRCA-mutant cancers. Nat Med. 2013;19(11):1381–8.

59. Nakagawa Y, et al. NF-kappaB signaling mediates acquired resistance after PARP inhibition. Oncotarget. 2015;6(6):3825–39.

60. Higuchi T, et al. CTLA-4 blockade synergizes therapeutically with PARP inhibition in BRCA1-deficient ovarian cancer. Cancer Immunol Res. 2015; 3(11):1257–68.

61. A Phase 1–2 Study of the Combination of Olaparib and Tremelimumab, in BRCA1 and BRCA2 Mutation Carriers With Recurrent Ovarian Cancer. 12/05/15]; Available from: https://clinicaltrials.gov/ct2/show/NCT02571725.

62. Phase 1 and 2 Study of MEDI4736 in Combination With Olaparib or Cediranib for Advanced Solid Tumors and Recurrent Ovarian Cancer. Available from: https://clinicaltrials.gov/ct2/show/NCT02484404.

63. Veliparib and Dinaciclib With or Without Carboplatin in Treating Patients With Advanced Solid Tumors. 9/2/2015]; Available from: https://clinicaltrials.gov/ct2/show/NCT01434316.

9

Metastatic small cell neuroendocrine carcinoma of the cervix treated with the PD-1 inhibitor, nivolumab: a case report

Sarah E. Paraghamian, Teresa C. Longoria and Ramez N. Eskander*

Abstract

Background: Nivolumab is an immune checkpoint inhibitor specific for the programmed death 1 (PD-1) receptor that has led to clinical responses in many cancer types. Identifying biomarkers predictive of response to PD-1 blockade is an area of active investigation.

Case presentation: We present a patient with recurrent, metastatic, PD-L1-negative small cell neuroendocrine carcinoma of the cervix (SCNEC) who experienced a complete response to nivolumab. Though nivolumab was discontinued over 4 months ago due to treatment-related adverse events, she continues to have no evidence of disease.

Conclusions: Immune checkpoint inhibitors may be active in neuroendocrine cervical cancer, with potential for dramatic responses in a modest subset of patients.

Keywords: Small cell neuroendocrine carcinoma, Cervical cancer, PD-1 inhibitor, Nivolumab, Immunotherapy

Background

Small cell neuroendocrine carcinoma of the cervix (SCNEC) is a rare and aggressive histology. It accounts for less than 2% of cervical cancers [1]. Unlike squamous cell and adenocarcinoma, SCNEC is more likely to have lymphovascular space invasion and lymph node involvement at the time of diagnosis [1, 2]. Patients frequently present with locally advanced tumors or distant metastases, resulting in poor oncologic outcomes with a 5-year survival rate estimated at 36.8% for early stage disease and less than 10% for advanced disease [1, 2]. Given these poor outcomes, as well as a lack of prospective data to guide treatment decisions, patients with SCNEC pose a therapeutic challenge.

SCNEC is morphologically similar to small cell lung cancer (SCLC) and treatment considerations draw on studies conducted in small cell lung cancer cohorts. For early stage disease, multimodal therapy with surgery followed by adjuvant cisplatin/etoposide with or without pelvic radiation is favored [1, 2]. More recently, results from the SCLC cohort of CheckMate 032 were published, describing durable responses in a pretreated patient population with single agent nivolumab or combination nivolumab and ipilimumab (Antonia, 2016 #2913) To date, there are no studies informing treatment of progressive or recurrent SCNEC after failure of platinum-based therapy [2]. There is an urgent, unmet clinical need to develop effective treatments.

Nivolumab is an immune checkpoint inhibitor that is specific for the programmed death 1 (PD-1) receptor. PD-1 can be expressed transiently or chronically on T cells depending on the duration of antigen exposure. The interaction of PD-1 with its ligand, PD-L1 or PD-L2, results in downstream signaling that inhibits T cell cytotoxicity and cytokine release. The rationale behind blockade of the PD-1 pathway is to abrogate an immunosuppressive mechanism present in the tumor microenvironment (TME). In this report, we present the clinical experience of a woman with recurrent, metastatic, SCNEC who had a complete response to treatment with nivolumab.

* Correspondence: eskander@uci.edu
Department of Obstetrics and Gynecology, Division of Gynecologic Oncology, University of California Irvine Medical Center, 33 City Blvd. West #1400, Orange, CA 92868, USA

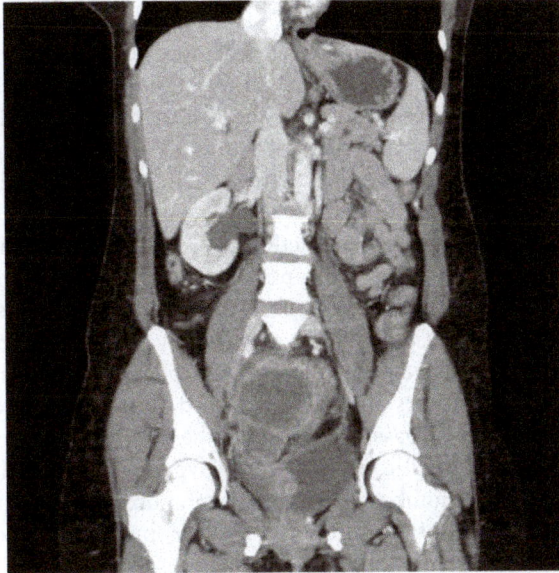

Fig. 1 Progressive recurrent pelvic disease resulting in hydronephrosis

Case presentation

A 38-year-old nulligravida with no history of abnormal pap smears presented to her primary gynecologist with complaint of malodorous brown vaginal discharge. A pap smear was performed, which returned positive for adenocarcinoma and high-risk human papillomavirus (HPV). She was subsequently referred to gynecologic oncology and diagnosed with a Federation of Gynecology and Obstetrics (FIGO) stage IB2 cervical cancer. Biopsies revealed a high-grade small cell neuroendocrine carcinoma, and positron emission tomography–computed tomography

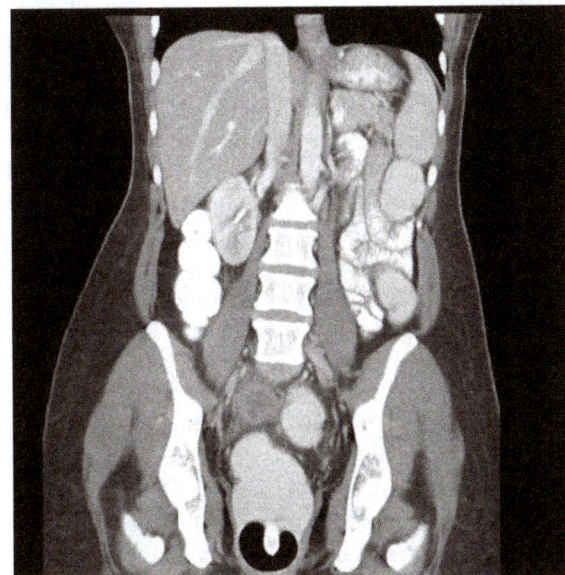

Fig. 2 Reduction in lesion size after starting nivolumab

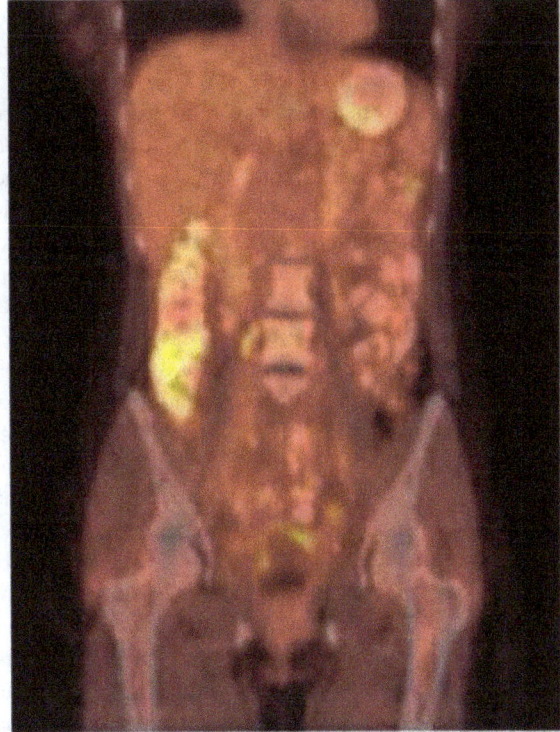

Fig. 3 Complete resolution of all lesions after 6th dose of nivolumab

(PET/CT) showed no evidence of metastatic disease. Plan was made for radical surgical excision followed by adjuvant chemotherapy and radiation.

The patient underwent radical abdominal hysterectomy, bilateral salpingo-oophorectomy and pelvic lymphadenectomy. Pathology was negative for involvement of the surgical margins, parametria or pelvic lymph nodes. The primary tumor was 4.5 by 3.3 cm in size and involved half of the cervical stroma, with lymphovascular space involvement. Her postoperative course was complicated by a pelvic abscess requiring re-exploration and washout. Following recovery, she was treated with 6 cycles of cisplatin 80 mg/m^2 intravenously (IV) on day 1 and etoposide 100 mg/m^2 IV on day 1, 2 and 3. Chemotherapy was well tolerated with only grade 1 nausea and fatigue.

One month after completion of chemotherapy, surveillance pelvic exam was significant for a 1.5-cm, firm, smooth anterior vaginal wall mass. PET/CT demonstrated interval development of multiple hypermetabolic mesenteric deposits, largest measuring 21 mm with a standard uptake value (SUV) of 10.6. Shortly thereafter, she was admitted for small bowel obstruction, with imaging revealing multifocal progression of the pelvic lesions (Fig. 1). Given disease distribution, systemic chemotherapy was favored over local radiotherapy, and she received 2 cycles of paclitaxel 135 mg/m^2 IV on day

1 and topotecan 0.75 mg/m^2 IV on day 1, 2 and 3. Following cycle 2 of therapy, the patient was admitted for progressive pelvic pain due disease progression resulting in obstructive uropathy (Fig. 1). While hospitalized, a right percutaneous nephrostomy tube was placed, and palliative pelvic radiation therapy was initiated. The patient ultimately received a total of 37.5 Gy in 15 fractions directed towards the obstructive lesion along the right pelvic side wall. The original tumor was sent for molecular testing to help inform future therapy and approval for the off-label use of nivolumab was requested from her insurance provider.

Nivolumab was initiated at a dose of 3 mg/kg IV every 2 weeks prior to molecular characterization of her tumor, which showed absent PD-L1 expression. After 2 doses, radiographic imaging demonstrated a decreased in size of all target lesions (Fig. 2). Concurrently, all cell counts began to decrease. After 4 doses, the patient reported vision changes and light sensitivity. She was evaluated by ophthalmology and diagnosed with severe dry eyes and pre-glaucoma. Despite standard topical therapies, her symptoms progressed and the decision was made to discontinue treatment for persistent grade 3 ocular toxicity after the 6th dose. PET/CT obtained 3 weeks after the final dose demonstrated complete resolution of all target and non-target lesions (Fig. 3). Cell counts nadired (grade 2 lymphocytopenia and thrombocytopenia, grade 3 anemia) 5 weeks after cessation of therapy and began to show significant recovery by week 7. Hematologic evaluation, inclusive of bone marrow biopsy, failed to identify an alternate source of her pancytopenia, which was attributed to nivolumab.

Discussion

We present a patient with recurrent, metastatic, PD-L1-negative SCNEC who experienced a complete response to nivolumab therapy. Though nivolumab was discontinued over 4 months ago due to treatment-related adverse events, she continues to have no evidence of disease.

From a therapeutics standpoint, orphan diseases such as SCNEC are traditionally unable to keep pace with more common malignancies. The low likelihood of achieving sufficient patient numbers for efficacy trials discourages scientific initiatives specifically designed for rare tumor types. The typical solution to this problem has been to extrapolate treatment strategies from more frequently encountered cancers of the same cell type, such as SCLC in the case of SCNEC. This practice assumes that cell origin or morphology is the key feature to predict response to treatment. The National Cancer Institute – Molecular Analysis for Therapy Choice (NCI-MATCH) trial is evidence that this thought process is changing. In this trial, treatment with various targeted therapies is directed by genetic testing. Patients

with solid tumors or lymphomas that have progressed following at least one line of standard treatment (or for which no agreed upon treatment approach exists) are assigned to a treatment arm based on the DNA sequencing results of their tumor. This strategy recognizes the heterogeneity that exists not only between different types of cancer but also between cancers of the same type.

In the search for predictive biomarkers to immune checkpoint inhibitors, the prevalence of somatic mutations has been the most promising. From the outset, mutagen-induced malignancies, namely melanoma and lung cancer, have had the greatest success in clinical trials. These cancers approach or exceed 10 somatic mutations per megabase, constituting the highest mutation frequencies of all cancers [3]. It is hypothesized that the greater the number of somatic mutations, the greater the number of neoantigens and the more immunogenic the tumor. This principle was assessed by Le and colleagues in a phase II trial designed to evaluate the clinical activity of pembrolizumab in patients with progressive metastatic carcinoma with or without mismatch-repair deficiency, which is associated with a difference of 10–100 times the number of somatic mutations [4]. They found an immune-related objective response rate of 40% and immune-related, 20-week progression-free survival rate of 78% in patients with mismatch repair–deficient colorectal cancers, compared to 0 and 11%, respectively, in patients with mismatch repair–proficient colorectal cancers. Patients with mismatch repair–deficient non-colorectal cancer had responses similar to those of patients with mismatch repair–deficient colorectal cancer.

The number of somatic mutations is unlikely to be the only determinant of tumor immunogenicity. Topalian and colleagues hypothesize that integrated oncogenic viruses are uniquely equipped to generate neoantigens that engage the immune system [5]. While point mutations or rearrangements of the tumor genome typically generate a single or limited number of T cell epitopes, the products of viral oncogenes are completely non-self and are likely to contain many more potential antigenic peptides for T cell recognition. Moreover, as drivers of tumorigenesis, products of viral oncogenes are less likely to be silenced or deleted as a mechanism of immune evasion. This theory has found support in a phase II trial of pembrolizumab in advanced Merkle-cell carcinoma [6]. Merkle-cell carcinoma, a rare but aggressive skin cancer, has been linked to 2 major causative factors, ultraviolet (UV) light and Merkle-cell polyomavirus (MCPyV), whose large T antigen is expressed in tumor cells and inactivates p53 and Rb. MCPyV-negative, UV-induced Merkel-cell carcinomas have a median of 1121 mutations per exome, which exceeds the mutational burden reported for cancers that have been most responsive to PD-1 blockade (i.e. melanoma, lung cancers, GU cancers). In contrast, MCPyV-positive Merkel-cell carcinomas, with a median of 12.5 mutations per exome, carry a mutational burden that is below cancers that have demonstrated a poor response to PD-1 blockade (i.e. prostate and pancreatic cancers). Among 25 patients assigned to pembrolizumab 2 mg per kg every 3 weeks, 44% (4 of 9 patients) of those with MCPyV-negative tumors and 62% (10 of 16 patients) of those with MCPyV-positive tumors had an objective response. In this trial, neither PD-L1 expression on tumor cells nor infiltrating immune cells was associated with clinical response to pembrolizumab.

The best correlate to Merkle-cell carcinoma in an HPV-associated cancer is head and neck squamous cell carcinoma (HNSCC). Just as in Merkle-cell carcinoma, HNSCC may be mutagen-driven (tobacco) or virus-driven, with the greater mutational burden found in the virus-negative tumors. In KEYNOTE-012, a phase Ib trial of pembrolizumab 10 mg per kg every 2 weeks in patients with PD-L1-positive recurrent or metastatic HNSCC, overall response rate (ORR) in all patients was 18% (8 of 45 patients), which consisted of 4 of 29 (14%) patients with HPV-negative tumors and 4 of 16 (25%) patients with HPV-positive tumors [7]. Similar results were found in an expansion cohort of PD-L1 positive or negative patients that received a fixed dose of pembrolizumab at a less frequent dosing schedule (200 mg IV every 3 weeks) [8]. Compared to 14% (15 of 104 patients) of patients with HPV-negative tumors, 32% (9 of 28 patients) of those with HPV-positive tumors had an objective response. Nivolumab has also performed well in recurrent or metastatic HNSCC. In CheckMate-141, a phase III trial, median overall survival (OS) was 7.5 months among patients who received nivolumab 3 mg per kg every 2 weeks compared to 5.1 months among patients who received single-agent systemic therapy [9]. There was a median OS difference of 4.7 months among patients with HPV-positive tumors (9.1 months in nivolumab group vs 4.4 months in standard-therapy group; hazard ratio for death, 0.56; 95% CI, 0.32–0.99) and a difference of 1.7 months among patients with HPV-negative tumors (7.5 months in nivolumab group versus 5.8 months in standard-therapy group; hazard ratio, 0.73; 95% CI, 0.42–1.25).

It remains to be seen whether integrated oncogenic viruses may ultimately be validated as a predictive biomarker for immune checkpoint inhibitors. While we await the results of additional trials examining checkpoint inhibition in subjects with virus-positive and virus-negative cervical cancer (NCT02488759, NCT02257528), it is important to note that complete responses and sustained responses remain rare. Of 177 patients in KEYNOTE-012 who were evaluated by central review, only 5 patients (2.8%), 4 of which where HPV-positive, demonstrated a complete response to therapy. In our patient, we hypothesize that radiotherapy may have served to sensitize or prime the immune system. Tumor-directed radiotherapy has been shown to stimulate the immune system by increasing antigen presentation and promoting a proinflammatory tumor microenvironment (TME), with well-documented changes in the cytokine milieu and expression of cell surface molecules [10]. These anti-tumor-specific immune responses may extend to distant, non-irradiated tumor sites, a phenomenon termed the abscopal effect. Using various mouse models, the combination of radiotherapy and immune checkpoint inhibitors has not only been shown to have synergistic effects on the TME [11] but also to extend survival [12, 13]. Dramatic responses to this combination have been reported in humans [14] and are being evaluated in the clinical trial setting (NCT02383212).

Conclusions

Unlike the more common histological types of cervical cancer, SCNEC is rarely cured, even when diagnosed at an early stage. Its resistance to traditional therapies, reflected in the heterogeneity of treatment sequence described in the literature, encourages oncologists to look to novel therapies. Immunotherapy has the capacity to turn the causative agent, high-risk HPV, into a feature that may be exploited for clinical benefit. Among recurrent, chemotherapy-resistant, metastatic cervical cancer patients treated with adoptive T-cell therapy (ACT) involving a single infusion of ex vivo–expanded tumor-infiltrating T cells, HPV reactivity of the infusion product positively correlated with clinical response [15]. More research is needed to evaluate whether HPV infection is a predictive biomarker for immune checkpoint inhibitors, which have the potential for dramatic responses in a modest subset of patients.

Abbreviations
FIGO: Federation of Gynecology and Obstetrics; HPV: Human papillomavirus; HSNCC: Head and neck squamous cell carcinoma; IV: Intravenously; MCPyV: Merkle-cell polyomavirus; ORR: Overall response rate; OS: Overall survival; PD-1: Programmed death 1; PET/CT: Positron emission tomography-computed tomography; SCLC: Small cell lung cancer; SCNEC: Small cell neuroendocrine carcinoma of the cervix; SUV: Standard uptake value; TME: Tumor microenvironment

Acknowledgements
Not applicable.

Funding
This study was supported by the Ruth L Kirschstein NRSA Institutional Training Research Grant, 2T32 CA06039611.

Authors' contributions

All authors contributed to the design, data acquisition, data analysis and interpretation and manuscript preparation (writing and assembly). All authors read and approved the final manuscript.

Competing interests

The authors declare that they have no competing interests.

References

1. Gardner GJ, Reidy-Lagunes D, Gehrig PA. Neuroendocrine tumors of the gynecologic tract: a society of gynecologic oncology (SGO) clinical document. Gynecol Oncol. 2011;122:190–8.
2. Satoh T, Takei Y, Treilleux I, Devouassoux-Shisheboran M, Ledermann J, Viswanathan AN, Mahner S, Provencher DM, Mileshkin L, Avall-Lundqvist E, Pautier P, Reed NS, Fujiwara K. Gynecologic Cancer InterGroup (GCIG) consensus review for small cell carcinoma of the cervix. Int J Gynecol Cancer. 2014;24:S102–8.
3. Alexandrov LB, Nik-Zainal S, Wedge DC, Aparicio SA, Behjati S, Biankin AV, Bignell GR, Bolli N, Borg A, Borresen-Dale AL, Boyault S, Burkhardt B, Butler AP, Caldas C, Davies HR, Desmedt C, Eils R, Eyfjord JE, Foekens JA, Greaves M, Hosoda F, Hutter B, Ilicic T, Imbeaud S, Imielinski M, Jager N, Jones DT, Jones D, Knappskog S, Kool M, Lakhani SR, Lopez-Otin C, Martin S, Munshi NC, Nakamura H, Northcott PA, Pajic M, Papaemmanuil E, Paradiso A, Pearson JV, Puente XS, Raine K, Ramakrishna M, Richardson AL, Richter J, Rosenstiel P, Schlesner M, Schumacher TN, Span PN, Teague JW, Totoki Y, Tutt AN, Valdes-Mas R, van Buuren MM, van Veer TL, Vincent-Salomon A, Waddell N, Yates LR, Zucman-Rossi J, Futreal PA, McDermott U, Lichter P, Meyerson M, Grimmond SM, Siebert R, Campo E, Shibata T, Pfister SM, Campbell PJ, Stratton MR. Signatures of mutational processes in human cancer. Nature. 2013;500:415–21.
4. Le DT, Uram JN, Wang H, Bartlett BR, Kemberling H, Eyring AD, Skora AD, Luber BS, Azad NS, Laheru D, Biedrzycki B, Donehower RC, Zaheer A, Fisher GA, Crocenzi TS, Lee JJ, Duffy SM, Goldberg RM, de la Chapelle A, Koshiji M, Bhaijee F, Huebner T, Hruban RH, Wood LD, Cuka N, Pardoll DM, Papadopoulos N, Kinzler KW, Zhou S, Cornish TC, Taube JM, Anders RA, Eshleman JR, Vogelstein B, Diaz Jr LA. PD-1 blockade in tumors with mismatch-repair deficiency. N Engl J Med. 2015;372:2509–20.
5. Topalian SL, Taube JM, Anders RA, Pardoll DM. Mechanism-driven biomarkers to guide immune checkpoint blockade in cancer therapy. Nat Rev Cancer. 2016;16:275–87.
6. Nghiem PT, Bhatia S, Lipson EJ, Kudchadkar RR, Miller NJ, Annamalai L, Berry S, Chartash EK, Daud A, Fling SP, Friedlander PA, Kluger HM, Kohrt HE, Lundgren L, Margolin K, Mitchell A, Olencki T, Pardoll DM, Reddy SA, Shantha EM, Sharfman WH, Sharon E, Shemanski LR, Shinohara MM, Sunshine JC, Taube JM, Thompson JA, Townson SM, Yearley JH, Topalian SL, Cheever MA. PD-1 blockade with pembrolizumab in advanced Merkel-cell carcinoma. N Engl J Med. 2016;374:2542–52.
7. Seiwert TY, Burtness B, Mehra R, Weiss J, Berger R, Eder JP, Heath K, McClanahan T, Lunceford J, Gause C, Cheng JD, Chow LQ. Safety and clinical activity of pembrolizumab for treatment of recurrent or metastatic squamous cell carcinoma of the head and neck (KEYNOTE-012): an open-label, multicentre, phase 1b trial. Lancet Oncol. 2016;17:956–65.
8. Chow LQ, Haddad R, Gupta S, Mahipal A, Mehra R, Tahara M, Berger R, Eder JP, Burtness B, Lee SH, Keam B, Kang H, Muro K, Weiss J, Geva R, Lin CC, Chung HC, Meister A, Dolled-Filhart M, Pathiraja K, Cheng JD, Seiwert TY. Antitumor activity of pembrolizumab in biomarker-unselected patients with recurrent and/or metastatic head and neck squamous cell carcinoma: results from the phase Ib KEYNOTE-012 expansion cohort. J Clin Oncol. 2016;34:3838–45.
9. Ferris RL, Blumenschein Jr G, Fayette J, Guigay J, Colevas AD, Licitra L, Harrington K, Kasper S, Vokes EE, Even C, Worden F, Saba NF, Iglesias Docampo LC, Haddad R, Rordorf T, Kiyota N, Tahara M, Monga M, Lynch M, Geese WJ, Kopit J, Shaw JW, Gillison ML. Nivolumab for recurrent squamous-cell carcinoma of the head and neck. N Engl J Med. 2016;375:1856–67.
10. Salama AK, Postow MA, Salama JK. Irradiation and immunotherapy: from concept to the clinic. Cancer. 2016;122:1659–71.
11. Deng L, Liang H, Burnette B, Beckett M, Darga T, Weichselbaum RR, Fu YX. Irradiation and anti-PD-L1 treatment synergistically promote antitumor immunity in mice. J Clin Invest. 2014;124:687–95.
12. Demaria S, Kawashima N, Yang AM, Devitt ML, Babb JS, Allison JP, Formenti SC. Immune-mediated inhibition of metastases after treatment with local radiation and CTLA-4 blockade in a mouse model of breast cancer. Clin Cancer Res. 2005;11:728–34.
13. Zeng J, See AP, Phallen J, Jackson CM, Belcaid Z, Ruzevick J, Durham N, Meyer C, Harris TJ, Albesiano E, Pradilla G, Ford E, Wong J, Hammers HJ, Mathios D, Tyler B, Brem H, Tran PT, Pardoll D, Drake CG, Lim M. Anti-PD-1 blockade and stereotactic radiation produce long-term survival in mice with intracranial gliomas. Int J Radiat Oncol Biol Phys. 2013;86:343–9.
14. Reynders K, Illidge T, Siva S, Chang JY, De Ruysscher D. The abscopal effect of local radiotherapy: using immunotherapy to make a rare event clinically relevant. Cancer Treat Rev. 2015;41:503–10.
15. Stevanovic S, Draper LM, Langhan MM, Campbell TE, Kwong ML, Wunderlich JR, Dudley ME, Yang JC, Sherry RM, Kammula US, Restifo NP, Rosenberg SA, Hinrichs CS. Complete regression of metastatic cervical cancer after treatment with human papillomavirus-targeted tumor-infiltrating T cells. J Clin Oncol. 2015;33:1543–50.

10

Opportunistic salpingectomy for ovarian cancer prevention

Gillian E. Hanley[1*], Jessica N. McAlpine[1], Janice S. Kwon[1] and Gillian Mitchell[2,3]

Abstract

Recently accumulated evidence has strongly indicated that the fallopian tube is the site of origin for the majority of high-grade serous ovarian or peritoneal carcinomas. As a result, recommendations have been made to change surgical practice in women at general population risk for ovarian cancer and perform bilateral salpingectomy at the time of hysterectomy without oophorectomy and in lieu of tubal ligation, a practice that has been termed opportunistic salpingectomy (OS). Despite suggestions that bilateral salpingectomy may be used as an interim procedure in women with BRCA1/2 mutations, enabling them to delay oophorectomy, there is insufficient evidence to support this practice as a safe alternative and risk-reducing bilateral salpingo-oophorectomy remains the recommended standard of care for high-risk women. While evidence on uptake of OS is sparse, it points toward increasing practice of OS during hysterectomy. The practice of OS for sterilization purposes, although expanding, appears to be less common. Operative and perioperative complications as measured by administered blood transfusions, hospital length of stay and readmissions were not increased with the addition of OS either at time of hysterectomy or for sterilization. Additional operating room time was 16 and 10 min for OS with hysterectomy and OS for sterilization, respectively. Short-term studies of the consequences of OS on ovarian function indicate no difference between women undergoing hysterectomy alone and hysterectomy with OS, but no long-term data exist. There is emerging evidence of effectiveness of excisional sterilization on reducing ovarian cancer rates from Rochester (OR = 0.36 95 % CI 0.13, 1.02), and bilateral salpingectomy from Denmark (OR = 0.58 95 % CI 0.36, 0.95) and Sweden (HR = 0.35, 95 % CI 0.17, 0.73), but these studies suffer from limitations, including that they were performed for pathological rather than prophylactic purposes. Initial cost-effectiveness modeling indicates that OS is cost-effective over a wide range of costs and risk estimates. While preliminary safety, efficacy, and cost-effectiveness data are promising, further research is needed (particularly long-term data on ovarian function) to firmly establish the safety of the procedure. The marginal benefit of OS compared with tubal ligation or hysterectomy alone needs to be established through large prospective studies of OS done for prophylaxis.

Keywords: Ovarian cancer, Bilateral salpingectomy, Cancer prevention, Fallopian tube

Introduction

Ovarian cancer is the leading cause of death due to gynecologic malignancy and the fifth most common cause of cancer deaths in developed countries. In the United States (US) and Canada, there are ~25,000 new diagnoses and ~16,000 deaths from the disease annually. While the general population lifetime risk of ovarian cancer is 1.4 % [1], women at high-risk of developing the disease due to their inheritance of a germline BRCA1 and BRCA2 mutation have an average cumulative risk of between 40 % to 75 % and 8 % to

34 %, respectively [2–5]. Inherited germline mutations of BRCA1 and BRCA2 account for approximately 11.7 to 15 % of all invasive ovarian carcinomas [6–9]. In both general population and high-risk women, screening for ovarian cancer is not recommended, as no mortality benefit has been demonstrated even with strict adherence to screening protocols [10–14]. Symptoms of ovarian cancer are non-specific and often do not arise until the cancer is in a late stage, the point at which the majority of women are diagnosed [15]. Five-year overall survival is less than 50 % and has not substantially changed in the last two decades [16, 17].

Ovarian cancer is a heterogeneous disease and itscellular origins remain an area of active debate [18, 19]. It has

* Correspondence: Gillian.hanley@vch.ca
[1]Department of Gynaecology and Obstetrics, Division of Gynaecologic Oncology, University of British Columbia, Vancouver, BC, Canada
Full list of author information is available at the end of the article

been postulated that ovarian cancers can arise from the ovarian surface epithelium, fallopian tube epithelium and ectopic endometrium and it appears likely that different histological subtypes have different origins. There are five main histological subtypes of ovarian carcinoma: high-grade serous (HGSC), low-grade serous (LGSC), endometrioid (ENOC), clear cell (CCOC) and mucinous cancers. Each has a distinct clinical characteristics and genetic landscape [20]. HGSC is the most common, accounting for approximately 70 % of invasive ovarian carcinomas [21]. It is usually diagnosed at an advanced stage, and, although it is initially highly responsive to chemotherapy, most women with HGSC ultimately relapse, develop resistance to chemotherapeutic agents and succumb to their disease.

Review

A new understanding of the role of the fallopian tube in ovarian cancer

The ovary is the most frequent site of the dominant tumor mass at the time of cancer diagnosis, and this, together with the epidemiological evidence that increasing parity is strongly related to a reduction in ovarian carcinoma risk led to the "incessant" ovulation hypothesis for the etiology of ovarian cancer [22] and to the focus on Mullerian-type cortical inclusion cysts (Mullerian-CICs) within the ovary as the probable source of the disease. Mullerian-CICs were postulated to arise from transformation of the ovarian surface epithelium (OSE) trapped within the ovary after ovulation. The first suggestion of fallopian tube involvement in ovarian cancer was made as early as 1896, with the case report of a primary fallopian tube cancer with pathological characteristics very similar to ovarian cancer [23]. More recently, examination of the fallopian tubes removed at risk-reducing bilateral salpingo-oophorectomy (RRBSO) from women with BRCA1 and BRCA2 mutations revealed the presence in the distal fallopian tube (the fimbriae) of occult/small cancers in 5–15 % of these high-risk women [24–26] and preinvasive lesions in the fimbriae (serous tubal intraepithelial cancers; STICs) in 1–6 % of the women [27–30]. In contrast, only one paper that conducted intensive study of the ovaries found a single case (1 of 28 women studied (3.5 %)) [27] of premalignant epithelial change [25, 27, 31–37].

The Sectioning and Extensive Examining of the Fimbria (SEE-FIM) protocol was developed to maximize the detection of ovarian cancer precursors or early fallopian tube cancers by sectioning and examining the fallopian tube fimbriae for pathology [35, 38]. This protocol has revealed tubal involvement in up to 70 % of unselected women diagnosed with ovarian or primary peritoneal HGSC (with and without BRCA 1/2) [18, 39–43], including the presence of fimbrial STICs in 40–60 % of these women [18, 43, 44]— a proportion that increased with more complete examination

of the fallopian tube [36, 42]. Importantly, STICs were not observed in women with non-gynecologic or benign conditions [37]. Based upon these findings, it has been proposed that tubal neoplasia is the primary lesion in HGSC and that these lesions spread to the ovary and peritoneum [18, 40].

Lending support to the theory that STICs are the precursor lesion to HGSC is the finding of identical TP53 mutations in STICs and concomitant ovarian and/or peritoneal cancers [39, 45]. It has been suggested that even earlier fallopian tube lesions precede STICs in the fallopian tube. The most well studies of these precursors is the 'p53 signature', defined as a focus of 12 or more cells with normal morphology, primarily localized at the fimbriated end of the fallopian tube, but with strong p53 immunostaining. Over 90 % of STICs have p53 signatures; p53 signatures have been reported in direct association or contiguous with STICs, and p53 signatures share identical TP53 mutations with both STICs and invasive cancers, all of which strongly suggests a clonal relationship among these tissues [45–47]. These data, along with the findings from the SEE-FIM protocol, underscore the fallopian tube as a clear target for prevention.

Current recommendations

In BRCA1/2 mutation carriers, RRBSO has been shown to be highly protective for ovarian cancer with a cancer risk reduction of 80 % and overall mortality reduction of 60 % following surgery, and is strongly recommended for prevention of ovarian cancers in this population [34, 48, 49]. Most high-risk women have been reported to experience a high quality of physical and mental well being following RRBSO, with significantly reduced cancer-related worries [50]. However, RRBSO is not recommended for the general population, as removal of the ovaries has been reported to be associated with increased total mortality, coronary heart disease, stroke, osteoporosis and colorectal cancer [51, 52]. While RRBSO has demonstrated a reduction in overall mortality in the high-risk population, prospective follow-up has been short (e.g. 6 years in Domchek et al.) [49] and longer follow-up will be necessary to ensure that non-cancer events do not ultimately overtake the overall mortality benefit from the cancer prevention effects. Bilateral salpingectomy may offer significant protection against ovarian cancer in the general population, and possibly in the high-risk population, while avoiding these downstream health risks.

Given the new understanding regarding the role of the fallopian tube in ovarian cancer, and the health risks associated with RRBSO which make it an inappropriate candidate for prevention in the general population, recommendations were made regarding the treatment of the fallopian tube in common gynecologic surgeries. In September 2010 the Ovarian Cancer Research team (OVCARE) recommended to all gynecologic surgeons in the province of British Columbia (BC) Canada that, when operating on women at general population risk for ovarian cancer, they should consider: 1) performing bilateral salpingectomy at the time of hysterectomy (even when the ovaries are being preserved); and 2) performing bilateral salpingectomy in place of tubal ligation for sterilization—herein referred to as opportunistic salpingectomy (OS). The surgical practice changes were presented as a cancer prevention strategy of unproven efficacy. The Society of Gynecologic Oncology of Canada acknowledged BC's campaign and officially endorsed BC's cancer prevention strategy in 2011 issuing a statement recommending that the "physician discuss the risks and benefits of bilateral salpingectomy with patients undergoing hysterectomy or requesting permanent irreversible contraception" [53]. Two years later the US Society for Gynecologic Oncology followed suit and made a similar recommendation [54]. Most recently the American College of Obstetricians and Gynecologists published a statement supporting the recommendation that "surgeons and patients discuss the potential benefits of the removal of fallopian tubes during hysterectomy in women at population risk of ovarian cancer who are not having an oophorectomy" and that "when counselling women about laparoscopic sterilization methods, clinicians can communicate that bilateral salpingectomy can be considered a method that provides effective contraception". These recommendations were made because "prophylactic salpingectomy may offer clinicians the opportunity to prevent ovarian cancer in their patients" [55].

Numbers of hysterectomies and tubal sterilizations in North America

There are approximately 430,000 and 41,000 hysterectomies performed annually in the US and Canada, respectively [56, 57]. In the US, between 50 and 55 % of women who had a hysterectomy also had a bilateral oophorectomy, while this number appears to be around 45 % of hysterectomies in Canada [58, 59]. This means that there are approximately 240,000 women of general ovarian cancer risk undergoing hysterectomies annually in the US and Canada who would likely be eligible for OS for ovarian cancer prevention.

Approximately 350,000 and 25,000 tubal sterilizations are done annually in the US and Canada, respectively [60, 61]. Approximately half of these annual tubal sterilizations occur after delivery, typically at the time of caesarean delivery or within 24 h after a vaginal delivery [62]. Salpingectomy as a primary method of sterilization has not been considered routinely until the past few years. However, for individuals in whom tubal sterilization fails, bilateral salpingectomy has long been considered the preferred method to ensure definitive treatment [63]. Combining these women with the women undergoing hysterectomy

without oophorectomy results in approximately 590,000 women who are potentially eligible for OS for ovarian cancer prevention purposes annually in the US and Canada.

Women at high-risk for ovarian cancer (those with BRCA1 and BRCA1 mutations) are strongly advised to have prophylactic RRBSO once child-bearing is complete based on the good short term data indicating the improvement in mortality in this cohort [49]. However, the long-term effects of premature menopause on mortality and morbidity in this cohort are largely unknown, and concerns regarding these effects have led to discussion of a staged approach of initial bilateral salpingectomy once childbearing is complete, followed by an oophorectomy closer to natural menopause [64–66]. While this presents a potentially promising alternative to premature menopause and the resulting health consequences, we do not yet have the prospective evidence demonstrating that a staged approach is not inferior to upfront RRBSO. RRBSO has an important impact on breast cancer risk in this population; the 50 % reduction in breast cancer incidence associated with premenopausal RRBSO in high-risk women [49] would also need to be considered in these prospective studies before changing clinical practice for ovarian cancer prevention among BRCA1/2 mutation carriers.

Opportunistic salpingectomy in the general population
Uptake
The uptake of OS has been studied in depth in British Columbia where the campaign was first initiated and was then adopted across Canada more widely. To examine rates of OS in BC we examined all hospitalizations in the province using the Discharge Abstract Database, which captures demographic, administrative and clinical information for all hospital discharges (inpatient and days surgeries) [67] beginning from the calendar year two years prior the educational campaign (Sept 2010) and continuing two years after. We reported that the proportion of hysterectomies with an associated OS (excluding hysterectomies where ovaries were removed) increased from 8 % in 2008 to 63 % in 2011, and the proportion of sterilizations by salpingectomy increased from 0.5 % in 2008 to 33 % in 2011 [59]. We have recently extended this analysis to 2013 and found that 75 % of all hysterectomies without oophorectomy included a bilateral salpingectomy and 48 % of all sterilizations were done by salpingectomy in 2013. While the rate of uptake in the rest of Canada has not been as dramatic, rates of hysterectomy with OS are significantly increasing from less than 1 % of all hysterectomies in 2006 to more than 11 % in 2011 [68]. There is less known about uptake of OS in the United States and while a

large nationally representative study is needed, there are indications that OS is being performed in parts of the United States [69]. We expect that rates of OS will increase in the US following the ACOG's January 2015 recommendation to discuss opportunistic salpingectomy with patients undergoing hysterectomy or tubal sterilization [55].

There have also been several surveys assessing physician attitudes towards OS. A Canadian survey of obstetrician-gynecologists revealed that 90 % had heard of OS, but 37 % were unaware of the evidence supporting the hypothesis that HGSC originates in the fallopian tube and 38 % were unsure whether there would be any population benefit to performing OS [70]. A survey of physicians in American institutions with Obstetrics & Gynecology residency programs reported that 54 % of physicians perform OS with hysterectomy. The 46 % of physicians who did not commonly perform OS reported that they did not believe there was any benefit [71]. While 58 % of practitioners believed it was the most effective method of sterilization after age 35 they only chose this method in patients in whom a previous tubal sterilization has failed or because of tubal disease [71]. Finally, a similar survey of Irish Obstetricians and Gynecologists reported that 90 % would consider OS at the time of abdominal hysterectomy and 73 % would consider OS for female sterilization [72].

Safety

The operative and perioperative complications of OS have been studied in British Columbia. We reported that OS with hysterectomy requires an additional 16 min of OR time while OS for sterilization requires an additional 10 min of OR time compared with hysterectomy alone and tubal ligation, respectively. We found no increased risks associated with OS when examining length of stay in hospital, or the likelihood of hospital readmission or blood transfusion—both of which were raised as concerns by gynecologic surgeons at the time of the educational campaign in BC [70]. The BC study indicated that OS was performed by open, laparoscopic, and vaginal routes, the latter of which accounted for 18 % of hysterectomies with OS. Compared with open approach, the vaginal approach for hysterectomy with OS was associated with significantly shorter length of stay in hospital and decreased risk for hospital readmission (OR = 0.51, 95%CI 0.37, 0.70) [59]. Vaginal approach for hysterectomy with OS appears to be both safe and feasible making hysterectomy with OS an option in both high and low resource settings.

OS also eliminates the risk of subsequent hydrosalpinx and, in the case of tubal sterilization, ectopic pregnancy—an advantage over conventional tubal sterilization methods such as partial salpingectomy, banding or coagulation. Hydrosalpinx is the most frequent complication

following hysterectomy without OS, and occurs in 35.5 % of patients requiring revision surgery in 7.8 % of patients [73, 74]. Other complications following retained tubes after hysterectomy and sterilization include pelvic inflammatory disease, salpingitis, benign fallopian tube tumors, and tube prolapse [75–80]—many of which are definitively treated with salpingectomy and could be avoided by performing OS at the time of hysterectomy and in lieu of tubal ligation. A concern raised regarding OS in lieu of tubal ligation is the inability to reverse the procedure for women who subsequently wish to regain their fertility who will then be reliant on an in vitro fertilization approach. Recommendations regarding tubal reversal surgery post TL versus proceeding to in vitro fertilization (IVF) vary greatly across the globe, often reflecting public health or insurance cost coverage (for surgical procedures, for IVF) and dependent on the presence of skilled surgeons who are willing to perform tubal microsurgery for reversals. The overall cost of a single IVF cycle compared with tubal microsurgery may be comparable but successful tubal reversal would allow multiple attempts at child bearing as compared to a single round of IVF. In areas where IVF coverage is free or heavily subsidized, or where women may have additional factors that would make natural conception challenging (eg. decreased ovarian reserve, male factor infertility) IVF may be the first choice of management thus her options would be no different than for women who had undergone OS.

Salpingectomy, when performed correctly, should not impact the ovarian blood supply and, therefore, should not have an impact on ovarian function (hormonal production, ovulation, age of menopause). Hysterectomy with ovarian conservation has been associated with decreased ovarian function [81] and earlier onset of menopause in prospective studies [81, 82]. Thus, studies examining ovarian function after hysterectomy with and without OS tend to examine differences between the groups according to OS status rather than differences from baseline. Encouragingly, a retrospective series involving ~160 premenopausal women who had total laparoscopic hysterectomy with or without bilateral salpingectomy showed small differences in ovarian sonographic and hormonal parameters from baseline in both groups and no difference between the groups. Anti-Mullerian hormone (AMH) levels (a measure of ovarian reserve) were slightly lower in both groups (which is consistent with the research reporting decreased ovarian function following hysterectomy) but the addition of salpingectomy to the procedure did not worsen the effect [83]. The lack of a hormonal difference between the groups was also reported in a recent pilot randomized controlled trial examining the short-term effects of salpingectomy during laparoscopic hysterectomy on ovarian reserve among thirty premenopausal women. Again AMH levels following surgery were lower from baseline in both groups, but there were no difference in postoperative AMH levels between the group randomized to undergo opportunistic salpingectomy at the time of hysterectomy and the group retaining their fallopian tubes [84]. The long-term effects, such as the timing of menopause, have not been analysed systematically after hysterectomy with OS or OS for sterilization. This requires further study, as it is possible that if OS reduces the age of menopause, the ovarian cancer mortality benefit may be entirely offset by the increase in all cause mortality from the earlier age of onset of menopause. While the short-term data indicating hormonal equivalence between the OS and hysterectomy alone is somewhat reassuring , no long-term studies have been published to date.

Effectiveness

We have long had epidemiologic evidence supporting the importance of the fallopian tube in ovarian cancer in the form of the reduced risk associated with tubal ligation (TL). TL appears to decrease the risk of ovarian cancer by 29 % overall [85, 86], but there are differences in this effect across histologic subtype with the greatest reduction in risk found for ENOC (52 %), followed by CCOC (48 %), and a 20 % reduction in risk of HGSC [86]. There is also encouraging data on a small number of excisional tubal ligation cases (defined as complete salpingectomy, distal fimbriectomy, or partial salpingectomy) from Minnesota. Researchers from the Rochester epidemiology project reported a 64 % reduction in the risk of ovarian cancer after excisional tubal sterilization compared to those without sterilization or with non-excisional tubal sterilization (OR = 0.36, 95 % CI 0.13, 1.02) [69]. While this study was small and did not distinguish bilateral salpingectomy from other forms of excisional tubal sterilization, the results are promising.

Danish researchers used a national database to study the relationship between bilateral salpingectomy and ovarian cancer in a retrospective cohort study [87]. They reported that bilateral salpingectomy reduced the risk for ovarian cancer by 42 % (OR = 0.58, 95 % CI 0.36, 0.95); however, their distribution of ovarian cancers by histologic subtype revealed a much smaller than usual proportion of HGSCs (46 % versus the standard 70 %). This suggests the possibility of some form of contamination of the cases, which would likely have decreased their estimate of risk reduction.

The most recent, largest and most rigorous study of the relationship between ovarian cancer and bilateral salpingectomy to date was a population-based retrospective Swedish study using health registers incorporating more than 5.5 million women and 30,000 ovarian cancer cases [88]. The authors identified the four gynecologic surgical procedures of interest (hysterectomy, hysterectomy with concomitant BSO, salpingectomy, sterilization). There

were so few hysterectomies with concomitant salpingectomies (n = 2646) that these women were excluded from analyses. The authors examined the potential impact of one- vs. two-sided salpingectomy, but for codes ocurring after 1997, the consistency in reporting one- or two-sided procedures was poor, so the study was restricted to the calendar years 1973 to 1996. While they were able to control for parity and education level, they did not control for use of oral contraceptive pills (an important protective factor) [89]. They reported that hysterectomy with BSO resulted in an almost complete risk cessation (HR = 0.06, 95 % CI 0.03 to 0.12). One-sided salpingectomy was associated with a reduction of risk of 29 % (HR = 0.71, 95 % CI–0.56 to 0.91) while bilateral salpingectomy was associated with a 65 % reduction in risk (HR = 0.35, 95 % CI 0.17, 0.73). They also reported a reduction in risk associated with hysterectomy alone (HR = 0.79, 95 % CI 0.70 to 0.89) [88].

While this study illustrates that women who have had a bilateral salpingectomy more than halved their risk for ovarian cancer, there are important limitations that need to be addressed in future research. The cohort of women undergoing bilateral salpingectomy was small (n = 3051) since bilateral salpingectomy was a fairly uncommon procedure and historically has not been performed for prophylactic purposes. Salpingectomy was done for the indications of hydrosalpinx, infections (primarily pelvic inflammatory disease), ectopic pregnancy, and endometriosis—all conditions resulting in considerable inflammation. Both PID and endometriosis are risk factors for ovarian cancer [90, 91], suggesting that the group of women who underwent salpingectomy in this historical cohort may have already been at increased risk for ovarian cancer. It is also plausible that salpingectomies performed for prophylactic reasons may confer more protection than those done for other indications, as surgeons will be more careful to remove the entire distal end of the fallopian tube. For both of these reasons, OS may be more protective against ovarian cancer than the results on bilateral salpingectomy reported by Falconer et al. suggest. They also report the reduction of risk conferred by bilateral salpingectomy compared with women unexposed to any of the gynecologic surgeries of interest. As recommendations suggest performing OS with hysterectomy or in lieu of tubal ligation and hysterectomy alone and tubal ligation both reduce ovarian cancer risk [85], it will be important to understand the marginal benefit of performing OS in terms of the additional cancer cases prevented. It is also important to note that none of the studies summarized above reports any data on BRCA1 or BRCA2 mutation carriers and the results should only be generalized to women at population-level risk for ovarian cancer.

Cost-effectiveness

Given the 590,000 women undergoing hysterectomy without oophorectomy and tubal sterilization annually in the US and Canada, implications of widespread performance of OS on health care system costs warrant further study and concerns have been raised [92]. While an accurate understanding of the effectiveness of OS in preventing ovarian cancer, as well as data on the long-term risks associated with this procedure is imperative to understand the implications of OS on our health care systems, in the absence of these data, we have used a decision analytic model to estimate the cost-effectiveness of OS as an ovarian cancer prevention strategy for the general population [61]. Using the assumptions that OS, BSO, hysterectomy, and tubal ligation each confer a 50 %, 90 %, 20 %, and 30 % reduction in risk for ovarian cancer, OS was found to be cost-effective. This result held over a wide range of costs and risk estimates. The model reported that hysterectomy with OS was less costly than hysterectomy alone or with bilateral salpingo-oophorectomy (BSO) but more effective with average comparative life expectancy gains of 1 week and 2 months (in the absence of routine hormone replacement after BSO), respectively. For sterilization, OS was more costly than tubal ligation but more effective with an average life expectancy gain of 1 week. While these average life expectancy gains appear insignificant, it represents a very large gain for women who would have died prematurely as a result of ovarian cancer averaged across many women in the population who receive no gain as they were never going to be diagnosed with ovarian cancer. The average life expectancy gain of 1 week is comparable to that of cervical cancer screening every 2 years compared to every 5 years [93]. The model suggested that the number of hysterectomies with OS needed to prevent one case of ovarian cancer was 273 and the corresponding NNT for salpingectomies for sterilization was 366—numbers that are in line with the number needed to vaccinate against human papilloma virus of 324 to prevent one case of cervical cancer [94]. As we learn more about OS, this model will be updated and improved, but these preliminary results suggest that OS may be cost saving in the long-term.

Conclusions

Our understanding of the pathogenesis of ovarian cancer has improved drastically with the understanding that HGSC can originate in the fallopian tube and, as a result, our approach to ovarian cancer prevention has fundamentally changed for women in the general population and is being challenged for women at high risk of developing the disease. For women at population risk of ovarian cancer, opportunistic salpingectomy presents a promising approach to reducing incidence and mortality from ovarian cancer, and recommendations to integrate it into routine gynecologic practice are increasingly common. While preliminary safety and efficacy data are very reassuring, there remain some unanswered questions. Specifically, we need more data on the impact of OS on ovarian function, which is being examined both through planned randomized controlled trials and a cohort study in BC in order to determine if OS accelerates menopause. In addition, the interaction of OS with other risk-reducing measures including oral contraceptive use will require a greater number of patients to define. OS remains an exciting ovarian cancer prevention strategy in women at general population risk for ovarian cancer undergoing routine gynecologic surgeries and is increasingly being performed vaginally, laparoscopically and robotically. To be clear, we are not advocating surgical intervention solely for the purposes of salpingectomy nor change in surgical approach if the planned route for the required gynecologic surgery cannot achieve salpingectomy.

For women at high risk of ovarian cancer, such as women with germline BRCA 1/2 mutations, who are advised to consider RRBSO from age 35, the possibility of ameliorating some of the effects of premature menopause by either bilateral salpingectomy alone or a staged approach of early bilateral salpingectomy followed by bilateral oophorectomy closer to the age of natural menopause, is attractive. This two-staged approach appears to be most effective in terms of quality-adjusted life expectancy, and is cost-effective [65] providing the tubal hypothesis of serous ovarian cancer is correct. Although most BRCA-associated ovarian cancers likely arise in the fallopian tube, there are four important reasons why oophorectomy, either concurrent with bilateral salpingectomy or delayed, is still recommended in this population: (1) some of these cancers still appear to originate in the ovary, (2) oophorectomy prior to menopause is known to reduce breast cancer risk in this high-risk population by 50 % [95], (3) even when incorporating the increased morbidity associated with surgical menopause, there is still a significant reduction in all-cause mortality associated with RRBSO among high-risk women [49], and (4) while bilateral salpingectomy may reduce ovarian cancer risk, the degree of protective effect on ovarian cancer is unknown. For these reasons we do not consider that it is yet appropriate to routinely advise young high-risk women (BRCA1 or 2 mutation carriers) to have bilateral salpingectomy as a prevention strategy either as a sole or staged procedure with a delayed oophorectomy; bilateral salpingo-oophorectomy on completion of childbearing still has to be the standard of care. However, bilateral salpingectomy may be an option for a well counselled woman if they are not yet prepared to undergo oophorectomy ie., vs. no intervention at all. Before bilateral salpingectomy, with or without, later bilateral oophorectomy can be routinely offered to high-risk women, we need to know that it is effective and does not abrogate the cancer incidence and mortality benefits proven for RRBSO. This will likely require an international effort over many years in order to recruit a large enough sample of these highly selected patients, most likely in the form of a registry rather than a randomised trial to compare outcomes between bilateral salpingectomy and RRBSO [96].

In summary, opportunistic salpingectomy is a safe intervention in the short term, when done concurrently with hysterectomy or instead of tubal ligation. It has the potential to reduce the incidence and mortality from ovarian cancer, and it may have an important role as a temporizing measure in high-risk women with BRCA mutations who are unwilling to undergo standard risk reducing surgery (bilateral salpingo-oophorectomy) at an early age. It will still be essential to evaluate long-term safety and efficacy outcomes to support the ongoing use of this intervention in the general population as well as the high-risk setting.

Abbreviations
HGSC: High Grade Serous ovarian cancer; LGSC: Low Grade Serous ovarian cancer; ENOC: Endometrioid ovarian cancer; CCOC: Clear cell ovarian cancer; BC: British Columbia; RRBSO: Risk Reducing bilateral salpingo-oophorectomy; OS: Opportunistic Salpingectomy; BSO: Bilateral salpingo-oophorectomy; TL: Tubal ligation; IVF: In vitro fertilization; ACOG: American College of Obstetrics & Gynecology; STICs: Serous tubal intraepithelial cancers.

Competing interests
The authors declare that they have no competing interests.

Authors' contributions
GH and GM were responsible for initial conception and design of the article. GH drafted the article. GH, JM, JK, and GM were all involved in editing and finalizing the article. All authors approved the final version of the manuscript.

Acknowledgments
Gillian Hanley is funded by the Canadian Cancer Society (grant #702786).

Author details
[1]Department of Gynaecology and Obstetrics, Division of Gynaecologic Oncology, University of British Columbia, Vancouver, BC, Canada. [2]Hereditary Cancer Program, BC Cancer Agency, Vancouver, BC, Canada. [3]Department of Medicine, University of British Columbia, Vancouver, BC, Canada.

References
1. Canadian Cancer Society. Canadian cancer statistics 2014. Toronto: 2014
2. Mavaddat N, Peock S, Frost D, Ellis S, Platte R, Fineberg E, et al. Cancer risks for BRCA1 and BRCA2 mutation carriers: results from prospective analysis of EMBRACE. J Natl Cancer Inst. 2013;105(11):812–22.
3. Boyd J. Specific keynote: hereditary ovarian cancer: what we know. Gynecol Oncol. 2003;88(1 Pt 2):S8–10. discussion S1-3.
4. King MC, Marks JH, Mandell JB, New York Breast Cancer Study G. Breast and ovarian cancer risks due to inherited mutations in BRCA1 and BRCA2. Science. 2003;302(5645):643–6.
5. Prat J, Ribe A, Gallardo A. Hereditary ovarian cancer. Hum Pathol. 2005;36(8):861–70.
6. Risch HA, McLaughlin JR, Cole DE, Rosen B, Bradley L, Fan I, et al. Population BRCA1 and BRCA2 mutation frequencies and cancer penetrances: a kin-cohort study in Ontario, Canada. J Natl Cancer Inst. 2006;98(23):1694–706.
7. Pal T, Permuth-Wey J, Betts JA, Krischer JP, Fiorica J, Arango H, et al. BRCA1 and BRCA2 mutations account for a large proportion of ovarian carcinoma cases. Cancer. 2005;104(12):2807–16.
8. Risch HA, McLaughlin JR, Cole DE, Rosen B, Bradley L, Kwan E, et al. Prevalence and penetrance of germline BRCA1 and BRCA2 mutations in a

population series of 649 women with ovarian cancer. Am J Hum Genet. 2001;68(3):700–10.
9. Alsop K, Fereday S, Meldrum C, deFazio A, Emmanuel C, George J, et al. BRCA mutation frequency and patterns of treatment response in BRCA mutation-positive women with ovarian cancer: a report from the Australian Ovarian Cancer Study Group.[Erratum appears in J Clin Oncol. 2012 Nov 20;30(33):4180]. J Clin Oncol. 2012;30(21):2654–63.
10. Rosenthal AN, Fraser L, Manchanda R, Badman P, Philpott S, Mozersky J, et al. Results of annual screening in phase I of the United Kingdom familial ovarian cancer screening study highlight the need for strict adherence to screening schedule. J Clin Oncol. 2013;31(1):49–57.
11. Buys SS, Partridge E, Black A, Johnson CC, Lamerato L, Isaacs C, et al. Effect of screening on ovarian cancer mortality: the Prostate, Lung, Colorectal and Ovarian (PLCO) Cancer Screening Randomized Controlled Trial. JAMA. 2011;305(22):2295–303.
12. Kobayashi H, Yamada Y, Sado T, Sakata M, Yoshida S, Kawaguchi R, et al. A randomized study of screening for ovarian cancer: a multicenter study in Japan. Int J Gynecol Cancer. 2008;18(3):414–20.
13. Menon U, Gentry-Maharaj A, Hallett R, Ryan A, Burnell M, Sharma A, et al. Sensitivity and specificity of multimodal and ultrasound screening for ovarian cancer, and stage distribution of detected cancers: results of the prevalence screen of the UK Collaborative Trial of Ovarian Cancer Screening (UKCTOCS). Lancet Oncol. 2009;10(4):327–40.
14. Menon U, Ryan A, Kalsi J, Gentry-Maharaj A, Dawnay A, Habib M, et al. Risk Algorithm Using Serial Biomarker Measurements Doubles the Number of Screen-Detected Cancers Compared With a Single-Threshold Rule in the United Kingdom Collaborative Trial of Ovarian Cancer Screening. J Clin Oncol. 2015;33(18):2062–71.
15. Lim AWW, Mesher D, Gentry-Maharaj A, Balogun N, Widschwendter M, Jacobs I, et al. Time to diagnosis of Type I or II invasive epithelial ovarian cancers: a multicentre observational study using patient questionnaire and primary care records. BJOG. 2015:n/a-n/a
16. Surveillance Epidemiology and End Results Program. Ovary Cancer Survival Statistics [cited 2014 August 25]. Available from: http://seer.cancer.gov/statfacts/html/ovary.html.
17. Tone AA, Salvador S, Finlayson SJ, Tinker AV, Kwon JS, Lee CH, et al. The role of the fallopian tube in ovarian cancer. Clin Adv Hematol Oncol. 2012;10(5):296–306.
18. Kindelberger DW, Lee Y, Miron A, Hirsch MS, Feltmate C, Medeiros F, et al. Intraepithelial carcinoma of the fimbria and pelvic serous carcinoma: Evidence for a causal relationship. Am J Surg Pathol. 2007;31(2):161–9.
19. Kobel M, Kalloger SE, Boyd N, McKinney S, Mehl E, Palmer C, et al. Ovarian carcinoma subtypes are different diseases: implications for biomarker studies. PLoS Med. 2008;5(12):e232.
20. Gilks CB. Molecular abnormalities in ovarian cancer subtypes other than high-grade serous carcinoma. J Oncol. 2010;2010:740968.
21. Kobel M, Kalloger SE, Huntsman DG, Santos JL, Swenerton KD, Seidman JD, et al. Differences in tumor type in low-stage versus high-stage ovarian carcinomas. Int J Gynecol Pathol. 2010;29(3):203–11.
22. Fathalla MF. Incessant ovulation–a factor in ovarian neoplasia? Lancet. 1971;2(7716):163.
23. Doran A. An unreported case of primary cancer in the fallopian tubes in 1847, with notes on primary tubal cancers. Trans Obstet Soc Lond. 1896;38:322–6.
24. Lamb JD, Garcia RL, Goff BA, Paley PJ, Swisher EM. Predictors of occult neoplasia in women undergoing risk-reducing salpingo-oophorectomy. Am J Obstet Gynecol. 2006;194(6):1702–9.
25. Leeper K, Garcia R, Swisher E, Goff B, Greer B, Paley P. Pathologic findings in prophylactic oophorectomy specimens in high-risk women. Gynecol Oncol. 2002;87(1):52–6.
26. Lu KH, Garber JE, Cramer DW, Welch WR, Niloff J, Schrag D, et al. Occult ovarian tumors in women with BRCA1 or BRCA2 mutations undergoing prophylactic oophorectomy. J Clin Oncol. 2000;18(14):2728–32.
27. Powell CB, Chen LM, McLennan J, Crawford B, Zaloudek C, Rabban JT, et al. Risk-reducing salpingo-oophorectomy (RRSO) in BRCA mutation carriers: experience with a consecutive series of 111 patients using a standardized surgical-pathological protocol. Int J Gynecol Cancer. 2011;21(5):846–51.
28. Powell CB, Swisher EM, Cass I, McLennan J, Norquist B, Garcia RL, et al. Long term follow up of BRCA1 and BRCA2 mutation carriers with unsuspected neoplasia identified at risk reducing salpingo-oophorectomy. Gynecol Oncol. 2013;129(2):364–71.

29. Reitsma W, de Bock GH, Oosterwijk JC, Bart J, Hollema H, Mourits MJ. Support of the 'fallopian tube hypothesis' in a prospective series of risk-reducing salpingo-oophorectomy specimens. Eur J Cancer. 2013;49(1):132–41.

30. Wethington SL, Park KJ, Soslow RA, Kauff ND, Brown CL, Dao F, et al. Clinical outcome of isolated serous tubal intraepithelial carcinomas (STIC). Int J Gynecol Cancer. 2013;23(9):1603–11.

31. Callahan MJ, Crum CP, Medeiros F, Kindelberger DW, Elvin JA, Garber JE, et al. Primary fallopian tube malignancies in BRCA-positive women undergoing surgery for ovarian cancer risk reduction. J Clin Oncol. 2007;25(25):3985–90.

32. Cass I, Holschneider C, Datta N, Barbuto D, Walts AE, Karlan BY. BRCA-mutation-associated fallopian tube carcinoma: a distinct clinical phenotype? Obstet Gynecol. 2005;106(6):1327–34.

33. Colgan TJ, Murphy J, Cole DE, Narod S, Rosen B. Occult carcinoma in prophylactic oophorectomy specimens: prevalence and association with BRCA germline mutation status. Am J Surg Pathol. 2001;25(10):1283–9.

34. Finch A, Beiner M, Lubinski J, Lynch HT, Moller P, Rosen B, et al. Salpingo-oophorectomy and the risk of ovarian, fallopian tube, and peritoneal cancers in women with a BRCA1 or BRCA2 Mutation. JAMA. 2006;296(2):185–92.

35. Medeiros F, Muto MG, Lee Y, Elvin JA, Callahan MJ, Feltmate C, et al. The tubal fimbria is a preferred site for early adenocarcinoma in women with familial ovarian cancer syndrome. Am J Surg Pathol. 2006;30(2):230–6.

36. Shaw PA, Rouzbahman M, Pizer ES, Pintilie M, Begley H. Candidate serous cancer precursors in fallopian tube epithelium of BRCA1/2 mutation carriers. Mod Pathol. 2009;22(9):1133–8.

37. Yates MS, Meyer LA, Deavers MT, Daniels MS, Keeler ER, Mok SC, et al. Microscopic and early-stage ovarian cancers in BRCA1/2 mutation carriers: building a model for early BRCA-associated tumorigenesis. Cancer Prev Res. 2011;4(3):463–70.

38. Powell CB, Kenley E, Chen LM, Crawford B, McLennan J, Zaloudek C, et al. Risk-reducing salpingo-oophorectomy in BRCA mutation carriers: role of serial sectioning in the detection of occult malignancy. J Clin Oncol. 2005;23(1):127–32.

39. Carlson JW, Miron A, Jarboe EA, Parast MM, Hirsch MS, Lee Y, et al. Serous tubal intraepithelial carcinoma: its potential role in primary peritoneal serous carcinoma and serous cancer prevention. J Clin Oncol. 2008;26(25):4160–5.

40. Gao FF, Bhargava R, Yang H, Li Z, Zhao C. Clinicopathologic study of serous tubal intraepithelial carcinoma with invasive carcinoma: is serous tubal intraepithelial carcinoma a reliable feature for determining the organ of origin? Hum Pathol. 2013;44(8):1534–43.

41. Przybycin CG, Kurman RJ, Ronnett BM, Shih Ie M, Vang R. Are all pelvic (nonuterine) serous carcinomas of tubal origin? Am J Surg Pathol. 2010;34(10):1407–16.

42. Seidman JD, Zhao P, Yemelyanova A. "Primary peritoneal" high-grade serous carcinoma is very likely metastatic from serous tubal intraepithelial carcinoma: assessing the new paradigm of ovarian and pelvic serous carcinogenesis and its implications for screening for ovarian cancer. Gynecol Oncol. 2011;120(3):470–3.

43. Tang S, Onuma K, Deb P, Wang E, Lytwyn A, Sur M, et al. Frequency of serous tubal intraepithelial carcinoma in various gynecologic malignancies: a study of 300 consecutive cases. Int J Gynecol Pathol. 2012;31(2):103–10.

44. Salvador S, Rempel A, Soslow RA, Gilks B, Huntsman D, Miller D. Chromosomal instability in fallopian tube precursor lesions of serous carcinoma and frequent monoclonality of synchronous ovarian and fallopian tube mucosal serous carcinoma. Gynecol Oncol. 2008;110(3):408–17.

45. Kurman RJ, Shih IM. Molecular pathogenesis and extraovarian origin of epithelial ovarian cancer–shifting the paradigm. Hum Pathol. 2011;42(7):918–31.

46. Lee Y, Miron A, Drapkin R, Nucci MR, Medeiros F, Saleemuddin A, et al. A candidate precursor to serous carcinoma that originates in the distal fallopian tube. J Pathol. 2007;211(1):26–35.

47. Folkins AK, Jarboe EA, Saleemuddin A, Lee Y, Callahan MJ, Drapkin R, et al. A candidate precursor to pelvic serous cancer (p53 signature) and its prevalence in ovaries and fallopian tubes from women with BRCA mutations. Gynecol Oncol. 2008;109(2):168–73.

48. Kauff ND, Domchek SM, Friebel TM, Robson ME, Lee J, Garber JE, et al. Risk-reducing salpingo-oophorectomy for the prevention of BRCA1- and BRCA2-associated breast and gynecologic cancer: a multicenter, prospective study. J Clin Oncol. 2008;26(8):1331–7.

49. Domchek SM, Friebel TM, Singer CF, Evans DG, Lynch HT, Isaacs C, et al. Association of risk-reducing surgery in BRCA1 or BRCA2 mutation carriers with cancer risk and mortality. JAMA. 2010;304(9):967–75.

50. Finch A, Metcalfe KA, Chiang J, Elit L, McLaughlin J, Springate C, et al. The impact of prophylactic salpingo-oophorectomy on quality of life and psychological distress in women with a BRCA mutation. Psychooncology. 2013;22(1):212–9.

51. Parker WH, Broder MS, Chang E, Feskanich D, Farquhar C, Liu Z, et al. Ovarian conservation at the time of hysterectomy and long-term health outcomes in the nurses' health study. Obstet Gynecol. 2009;113(5):1027–37.

52. Parker WH, Feskanich D, Broder MS, Chang E, Shoupe D, Farquhar CM, et al. Long-term mortality associated with oophorectomy compared with ovarian conservation in the nurses' health study. Obstet Gynecol. 2013;121(4):709–16.

53. The Society of Gynecologic Oncology of Canada. GOC Statement regarding salpingectomy and ovarian cancer prevention. 2011. http://www.g-oc.org/uploads/11sept15_gocevidentiarystatement_final_en.pdf.

54. Society of Gynecologic Oncology. SGO Clinical Practice Statement: Salpingectomy for Ovarian Cancer. 2013. https://www.sgo.org/clinicalpractice/guidelines/sgo-clinical-practice-statement-salpingectomy-for-ovarian-cancer-prevention/.

55. American College of Obstetrics & Gynecology. Committee opinion no. 620: salpingectomy for ovarian cancer prevention. Obstet Gynecol. 2015;125(1):279–81.

56. Canadian Institutes for Health Information. Number, Percentage and Average length of stay for Top 10 High-Volume Inpatient Surgeries by Province/Territory, HMBD, 2014,2014. Ottawa, Canada: Canadian Insitutes of Health Information; 2015.

57. Wright JD, Herzog TJ, Tsui J, Ananth CV, Lewin SN, Lu YS, et al. Nationwide trends in the performance of inpatient hysterectomy in the United States. Obstet Gynecol. 2013;122(2 Pt 1):233–41.

58. Whiteman MK, Hillis SD, Jamieson DJ, Morrow B, Podgornik MN, Brett KM, et al. Inpatient hysterectomy surveillance in the United States, 2000–2004. Am J Obstet Gynecol. 2008;198(1):34 e1–7.

59. McAlpine JN, Hanley GE, Woo MM, Tone AA, Rozenberg N, Swenerton KD, et al. Opportunistic salpingectomy: uptake, risks, and complications of a regional initiative for ovarian cancer prevention. Am J Obstet Gynecol. 2014;210(5):471 e1–11.

60. Mosher WD, Jones J. Use of contraception in the United States: 1982–2008. Vital Health Stat 23. 2010(29):1–44

61. Kwon JS, McAlpine JN, Hanley GE, Finlayson S, Cohen T, Miller D, et al. Costs and benefits of opportunistic salpingectomy as an ovarian cancer prevention strategy. Obstet Gynecol. 2014;In Press.

62. Chan LM, Westhoff CL. Tubal sterilization trends in the United States. Fertil Steril. 2010;94(1):1–6.

63. Chakravarti S, Shardlow J. Tubal pregnancy after sterilization. Br J Obstet Gynaecol. 1975;82(1):58–60.

64. Anderson CK, Wallace S, Guiahi M, Sheeder J, Behbakht K, Spillman MA. Risk-reducing salpingectomy as preventative strategy for pelvic serous cancer. Int J Gynecol Cancer. 2013;23(3):417–21.

65. Kwon JS, Tinker A, Pansegrau G, McAlpine J, Housty M, McCullum M, et al. Prophylactic salpingectomy and delayed oophorectomy as an alternative for BRCA mutation carriers. Obstet Gynecol. 2013;121(1):14–24.

66. Leblanc E, Narducci F, Farre I, Peyrat JP, Taieb S, Adenis C, et al. Radical fimbriectomy: a reasonable temporary risk-reducing surgery for selected women with a germ line mutation of BRCA 1 or 2 genes? Rationale and preliminary development. Gynecol Oncol. 2011;121(3):472–6.

67. Juurlink D, Preyra C, Croxford R, Chong A, Austin P, Tu J, et al. Canadian Institute for Health Information Discharge Abstract Database: A validation study. Toronto: Institute for Clinical Evaluative Sciences; 2006.

68. Sandoval C, Fung-Kee-Fung M, Gilks B, Murphy KJ, Rahal R, Bryant H. Examining the use of salpingectomy with hysterectomy in Canada. Curr Oncol. 2013;20(3):173–5.

69. Lessard-Anderson CR, Handlogten KS, Molitor RJ, Dowdy SC, Cliby WA, Weaver AL, et al. Effect of tubal sterilization technique on risk of serous epithelial ovarian and primary peritoneal carcinoma. Gynecol Oncol. 2014;135(3):423–7.

70. Reade CJ, Finlayson S, McAlpine J, Tone AA, Fung-Kee-Fung M, Ferguson SE. Risk-reducing salpingectomy in Canada: a survey of obstetrician-gynaecologists. J Obstet Gynaecol Can. 2013;35(7):627–34.

71. Gill SE, Mills BB. Physician opinions regarding elective bilateral salpingectomy with hysterectomy and for sterilization. J Minim Invasive Gynecol. 2013;20(4):517–21.

72. Kamran MW, Vaughan D, Crosby D, Wahab NA, Saadeh FA, Gleeson N. Opportunistic and interventional salpingectomy in women at risk: a strategy

for preventing pelvic serous cancer (PSC). Eur J Obstet Gynecol Reprod Biol. 2013;170(1):251–4.

73. Morse AN, Schroeder CB, Magrina JF, Webb MJ, Wollan PC, Yawn BP. The risk of hydrosalpinx formation and adnexectomy following tubal ligation and subsequent hysterectomy: a historical cohort study. Am J Obstet Gynecol. 2006;194(5):1273–6.

74. Repasy I, Lendvai V, Koppan A, Bodis J, Koppan M. Effect of the removal of the Fallopian tube during hysterectomy on ovarian survival: the orphan ovary syndrome. Eur J Obstet Gynecol Reprod Biol. 2009;144(1):64–7.

75. Basu D, Ward SJ. Post-hysterectomy fallopian tube prolapse–a diagnostic pitfall. J Obstet Gynaecol. 2007;27(3):324.

76. Ghezzi F, Cromi A, Siesto G, Bergamini V, Zefiro F, Bolis P. Infectious morbidity after total laparoscopic hysterectomy: does concomitant salpingectomy make a difference? BJOG. 2009;116(4):589–93.

77. Piacenza JM, Salsano F. Post-hysterectomy fallopian tube prolapse. Eur J Obstet Gynecol Reprod Biol. 2001;98(2):253–5.

78. Rezvani M, Shaaban AM. Fallopian tube disease in the nonpregnant patient. Radiographics. 2011;31(2):527–48.

79. Singla A. An unusual case of torsion hydrosalpinx after hysterectomy: a case report. Aust N Z J Obstet Gynaecol. 2007;47(3):256–7.

80. Timor-Tritsch IE, Monteagudo A, Tsymbal T. Three-dimensional ultrasound inversion rendering technique facilitates the diagnosis of hydrosalpinx. J Clin Ultrasound. 2010;38(7):372–6.

81. Moorman PG, Myers ER, Schildkraut JM, Iversen ES, Wang F, Warren N. Effect of hysterectomy with ovarian preservation on ovarian function. Obstet Gynecol. 2011;118(6):1271-9.

82. Farquhar CM, Sadler L, Harvey SA, Stewart AW. The association of hysterectomy and menopause: a prospective cohort study. BJOG. 2005;112(7):956-62.

83. Morelli M, Venturella R, Mocciaro R, Di Cello A, Rania E, Lico D, et al. Prophylactic salpingectomy in premenopausal low-risk women for ovarian cancer: primum non nocere. Gynecol Oncol. 2013;129(3):448–51.

84. Findley AD, Siedhoff MT, Hobbs KA, Steege JF, Carey ET, McCall CA, et al. Short-term effects of salpingectomy during laparoscopic hysterectomy on ovarian reserve: a pilot randomized controlled trial. Fertil Steril. 2013;100(6):1704–8.

85. Rice MS, Murphy MA, Tworoger SS. Tubal ligation, hysterectomy and ovarian cancer: A meta-analysis. J Ovarian Res. 2012;5(1):13.

86. Sieh W, Salvador S, McGuire V, Weber RP, Terry KL, Rossing MA, et al. Tubal ligation and risk of ovarian cancer subtypes: a pooled analysis of case–control studies. Int J Epidemiol. 2013;42(2):579–89.

87. Madsen C, Baandrup L, Dehlendorff C, Kjaer SK. Tubal ligation and salpingectomy and the risk of epithelial ovarian cancer and borderline ovarian tumors: a nationwide case–control study. Acta Obstet Gynecol Scand. 2015;94(1):86–94.

88. Falconer H, Yin L, Gronberg H, Altman D. Ovarian cancer risk after salpingectomy: a nationwide population-based study. J Natl Cancer Inst. 2015;107(2).

89. McGuire V, Felberg A, Mills M, Ostrow KL, DiCioccio R, John EM, et al. Relation of contraceptive and reproductive history to ovarian cancer risk in carriers and noncarriers of BRCA1 gene mutations. Am J Epidemiol. 2004;160(7):613–8.

90. Lin HW, Tu YY, Lin SY, Su WJ, Lin WL, Lin WZ, et al. Risk of ovarian cancer in women with pelvic inflammatory disease: a population-based study. Lancet Oncol. 2011;12(9):900–4.

91. Pearce CL, Templeman C, Rossing MA, Lee A, Near AM, Webb PM, et al. Association between endometriosis and risk of histological subtypes of ovarian cancer: a pooled analysis of case–control studies. Lancet Oncol. 2012;13(4):385–94.

92. Herzog TJ, Dinkelspiel HE. Fallopian tube removal: "stic-ing" it to ovarian cancer: what is the utility of prophylactic tubal removal? Curr Oncol. 2013;20(3):148–51.

93. van den Akker-van Marle ME, van Ballegooijen M, van Oortmarssen GJ, Boer R, Habbema JDF. Cost-Effectiveness of Cervical Cancer Screening: Comparison of Screening Policies. J Natl Cancer Inst. 2002;94(3):193–204.

94. Brisson M, Van de Velde N, De Wals P, Boily MC. Estimating the number needed to vaccinate to prevent diseases and death related to human papillomavirus infection. CMAJ. 2007;177(5):464–8.

95. Rebbeck TR, Kauff ND, Domchek SM. Meta-analysis of risk reduction estimates associated with risk-reducing salpingo-oophorectomy in BRCA1 or BRCA2 mutation carriers. J Natl Cancer Inst. 2009;101(2):80–7.

96. Foulkes WD. Preventing ovarian cancer by salpingectomy. Curr Oncol. 2013;20(3):139–42.

11

Updates on drug discovery in ovarian cancer

Steven J Gibson[1,2], Krishnansu S Tewari[3], Bradley J Monk[1,2] and Dana M Chase[1,2]*

Abstract

Drug discovery in the ovarian cancer arena continues to launch important new clinical trials. Many biologic agents are being studied in phase II and phase III clinical trials for recurrent disease. These agents include compounds that disrupt angiogenesis through a variety of mechanisms. Other oncogenic pathways are also specifically targeted such as PARP, MEK, and topoisomerase inhibitors which are currently being studied in phase III trials. Various cytotoxic agents, as well as therapeutic vaccines, are also under investigation, and continue to demonstrate promising new data. The relevant agents in the treatment of ovarian cancer which have demonstrated positive phase II activity will be discussed.

Keywords: Ovarian cancer, Chemotherapy, Targeted therapy, Angiogenesis, Recurrent cancer, Clinical trials

Review

Remissions after primary therapy in ovarian cancer are usually short-lived. Although intially responsive to a platinum and taxane-based therapy, recurrent disease is difficult to treat. Furthermore, there are few approved agents to treat recurrent ovarian cancer. Although patients that recur after 6 to 12 months of initial treatment may be retreated with a platinum plus taxane, those who relapse earlier or develop significant toxicity, may be given pegalated lipsomal doxorubicin, gemcitabine (in combination with platinum), etoposide, alkeran, topotecan, and/or hexamethylmelamine [1]. Unfortunately the response rate to these agents is generally less than 30%, and demonstrable survival benefits have not been shown. With the introduction of targeted drugs, such as trastuzumab in breast cancer, strategies in drug development have focused on the development of biologic agents that demonstrate selectivity for tumor tissue.

Introduction

In 2010, we published on recent advances in drug discovery for ovarian cancer [1]. Since then, multiple drugs have either failed to advance into further development, have newly been developed, or have demonstrated activity in phase III trials. For example, with respect to

* Correspondence: Dana.chase@chw.edu
[1]The Division of Gynecologic Oncology, University of Arizona Cancer Center, 500 West Thomas Road, Suite 600, Phoenix, AZ 85013, USA
[2]Creighton University School of Medicine, St. Joseph's Hospital and Medical Center, A Dignity Health Member, 500 West Thomas Road, Suite 600, Phoenix, AZ 85013, USA
Full list of author information is available at the end of the article

bevacizumab, several positive phase III trials have supported the use of this drug in upfront and recurrent ovarian cancer cases yet FDA approval is pending. Another example includes a 940 patient, phase III AGO-OVAR16 study which proved advantageous in ovarian cancer treatment with pazopanib, increasing median progression-free survival (PFS) by about 5.6 months [2]. In addition, trabectedin was previously discussed and positive phase III activity was reported, improving PFS, and overall response rate in a 672 patient study [3]. Lastly, phase III results from the TRINOVA-1 trial of over 900 patients found that trebananib (AMG 386) increased PFS as well as reduced disease progression and death by 34% when combined with paclitaxel. Unfortunately, several of the drugs previously described have been found to be inactive, or with disappointing clinical outcomes. This review will thus highlight new drugs for ovarian cancer that have recently demonstrated positive phase II activity (Table 1). The ultimate goal with this type of drug development is to achieve prolonged remission and improved quality of life (QOL), for patients with recurrent ovarian cancer.

Targeted agents
Angiogenesis inhibitors
VEGF-dependent

Vascular endothelial growth factor (VEGF) is a signaling molecule involved in triggering the growth of blood vessels within cancers. The VEGF mechanism of action encompasses binding to tyrosine kinase transmembrane

Table 1 Updates in ovarian cancer drug discovery demonstrating positive phase II activity

Category		Agent/patent (manufacturer)	Mechanism of action
Targeted agents	VEGF-dependent angiogenesis inhibition	**Cediranib** (AZD2171)/US20070135462 (AstraZeneca)	Oral VEGFR-1,-2,-3 tyrosine kinase inhibitor
		Nintedanib (BIBF1120)/US20140018405 (Boehringer Ingelheim)	Oral VEGFR, PDGFR, FGFR tyrosine kinase inhibitor
	PARP inhibitors	**Olaparib** (AZD2281)/US2010098763 (AstraZeneca)	Oral Poly (ADP-ribose) polymerase-1,-2 inhibitor
		Rucaparib (CO-338)/US8765751 (Clovis Oncology)	Oral Poly (ADP-ribose) polymerase-1,-2 inhibitor
		Niraparib (MK-4827)/US20120035244 (Merck)	Oral Poly (ADP-ribose) polymerase-1,-2 inhibitor
	MEK inhibitors	**Selumetinib** (AZD6244)/US8193229 (Array BioPharma/AstraZeneca)	Oral inhibitor of MEK-1,-2
		Binimetinib (MEK162)/US20130273061 (Array BioPharma/Novartis)	Oral inhibitor of MEK-1,-2
Cytotoxic agents		**Etirinotecan pegol** (NKTR-102)/US20090074704 (Nektar)	Inhibits Topoisomerase I (IV)
		Paclitaxel poliglumex (CT2103)/US20070167349 (CTI BioPharma)	Mitotic inhibitor (IV)
		Lurbinectedin (PM1183)/US20130266666 (PharmaMar)	Marine-derived DNA minor groove binder (IV)
Therapeutic vaccines		**Catumaxomab**/US20120095192 (Trion Pharma)	Oral tri-functional antibody binds EpCAM, CD3, and Fc receptor

receptors (VEGFR), found on tumor endothelial cells, initiating angiogenesis (Figure 1) [4]. VEGFR-2 regulates cellular VEGF interactions, making it a crucial component in the angiogenic process. Modulating VEGF has become a highlighted area of study with potential in therapeutic interventions.

VEGFR-1,-2,-3 inhibitor: cediranib (AZD2171)
While multiple phase III trials of cediranib (Recentin™) may have been disappointing for colon cancer drug discovery, the drug has gained noticeable attention in the treatment of ovarian cancer [5,6]. Cediranib is a potent anti-angiogenesis agent that acts by blocking the VEGF signaling cascade via the inhibition of all three VEGFR tyrosine kinases, thus preventing the formation of tumor vasculature [7].

Cediranib was evaluated in combination with the PARP inhibitor, olaparib, in the first ovarian cancer trial to utilize two orally-administered investigational drugs [8]. The multi-center, phase II study comparing olaparib

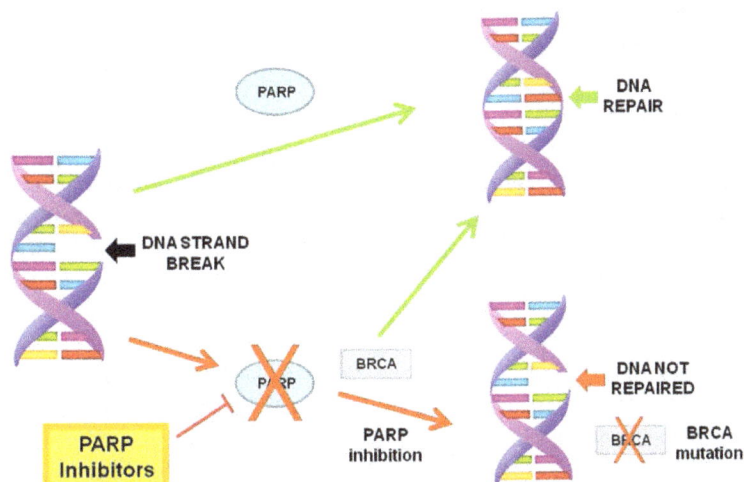

Figure 1 Poly(ADP-Ribose) polymerase (PARP) inhibitors.

(400 mg twice daily) to cediranib (30 mg daily) plus olaparib (200 mg twice daily) found that the combination had nearly doubled PFS (9 vs 17.7 months). Of the 90 platinum-sensitive or BRCA-mutation patients in the study, significantly more had an objective response rate (ORR) in the combination group (56% vs 84%). With these improvements in PFS and ORR came an increase in grade 3/4 toxicities, with about ten times as many observed with the combination (7% vs 70%) [9]. The ICON6 phase III European trial found similar improvements in PFS and overall survival (OS) when cediranib was combined with platinum-based chemotherapy [10]. With these encouraging results, the planning of a phase III cediranib and olaparib combination trial is underway [8].

VEGF receptor, platelet-derived and fibroblast growth factor receptor: Nintedanib (BIBF 1120)

The additional targeting of proangiogenic receptors continues to be of interest, and has been proposed to improve the efficacy of VEGF blockade. Nintedanib is a triple angiokinase inhibitor that simultaneously blocks the VEGF, platelet-derived, and fibroblast growth factor receptors [11]. When studied in animal tumor models, nintedanib effectively reduced tumor blood vessel density and integrity [12].

A randomized, placebo-controlled phase II trial evaluated nintedanib maintenance therapy (250 mg for 36 weeks), after chemotherapy in patients with relapsed ovarian cancer. Eighty-three women were enrolled and following the treatment cycle, the PFS was 16.3% for nintedanib patients and 5% for placebo patients. Nintedanib patients experienced a much higher rate of grade 3 or 4 hepatotoxicity (51.2%), compared to that of the placebo group (7.5%) [13]. The potential effect of nintedanib nearly tripling PFS, when compared to the placebo, has warranted a 1,300 patient, phase III study of this drug in the LUME-Ovar 1 trial [14]. Phase III trials of nintedanib are also currently underway for non-small cell lung cancer and being planned for hepatocellular, renal, and colorectal cancers [12].

Poly (ADP-ribose) polymerase inhibitor
Olaparib (AZD2281)

Poly(ADP-ribose) polymerases (PARPs) are proteins involved in the repair of DNA [15]. PARPs assist in the repair of DNA single-strand breaks by repairing base excisions. BRCA1 and BRCA2 proteins involved in DNA recombination play crucial roles in repairing double-strand breaks, and can do so in the setting of PARP inhibition. However, PARP inhibition in BRCA-deficient cells results in the incapability to repair DNA damage induced by chemotherapy. In a BRCA-deficient environment, cell death can manifest when DNA breakage is not repaired, and the cell is exposed to such agents as PARP inhibitors that hinder single-strand break repair (Figure 1) [16].

BRCA mutations represent a minority of breast and ovarian cancers. These homozygous mutations, that are unique to the tumor cells, result in the inability to repair DNA which then can be exclusively targeted by a PARP inhibitor, preserving the patient's non-tumor cells. Preclinical studies discussed by Fong et al. [17] demonstrate that BRCA-deficient cells were 1000-fold more sensitive to PARP inhibitors. Ledermann et al. supported these findings in subgroup analysis of a 265 patient study evaluating olaparib (400 mg) maintenance therapy in platinum-sensitive, relapsed ovarian cancer. The original phase II study found PFS to be significantly longer with olaparib maintenance than placebo (8.4 vs. 4.8 months, respectively) [18]. A preplanned, subgroup analysis showed patients with a BRCA mutation (BRCAm) had the greatest clinical benefit, specifically germline BRCAm which had a 7.1 month increase in PFS and significant improvement in QOL. They found an average 6.9 month increase in PFS, an 8.5 month improvement in time to second disease progression, and a three month increase in OS in BRCAm patients when compared with placebo [19].

These results have initiated two phase III (SOLO) trials [20]. The U.S.-based SOLO1 trial, will examine olaparib (300 mg twice daily) as maintenance therapy in 2,500 BRCAm ovarian cancer patients following first-line platinum chemotherapy [21]. The European-based SOLO2 trail will examine the same dosage of olaparib maintenance therapy but instead in 440 BRCAm patients with platinum-sensitive, relapsed, or recurrent ovarian cancer [22].

A separate, randomized, phase II study also found significant improvement in PFS with the addition of olaparib to paclitaxel and carboplatin followed by subsequent maintenance therapy (12.2 vs. 9.6 months placebo). The ORR remained fairly similar (64% vs. 58%), and the most common adverse events reported in the combination phase were alopecia, nausea, and fatigue [23].

Rucaparib (CO-338)

Rucaparib is an inhibitor of poly(ADP-ribose) polymerases 1 and 2, and works via the same mechanism as olaparib described above and illustrated in Figure 1. Data suggests that PARP inhibitors are especially effective in patients with mutations in DNA repair mechanisms, such as those carrying BRCA mutations [24]. The ARIEL2 trial is investigating specific biomarkers like these to evaluate which, if any, subgroups of the 180 ovarian cancer patients may be sensitive to rucaparib treatment [25]. This data will be incorporated into ARIEL3, a current, randomized, double-blind study phase III trial comparing rucaparib treatment to placebo in 540 ovarian cancer patients [26].

Niraparib (MK-4827)

Niraparib, like the other PARP inhibitors above in Figure 1, blocks poly(ADP-ribose) polymerases 1 and 2 from repairing single-strand breaks in damaged DNA. While most PARP inhibitors exhibit similar catalytic inhibitory properties, it is important to note the differences in potency among drugs in this class [27]. Many propose this discrepancy is due to each drug's individual ability to trap the PARPs at the damaged DNA site. Interestingly, the trapped PARP-DNA complex that forms is more cytotoxic than the single-strand DNA break itself, associating the potency of PARP inhibitors to their ability to form these complexes [27,28]. Murai, et al. demonstrated that niraparib was the most potent of the PARP inhibitors due to its superior ability in forming the trapped PARP-DNA complex [28].

A large, 100 patient, phase I trial evaluated niraparib in BRCA 1/2 mutation-carrying (BRCA-MC) patients with high-grade serous ovarian cancer (HGSOC) (n = 49), among others cancers. Of these ovarian cancer patients, 45% had a partial response from niraparib (60 mg daily). The platinum-sensitive HGSOC subgroup had a response rate almost double that of the platinum-resistant group (60% vs. 33%, respectively), with a median time of response of 429 compared to 340 days. The most common adverse events were grade 1/2 anemia (48%), fatigue (42%), nausea (42%), and thrombocytopenia (35%). The maximum tolerated dose was determined to be 300 mg daily [29]. Niraparib is currently being studied as maintenance therapy in the randomized, phase III NOVA trial evaluating daily niraparib (300 mg) in 360 patients with high grade serous, platinum sensitive, relapsed ovarian cancer [30].

MAPK kinase (MEK-1 and −2) inhibitors
Selumetinib (AZD6244)

Selumetinib is a mitogen-activated protein kinase inhibitor that shows preclinical benefit in targeting the MEK oncogenic pathway. The small molecular agent is a protein regulator in activated oncogenic pathways expressed in ovarian cancer patients. Results from a phase II study indicate positive activity in the treatment of ovarian cancer. Fifty-two women received two doses of selumetinib (100 mg daily) in the clinical trial, and grade 4 adverse events were only observed in 3 patients (6%). Thirty-four (63%) of the women in the study had a PFS of more than 6 months, with a median OS of 11 months [31]. Larger phase III studies are being planned to further investigate the use of selumetinib as a viable treatment option in ovarian cancer.

Binimetinib (MEK162)

Binimetinib is an oral inhibitor of MEK-1 and MEK-2, both of which play an important role in cancer cell

proliferation and survival via the RAS/RAF/MEK/ERK signal cascade. Inhibiting this pathway is believed to interrupt growth-factor mediated cell signaling as well as inhibit the production of inflammatory cytokines [32]. Binimetinib is currently the subject of nearly twenty clinical trials, including three phase III trials in ovarian cancer and melanoma [33]. The MILO study is an international, randomized phase III study seeking to compare binimetinib to standard chemotherapy in 300 low-grade serous ovarian cancer (LGSOC) patients [34]. With LGSOC representing about 10% of all ovarian cancer diagnoses, chemotherapy response rates remain much lower in this group than in their high-grade counterparts. Even more so, less than 4% of recurrent LGSOC patients respond to additional chemotherapy [33]. The results of the MILO study are highly anticipated, as women with pretreated, recurrent LGSOC do not currently have a successful treatment option [35].

Topoisomerase I inhibitors
Etirinotecan pegol (NKTR-102)

Etirinotecan pegol is a next-generation topoisomerase I inhibitors. Topoisomerase I inhibitors are typically semi-synthetic derivatives of the plant extract camptothecin that prevent DNA from unwinding and therefore impede tumor cells from replicating [36]. When normal topoisomerase I inhibitors like irinotecan and belotecan are quickly dispersed within the body, they not only damage healthy tissues, but also have poor half-lives, and do not sufficiently expose the tumor to the concentrated therapeutic agent. Etirinotecan pegol, instead connects small cytotoxic agents to a macromolecular polymer, using specialized linkers. These linkers are then slowly metabolized, resulting in a continuous, controlled release of the chemotherapy, which works as previously described by inhibiting topoisomerase I, and thus, hindering the division of the tumor cells. Preclinical studies have shown a 300-fold increase in the chemotherapy concentration, within the tumor, when compared to other topoisomerase I inhibitors. Along with this, increased effectiveness in tumor concentrations, the half-life of this agent has improved to 50 days, with activity in circulation throughout the entire cell cycle [37].

Clinical trials are under investigation for the use of this agent in various cancers, including ovarian cancer. One phase II, open-label study evaluated etirinotecan pegol (145 mg/m^2), every 14 or 21 days in 71 women with platinum-resistant or refractory ovarian cancer. Of patients receiving the drug every 14 days, 27% had a RECIST response compared to 22% for those receiving it every 21 days. CA-125 responses were 61% and 52%, respectively, with a median time of 31 days to 50% decline in CA-125. The most common grade 3/4 toxicities included diarrhea (22% vs. 11%, respectively), dehydration (14% vs. 6%, respectively), and hypokalemia (14% vs. 6%, respectively) [38]. Further investigation was encouraged by the activity observed in these heavily pretreated patients.

A different randomized, multicenter, phase II trial evaluated etirinotecan pegol (145 mg/m^2) every 14 or 21 days in 71 women with platinum-resistant or refractory ovarian cancer. Patients who received the agent every 14 days had a slightly higher response rate and response duration (20% and 4.1 months, respectively) than those who received it every 21 days (19% and 4.0 months, respectively). Median PFS and overall response rates were higher in patients receiving the drug every 21 days (5.3 and 11.7 months, respectively) than those receiving it every 14 days (4.1 and 10.0 months, respectively). The drug was well tolerated with grade 3/4 toxicities including dehydration (24%) and diarrhea (23%). Planning for a phase III investigation of etirinotecan pegol (145 mg/m^2) every 21 days is currently underway [39]. Phase III investigation in ovarian cancer has also been encouraged by the recent, positive interim efficacy analysis in the phase III BEACON trial for metastatic breast cancer [40].

Cytotoxic agents
Mitotic Inhibitor
Paclitaxel poliglumex (CT2103)
Paclitaxel poliglumex is an agent that utilizes polyglutamate drug delivery technology, similar to that described in etirinotecan pegol above. These polyglutamate molecules are much larger than standard paclitaxel molecules, allowing them to lodge themselves in tumor tissue through leaky tumor vasculature. The drug remains inactive in the bloodstream and is too large to fit through normal vasculature, so it specifically targets only tumor cells. Once inside the tumor tissue, the agent is slowly metabolized by the tumor cells, resulting in the controlled release of the cytotoxic agent. This process reduces toxicity to healthy tissues while simultaneously increasing efficacy [41]. Paclitaxel poliglumex falls into the mitotic inhibitor drug class and is under investigation in the treatment of ovarian cancer [42].

Paclitaxel poliglumex (OPAXIO™) has completed enrollment in a 1,100 patient, randomized phase III trial comparing 12 cycles of maintenance therapy paclitaxel poliglumex or paclitaxel versus no treatment [43]. The previous phase II data that encouraged this phase III trial came nearly 10 years ago in the study of carboplatin with paclitaxel poliglumex in 82 ovarian cancer patients. The study reported 98% of patients having a major tumor response with reduction in CA-125 levels, complete responses occurring in 85% of patients, and partial response in 12%. The most common adverse events were grade 3/4 neutropenia (92%), thrombocytopenia (55%), and neuropathy (23%) [44].

DNA minor groove binders
Lurbinectedin (PM1183)
Lurbinectedin is a synthetic analogue of trabectedin (previously discussed) [1]. Positive phase III results were reported for the combination of trabectedin with pegylated liposomal doxorubicin, increasing PFS and overall response rate in women with relapsed ovarian cancer [45]. Trabectedin became the first marine-derived cancer drug, derived from the colonial tunicate, *Ecteinascidia turbinate*, and marketed in Europe and Japan as Yondelis® [46]. Lurbinectedin has the same structure as trabectedin, differing only in the C subunit. Soares et al. found that the modified C subunit did not significantly alter lurbinectedin activity or cytotoxicity, and suggested the new analogue may be useful for altering dosages to increase antitumor activity [47]. Lurbinectedin works by covalently binding the minor groove in DNA. This binding causes the DNA strand to bend, increasing the incidence of double-strand breaks while also interfering with cell cycle processes and the nucleotide excision repair pathway [48].

Early *in vivo* mouse models demonstrated that single-agent lurbinectedin was effective in treating cisplatin-sensitive and cisplatin-resistant ovarian tumor models. Preclinical data also suggested that the combination of lurbinectedin with cisplatin-combined therapy was especially effective in the cisplatin-resistant tumors [49]. A randomized, phase II study of 81 platinum-resistant/refractory ovarian cancer patients compared lurbinectedin to topotecan and found that lurbinectedin had significantly improved OS (10.6 vs 5.7 months), PFS (3.9 vs 2.0 months), and the overall response rate (22%). In the lurbinectedin treatment arm, 85% of patients experienced grade 3/4 neutropenia, which was found to be preventable by using a G-CSF blood stimulating factor [50]. With this encouraging data and the success of trabectedin, lurbinectedin has received Orphan Drug status from the FDA and phase III trials in platinum-resistant patients have been planned [48,50].

Therapeutic vaccines
EpCAM, CD3, and Fc receptor antibody
Catumaxomab
Catumaxomab (Removab®) is classified as a trifunctional antibody, with a structure comprised of an anti-EpCAM antibody and an anti-CD3 antibody. This allows catumaxomab to bind to the antigen EpCAM on tumor cells, the CD3 molecules on T cells, and to the Fc receptor on accessory cells, and in doing so, trigger an antitumor immune response [51]. Catumaxomab was approved in Europe in 2009 for the intraperitoneal treatment of malignant ascites in EpCAM-positive cancer patients, and it is currently in clinical trials in the U.S. [52]. Approximately 10% of ascites, which is the

accumulation of fluid in the peritoneal cavity, is caused by cancer and called malignant ascites [53].

An open-label, phase II study of catumaxomab in patients with malignant ascites enrolled 32 women and found almost one-fourth (22.6%) of patients had at least a 400% increase in their platinum-free interval after catumaxomab treatment. Patients received catumaxomab (10, 20, 50, 150 μg) on days 0, 3, 7, and 10. The median OS was 3.6 months, with toxicities that were tolerable and consistent with what would be expected for this type of antibody [54]. Another single-arm phase II study administered one intraoperative (10 μg) and four postoperative (10, 20, 50, 150 μg) doses of catumaxomab on days 7, 10, 13, and 16. The study found a 3-year survival benefit in patients who received catumaxomab when compared to a match-pair control group (respective survival rates of 85.4% and 63.4%) [55]. This favorable survival data initiated a phase III trial of 258 EpCAM-positive cancer patients with malignant ascites [56].

Conclusions

As the inclusion of unconventional agents are increasingly incorporated into clinical trials and practice, the hope is that drug discovery will be encouraged in all areas of cancer therapy, from improving our ability to predict response to chemotherapy, to enhancing the delivery of drugs to targeted tissues. As stated previously in an earlier review [1], with the future of cancer treatment moving towards a more personalized approach, the goal is that an individual profile will be determined, and thus agents used that target key pathways in this individual's cancer.

Competing interests
Dr. Tewari reports that he does have contracted research with Biogen Idec, Amgen, Genentech, US Biotest, and Precision Therapeutics. Dr. Monk discloses that his institution has received research grants from Novartis, Amgen, Genentech, Lilly, Janssen/Johson & Johnson, Array, and TESARO. Additionally, Dr. Monk reports that he has received honoraria from Roche/Genentech as well are consulting fees from Roche/Genentech, GlaxoSmithKline, Merck, TESARO, Boehringer Ingelheim, and AstraZeneca.

Authors' contributions
DMC, BJM, and KST all provided writing assistance and general support to SJG in the preparation of the tables, figures, and drafting of the manuscript. All authors read and approved the final manuscript.

Acknowledgements
The authors would like to thank Daniele A. Sumner, BA for her assistance in editing the manuscript. The authors are solely responsible for the preparation and content of the manuscript.

Author details
[1]The Division of Gynecologic Oncology, University of Arizona Cancer Center, 500 West Thomas Road, Suite 600, Phoenix, AZ 85013, USA. [2]Creighton University School of Medicine, St. Joseph's Hospital and Medical Center, A Dignity Health Member, 500 West Thomas Road, Suite 600, Phoenix, AZ 85013, USA. [3]The Division of Gynecologic Oncology, Department of Obstetrics & Gynecology, The Chao Family Comprehensive Cancer Center, University of California, Irvine Medical Center, 101 The City Drive South, Building 56, Room 275, Orange, CA 92868, USA.

References
1. Chase DM, Mathur N, Tewari KS: Drug discovery in ovarian cancer. *Recent Pat Anticancer Drug Discov* 2010, **5**:251–260.
2. Du Bois A, Floquet A, Kim JW, Rau J, Del Campo JM, Friedlander M, Pignata S, Fujiwara K, Vergote I, Colombo N, Mirza MR, Monk BJ, Wimberger P, Ray-Coquard I, Zang R, Diaz-Padilla I, Baumann KH, Kim JH, Harter P: Randomized, double-blind, phase III trial of pazopanib versus placebo in women who have not progressed after first-line chemotherapy for advanced epithelial ovarian, fallopian tube, or primary peritoneal cancer (AEOC): Results of an international Intergroup trial (AGO-OVAR16). *J Clin Oncol* 2013, **31**:LBA5503.
3. Krasner CN, Poveda A, Herzog TJ, Vermorken JB, Kaye SB, Nieto A, Claret PL, Park YC, Parekh T, Monk BJ: Patient-reported outcomes in relapsed ovarian cancer: results from a randomized Phase III study of trabectedin with pegylated liposomal doxorubicin (PLD) versus PLD alone. *Gynecol Oncol* 2012, **127**:161–167.
4. Li JL, Harris AL: Crosstalk of VEGF and Notch pathways in tumour angiogenesis: therapeutic implications. *Front Biosci* 2009, **14**:3094–3110.
5. Hoff PM, Hochhaus A, Pestalozzi BC, Tebbutt NC, Li J, Kim TW, Koynov KD, Kurteva G, Pintér T, Cheng Y, van Eyll B, Pike L, Fielding A, Robertson JD, Saunders MP: Cediranib Plus FOLFOX/CAPOX Versus Placebo Plus FOLFOX/CAPOX in Patients With Previously Untreated Metastatic Colorectal Cancer: A Randomized, Double-Blind, Phase III Study (HORIZON II). *JCO* 2012, **30**:3596–3603.
6. Schmoll HJ, Cunningham D, Sobrero A, Karapetis CS, Rougier P, Koski SL, Kocakova I, Bondarenko I, Bodoky G, Mainwaring P, Salazar R, Barker P, Mookerjee B, Robertson J, Van Cutsem E: Cediranib With mFOLFOX6 Versus Bevacizumab With mFOLFOX6 As First-Line Treatment for Patients With Advanced Colorectal Cancer: A Double-Blind, Randomized Phase III Study (HORIZON III). *JCO* 2012, **30**:3588–3595.
7. NCI Drug Dictionary: *cediranib maleate*. National Cancer Institute at the National Institutes of Health.
8. AstraZeneca Press Release: *AstraZeneca welcomes positive data on the combination of olaparib and cediranib for the treatment of ovarian cancer patients*; 2014.
9. Liu J, Barry WT, Birrer MJ, Lee JM, Buckanovich RJ, Fleming GF, Rimel BJ, Buss MK, Nattam SR, Hurteau J, Luo W, Quy P, Obermayer E, Whalen C, Lee H, Winer EP, Kohn EC, Ivy SP, Matulonis U: A randomized phase 2 trial comparing efficacy of the combination of the PARP inhibitor olaparib and the antiangiogenic cediranib against olaparib alone in recurrent platinum-sensitive ovarian cancer. *J Clin Oncol* 2014, **32**:5s.
10. ICON6: *Cediranib in Ovarian Cancer.* http://www.icon6.org.
11. Hilberg F, Roth GJ, Krssak M, Kautschitsch S, Sommergruber W, Tontsch-Grunt U, Garin-Chesa P, Bader G, Zoephel A, Quant J, Heckel A, Rettig WJ: BIBF 1120: triple angiokinase inhibitor with sustained receptor blockade and good antitumor efficacy. *Cancer Res* 2008, **68**:4774–4782.
12. Nintedanib (BIBF 1120): *Boehringer Ingelheim*; 2012.
13. Ledermann JA, Hackshaw A, Kaye S, Jayson G, Gabra H, McNeish I, Earl H, Perren T, Gore M, Persic M, Adams M, James L, Temple G, Merger M, Rustin G: Randomized phase II placebo-controlled trial of maintenance therapy using the oral triple angiokinase inhibitor BIBF 1120 after chemotherapy for relapsed ovarian cancer. *J Clin Oncol* 2011, **29**:3798–3804.
14. LUME-Ovar 1: *Nintedanib (BIBF 1120) or Placebo in Combination With Paclitaxel and Carboplatin in First Line Treatment of Ovarian Cancer.* http://clinicaltrials.gov/show/NCT01015118.
15. Beaton G, Moree WJ, Rueter JK, Dahl RS, McElligott DL, Goldman P, DeMaggio AJ, Christenson E, Herendeen D, Fowler KW, Huang D, Bertino JE, Bourdon LH, Fairfax DJ, Jiang Q, Reisch HA, Song RH, Zhichkin PE: *PARP inhibitors.* 2005. US6924284.
16. De Lartigue J: *New Life for PARP Inhibitors: Emerging Agents Leave Mark at ASCO.* OncLive; 2013. http://www.onclive.com/publications/Oncology-live/2013/August-2013/New-Life-for-PARP-Inhibitors-Emerging-Agents-Leave-Mark-at-ASCO.
17. Fong PC, Boss DS, Yap TA, Tutt A, Wu P, Mergui-Roelvink M, Mortimer P, Swaisland H, Lau A, O'Connor MJ, Ashworth A, Carmichael J, Kaye SB, Schellens JH, de Bono JS: Inhibition of poly(ADP-ribose) polymerase in tumors from BRCA mutation carriers. *N Engl J Med* 2009, **361**:123–134.

18. Ledermann J, Harter P, Gourley C, Friedlander M, Vergote I, Rustin G, Scott C, Meier W, Shapira-Frommer R, Safra T, Matei D, Macpherson E, Watkins C, Carmichael J, Matulonis U: **Olaparib maintenance therapy in platinum-sensitive relapsed ovarian cancer.** *N Engl J Med* 2012, 366:1382–1392.

19. Goodman A: *Olaparib Shows Robust Progression-Free Survival Benefit in Patients With BRCA Mutations.* The ASCO Post; 2013. http://www.ascopost.com/issues/september-1,-2013/olaparib-shows-robust-progression-free-survival-benefit-in-patients-with-brca-mutations.aspx; http://ovariancancertrials.com/ovarian-cancer-studies/solo-2/.

20. *Studies of olaparib in ovarian cancer (SOLO).* AstraZeneca; 2014. http://ovariancancertrials.com/.

21. *Olaparib Monotherapy in Patients With BRCA Mutated Ovarian Cancer Following First Line Platinum Based Chemotherapy.* http://clinicaltrials.gov/show/NCT01844986.

22. *Olaparib Treatment in BRCA Mutated Ovarian Cancer Patients After Complete or Partial Response to Platinum Chemotherapy.* http://clinicaltrials.gov/show/NCT01874353.

23. Oza AM, Cibula D, Oaknin A, Poole CJ, Mathijssen RHJ, Sonke GS, Colombo N, Spacek J, Vuylsteke P, Hirte HW, Mahner S, Plante M, Schmalfeldt B, Mackay H, Rowbottom J, Tchakov I, Friedlander M: **Olaparib plus paclitaxel plus carboplatin (P/C) followed by olaparib maintenance treatment in patients (pts) with platinum-sensitive recurrent serous ovarian cancer (PSR SOC): A randomized, open-label phase II study.** *J Clin Oncol* 2012, 30:5001.

24. ARIEL2/ARIEL3: *New Clinical Trials for Ovarian Cancer.* http://www.arielstudy.com.

25. *A Study of Rucaparib in Patients With Platinum-Sensitive, Relapsed, High-Grade Epithelial Ovarian, Fallopian Tube, or Primary Peritoneal Cancer (ARIEL2).* http://clinicaltrials.gov/show/NCT01891344.

26. *A Study of Rucaparib as Switch Maintenance Following Platinum-Based Chemotherapy in Patients With Platinum-Sensitive, High-Grade Serous or Endometrioid Epithelial Ovarian, Primary Peritoneal or Fallopian Tube Cancer (ARIEL3).* http://clinicaltrials.gov/show/NCT01968213.

27. BioMarin Press Release: *Five Data Presentations on BioMarin's BMN 673 PARP Inhibitor at the 2013 AACR-NCI-EORTC International Conference on Molecular Targets and Cancer Therapeutics;* 2013.

28. Murai J, Huang SY, Das BB, Renaud A, Zhang Y, Doroshow JH, Ji J, Takeda S, Pommier Y: **Trapping of PARP1 and PARP2 by Clinical PARP Inhibitors.** *Cancer Res* 2012, 72:5588–5599.

29. Michie CO, Sandhu SK, Schelman WR, Molife LR, Wilding G, Omlin AG, Kansra V, Brooks DG, Martell RE, Kaye SB, De Bono JS, Wenham RM: **Final results of the phase I trial of niraparib (MK4827), a poly(ADP)ribose polymerase (PARP) inhibitor incorporating proof of concept biomarker studies and expansion cohorts involving BRCA1/2 mutation carriers, sporadic ovarian, and castration resistant prostate cancer (CRPC).** *J Clin Oncol* 2013, 31:abstr 2513.

30. *A Maintenance Study With Niraparib Versus Placebo in Patients With Platinum Sensitive Ovarian Cancer.* http://clinicaltrials.gov/show/NCT01847274.

31. Array BioPharma Press Release: *Encouraging Selumetinib Results Announced for Phase 2 Trial in Ovarian Cancer;* 2012.

32. NCI Drug Dictionary: *binimetinib.* National Cancer Institute at the National Institutes of Health.

33. Array BioPharma 2013 Annual Report: *Low Grade Serous Ovarian Cancer (MEK162 – MEK Inhibitor);* 2013.

34. Monk BJ, Grisham RN, Marth C, Banerjee SN, Hilpert F, Coleman RL, Pujade-Lauraine E, Pignata S, Mirza MR, Oza AM, Del Campo JM, Oehler MK, James A, Christy-Bittel J, Barrett E, Boyd A, Vergote I: **The MEK Inhibitor in Low-Grade Serous Ovarian Cancer (MILO)/ENGOT-ov11 study: A multinational, randomized, open-label phase 3 study of binimetinib (MEK162) versus physician's choice chemotherapy in patients with recurrent or persistent low-grade serous carcinomas of the ovary, fallopian tube, or primary peritoneum.** *J Clin Oncol* 2014, 32:5s.

35. Array BioPharma 2013 Annual Report: *Our Product Pipeline;* 2013.

36. Ewesuedoa RB, Ratain MJ: **Topoisomerase I Inhibitors.** *Oncologist* 1997, 2:359–364.

37. NEKTAR: R&D Pipeline: *Etirinotecan pegol (NKTR-102);* 2014.

38. Vergote IB, Micha JP, Pippitt CH Jr, Rao GG, Spitz DL, Reed N, Dark GG, Garcia A, Maslyar DJ, Rustin GJ: **Phase II study of NKTR-102 in women with platinum-resistant/refractory ovarian cancer.** *J Clin Oncol* 2010, 28:5013.

39. Vergote IB, Garcia A, Micha JP, Pippitt CH, Bendell J, Spitz D, Reed N, Dark G, Fracasso PM, Ibrahim EN, Armenio VA, Duska L, Poole C, Gennigens C, Dirix LY, Leung AC, Zhao C, Soufi-Mahjoubi R, Rustin G: **Randomized Multicenter Phase II Trial Comparing Two Schedules of Etirinotecan Pegol (NKTR-**

40. Nektar Therapeutics (NKTR) News: *Etirinotecan Pegol (NKTR-102) Passes Interim Efficacy Analysis for BEACON Pivotal Phase 3 Clinical Study in Patients with Metastatic Breast Cancer;* 2014.

41. CTI BioPharma: *Development: About paclitaxel poliglumex;* 2014.

42. NCI Drug Dictionary: *paclitaxel polyglutamate.* National Cancer Institute at the National Institutes of Health.

43. *Paclitaxel or Polyglutamate Paclitaxel or Observation in Treating Patients With Stage III or Stage IV Ovarian Epithelial or Peritoneal Cancer or Fallopian Tube Cancer.* http://clinicaltrials.gov/show/NCT00108745.

44. PRNewswire: *XYOTAX in Combination with Carboplatin Produces Major Tumor Response in 98 Percent of First-line Ovarian Cancer Patients;* 2005.

45. Amgen Press Release: *Amgen Announces Top-Line Results Of Phase 3 Trebananib (AMG 386) TRINOVA-1 Trial In Recurrent Ovarian Cancer;* 2013.

46. Kroll D: *Drug From Sea Creature Proves Promising Against Ovarian Cancer.* Forbes; 2014. http://www.forbes.com/sites/davidkroll/2014/06/10/under-the-sea-pharmamars-lurbinectedin-beats-topotecan-in-platinum-resistant-ovarian-cancer/.

47. Soares DG, Machado MS, Rocca CJ, Poindessous V, Ouaret D, Sarasin A, Galmarini CM, Henriques JA, Escargueil AE, Larsen AK: **Trabectedin and Its C Subunit Modified Analogue PM01183 Attenuate Nucleotide Excision Repair and Show Activity toward Platinum-Resistant Cells.** *Mol Cancer Ther* 2011, 10:1481.

48. PharmaMar (Zeltia Group) Press Release: *ZELTIA NEWS: Aplidin®, Yondelis®, PM01183 and PM060184 highlighted at the 2014 Annual Meeting of the American Association for Cancer Research (AACR);* 2014.

49. Vidal A, Muñoz C, Guillén MJ, Moretó J, Puertas S, Martínez-Iniesta M, Figueras A, Padullés L, García-Rodriguez FJ, Berdiel-Acer M, Pujana MA, Salazar R, Gil-Martin M, Martí L, Ponce J, Molleví DG, Capella G, Condom E, Viñals F, Huertas D, Cuevas C, Esteller M, Avilés P, Villanueva A: **Lurbinectedin (PM01183), a new DNA minor groove binder, inhibits growth of orthotopic primary graft of cisplatin-resistant epithelial ovarian cancer.** *Clin Cancer Res* 2012, 18:5399–5411.

50. Poveda A, Berton-Rigaud D, Ray-Coquard IL, Alexandre J, Provansal M, Soto A, Kahatt CM, Szyldergemajn SA, Nieto A, Fernandez C, Alia EG, Casado A, Gonzalez-Martin A, Del Campo JM: **Lurbinectedin (PM01183), an active compound in platinum-resistant/refractory ovarian cancer (PRROC) patients: Results of a two-stage, controlled phase II study.** *J Clin Oncol* 2014, 32:5s.

51. Chelius D, Ruf P, Gruber P, Plöscher M, Liedtke R, Gansberger E, Hess J, Wasiliu M, Lindhofer H: **Structural and functional characterization of the trifunctional antibody catumaxomab.** *MAbs* 2010, 2:309–319.

52. Fresenius SE: *Life Sciences Online;* 2009. TRION Pharma: Trifunctional Antibody Catumaxomab Kills Cancer Stem Cells.

53. Cancer.net: *Fluid in the Abdomen or Ascites;* 2014.

54. Berek JS, Edwards RP, Parker L, DeMars LR, Herzog TJ, Lentz SS, Morris R, Akerley WL, Holloway RW, Method M, Plaxe SC, Walker JL, Schindler T, Schulze E, Krasner CN: **Catumaxomab treatment of malignant ascites in patients with chemotherapy-refractory ovarian cancer: A phase II study.** *J Clin Oncol* 2011, 29:5048.

55. Pietzner K, Chekerov R, Reinthaller A, Reimer D, Reimer T, Angleitner-Boubenizek L, Tschirschmann M, Lindhofer H, Braicu EI, Fotopoulou C, Sehouli J: **A matched pair analysis of intra- and postoperative catumaxomab in patients with ovarian cancer from a multicenter, single-arm phase II trial versus a consecutive single-center collective of ovarian cancer patients without immunotherapy.** *J Clin Oncol* 2012, 30:5080.

56. *Study in EpCAM Positive Patients With Symptomatic Malignant Ascites Using Removab Versus an Untreated Control Group.* http://clinicaltrials.gov/ct2/show/NCT00836654.

102) in Women With Recurrent Platinum-Resistant/Refractory Epithelial Ovarian Cancer. *J Clin Oncol* 2013, 45:1278.

12

Homologous recombination deficiency (HRD) testing in ovarian cancer clinical practice: a review of the literature

Melissa K. Frey[1] and Bhavana Pothuri[2]* (iD)

Abstract

Until recently our knowledge of a genetic contribution to ovarian cancer focused almost exclusively on mutations in the *BRCA1/2* genes. However, through germline and tumor sequencing an understanding of the larger phenomenon of homologous recombination deficiency (HRD) has emerged. HRD impairs normal DNA damage repair which results in loss or duplication of chromosomal regions, termed genomic loss of heterozygosity (LOH). The list of inherited mutations associated with ovarian cancer continues to grow with the literature currently suggesting that up to one in four cases will have germline mutations, the majority of which result in HRD. Furthermore, an additional 5–7% of ovarian cancer cases will have somatic HRD. In the near future, patients with germline or somatic HRD will likely be candidates for a growing list of targeted therapies in addition to poly (ADP-ribose) polymerase (PARP) inhibitors, and, as a result, establishing an infrastructure for widespread HRD testing is imperative. The objective of this review article is to focus on the current germline and somatic contributors to ovarian cancer and the state of both germline and somatic HRD testing. For now, germline and somatic tumor testing provide important and non-overlapping clinical information. We will explore a proposed testing strategy using somatic tumor testing as an initial triage whereby those patients found with somatic testing to have HRD gene mutations are referred to genetics to determine if the mutation is germline. This strategy allows for rapid access to genomic information that can guide targeted treatment decisions and reduce the burden on genetic counselors, an often limited resource, who will only see patients with a positive somatic triage test.

Keywords: Ovarian cancer, Genetics, Tumor testing

Background

Ovarian cancer is the fifth leading cause of death in women in the United States with an estimated 22,280 new cases and 14,240 deaths in 2016 [1]. The majority of women with epithelial ovarian cancer (EOC) are diagnosed with advanced disease. Standard therapy includes surgical debulking and platinum and taxane-based chemotherapy, resulting in complete clinical remission in up to 75% of patients, however only 30% of patients will be cured. Once recurrent, ovarian cancer generally does not exhibit the same level of chemo-sensitivity, highlighting the need for rational therapies directed toward specific molecular targets [2, 3]. The advent of next-generation sequencing

(NGS) has allowed for the systematic investigation of the genomic and molecular alterations in EOC which can identify patients as candidates for individualized targeted therapy. EOC tumors with deficient homologous recombination (HR) repair represent such a group and have demonstrated sensitivity to poly(ADP-ribose)polymerase (PARP) inhibitors [4–6]. The majority of homologous recombination deficient (HRD) tumors will occur in patients with germline *BRCA1* and *BRCA2* mutations. However, there also are patients with germline mutations in other HR pathway genes and patients who do not carry an inherited germline mutation but have tumors with sporadic HRD mutations. Data from the Cancer Genome Atlas (TCGA) demonstrates that approximately fifty percent of high grade serous ovarian cancers have aberrations in HR repair [7]. Patients and physicians now have access to NGS analysis of both germline samples and somatic tumor

* Correspondence: Bhavana.Pothuri@nyumc.org
[2]Division of Gynecologic Oncology, New York University Langone Medical Center, 240 E. 38th St, 19th floor, New York, NY 10016, USA
Full list of author information is available at the end of the article

tissue. The objective of this review article is to focus on the current germline and somatic contributors to ovarian cancer and the state of germline and somatic HRD testing.

Homologous recombination (HR)

DNA damage is a constantly occurring phenomenon that necessitates a complex network of molecular repair pathways in order to maintain genomic integrity and prevent cell death. HR is an important pathway that allows repair of double-stranded DNA breaks. HR operates during the S and G2 phases of the cell cycle and relies on many proteins including *BRCA1* and *BRCA2*, proteins of the MNR complex (*MRE11/RAD50/NBS1*), CtIP, MRE11, RAD51, ATM, H2AX, PALB2, RPA, RAD52 and proteins of the Fanconi anemia pathway [8, 9]. When cells have nonfunctioning HR, for example due to *BRCA1* or *BRCA2* deficiency, they rely on other repair pathways like non-homologous end-joining (NHEJ), which is less precise and more error-prone [10]. NHEJ results in the accumulation of additional mutations and chromosomal instability, increasing the risk that a cell undergoes malignant transformation [10, 11].

Until recently, hereditary EOC was thought to be caused almost exclusively by mutations in *BRCA1* and *BRCA2*, with a small contribution from mutations in the DNA mismatch repair (MMR) genes [12]. TCGA, however, has shown that about half of high grade serous ovarian cancers, the most common histologic subtype, have aberrations in HR repair. Further investigation of the HR pathway highlights multiple other protein co-factors that are necessary for successful HR repair including *RAD51C*, *RAD51D*, *BRIP1*, *PALB2*, *BARD1* and the MMR genes [12, 13]. This group of genes is collectively referred to as the HRD genes [14].

Germline mutations in EOC

When considering the genetic contribution to carcinogenesis, an important distinction is whether a mutation is germline or somatic. Germline implies that the mutation was inherited and is therefore present in all of the individuals' cells. Somatic mutations are those mutations that are acquired and therefore occur exclusively in the tumor cells. *BRCA1* and *BRCA2* are the most well-known ovarian cancer susceptibility genes, with germline genetic testing available since the 1990s [15]. *BRCA* mutation-associated ovarian cancers have multiple distinct clinical features including earlier age at diagnosis, visceral distribution of disease, improved survival, enhanced sensitivity to platinum-based chemotherapies and sensitivity to PARP inhibitors [16–18]. The prevalence of *BRCA1/2* germline mutations in patients with epithelial ovarian cancer is estimated to be about 11–15% [19–21].

In June 2013 the Supreme Court ruled unanimously against Myriad Genetics, invalidating the exclusive license rights to *BRCA1* and *BRCA2* testing in the United States. Following this decision, many other clinical laboratories began offering *BRCA1* and *BRCA2* testing, both as single gene tests and in the form of comprehensive genetic panels [22]. Although used for many hereditary cancer syndromes, multigene panels have been particularly interesting in ovarian cancer. Recent literature suggests that up to 24% of ovarian cancers are associated with germline mutations, and of these, 29% have mutations in genes other than *BRCA1* or *BRCA2* [12, 13, 23, 24] (Table 1).

Somatic mutations in EOC

Several publications have reported the presence of somatic *BRCA1/2* mutations in ovarian cancer, highlighting that both germline and somatic mutations in HRD genes can result in ovarian cancer. TCGA sequenced 316 high grade serous EOCs and matched germline patient DNA. Germline *BRCA1* mutations were discovered in 9% of patients and *BRCA2* mutations in 8%. Evaluation of tumor tissue found additional somatic mutations in *BRCA1/2* (3%), *EMSY* (8%), *PTEN* (7%), *RAD51C* (3%), *ATM/ATR* (2%) and Fanconi anemia genes (5%) [7]. Hennessy et al. [25] performed *BRCA1* and *BRCA2* sequencing of 235 unselected ovarian cancer tumors and found mutations in 19% of cases (31 mutations in *BRCA1* and 13 in *BRCA2*). Germline DNA specimens

Table 1 Genes associated with hereditary ovarian cancer

Hereditary breast and ovarian cancer syndrome
BRCA1
BRCA2
Fanconi anemia pathway
RAD51C
RAD51D
RAD50
BRIP1
BARD1
CHEK2
MRE11A
NBN
PALB2
Mismatch repair
MLH1
MSH2
MSH6
PMS2
Other
TP53

were available for 28 of the patients harboring a *BRCA1* or *BRCA2* tumor mutation. Eleven (39.3%) of the mutations present in the EOC tumor were found to be somatic and 17 germline (60.7%) [25]. When evaluating 367 ovarian carcinomas, Pennington et al.[26] discovered that 24% patients carried a germline mutations in HRD genes and 9% of patients had a somatic tumor mutation. Finally, Cunningham et al. [27] evaluated 279 EOC patients and found that 3.5% of patients had somatic mutations in *BRCA1* (2.1%) and *BRCA2* (1.4%). (Table 2). The variable rates of somatic mutations reported in the literature likely reflect differences in patient selection (e.g., histologic subtype) and scope of testing (e.g.,

number of genes included on the NGS panel). Currently, the true prevalence of somatic mutations remains unknown, however it has been estimated as somewhere between 5 and 7% of cases. This implies that for every 4–5 ovarian cancer patients with a germline BRCA mutation there will be one patient with a somatic mutation [8].

Genetic evaluation
Germline testing

Genetic testing for germline mutations is recommended for all women with non-mucinous epithelial ovarian cancer by multiple professional societies including the American College of Medical Genetics and Genomics (ACMG) [28], the American Society of Clinical Oncology (ASCO) [29], the National Cancer Comprehensive Network (NCCN) [30], the National Society of Genetic Counselors (NSGC) [28] and the Society of Gynecologic Oncology (SGO) [31]. Multigene panels can assess a virtually unlimited number of genes in a method that is both time- and cost-effective when compared to the prior standard of single gene Sanger sequencing. The availability of NGS technology combined with the Supreme Court ruling invalidating exclusive gene patent rights has resulted in rapid uptake of multigene panels [32]. The scope of available testing ranges from screening for founder mutations, to sequencing *BRCA1* and *BRCA2*, to full panel testing of multiple cancer-associated genes.

Currently, the guidelines that recommend germline testing do not make specific recommendations regarding which of the many available platforms to utilize [14]. Cancer genetic counselors play an integral role both in helping patients choose the specific method of testing and analyzing the results, which are becoming increasingly complex. While adding additional genes to panels increases the chance of finding deleterious mutations it also increases the likelihood of finding variants of uncertain significance (VUS) and non-actionable mutations defined as mutations for which the clinical relevance is unclear and clinical management guidelines do not exist. Finding VUS and non-actionable mutations does not improve patient outcomes but can result in patient and physician anxiety and unindicated and inappropriate interventions [33]. Pre- and post-test cancer genetic counseling has been recognized to benefit the individual tested and relatives, associated with improved adherence to cancer risk management, better informed surgical decision making, increased cancer genetics knowledge, improved patient satisfaction and cost savings [34–46].

Discovering a germline mutation in a patient with EOC has multiple significant clinical implications. As previously stated, *BRCA1/2*-associated ovarian cancer has multiple distinct features affecting age at diagnosis, disease distribution, chemosensitivity and survival. Patients with known mutations have access to targeted

Table 2 Germline and somatic HRD mutations in ovarian cancer

Study	Included histologic subtypes	Findings
TCGA [7]	High grade serous ovarian cancer (316)	Germline mutations (*N* = 316) BRCA1 – 9% BRCA2 – 8% Somatic mutations (*N* = 216) BRCA1/2–3% EMSY – 8% PTEN – 7% RAD51C – 3% ATM/ATR – 2% Fanconi anemia genes – 5%
Hennessy et al. [25]	Serous (186) Nonserous (13) Mixed (13) Unknown (22)	Tumor sequencing (*N* = 235) BRCA1 – 13% BRCA2 – 5.5% Germline testing from patients with tumors harboring BRCA1/2 mutations (*N* = 28) BRCA1/2 germline mutation – 61% BRCA1/2 somatic mutation – 39%
Pennington et al. [26]	High grade serous (249) Low grade serous (9) Poorly-differntiated NOS (48) Clear cell (19) High-grade endometrioid (20) Low-grade endometrioid (6) Carcinosarcoma (12) Other (4)	Germline mutations (*N* = 367) HRD genes – 24% (BRCA1 – 56%, BRCA2 – 19%, BARD1 – 2%, 4, BRIP1 – 4.5%, CHEK1 – 1%, CHEK2 – 3%, FAM175A – 2%, NBN – 1%, PALB2 – 2%, RAD51C – 3%, RAD51D – 4.5%) Somatic Mutations (*N* = 367) HRD genes – 9% (BRCA1 – 54%, BRCA2 – 17%, ATM – 9%, BRIP1 – 6%, CHEK2 – 9%, MRE11A – 3%, RAD51C – 3%)
Cunningham et al. [27]	High grade serous (735) High grade endometrioid (73) Low grade endometrioid (67) Clear cell (69) Low-grade serous (34) Mucinous (29) Other/Unknown (56)	Germline mutations (*N* = 899) BRCA1 – 3.5% BRCA2 – 3% RAD51C – 3% Somatic Mutations (*N* = 279) BRCA1 – 2% BRCA2 – 1.4%

therapy, for example PARP inhibitors for *BRCA1/2* mutation carriers. In December 2014, the U.S. Food and Drug Administration (FDA) granted olaparib accelerated approval for monotherapy in patients with germline *BRCA1/2* mutations and recurrent ovarian cancer with three or more prior lines of chemotherapy, making olaparib the first of the PARP inhibitors to receive FDA approval. On December 19, 2016 the FDA granted accelerated approval to rucaparib in patients with recurrent ovarian cancer with two or more prior lines of chemotherapy and either germline *BRCA1/2* mutations or somatic *BRCA1/2* mutations in the tumor detected by a next-generation sequencing-based companion diagnostic test. The European Commission granted marketing authorization for the PARP inhibitor olaparib as monotherapy in the maintenance treatment of adult patients with platinum-sensitive, relapsed *BRCA*-mutated (germline and/or somatic) high-grade serous epithelial ovarian, fallopian tube, or primary peritoneal cancer who are in complete response or partial response following platinum-based chemotherapy [47]. The recently published phase III data of Mirza et al. support the use of Niraparib in the maintenance setting for patients with platinum sensitive recurrent ovarian cancer. Patients with germline HRD mutations derived the greatest clinical benefit from this treatment [48].

In addition to treatment eligibility, many mutations are predictive of other cancers in addition to ovarian cancer, offering patients the opportunity for heightened awareness and screening. Finally, identifying a germline mutation can allow family members to undergo genetic counseling and testing, termed "cascade" testing. Informed relatives have the opportunity to pursue intensive cancer surveillance and risk-reducing options. Data from individuals with Lynch syndrome demonstrate that awareness of a mutation results in cancer prevention or early diagnosis of cancer, which can improve morbidity and prevent mortality [49–51].

Tumor profiling

In addition to germline testing, multiple companies now offer tumor genetic profiling for somatic mutations. There are methods using NGS similar to that done for germline DNA. There are also independent DNA-based measures of genomic instability reflecting underlying tumor HRD on the basis of loss of heterozygosity (LOH), telomeric allelic imbalance (TAI) and large-scale state transitions (LST). Each individual metric and the combination is significantly associated with *BRCA1/2* status and identifying HRD tumors [52–54]. Somatic mutation testing is more laborious and less reproducible than germline testing for several reasons. First, unlike germline testing, somatic testing utilizes a heterogeneous collection of cells. Different tumor types and specimens

will have varying quantities of normal cells and neoplastic cells in a sample. Multiple methods of DNA evaluation exist for tumor profiling. Obtaining high-quality tumor DNA extraction relies on an adequately sized specimen that has been well preserved. In contrast to germline testing which looks at DNA extracted from healthy cells to determine if a mutation was inherited, somatic testing evaluates the genetic composition of tumor cells. Once adequate high-quality DNA has been obtained the data analysis is also challenging. There is currently no standard method of interpreting results. Laboratories rely on databases such as COSMIC or in silico predictive software to attempt to predict pathogenicity of findings but neither is exhaustive [8]. Finally there is the issue of the stability of a somatic mutation. Data suggest that there is intra-tumor genetic heterogeneity resulting from clonal evolution and the emergence of subclonal tumor populations in high grade EOC, causing spatial and temporal heterogeneity [55]. While data from the ARIEL-2 trial has begun to address this issue, demonstrating a change in biomarker status over time, the phenomenon of tumor heterogeneity is not fully understood [56].

Early evidence suggests that a somatic *BRCA1/2* mutation is a predictive biomarker of PARP inhibitor activity however the number of patients with somatic mutations that have been analyzed is low. In a phase II study of olaparib, Gelmon et al. found that 24% of *BRCA*-negative patients with high grade serous or undifferentiated ovarian cancer achieved a radiological objective response [57]. In the recent publication by Mirza et al. [48] niraparib maintenance therapy had activity in all patients with platinum sensitive recurrent ovarian cancer, however there was improved progression free survival in patients with germline *BRCA1/2* mutations and without germline *BRCA1/2* mutations but with HRD. Swisher et al. [59] found that for patients with platinum sensitive recurrent ovarian cancer, rucaparib had activity in patients with germline *BRCA1/2* mutations and patients who were *BRCA1/2* wild-type but were found to be LOH high. LOH status was determined by next-generation sequencing using a cutoff of 14% or more of genomic LOH in pretreatment biopsy specimens to be considered LOH high. Studies that are currently ongoing or recently completed, and future planned studies will likely clarify this question, including SOLO-2 (NCT01874353) and ARIEL-3 (NCT01968213) [5, 60]. See Table 3 for a review of phase II/III trials of PARP inhibitors in ovarian cancer.

Somatic tumor testing has two important implications: 1) identifying patients for targeted therapies like PARP inihibitors, 2) identifying patients who should be referred for genetic counseling and offered genetic testing. Mutations that are purely somatic and not found in the germline DNA are not inherited, cannot be passed to offspring, and therefore do not warrant cascade genetic

Table 3 Phase II/III studies of PARP inhibitors in ovarian cancer

Study	Patient population	BRCA status of patient population	Treatment arms	Total accrual	Primary endpoint	Results — Objective Response Rate (ORR)	Progression free survival (PFS)	Pertinent Findings
Audeh MW et al. Lancet. 2010 [4].	Recurrent epithelial ovarian, primary peritoneal, or fallopian tube carcinoma	BRCA1/2 positive	Cohort 1: Olaparib 400 mg BID; Cohort 2: Olaparib 100 mg BID	57	ORR	Cohort 1: 33%; Cohort 2: 13%	Cohort 1: 5.8 months; Cohort 2: 1.9 months	Positive proof of concept of utility of PARP inhibitors from phase I data. Superior efficacy of 400 mg BID dosing.
Kaye SB et al. J Clin Oncol. 2012 [73].	Platinum resistent recurrent epithelial ovarian, primary peritoneal, or fallopian tube carcinoma	BRCA1/2 positive	Arm 1: Olaparib 200 mg BID; Arm 2: Olaparib 400 mg BID; Arm 3: PLD 50 mg/m2	97	PFS	Arm 1: 25%; Arm 2: 31%; Arm 3: 18%	Arm 1: 6.5 months; Arm 2: 8.8 months; Arm 3: 7.1 months	No significant difference in outcomes between 2 doses of olaparib and PLD.
Gelmon KA et al. Lancet Oncol 2011 [57].	Advanced metastatic or recurrent ovarian, primary peritoneal or fallopian tube cancer (high-grade serous and/or undifferentiated) or breast cancer	BRCA1/2 positive AND BRCA1/2 negative	Olaparib 400 mg BID	91 (65 with gynecologic cancer)	ORR	BRCA1/2 positive: 41%; BRCA1/2 negative: 24%; BRCA1/2 positive + platinum sensitive: 60%; BRCA1/2 negative + platinum sensitive: 50%; BRCA1/2 positive + platinum resistant: 33%; BRCA1/2 negative + platinum resistant: 4%	BRCA1/2 positive: 221 days; BRCA1/2 negative: 192 days	Olaparib has activity in BRCA1/2 positive and negative populations.
Ledermann J et al. Lancet Oncol. 2014 [5].	Platinum sensitive recurrent high grade serous epithelial ovarian, primary peritoneal, or fallopian tube carcinoma	BRCA1/2 positive AND BRCA1/2 negative	(Maintenance therapy following platinum-based chemotherapy) Arm 1: Olaparib 400 mg BID; Arm 2: Placebo	265	PFS		Arm 1: 8.4 months; Arm 2: 4.8 months; Olaparib + BRCA1/2 positive: 11.2 months; Olaparib + BRCA1/2 negative: 5.6 months; Placebo + BRCA1/2 positive: 4.3 months; Placebo + BRCA1/2 negative: 5.5 months	Olaparib maintenance associated with improved PFS. No diffrence in OS.
Oza AM et al. Lancet Oncol. 2015 [74].	Platinum sensitive recurrent serous ovarian cancer	BRCA1/2 positive AND BRCA1/2 negative	Arm 1: Olaparib 200 mg BID + Paclitaxel 175 mg/m2 + Carboplatin AUC 4 × 6 cycles followed by olaparib 400 mg BID maintenance	162	PFS	Arm 1: 64%; Arm 2: 58%	Arm 1: 12.2 months; Arm 2: 9.6 months	Olaparib associated with improved PFS.

Table 3 Phase II/III studies of PARP inhibitors in ovarian cancer *(Continued)*

Study	Population	BRCA status	Treatment	N	Endpoint	Result	Median	Conclusion
			Arm 2: Paclitaxel 175 mg/m2 + Carboplatin AUC 4 × 6 cycles					
Coleman RL et al. Gynecol Oncol. 2015 [75].	Recurrent or persistent ovarian, primary peritoneal or fallopian tube cancer	BRCA1/2 positive	Veliparib 400 mg BID	52	ORR	Total population – 26% Platinum resistant – 20% Platinum sensitive – 35% BRCA1 – 26% BRCA2 – 27%	8.11 months	Veliparib has single agent acitivity in platinum resistent disease.
Kaufman B et al. J Clin Oncol. 2015 [76].	Platinum resistant recurrent ovarian, primary peritoneal or fallopian tube cancer	BRCA1/2 positive	Olaparib 400 mg BID	193	ORR	31%	225 days	Olaparib has single agent acitivity in BRCA1/2 positive platinum resistent disease.
Kumrar S et al. Clin Cancer Res 2015 [58].	Recurrent ovarian cancer or recurrent primary peritoneal, fallopian tube or high-grade serous ovarian cancers	BRCA1/2 positive AND BRCA1/2 negative	Arm 1: Cyclophosphamide 50 mg daily Arm 2: Cyclophosphamide 50 mg daily + Veliparib 60 mg daily	75	ORR	Arm 1: (n = 38) 1 complete response, 6 partial responses Arm 2: (n = 37) 1 complete response, 3 partial responses	Arm 1: 2.3 months Arm 2: 2.1 months	The addition of veliparib to cyclophosphamide did not improve the response rate or the median PFS.
Mirza MR et al. N Engl J Med 2016 [48].	Platinum sensitive recurrent ovarian cancer or recurrent primary peritoneal, fallopian tube or high-grade serous ovarian cancers	BRCA1/2 positive AND BRCA1/2 negative	Niraparib 300 mg daily vs. placebo daily	553	PFS		gBRCA cohort - Niraparib: 21.0 months - Placebo: 5.5 months non-gBRCA with HRD cohort - Niraparib: 12.9 months - Placebo: 3.8 months non-gBRCA cohort - Niraparib: 9.3 months - Placebo: 3.9 months	Niraparib maintenance therapy has activity for platinum-sensitive recurrent ovarian cancer regardles of the presence or absense of gBRCA mutations or HRD status.
Swisher EM, et al. Lancet Oncol 2017 [59].	Platinum sensitive recurrent ovarian cancer or recurrent primary peritoneal, fallopian tube or high-grade ovarian cancers	BRCA1/2 positive AND BRCA1/2 negative	Rucaparib 600 mg BID	206	PFS	BRCA 1/2 positive – 80% BRCA1/2 wild-type and LOH high – 29% BRCA1/2 wild-type and LOH low – 10%	BRCA 1/2 positive: 12.8 months BRCA1/2 wild-type and LOH high: 5.7 months BRCA1/2 wild-type and LOH low: 5.2 months	Rucaparib activity in BRCA1/2 mutant and BRCA wild-type LOH high platinum sensitive recurrent disease.

gBRCA Germline BRCA mutation, *non-gBRCA* Non-germline BRCA mutation, *LOH* Loss of heterozygosity

counseling and testing. If a patient is found to have a mutation on tumor profiling, the only way to definitively classify it as a germline versus somatic mutation is through germline testing. As described previously, Hennessy et al. [25] found that among 28 tumors with *BRCA1/2* mutations, 61% were the result of germline inherited mutations. This presents an important ethical consideration regarding patient counseling and informed consent. Thorough genetic counseling and informed consent are required prior to germline genetic testing however this is not the case with tumor profiling. This is important given that almost two-thirds of patients with a mutation found on tumor profiling will have a germline mutation which carries significant clinical implications for the patient and her family members.

Tumor profiling vs. germline testing?

It has become clear that both somatic and germline mutation testing provide important information for patients with EOC. The question is whether or not both are necessary and if so what is the ideal chronology of testing. Table 4 outlines the advantages of each testing method. Germline testing is more well established with more robust data linking results to valuable prognostic and predictive information. Germline testing can also identify other cancers for which a patient is at risk and can initiate cascade testing of family members. Somatic testing will capture a larger number of patients with HRD who can potentially receive targeted therapy and does not require access to a genetic counselor, which is limited in many clinical settings.

This issue of genetic counseling as a limited resource is an important one. The exponential growth in diagnostic and treatment options that utilize genetic and genomic sequencing information coupled with public coverage of celebrity *BRCA* mutation status has led to an increasing demand for genetic counselors [61, 62]. A study of 3765 patients in the U.S. with epithelial ovarian cancer found that only 50% of patients meeting substantial-risk criteria for *BRCA1/2* mutations were referred to genetics [63]. Another study of 416 patients in Ontario with epithelial ovarian cancer found that only 19% of patients had undergone clinical genetic testing for *BRCA1/2* [64]. There currently are not enough genetic counselors and geneticists to meet this demand and alternative service delivery models are being evaluating including telephone counseling, videoconferencing, group counseling and direct-to-consumer testing [65]. Video-assisted genetic counseling has been found to significantly increase the percentage of patients undergoing testing compared to traditional referral to genetic counseling (31% vs. 55%) however this method has not yet been tested in a prospective manor [66].

Table 4 Advantages of germline versus somatic tumor testing of HRD genes

Advantages of germline testing
1. Germline testing is a more well established technique.
DNA extraction is easier.
The results are highly accurate and reproducible.
2. Germline mutations have prognostic and predictive value.
There is robust data supporting the prognostic and predictive value of germline *BRCA1/2* mutations.
Such data is limited for somatic mutations.
3. Germline mutations can offer knowledge of risk for other associated cancers.
As germline mutations often increase the risk for multiple cancers, awareness of germline mutations allows patients to pursue risk-reducing interventions for other cancers.
4. Germline mutation identification is clinically relevant for family members and allows for cascade testing.

Advantages of somatic testing
1. Somatic testing with NGS will identify a larger number of patients with HRD who can be therapeutically targeted.
Including patients with somatic (and not germline) mutations who would be missed with germline testing alone.
2. Somatic testing can help patients understand the magnitude of clinical benefit from targeted therapy in the context of risks and side effects of particular therapeutic agents.
3. Somatic testing does not require genetic counseling which is often a limited resource.
4. Somatic testing can serve as a triage for germline testing.
Patients found to have a somatic mutation can then be referred to clinical genetics for germline testing, allowing for better utilization of genetic counselors and geneticists.

The recent approval of rucaparib for BRCA positive (germline or somatic) patients with recurrent ovarian cancer who have had two or more lines of therapy would argue for tumor testing to screen for therapeutic options and as a triage for germline testing. However, the success of niraparib in significantly extending the duration of progression-free survival in all platinum-sensitive recurrent ovarian cancer patienrs, (those with and without *BRCA1/2* mutations) indicates a great expansion of the population who can benefit from PARP inhibitors. Interestingly Mirza et al. even found efficacy in the non-germline BRCA mutation and HRD-negative group (HR 0.58, $P = 0.02$). In an exploratory analysis of ARIEL2 Part 1, Swisher et al. [59] found that among BRCA wild-type tumors, genomic LOH was a more sensitive predictor of response than was mutation of other HR genes and gene methylation. In the near future PARP inhibitors may be available to all patients with ovarian cancer regardless of their genetic profile for treatment and maintenance therapy. With this expanded information about germline mutations, somatic mutations and LOH status may serve a new role, no longer as an indicator of who is eligible for treatment with this class of drugs but instead as a biomarker for treatment efficacy. This information would allow individualized patient counseling where the provider can offer information about the magnitude of benefit given the patient's genetic profile in the context of risk of side effects.

In summary both somatic and germline testing offer clinically important and not entirely overlapping information. One strategy is to start with somatic tumor testing and use this to triage additional testing. Those patients found to have HRD gene mutations on somatic testing can be referred to genetics to establish whether the mutation is somatic or germline. This strategy would allow for rapid access to genomic information that can guide targeted treatment decisions especially with the recent approval of rucaparib for BRCA mutation carriers, and reduce the burden on genetic counselors who would then only see patients with positive somatic testing. Whether this proposed strategy is feasible based on availability of testing resources and cost is unknown and must be examined in future studies. Furthermore, given recent niraparib data this strategy may not be needed as therapeutic benefit was noted in the maintenance setting in all patients with ovarian cancer regardless of BRCA or HRD status.

Future directions, can somatic testing replace germline testing?

Currently, as stated above, somatic tumor testing can provide information only about genetic aberrations in the tumor, however as NGS continues to become increasing widespread its applications will likely broaden. Stadler et al. [67] recently published their experience with tumor genomic profiling via NGS panels in 224 patients with colorectal cancer. Previously in colorectal cancer NGS panels were used to identify *KRAS*, *NRAS* and *BRAF* somatic mutations and parallel MMR protein assessment via ether immunohistochemistry (IHC) or microsatellite instability (MSI) analysis was used for initial screening of Lynch syndrome. Mismatch repair deficiency (MMR-D) occurs in 15–20% of colorectal tumors with one-quarter resulting from Lynch syndrome [68]. Stadley and colleagues discovered that by utilizing an expanded NGS panel with 341-genes, a specific mutational load cutoff could reliably identify tumors with DNA MMR-D. This was not surprising given that a deficiency in the DNA MMR apparatus would be expected to result in more uncorrected mismatched bases and thus a greater rate of mutations. The authors concluded that the use of multigene tumor panels may obviate the need for parallel MMR protein assessment and thus make the molecular work-up patients with colorectal cancer more efficient and cost-effective. Identifying MMR-D is becoming particularly important as it may serve as a biomarker for

response to immunotherapy with checkpoint inhibitors in colorectal and endometrial cancer [69, 70].

If somatic tumor profiling can replace MMR assessment, the next question is whether or not somatic tumor profiling can replace germline testing altogether. Currently none of the tumor profiling platforms offer information on germline mutational status however this may change. The feasibility of this question was evaluated with a study comparing deep, uniform NGS sequencing of tumor tissue compared to Clinical Laboratory Improvement Amendments (CLIA)-certified, NGS-based germline exon sequencing of 236-cancer related genes. A computational method could predict the somatic status of mutations from tumor tissue without the need for a matched normal control with an accuracy of greater than 95%. As tumor profiling for this indication is permitted under investigational use only and is not CLIA-certified, the authors concluded that NGS tumor sequencing can indicate which patients require additional work-up for germline testing [71]. However, with further analysis and certification, clinicians will likely be able to use somatic testing to definitively predict germline status. While this approach to testing may not make sense for cancers with a low prevalence of hereditary causation, it is very applicable and exciting in ovarian cancer where up to a quarter of patients carry a germline mutation. The FDA accelerated approvals of olaparib and rucaparib came with specified companion diagnostic tests however there are multiple available next-generation sequencing assays and algorithms for defining LOH. Whether or not approval for specific targeted therapies will mandate a specific companion test and how physicians choose the most appropriate diagnostic test remains unclear. Methods to combine assays and validate data across the various PARP inhibitors, so one cost-effective test can be utilized makes logical sense.

Finally, an important remaining area of uncertainty is the role of epigenetic alterations in EOC. HRD can result from genomic processes that are distinct from germline and somatic mutations in HR genes. For example *BRCA1/2* silencing can occur via indirect mechanisms including promoter methylation and interactions with other proteins involved in DNA repair. The clinical implications of epigenetic changes remain unclear with conflicting data in the literature. Chiang et al. [72] found that *BRCA1* promoter hypermethylation resulted in significantly shorter survival when compared to *BRCA1* germline mutations and *BRCA1* wild-type without promoter hypermethylation. In contrast, TCGA found no survival difference with *BRCA1* hypermethylation [7] and Cunningham et al. [27] observed that *BRCA1* methylated cases had a survival benefit compared to germline wild-type and similar to that of the germline mutation cases. Prospective studies are necessary to better address the clinical significance of epigenetic alterations in the HR pathway.

Conclusions

It is clear that the knowledge of both germline and somatic mutation status is becoming increasingly important in the management of patients with ovarian cancer. The experience with PARP inhibitors in ovarian cancer clinical trials demonstrates that the targeted therapeutic effect is beyond just BRCA germline mutations and more widely applicable to HRD. Whether epigenetic modifications to HRD genes confer the same therapeutic sensitivity remains unclear however future studies will likely allow for a better understanding of their underlying mechanisms and clinical significance. The list of ovarian cancer-associated genes continues to grow and the literature currently suggests that up to one in four women with ovarian cancer will have a germline HR deficiency and an additional 5–7% will have a somatic HR deficiency. Currently, these patients with recurrent disease are candidates for approved therapy with PARP inhibitors, however in the near future there will likely be a growing list of targeted therapies available for ovarian cancer patients. As a result, infrastructure for widespread somatic HRD testing in routine clinical practice, as is the case for HER2 in breast cancer and epidermal growth factor receptor in lung cancer, should be supported [8]. Furthermore, in the maintenance setting where PARP inhibitors may be useful in all patients as noted the NOVA trial, HRD testing maybe useful for counseling to understand the magnitude of the benefit in context with the risks of side effects. Both germline and somatic tumor testing provide important and nonoverlapping clinical information. Further research is necessary to address whether somatic testing can completely replace germline testing or if the practice of universal somatic tumor testing followed by directed germline confirmation should be implemented.

Abbreviations
ACMG: American College of Medical Genetics and Genomics; ASCO: American Society of Clinical Oncology; CLIA: Clinical Laboratory Improvement Amendments; EOC: Epithelial ovarian cancer; HRD: Homologous recombination deficiency; IHC: Immunohistochemistry; LOH: Loss of heterozygosity; LST: Large scale transitions; MMR: Mismatch repair; MMR-D: Mismatch repair deficiency; MSI: Microsatellite instability; NCCN: National Comprehensive Cancer Network; NGS: Next generation sequencing; NHEJ: Non-homologous end-joining; NSGC: National Society of Genetic Counselors; PARP: Poly(ADP-ribose)polymerase; SGO: Society of Gynecologic Oncology; TCGA: The Cancer Genome Atlas; VUS: Variants of uncertain significance

Acknowledgements
Not applicable.

Funding
Not applicable.

Authors' contributions
All authors worked together to research and draft the manuscript. All authors read and approved the final manuscript.

Competing interests
The authors declare that they have no competing interests.

Author details
[1]Division of Gynecologic Oncology, Weill Cornell Medicine, 525 East 68th Street, Suite J-130, New York, NY 10065, USA. [2]Division of Gynecologic Oncology, New York University Langone Medical Center, 240 E. 38th St, 19th floor, New York, NY 10016, USA.

References
1. American Cancer Society: Cancer Statistics Center. 2016. p. https://cancerstatisticscenter.cancer.org/.
2. Covens A, Carey M, Bryson P, Verma S, Fung Kee Fung M, Johnston M. Systematic review of first-line chemotherapy for newly diagnosed postoperative patients with stage II, III, or IV epithelial ovarian cancer. Gynecol Oncol. 2002;85:71–80.
3. Gadducci A, Sartori E, Maggino T, Zola P, Landoni F, Fanucchi A, et al. Analysis of failures after negative second-look in patients with advanced ovarian cancer: an Italian multicenter study. Gynecol Oncol. 1998;68:150–5.
4. Audeh MW, Carmichael J, Penson RT, Friedlander M, Powell B, Bell-McGuinn KM, et al. Oral poly(ADP-ribose) polymerase inhibitor olaparib in patients with BRCA1 or BRCA2 mutations and recurrent ovarian cancer: a proof-of-concept trial. Lancet. 2010;376:245–51.
5. Ledermann J, Harter P, Gourley C, Friedlander M, Vergote I, Rustin G, et al. Olaparib maintenance therapy in patients with platinum-sensitive relapsed serous ovarian cancer: a preplanned retrospective analysis of outcomes by BRCA status in a randomised phase 2 trial. Lancet Oncol. 2014;15:852–61.
6. Fong PC, Yap TA, Boss DS, Carden CP, Mergui-Roelvink M, Gourley C, et al. Poly(ADP)-ribose polymerase inhibition: frequent durable responses in BRCA carrier ovarian cancer correlating with platinum-free interval. J Clin Oncol. 2010;28:2512–9.
7. Cancer Genome Atlas Research N. Integrated genomic analyses of ovarian carcinoma. Nature. 2011;474:609–15.
8. Moschetta M, George A, Kaye SB, Banerjee S. BRCA somatic mutations and epigenetic BRCA modifications in serous ovarian cancer. Ann Oncol. 2016;27:1449–55.
9. Lupo B, Trusolino L. Inhibition of poly(ADP-ribosyl)ation in cancer: old and new paradigms revisited. Biochim Biophys Acta. 1846;2014:201–15.
10. Wang M, Wu W, Wu W, Rosidi B, Zhang L, Wang H, et al. PARP-1 and Ku compete for repair of DNA double strand breaks by distinct NHEJ pathways. Nucleic Acids Res. 2006;34:6170–82.
11. Hoeijmakers JH. Genome maintenance mechanisms for preventing cancer. Nature. 2001;411:366–74.
12. Pennington KP, Swisher EM. Hereditary ovarian cancer: beyond the usual suspects. Gynecol Oncol. 2012;124:347–53.
13. Norquist BM, Harrell MI, Brady MF, Walsh T, Lee MK, Gulsuner S, et al. Inherited mutations in women with ovarian carcinoma. JAMA Oncol. 2015:1–9.
14. Randall LM, Pothuri B. The genetic prediction of risk for gynecologic cancers. Gynecol Oncol. 2016;141:10–6.
15. Hall JM, Lee MK, Newman B, Morrow JE, Anderson LA, Huey B, et al. Linkage of early-onset familial breast cancer to chromosome 17q21. Science. 1990;250:1684–9.
16. Alsop K, Fereday S, Meldrum C, DeFazio A, Emmanuel C, George J, et al. BRCA mutation frequency and patterns of treatment response in BRCA mutation-positive women with ovarian cancer: a report from the Australian Ovarian Cancer Study Group. J Clin Oncol. 2012;30:2654–63.
17. Gourley C, Michie CO, Roxburgh P, Yap TA, Harden S, Paul J, et al. Increased incidence of visceral metastases in scottish patients with BRCA1/2-defective

ovarian cancer: an extension of the ovarian BRCAness phenotype. J Clin Oncol. 2010;28:2505–11.

18. Tan DS, Yap TA, Hutka M, Roxburgh P, Ang J, Banerjee S, et al. Implications of BRCA1 and BRCA2 mutations for the efficacy of paclitaxel monotherapy in advanced ovarian cancer. Eur J Cancer. 2013;49:1246–53.

19. Risch HA, McLaughlin JR, Cole DE, Rosen B, Bradley L, Fan I, et al. Population BRCA1 and BRCA2 mutation frequencies and cancer penetrances: a kin-cohort study in Ontario, Canada. J Natl Cancer Inst. 2006;98:1694–706.

20. Risch HA, McLaughlin JR, Cole DE, Rosen B, Bradley L, Kwan E, et al. Prevalence and penetrance of germline BRCA1 and BRCA2 mutations in a population series of 649 women with ovarian cancer. Am J Hum Genet. 2001;68:700–10.

21. Pal T, Permuth-Wey J, Betts JA, Krischer JP, Fiorica J, Arango H, et al. BRCA1 and BRCA2 mutations account for a large proportion of ovarian carcinoma cases. Cancer. 2005;104:2807–16.

22. Walsh CS. Two decades beyond BRCA1/2: Homologous recombination, hereditary cancer risk and a target for ovarian cancer therapy. Gynecol Oncol. 2015;137:343–50.

23. Walsh T, Casadei S, Lee MK, Pennil CC, Nord AS, Thornton AM, et al. Mutations in 12 genes for inherited ovarian, fallopian tube, and peritoneal carcinoma identified by massively parallel sequencing. Proc Natl Acad Sci U S A. 2011;108:18032–7.

24. Song H, Dicks E, Ramus SJ, Tyrer JP, Intermaggio MP, Hayward J, et al. Contribution of Germline Mutations in the RAD51B, RAD51C, and RAD51D Genes to Ovarian Cancer in the Population. J Clin Oncol. 2015;33:2901–7.

25. Hennessy BT, Timms KM, Carey MS, Gutin A, Meyer LA, Flake 2nd DD, et al. Somatic mutations in BRCA1 and BRCA2 could expand the number of patients that benefit from poly (ADP ribose) polymerase inhibitors in ovarian cancer. J Clin Oncol. 2010;28:3570–6.

26. Pennington KP, Walsh T, Harrell MI, Lee MK, Pennil CC, Rendi MH, et al. Germline and somatic mutations in homologous recombination genes predict platinum response and survival in ovarian, fallopian tube, and peritoneal carcinomas. Clin Cancer Res. 2014;20:764–75.

27. Cunningham JM, Cicek MS, Larson NB, Davila J, Wang C, Larson MC, et al. Clinical characteristics of ovarian cancer classified by BRCA1, BRCA2, and RAD51C status. Sci Rep. 2014;4:4026.

28. Hampel H, Bennett RL, Buchanan A, Pearlman R, Wiesner GL. Guideline Development Group ACoMG, et al. A practice guideline from the American College of Medical Genetics and Genomics and the National Society of Genetic Counselors: referral indications for cancer predisposition assessment. Genet Med. 2015;17:70–87.

29. Lu KH, Wood ME, Daniels M, Burke C, Ford J, Kauff ND, et al. American Society of Clinical Oncology Expert Statement: collection and use of a cancer family history for oncology providers. J Clin Oncol. 2014;32:833–40.

30. Daly MB, Pilarski R, Axilbund JE, Berry M, Buys SS, Crawford B, et al. Genetic/familial high-risk assessment: breast and ovarian, version 2.2015. J Natl Compr Canc Netw. 2016;14:153–62.

31. Lancaster JM, Powell CB, Chen LM, Richardson DL, Committee SGOCP. Society of Gynecologic Oncology statement on risk assessment for inherited gynecologic cancer predispositions. Gynecol Oncol. 2015;136:3–7.

32. Blackburn HL, Schroeder B, Turner C, Shriver CD, Ellsworth DL, Ellsworth RE. Management of incidental findings in the era of next-generation sequencing. Curr Genomics. 2015;16:159–74.

33. Norquist BM, Swisher EM. More genes, more problems? Benefits and risks of multiplex genetic testing. Gynecol Oncol. 2015;139:209–10.

34. Collins VR, Meiser B, Ukoumunne OC, Gaff C, St John DJ, Halliday JL. The impact of predictive genetic testing for hereditary nonpolyposis colorectal cancer: three years after testing. Genet Med. 2007;9:290–7.

35. Watson M, Kash KM, Homewood J, Ebbs S, Murday V, Eeles R. Does genetic counseling have any impact on management of breast cancer risk? Genet Test. 2005;9:167–74.

36. Pal T, Lee JH, Besharat A, Thompson Z, Monteiro AN, Phelan C, et al. Modes of delivery of genetic testing services and the uptake of cancer risk management strategies in BRCA1 and BRCA2 carriers. Clin Genet. 2014;85:49–53.

37. Hadley DW, Jenkins JF, Dimond E, de Carvalho M, Kirsch I, Palmer CG. Colon cancer screening practices after genetic counseling and testing for hereditary nonpolyposis colorectal cancer. J Clin Oncol. 2004;22:39–44.

38. Schwartz MD, Lerman C, Brogan B, Peshkin BN, Halbert CH, DeMarco T, et al. Impact of BRCA1/BRCA2 counseling and testing on newly diagnosed breast cancer patients. J Clin Oncol. 2004;22:1823–9.

39. Calzone KA, Prindiville SA, Jourkiv O, Jenkins J, DeCarvalho M, Wallerstedt DB, et al. Randomized comparison of group versus individual genetic

40. Armstrong J, Toscano M, Kotchko N, Friedman S, Schwartz MD, Virgo KS, et al. Utilization and outcomes of BRCA genetic testing and counseling in a national commercially insured population: the ABOUT study. JAMA Oncol. 2015;1:1251–60.

41. Hilgart JS, Coles B, Iredale R. Cancer genetic risk assessment for individuals at risk of familial breast cancer. Cochrane Database Syst Rev. 2012;15.

42. Braithwaite D, Emery J, Walter F, Prevost AT, Sutton S. Psychological impact of genetic counseling for familial cancer: a systematic review and meta-analysis. J Natl Cancer Inst. 2004;96:122–33.

43. DeMarco TA, Peshkin BN, Mars BD, Tercyak KP. Patient satisfaction with cancer genetic counseling: a psychometric analysis of the Genetic Counseling Satisfaction Scale. J Genet Couns. 2004;13:293–304.

44. Miller CE, Krautscheid P, Baldwin EE, Tvrdik T, Openshaw AS, Hart K, et al. Genetic counselor review of genetic test orders in a reference laboratory reduces unnecessary testing. Am J Med Genet A. 2014;164A:1094–101.

45. Cragun D, Camperlengo L, Robinson E, Caldwell M, Kim J, Phelan C, et al. Differences in BRCA counseling and testing practices based on ordering provider type. Genet Med. 2015;17:51–7.

46. Weitzel JN, McCaffrey SM, Nedelcu R, MacDonald DJ, Blazer KR, Cullinane CA. Effect of genetic cancer risk assessment on surgical decisions at breast cancer diagnosis. Arch Surg. 2003;138:1323–8. discussion 9.

47. Lynparza prescribing information. Lynparza [package insert]. Wilmington, DE: AstraZeneca Pharmaceuticals LP. 2014. Available at http://www.azpicentral.com/Lynparza/pi_lynparza.pdf#page=1.

48. Mirza MR, Monk BJ, Herrstedt J, Oza AM, Mahner S, Redondo A, et al. Niraparib maintenance therapy in platinum-sensitive, recurrent ovarian cancer. N Engl J Med. 2016;375:2154-2164.

49. Vasen HF, Abdirahman M, Brohet R, Langers AM, Kleibeuker JH, van Kouwen M, et al. One to 2-year surveillance intervals reduce risk of colorectal cancer in families with Lynch syndrome. Gastroenterology. 2010;138:2300–6.

50. Schmeler KM, Lynch HT, Chen LM, Munsell MF, Soliman PT, Clark MB, et al. Prophylactic surgery to reduce the risk of gynecologic cancers in the Lynch syndrome. N Engl J Med. 2006;354:261–9.

51. Engel C, Rahner N, Schulmann K, Holinski-Feder E, Goecke TO, Schackert HK, et al. Efficacy of annual colonoscopic surveillance in individuals with hereditary nonpolyposis colorectal cancer. Clin Gastroenterol Hepatol. 2010;8:174–82.

52. Abkevich V, Timms KM, Hennessy BT, Potter J, Carey MS, Meyer LA, et al. Patterns of genomic loss of heterozygosity predict homologous recombination repair defects in epithelial ovarian cancer. Br J Cancer. 2012; 107:1776–82.

53. Birkbak NJ, Wang ZC, Kim JY, Eklund AC, Li Q, Tian R, et al. Telomeric allelic imbalance indicates defective DNA repair and sensitivity to DNA-damaging agents. Cancer Discov. 2012;2:366–75.

54. Popova T, Manie E, Rieunier G, Caux-Moncoutier V, Tirapo C, Dubois T, et al. Ploidy and large-scale genomic instability consistently identify basal-like breast carcinomas with BRCA1/2 inactivation. Cancer Res. 2012;72:5454–62.

55. Schwarz RF, Ng CK, Cooke SL, Newman S, Temple J, Piskorz AM, et al. Spatial and temporal heterogeneity in high-grade serous ovarian cancer: a phylogenetic analysis. PLoS Med. 2015;12:e1001789.

56. Lin K, Sun J, Maloney L, Goble S, Oza A, Coleman R, Scott C, Robillard L, Mann E, Isaacson J, Harding T. 2710 Quantification of genomic loss of heterozygosity enables prospective selection of ovarian cancer patients who may derive benefit from the PARP inhibitor rucaparib. Eur J Cancer. 2015;51:S531–2.

57. Gelmon KA, Tischkowitz M, Mackay H, Swenerton K, Robidoux A, Tonkin K, et al. Olaparib in patients with recurrent high-grade serous or poorly differentiated ovarian carcinoma or triple-negative breast cancer: a phase 2, multicentre, open-label, non-randomised study. Lancet Oncol. 2011;12:852–61.

58. Kummar S, Oza AM, Fleming GF, Sullivan DM, Gandara DR, Naughton MJ, et al. Randomized Trial of Oral Cyclophosphamide and Veliparib in High-Grade Serous Ovarian, Primary Peritoneal, or Fallopian Tube Cancers, or BRCA-Mutant Ovarian Cancer. Clin Cancer Res. 2015;21:1574–82.

59. Swisher EM, Lin KK, Oza AM, Scott CL, Giordano H, Sun J, et al. Rucaparib in relapsed, platinum-sensitive high-grade ovarian carcinoma (ARIEL2 Part 1): an international, multicentre, open-label, phase 2 trial. Lancet Oncol. 2017; 18:75–87.

60. Ledermann J, Harter P, Gourley C, Friedlander M, Vergote I, Rustin G, et al. Olaparib maintenance therapy in platinum-sensitive relapsed ovarian cancer. N Engl J Med. 2012;366:1382–92.

61. Collins FS, Varmus H. A new initiative on precision medicine. N Engl J Med. 2015;372:793–5.

62. Borzekowski DL, Guan Y, Smith KC, Erby LH, Roter DL. The Angelina effect: immediate reach, grasp, and impact of going public. Genetics Med. 2014;16:516–21.

63. Meyer LA, Anderson ME, Lacour RA, Suri A, Daniels MS, Urbauer DL, et al. Evaluating women with ovarian cancer for BRCA1 and BRCA2 mutations: missed opportunities. Obstet Gynecol. 2010;115:945–52.

64. Metcalfe KA, Fan I, McLaughlin J, Risch HA, Rosen B, Murphy J, et al. Uptake of clinical genetic testing for ovarian cancer in Ontario: a population-based study. Gynecol Oncol. 2009;112:68–72.

65. Buchanan AH, Rahm AK, Williams JL. Alternate service delivery models in cancer genetic counseling: a mini-review. Front Oncol. 2016;6:120.

66. Watson MU CH, Tillmanns T, Reed ME, Smiley L, Covington R. The implementation of video-assisted genetic counseling for ovarian, fallopian, and peritoneal cancer patients Society of Gynecologic Oncology Annual Meeting on Women's Cancer San Diego. 2016.

67. Stadler ZK, Battaglin F, Middha S, Hechtman JF, Tran C, Cercek A, et al. Reliable detection of mismatch repair deficiency in colorectal cancers using mutational load in next-generation sequencing panels. J Clin Oncol. 2016; 34:2141–7.

68. Hampel H, Frankel WL, Martin E, Arnold M, Khanduja K, Kuebler P, et al. Screening for the Lynch syndrome (hereditary nonpolyposis colorectal cancer). N Engl J Med. 2005;352:1851–60.

69. Le DT, Uram JN, Wang H, Bartlett BR, Kemberling H, Eyring AD, et al. PD-1 blockade in tumors with mismatch-repair deficiency. N Engl J Med. 2015; 372:2509–20.

70. A.N. Fader LAD, D.K. Armstrong, E.J. Tanner III, J. Uram, A. Eyring, H. Wang, G. Fisher, T. Greten and D. Le. Preliminary results of a phase II study: PD-1 blockade in mismatch repair–deficient, recurrent or persistent endometrial cancer. Society of Gynecologic Oncology Annual Meeting on Women's Cancer: Late-breaking abstract sessions 3; 2016.

71. James X. Sun GF, Kai Wang, Jeffrey S. Ross, Vincent A. Miller, Philip J. Stephens, Doron Lipson, Roman Yelensky. Abstract 1893: A computational method for somatic versus germline variant status determination from targeted next-generation sequencing of clinical cancer specimens without a matched normal control. Proceedings of the 105th Annual Meeting of the American Association for Cancer Research; 2014 Apr 5–9. San Diego, CA 2014.

72. Chiang JW, Karlan BY, Cass L, Baldwin RL. BRCA1 promoter methylation predicts adverse ovarian cancer prognosis. Gynecol Oncol. 2006;101:403–10.

73. Kaye SB, Lubinski J, Matulonis U, Ang JE, Gourley C, Karlan BY, et al. Phase II, open-label, randomized, multicenter studycomparing the efficacy and safety of olaparib, a poly (ADP-ribose) polymerase inhibitor, and pegylated liposomal doxorubicin in patients with BRCA1 or BRCA2mutations and recurrent ovarian cancer. J Clin Oncol. 2012;30:372–9.

74. Oza AM, Cibula D, Benzaquen AO, Poole C, Mathijssen RH, Sonke GS, et al. Olaparib combined with chemotherapy for recurrent platinum-sensitive ovarian cancer: a randomised phase 2 trial. Lancet Oncol. 2015;16:87–97.

75. Coleman RL, Sill MW, Bell-McGuinn K, Aghajanian C, Gray HJ, Tewari KS, et al. A phase II evaluation of the potent, highly selective PARP inhibitor veliparib in the treatment of persistent or recurrent epithelial ovarian, fallopian tube, or primary peritoneal cancer in patients who carry a germline BRCA1 or BRCA2 mutation - An NRG Oncology/Gynecologic Oncology Group study. Gynecol Oncol. 2015;137:386–91.

76. Kaufman B, Shapira-Frommer R, Schmutzler RK, Audeh MW, Friedlander M, Balmaña J, et al. Olaparib monotherapy in patients with advanced cancer and a germline BRCA1/2 mutation. J Clin Oncol. 2015; 33:244–50.

13

Clinico-epidemiological profile of molar pregnancies in a tertiary care centre of Eastern Nepal: a retrospective review of medical records

Nimisha Agrawal[1], Reshu Agrawal Sagtani[2], Shyam Sundar Budhathoki[2] and Hanoon P. Pokharel[1*]

Abstract

Background: The incidence of molar pregnancy has demonstrated marked geographic and ethnic differences. The reported data in Nepal is inconsistent with minimal published literature. Thus, we designed a study to determine prevalence of molar pregnancies and demonstrate clinical and epidemiological characteristics of the patients attending a tertiary care center in eastern Nepal.

Methods: A retrospective review of medical records was conducted to determine the prevalence of molar pregnancies at the B.P. Koirala Institute of Health Sciences (BPKIHS) from the year 2008 to 2012. Secondary data from the medical records were analyzed. Annual and 5-year prevalence of molar pregnancy per 1000 live births was calculated. Demographic characteristics, clinical presentation, management methods and complications of molar pregnancy were studied.

Results: The 5- year prevalence of molar pregnancy at BPKIHS is 4.17 per 1000 live births with annual prevalence ranging 3.8–4.5 per 1000 live births. More than one third of the patients were in the age group of 20–35 years and majority of them were of Hindu religion. For more than one third (41.7 %) of the patients, it was their first pregnancy while about 10 % gave a positive past history of molar pregnancy. Abnormal uterine bleeding (86.3 %) was the most frequent complaint, suction evacuation was the most common method of treatment and more than half of the patients required prolonged care after initial management.

Conclusion: There is a need for studies at country level which will give us a national figure on molar pregnancies. Thus, a standardized clinic-epidemiological profile of molar pregnancy in Nepal can be created.

Keywords: *Molar pregnancy, Hydatidiform mole profile, Retrospective, Nepal*

Background

The management of gestational trophoblastic disease (GTD) depicts one of the success stories of modern medicine. As the majority, if not all, GTDs are potentially curable with the retention of reproductive function, once the correct diagnosis is made and treatment is commenced early enough [1–4] GTD constitutes a spectrum of tumors and tumor-like conditions characterized by abnormal proliferation of pregnancy associated tropho-blastic tissues of varying propensities for invasion and spread [4–7].

They include complete and partial hydatidiform mole, invasive mole, placental-site trophoblastic tumor (PSTT), and choriocarcinoma. Hydatidiform mole is the most common GTD [5, 7].

The incidence of GTD varies greatly in different parts of the world, with 0.4 per 1000 birth in United States of America to 12.5 per 1000 births in Taiwan [8]. In Nepal, hospitals in Kathmandu valley have recorded its incidence as 5.1, 2.9, 2.8, and 4.1 per 1000 live births [9]. These 10–20-fold variations in the incidence of molar

* Correspondence: hanoon.pokharel@bpkihs.edu
Principal Author: Nimisha Agrawal
[1]Department of Obstetrics and Gynaecology, B.P. Koirala Institute of Health Sciences, Dharan, Nepal
Full list of author information is available at the end of the article

pregnancy might be overestimated by reporting biases, such as population-based and hospital-based data [2]. Published literature on incidence of hydatidiform mole from this part of the world is rather minimal.

Maternal age is the most consistent risk factor for GTD in geographical regions and ethnic groups. Commonly affecting women in the reproductive age group, GTD has the propensity to become malignant but relatively easy to identify, diagnose and treat. Clinically hydatidiform mole presents with amenorrhoea, painless vaginal bleeding and spontaneous passage of grape-like vesicles, high serum and urinary β human chorionic gonadotrophin (βHCG) levels. There may also be hyperemesis gravidarum, doughy uterus, inappropriate uterine size, bilateral theca lutein cyst and rarely, features of thyrotoxicosis and pre-eclampsia in the first half of pregnancy [10–12]. Hydatidiform mole is a relatively common gynecological problem which could present like spontaneous abortion, one of the most common gynecological emergencies. Ultrasonography is a simple non-invasive examination which can correctly identify the placental molar transformations in-utero. Currently with widespread use of first trimester ultrasonography a significant proportion of patients with molar pregnancy are asymptomatic at the time of diagnosis. Careful and reliable human chorionic gonadotropin monitoring is essential for the early detection of post molar persistent gestational trophoblastic tumor.

Studies concerning the epidemiological characteristics, clinical presentation, management practices and outcome of molar pregnancy are rarely published from Nepal apart from a few case reports. Considering the relative lack of published epidemiology studies on hydatidiform mole from Nepal and considering the varied incidence rates reported from Asian countries, there is a need to determine the incidence rate in eastern Nepalese population in a well designed epidemiological study. With this background, we analyzed the past medical records of 5 years to determine the prevalence of molar pregnancy, evaluate the management practices and determine the outcome of hydatidiform mole at B P Koirala Institute of Health Sciences (BPKIHS), a tertiary care centre in eastern part of Nepal.

Methods

A retrospective review of medical records was conducted at B. P. Koirala Institute of Health Sciences (BPKIHS) to develop a clinio—epidmiological profile of molar pregnancy. All women who are diagnosed with molar pregnancy/ hydatidiform mole (complete or partial) sonologically or histopathologically, and reporting to BPKIHS for treatment during the study period i.e. between 2008–2012 were included in the study. The data for total deliveries conducted in the hospital during the study period was also taken from the hospital registries. In-patient medical records from the medical records section of BPKIHS from the year 2008 to 2012 were reviewed and information of the current study was acquired.

The current study was approved by the Institutional Ethical Review Board (IERB), BPKIHS. Permission from the Hospital authority was taken to access the medical records was taken. All information collected from the hospital records were kept confidential. The details of maternal characteristics like maternal age, parity and period of gestation at the time of presentation, clinical presentation, diagnostic tools, management and complications was noted for each of cases. Details of past obstetric history such as previous history of molar pregnancy was noted as well as complications of molar pregnancy occurring during the hospital stay, need for blood transfusion or intensive care unit stay was noted. Anemia is classified according to the WHO criteria for anemia during pregnancy [13].

Descriptive statistics were used to summarize the continuous and categorical variables. Period prevalence was calculated by the number of cases of molar pregnancies reported to the institution for treatment during the study period for every 1000 live births delivered during the same period. All statistical analyses were performed using SPSS version 11.5.

Results

A total of 48,805 live births took place in BPKIHS during from 2008 and 2012 with 204 molar pregnancies. The 5- year prevalence of molar pregnancy at BPKIHS is 4.17 per 1000 live births. The annual prevalence of molar pregnancies during the study period ranged from 3.8–4.5 per 1000 live births as shown in Table 1.

Table 2 shows the clinical profile of the patients reporting to BPKIHS for treatment of molar pregnancy. A total of 204 cases of molar pregnancy were included in this study. More than one third of the patients were in the age group of 20–35 years with a range of 16–51 and mean age 23.9 years. Majority of the patients belonged to Hindu religion. More than one third (41.7 %) of the patients were primigravida and about ten per cent gave a positive past history of molar pregnancy. The period of gestation ranged from 8 to 34 weeks with a major proportion (66.4 %) having period of gestation more or equal to 13 weeks with average uterine height of 17.8 weeks. About a quarter (24.5 %) of the patients gave a positive history of contraceptives with injectables (66 %) being the most frequently used followed by oral contraceptives (26 %). More than one third (38.7 %) of patients had pallor on examination. The Ultra-sonography (USG) findings suggest that more than one fifth (20.6 %) of pregnant women had theca lutein cysts. The blood grouping found A positive to be

Table 1 Prevalence of molar pregnancy per 100 live births at BPKIHS, Nepal

Year	No. of molar pregnancies/year	Percentage (%)	Number of live births/year	Prevalence/ 1000
2008	38	18.6	8976	4.2/1000
2009	38	18.6	9866	3.8/1000
2010	42	20.6	10234	4.1/1000
2011	44	21.6	9651	4.6/1000
2012	42	20.6	10078	4.2/1000
Total	204	100.0	48805	4.2/1000

the most common blood group followed by O positive and B positive.

The hCG level of patients on an average was 18644.70 IU/ml while post management during the follow up after 1 week was 4156.84 IU/ml.

There were 28 (13.7 %) patients who had come to our hospital for regular ANC checkup, who were later diagnosed molar pregnancy. The rest 176 (86.3 %) cases presented with one or more complaints. Abnormal uterine bleeding (86.3 %) was the most frequent complaint of the patients coming to our center with molar pregnancy followed by, pain per abdomen (33.8 %), hyper emesis (26.5 %) and passage of grape like cysts (11.8 %). The various treatment modalities for molar pregnancy were

Table 2 Clinico-epidemiological profile of patients with molar pregnancy attending BPKIHS, Nepal

Variables	Categories	Number	Percentage
Age group in years	≤20	51	25.0 %
	20–35	143	70.1 %
	≥35	10	04.9 %
Mean age ± sd = 23.9 ± 6.6 Range = 16–51 years			
Religion	Hindu	174	85.8 %
	Kirat	24	11.8 %
	Buddhist	03	01.5 %
	Muslim	02	01.0 %
Parity	Primigravida	85	41.7 %
	Multigravida	119	58.3 %
Previous history of molar pregnancy	Yes	18	08.8 %
	No	186	91.2 %
Period of gestation	≥13 weeks	131	64.2 %
	<13 weeks	73	35.8 %
Period of gestation (in weeks) Mean age ± sd = 15.9 ± 5.8 weeks; Range = 6–34 weeks			
Previous history of contraceptive usage	Yes	50	24.5 %
	No	154	75.5 %
Type of contraceptive use	Oral contraceptives	13	26.0 %
	Injectable (Depo)	33	66.0 %
	IUCD (Copper-T)	03	06.0 %
	Intra dermal patch(Norplant)	01	02.0 %
Mean ± Sd (uterine size in weeks) 17.8 ± 6.5 weeks; Range: 06–36 weeks			
Pallor	Presence	79	38.7 %
	Absence	125	61.3 %
Theca lutein cyst on USG	Presence	42	20.6 %
	Absence	162	79.4 %
Blood group	A positive	80	39.2 %
	O positive	63	30.9 %
	B positive	52	25.5 %
	AB positive	07	03.4 %
	B negative	02	01.0 %

used. Suction evacuation was the most common method of treatment followed by chemotherapy and manual vacuum extraction. Combined treatment modalities were used among 6.8 % of patients (Table 3).

Table 4 shows that 56.4 % of patients suffered complications during management of cases. Blood transfusion was required among 45.6 % of patients, and anemia was seen among 40.2 % of the patients. There were 11.8 % were admitted in Intensive Care Unit (ICU) for post management care, fever was seen among 6.4 % of cases and Gestational Trophoblastic Neoplasia (GTN) was diagnosed in 5.9 % of cases.

Discussion

The 5- year prevalence of molar pregnancy at BPKIHS from 2008–2012 was 4.17 per 1000 live birth with range of annual prevalence of molar pregnancies during the study period between 3.85–4.50 per 1000 live births. A study reports a lower prevalence among Asian population of about 2.58 per 1000 live births [14]. As BPKIHS is the tertiary referral hospital for the whole of Eastern Nepal, the cases and the deliveries represent a large proportion of cases that show up at a hospital for treatment. However the prevalence may be different, as deliveries also happen at home or at birthing centers at governmental and private health institutions in eastern Nepal. Half of the delivery takes place at home in Nepal [15].

There are wide geographical variations in the incidence of gestational trophoblastic disease as a result of differences in methodology, classifications of mole, case detection [14]. Similarly, the epidemiology of trophoblastic disease in Nepal remains unknown as there are inconsistent findings from many centers. A study done from maternity hospital of Kathmandu reported annual incidence of 2.84 and 3.24 per 1000 live births while in another teaching hospital the incidence of trophoblastic disease ranged from 7.07 per 1000 pregnancies to 8.04 per 1000 deliveries [16]. A study done to compare GTD among Asian women of North England and North Wales showed that Asian women are at increased risk of having molar pregnancies compared to the western populations [14].

While in the current study, more than one third of the patients were in the age group of 20–35 years with a range of 16–51 and mean age of 23.7 years. Prevalence of molar pregnancy was found to be higher in women younger than 29 years (80 %) in another 8 year retrospective study done in Kathmanudu [9]. In other studies, it has been found that there is a relationship between risk of molar pregnancy and both upper and lower extremes of maternal age. Furthermore, the extent of risk is much greater with older rather than younger maternal ages, and it is only at the true extremes of maternal age (15 and 45 years) that the increase in risk sharply rises

Table 3 Presenting complaints and subsequent management of molar pregnancies at BPKIHS, Nepal

Symptoms and management		Number (n = 204)	Percentage (%)
Symptoms (multiple responses)	Abnormal uterine bleeding	176	86.3 %
	Lower Abdominal Pain	69	33.8 %
	Hyperemesis	54	26.5 %
	Passage of grape like cysts	24	11.8 %
	Hemoptysis	14	06.9 %
	Mass per abdomen	08	03.9 %
	Shortness of breath	06	02.9 %
	Fever	06	02.9 %
	Nausea and Vomiting	03	01.5 %
	Chest pain	02	01.0 %
	Abdominal distension	01	0.5 %
	Shock	01	0.5 %
	No symptoms	28	13.7 %
Management methods	Suction and Evacuation	183	89.8 %
	Suction and Evacuation + Chemotherapy	12	5.8 %
	Chemotherapy	5	2.4 %
	Spontaneous abortion	1	0.5 %
	Manual vacuum extraction	1	0.5 %
	Suction and Evacuation + Manual Vacuum Extraction	1	0.5 %
	Manual vacuum extraction + Chemotherapy	1	0.5 %

Table 4 Complications (multiple responses) seen during and after management of molar pregnancies at BPKIHS, Nepal

Complications	Number	Percentage
Present	115	56.4 %
Absent	89	43.6 %
1. Blood transfusion	93	45.6 %
2. Anemia	82	40.2 %
3. Admission in ICU	24	11.8 %
4. Fever	13	6.4 %
5. Gestational Trophoblastic Neoplasia	12	5.9 %
6. Hemoptysis	10	4.9 %
7. Retain products of conception	06	2.9 %
8. Shortness of breath	05	2.5 %
9. Re-Manual Vaccum Aspiration	05	4.5 %
10. Edema	01	0.5 %
11. High blood pressure	01	0.5 %
12. Intravenous Iron therapy	01	0.5 %
13. Hyperthyroidism	01	0.5 %
14. Upper Respiratory tract Infection	01	0.5 %
15. Rise in Hcg	01	0.5 %
16. Septic abortion	01	0.5 %
17. Glossitis	01	0.5 %
18. Exploratory Laporotomy	01	0.5 %
19. Ventillation support	01	0.5 %
20. Invasive Mole	01	0.5 %

[17]. There is a need to look further about the association of age with molar pregnancies in future studies.

More than one third (41.7 %) of the patients were primigravida and about ten per cent gave a positive past history of molar pregnancy. In a descriptive case series from 2001 to 2007 in Bharatpur, Nepal showed that in 15.5 % of cases of molar pregnancy had occurred among primigravida and same proportion had positive past history of molar pregnancy [18] while large proportion (36.7 %) of primigravida suffered from molar pregnancy in another study [2]. However, studies have also shown that there is no real association of gravidity with molar pregnancy when corrected for age [19].

The period of gestation ranged from 8 to 34 weeks with a major proportion (66.4 %) having gestational age at time of evaluation more or equal to 13 weeks and the average uterine size at evaluation was 17.83 ± 6.54 weeks in the present study. A study from Sweden also reported the mean gestational age at the time of USG was 12.4 weeks similar to our study [20] while dissimilar findings was seen from the New England Trophoblastic Disease Centre [21]. According to their report, the mean estimated gestational age at evaluation was 11.8 weeks (range 6–22) and the mean uterine size at evaluation was 12.4 weeks (range 7–20 weeks) [21].

The mean level of pre-evacuation hCG of our patients was 18,644 IU/ml and after the management during the follow up after 1 week was 4156.84 IU/ml. This level was much lower compared to an Israeli study which reported The mean pre-evacuation β-hCG was 2,75,901 IU/l (range 2,011,000–9,19, 000 IU/l) [22]. The analysis of Hungarian patients in 2004 with uncomplicated hydatidiform mole, indicates that once undetectable serum hCG levels are attained relapse is unlikely. The follow up of uncomplicated partial moles and complete moles with weekly serum hCG levels until negative titers seems to be safe [23].

The USG findings among patients attending BPKIHS suggests that more than one fifth (20.6 %) of pregnant women had theca lutein cyst. USG service is available in some institutions of eastern Nepal. However, there are limited places in referral area with reliable recording and reporting done by ultrasonologists. Similar proportion (24.5 %) of theca lutein was reported by a study in another region of Nepal [18].

The patients presented to our center with abnormal uterine bleeding as the most frequent (86.3 %) complaint. The other presenting symptoms were pain (33.8 %), hyper emesis (26.5 %) and passage of grape like cysts (11.8 %) while 13.7 % did not report any symptoms and were diagnosed during routine examination. More than one third (38.7 %) of patients had pallor on examination.

Similar complaints were reported by patients with molar pregnancies in various studies. Vaginal bleeding was the most common presenting symptom while presence of excessive uterine size, anaemia, pre-eclampsia, hyperemesis and hyperthyroidism was significantly less common among current patients than in past cases at a centre [21].

A study from Israel showed that although vaginal bleeding was the most common presenting symptom while 41 % of their patients were asymptomatic. Furthermore, systemic manifestations such as hyperemesis, pre-eclampsia, clinical thyrotoxicosis and respiratory distress were exceedingly rare in this study [22]. It was seen from reports of a study done in Sweden that the current clinical presentation of complete mole has clearly changed compared to that of the classic type of mole with vaginal bleeding (77 %), abdominal pain (23 %) and hyperemesis (19 %) being the most commonly occurring symptoms. The clinical presentation of partial moles usually includes no typical symptoms. Rather, the signs and symptoms are those of incomplete abortion or missed abortion [23].

In the present study, the various management methods were suction evacuation, chemotherapy and manual vacuum extraction. Combined treatment modalities were used among 6.8 % of patients. At another center in Nepal, 13.3 % of patients were treated with suction evacuation, 62.2 % of patients underwent adjuvant chemotherapy among which 26.6 % received single agent chemotherapy and received EMA-CO regimen [18].

Gestational Trophoblastic Neoplasia (GTN) was diagnosed in 5.9 % of cases the cases could suggest that there may be over diagnosis of molar pregnancy in this center. This may need further investigation in the future.

A large proportion (56.4 %) of the patients in this study required extra attention and suffered some form (major or minor) complications during management of cases. This can be due to patients coming with more severe conditions and complaints in which management is aggressive and require long term attention and care. With anemia seen among 40.2 % of the patients, transfusion was done in 45.6 % of the patients. A high level of is reported by another study [21]. ICU admission and respiratory distress have been reported in other studies [24–26]. During the management of molar pregnancy, patients are required to pre arrange blood for transfusion. While those with anticipated hemorrhage are transfused, many don't require transfusion. Admissions in ICU included those patients with shortness of breath, septic abortion, exploratory laporotomy, patient requiring ventilation support, and those that are anticipated to required were kept in Intensive unit for observation for 24 to 48 h. However, since these are based on the medical records the practices could not be further explored in detail. There seems to be a need for a standard protocol for management of molar pregnancy in our hospital.

This study used a secondary data source and thus, validity and reliability of the data is of concern. Patients of molar pregnancy need follow up for at least 9 months, there was no data on follow up of patients which also an important issue. The study has limitations of not having the descriptions of the type of molar pregnancy. The medical records could not provide the findings dings on the histopathologic examinations (HPE) which could have given a more clearepicture molar pregnancy. There is a need to strengthen the recording and reporting system to include the comprehensive records in our hospital.

Conclusion

The 5-year prevalence of molar pregnancy at B.P. Koirala Insitute of Health Sciences—the only tertiary care center of eastern Nepal during the study period of 2008–2012 is 4.17 per 1000 live births. Similar studies in the future at a national level will help us to reach a national figure regarding prevalence and incidence of molar pregnancies in Nepal.

Competing interests
The authors declare that they have no competing interests.

Authors' contributions
NA, RAS, SSB & HPP, all contributed to the conception of the study. NA, RAS & HPP analyzed and interpreted the data of the work. Drafting of the manuscript and revising it critically for the important intellectual content was done by RAS, SSB & HPP. Manuscript preparation, editing and finalizing of the version to be published is the work of NA, RAS, SSB & HPP. All authors agree to be accountable for all aspects of the work related to the integrity of the work.

Acknowledgements
We would like to thank the medical records section of BPKIHS who facilitated data collection for conduction of the present study.

Author details
[1]Department of Obstetrics and Gynaecology, B.P. Koirala Institute of Health Sciences, Dharan, Nepal. [2]School of Public Health and Community Medicine, B.P. Koirala Institute of Health Sciences, Dharan, Nepal.

References
1. Chakrabarti BK, Mondal NR, Chatterjee T. Gestational trophoblastic tumor at a tertiary level cancer center: A retrospective study. J Reprod Med. 2006;51(11):875–8.
2. Garret LA, Garner EI, Feltmate CM, Goldstein DP, Berkowitz RS. Subsequent pregnancy outcomes in patients with molar pregnancy and persistent gestational trophoblastic neoplasia. J Reprod Med. 2008;53(7):481–6.
3. Ben-Arie A, Deutsch H, Volach V, Peer G, Husar M, Lavie O, et al. Reduction of postmolar gestational trophoblastic neoplasia by early diagnosis and treatment. J Reprod Med. 2009;54(3):151–4.
4. Mbamara SU, Obiechina NJA, Eleje GU, Akabuike CJ, Umeononihu OS. Gestational Trophoblastic Disease in a Tertiary Hospital in Nnewi, Southeast Nigeria. Niger Med J. 2009;50(4):87–9.
5. Nevin J, Bloch B, Dehaeck K, Soeters R. Gestational tropiblastic disease. Manual of Practical Gynaecological Oncology. London: Chapman and Hall; 1995. p. 130–46.
6. Berkowitz RS, Goldstein DP. Molar Pregnancy. N Engl J Med. 2009;360:1639–45.
7. Moore LE, Hernandez E. Hydatidiform Mole [Internet]. Medscape Reference, Web MD LLC. 2014 [cited 2014 Dec 10]. Available from: http://emedicine.medscape.com/article/254657-overview#showall
8. Chhabra A, Sinha P. Gestational Trophoblastic Disease – some observation. J Obs Gynecol India. 1988;38:590–3.
9. Thapa K, Shrestha M, Sharma S, Pandey S. Trend of complete Hydatidiform mole. J Nepal Med Assoc. 2010;49(1):10–3.
10. Goldstein DP, Berkowitz RS. Gestational trophoblastic neoplasms: Clinical principles of disgnosis and treatment. Philadelphia: W B Saunders; 1982. p. 1–301.
11. Bagshawe KD, Dent J, Webb J. Hydatidiform mole in England and Wales 1973–83. Lancet. 1986;328(8508):70–4.
12. Evans AC, Soper JT, Hammond CB. Clinical features of molar pregnancies and gestational trophoblastic tumours. Obstet Gynaecol. 2003;87:182–205.
13. Federation of Obstetric & Gynecological Societies of India. Good Clinical Practice Recommendations for Iron Deficiency Anemia in Pregnancy (IDA) in Pregnancy in India. J Obstet Gynecol India [Internet]. 2011;61(5):569–71. Available from: http://link.springer.com/10.1007/s13224-011-0097-5.
14. Tham BWL, Everard JE, Tidy JA, Drew D, Hancock BW. Gestational trophoblastic disease in the Asian population of Northern England and North Wales. BJOG An Int J Obstet Gynaecol. 2003;110(6):555–9.
15. Department of Health Services. Annual Report Department of Health Services 2070/71 [Internet]. Kathmandu; 2015. Available from: http://dohs.gov.np/wp-content/uploads/2014/04/Annual_Report_2070_71.pdf
16. Soma H, Malla D, Dali SM. Clinical experience with trophoblastic diseases in Nepal. Gan To Kagaku Ryoho. 1989;16(4 Pt 2–3):1577–781.
17. Sasaki S. Clinical presentation and management of molar pregnancy. Bailliere's Best Pract Res Clin Obstet Gynaecol. 2003;17(6):885–92.
18. Pariyar J. Gestational trophoblastic disease in Nepalese women managed in B. P. Koirala Memorial Cancer Hospital. J Clin Oncol 27, 2009 (suppl; abstr e16570).
19. Matalon M, Modan B. Epidemiologic aspects of hydatidiform mole in Israel. Am J Obstet Gynecol. 1972;112(1):107–12.
20. Lindholm H, Flam F. The diagnosis of molar pregnancy by sonography and gross morphology. Acta Obstet Gynecol Scand. 1999;78(1):6–9.
21. Soto-Wright V, Bernstein M, Goldstein DP, Berkowitz RS. The changing clinical presentation of complete molar pregnancy. Obstet Gynecol. 1995;86(5):775–9.
22. Gemer O, Segal S, Kopmar A, Sassoon E. The current clinical presentation of complete molar pregnancy. Arch Gynecol Obstet. 2000;264(1):33–4.
23. Batorfi J, Vegh G, Szepesi J, Szigetvari I, Doszpod J, Fulop V. How long should patients be followed after molar pregnancy? Analysis of serum hCG follow-up data. Eur J Obstet Gynecol Reprod Biol. 2004;112(1):95–7.

14

In vitro chemoresponse in metachronous pairs of gyneclologic cancers

Heather J Dalton[1], James Fiorica[2], Candace K McClure[3], Rodney P Rocconi[4], Fernando O Recio[5], John L Levocchio[6], Matthew O Burrell[7] and Bradley J Monk[8]*

Abstract

Background: While most gynecologic cancers respond to first-line cytotoxic chemotherapy, treatment of recurrent disease is frequently associated with acquired drug resistance. In order to find an in vitro surrogate of this clinical phenomenon, a tumor chemoresponse assay was studied.

Methods/Materials: Patients who had tissue submitted for repeated chemoresponse testing were identified through a retrospective search. Sixty-three patients met inclusion criteria (chemoresponse testing completed at primary diagnosis and upon recurrence of disease and assays completed ≥90 days apart). The Wilcoxon signed-rank test was used to compare chemoresponse, represented as a response index (RI), between primary and recurrent measurements. In a secondary analysis, response was categorized and coded as Responsive = 3, Intermediately Responsive = 2 and Non-Responsive = 1, and the paired t-test was used to compare chemoresponse between primary and recurrent measurement.

Results: Median time between primary and recurrent tumor testing was 309 days (IQR 208–422). Drugs tested included carboplatin, cisplatin, docetaxel, doxorubicin, gemcitabine, paclitaxel, topotecan, and combination carboplatin/gemcitabine and carboplatin/paclitaxel. There were no differences in chemoresponse between primary and recurrent measurement when chemoresponse was represented by RI scores; although a trend toward increased resistance to paclitaxel upon recurrence was noted. When chemoresponse was analyzed as a continuous variable corresponding to categorized response, a significant shift toward increased resistance to paclitaxel at recurrence, and a marginally significant trend toward increased resistance to carboplatin at recurrence, were observed.

Conclusions: We observed a trend toward increased chemoresistance at recurrence for paclitaxel, and a marginally significant trend toward increased chemoresistance to carboplatin, but no change in chemoresponsiveness between primary diagnosis and recurrence of disease for other common chemotherapy drugs, including common second-line agents such as doxorubicin, gemcitabine, and topotecan.

Keywords: Gynecologic cancer, Drug resistance, Recurrent ovarian, Chemotherapy, Cross-resistance

Background

It is estimated that in 2014, there were 21,980 new cases of ovarian cancer with 14,270 deaths [1]. The majority of patients present with advanced stage disease. While the majority of women will achieve complete clinical remission after cytoreductive surgery and platinum-based chemotherapy, approximately 30% of ovarian cancer patients do not have a complete response to front-line platinum-based

treatment [2-6]. Furthermore, the majority of ovarian cancer patients recur and response rates to second-line treatments are substantially lower. This may be due, in part, to acquired drug resistance [7]. In the recurrent population, empiric-based chemotherapy is associated with response rates ranging from only 5 to 20% with limited progression-free (PFS) and overall survival (OS) [8-11].

Since recurrence rates for ovarian cancer are high and the associated toxicity to chemotherapy can be significant, knowledge of potential tumor responses to chemotherapy a priori could be a useful tool in the selection of effective chemotherapy for patients with advanced or

* Correspondence: bradley.monk@chw.edu
[8]University of Arizona Cancer Center, Creighton University School of Medicine at Dignity Health St. Joseph's Hospital and Medical Center, 500 W. Thomas Road, Suite 600, Phoenix, AZ 85013, USA
Full list of author information is available at the end of the article

recurrent disease. Ineffective chemotherapy results in unnecessary toxicity and costs, delay of more effective treatment, and the potential development of acquired drug- and cross drug-resistance. An in vitro assay performed before therapy initiation to identify the drug(s) most likely to be effective for the individual patient would have clinical utility. Information provided by an in vitro assay, when integrated with clinical judgment, could lead to the identification of a potentially more effective treatment, thus eliminating toxicity due to ineffective treatments, avoiding a delay in the implementation of effective treatments, and potentially reducing treatment costs. Chemosensitivity and resistance assays are currently recognized in the National Comprehensive Cancer Network (NCCN®) Clinical Practice Guidelines for Oncology for ovarian, fallopian tube, and peritoneal cancers [12,13]. ChemoFx is a live cell platform-based drug response marker that was developed to overcome the technical limitations of earlier generations of chemotherapy sensitivity and resistance assays and to determine chemosensitivity as well as chemoresistance [14]. Studies of this assay in ovarian cancer indicate that ChemoFx results are predictive of PFS [15] and OS [16].

There is currently limited information on whether chemosensitivity changes throughout the course of adjuvant chemotherapy administration and upon recurrence of disease. Therefore, the primary objective of this study is to determine whether in vitro tumor response differs in metachronous gynecologic cancer specimens collected from the same patient upon primary diagnosis and upon recurrence.

Methods
Participants
Inclusion criteria were as follows: (1) tumor samples were submitted to Precision Therapeutics, Inc. (Pittsburgh, Pa) for ChemoFx testing between August 2, 2006 and May 31, 2010; (2) chemoresponse testing was completed at primary diagnosis and upon recurrence of disease; and (3) assays were completed at least 90 days apart. A total of 63 participants met the inclusion criteria. Thirty-six of these patients were enrolled in the ChemoFx Physician Reported Outcomes (ChemoFx PRO) study. The research protocol was reviewed by the Copernicus Group Institutional Review Board, and they determined that this study qualifies as exempt research under 45 CFR §46.101 (b) (4) before the initiation of the analysis. Existing de-identified (anonymized) clinical and pathological data were used to perform the analysis.

ChemoFx
Fresh tumor specimens preserved in McCoy's medium were received by the commercial laboratory, usually within 24 hours of removal. Tumor testing methods

were reported previously [15]. Briefly, tumor specimens were mechanically disrupted to release and establish malignant epithelial cells as monolayer cultures. The tumor sample was then tested against a series of 10 serial dilutions of each drug or drug combination. The range of drug concentrations tested for each drug(s) was as follows: carboplatin (1 μM-500 μM), cisplatin (0.2 μM-100 μM), docetaxel (0.1 nM-25 nM), doxorubicin (2 nM-1 μM), etoposide (20 nM- 2 μM), gemcitabine (1 nM- 50 nM), ifosfamide (0.2 μM- 100 μM), paclitaxel (0.2 nM-0.1 μM), and topotecan (0.4 nM- 0.2 μM), in addition to combination carboplatin/gemcitabine and carboplatin/paclitaxel. Combination drugs were tested as a 1:1 combination of each drug at each dose, for example, dose 1 of carboplatin-paclitaxel is dose 1 (1 μM) of carboplatin plus dose 1 (0.2 nM) of paclitaxel. After an incubation period of 72 hours, the cells were fixed with anhydrous ethanol (95% fixing grade) and stained with 4'6-diamidino-2-phenylindole (DAPI), a fluorescent DNA stain for imaging the nucleus (Sigma-Aldrich Corp, St Louis, MO, USA). Cells that remained attached after staining were imaged and counted using automated cell microscopy and cell-counting software. The percentages of cells remaining after drug treatment were used to determine survival fraction (SF = average cell count$_{dosex}$/average cell count$_{control}$), from which dose–response curves were plotted. Each dose–response curve was assigned a response index (RI) score ranging from 0 to 10. The RI score is a metric based on adjusted areas under the curve (aAUC); greater RI values represent greater sensitivity. Curves were smoothed using a logarithmic curve-fit tool (GraphPad Prism®, LaJolla, CA, USA). Based on the aAUC score, in vitro tumor response was then categorized into three groups: responsive (R), intermediately responsive (IR), or non-responsive (NR). The thresholds for these classifications were established based on the 25th and 75th aAUC percentiles. Drugs tested included carboplatin, cisplatin, docetaxel, doxorubicin, gemcitabine, paclitaxel, and topotecan, in addition to combination carboplatin/gemcitabine and carboplatin/paclitaxel.

Statistical methods
The Wilcoxon signed rank test was used to compare chemoresponse (RI score) between primary and recurrent measurement. In commercial reports, tumors are categorized as R, IR or NR to chemotherapies; we therefore completed a second analysis with code corresponding to R = 3, IR = 2 and NR =1, and utilized a two-tailed Wilcoxon signed rank test to compare chemoresponse between primary and recurrent measurement. Statistical significance was set at p < 0.05. All analyses were performed with SAS (version 9.2; SAS Institute, Cary, NC).

Results

The demographic characteristics of the 63 patients who met inclusion criteria are shown in Table 1. Of the 63 pairs, 44 (70%) were diagnosed with ovarian cancer, 6 (10%) with peritoneal cancer, 4 (6%) with fallopian tube cancer, and 9 (14%) with uterine cancer. Mean age of patients was 59 (±11) years. The majority of cases exhibited poor tumor grade (grade 3) and FIGO Stage III. In the subset of patients with known treatment information (those enrolled in the ChemoFx PRO study), all were treated with a platinum/taxane combination for at least one cycle between in vitro chemoresponse testing of their metachronous tumors. Treatment information in this subsample is shown in Table 2.

Because specific individual chemotherapy agents or combinations of agents tested in the assay were selected by the treating physician, determination of chemoresponse was not possible for every drug in each patient. Overall, median time between primary and recurrent assay testing was 309 days (IQR = 208,422; minimum 91; maximum 680).

When examined using the RI score, no significant differences were observed in chemoresponse between primary and recurrent assay results (Table 3); however, a trend toward increased resistance was observed for the drug paclitaxel (p = 0.08). When chemoresponse was examined using the commercially reported categories, a significant shift toward chemoresistance were observed for the drug paclitaxel (p = 0.04) and a marginally significant shift was observed for the drug carboplatin (p = 0.06) (Table 4). There were no statistically significant differences between primary and recurrent measurement in the remaining drugs tested.

Table 1 Characteristics of patients at diagnosis (N = 63)

Age (years)	59.8 ± 11
Cancer Type	
Fallopian Tube	4 (6%)
Ovarian	44 (70%)
Peritoneal	6 (10%)
Uterine	9 (14%)
Tumor Grade	
G1 Well	1 (2%)
G2 Moderate	6 (10%)
G3 Poor	24 (38%)
G4 Undifferentiated	10 (16%)
Unknown	22 (35%)
FIGO Stage	
I	4 (6%)
II	4 (6%)
III	47 (75%)
IV	7 (11)
Unknown	1 (2%)

Table 2 Treatment administered to the subset of patients enrolled in the ChemoFx (Precision Therapeutics, Inc., Pittsburgh, PA) Physician Reported Outcomes Study between assays

	N = 36
Bevacizumab/Carboplatin/Paclitaxel	2 (6%)
Carboplatin/Cisplatin/Paclitaxel	7 (19%)
Carboplatin/Gemcitabine/Paclitaxel	1 (3%)
Carboplatin/Docetaxel	2 (6%)
Carboplatin/Paclitaxel	22 (61%)
Cisplatin/Docetaxel/Paclitaxel	1 (3%)
Cisplatin/Paclitaxel	1 (3%)

Discussion

Our results suggest that chemoresponsiveness does not change between primary diagnosis of disease and recurrence of disease for the majority of drugs in patients with gynecologic cancer who experienced recurrence within approximately one year. These results are consistent with a large analysis of 334 metachronous pairs of epithelial ovarian cancer specimens performed by Tewari et al. Their analysis failed to show a significant difference in the drug resistance profile of primary tumors and matched recurrences in the same patient [17]. These findings, in addition to ours, may be unexpected but not inexplicable. Furthermore, these results are consistent with observations of biomarker expression in metachronous pairs of epithelial ovarian cancer. No significant changes in the expression of MDR1, p53, or HER2 were noted between primary diagnosis and relapse of disease in 66 patients [18].

A possible explanation for continued chemosensitivity following exposure to chemotherapy, as observed in our primary analysis, has been offered by Tewari et al. They

Table 3 Chemoresponse assay results (expressed as a continuous variable (RI score)) for metachronous tumor pairs

	Number of pairs	Primary median (IQR) RI SCORE	Recurrent median (IQR) RI SCORE	p
Carboplatin	46	5.59(4.89,6.09)	5.32(4.94,5.80)	0.28
Carboplatin/ Gemcitabine	35	5.71(5.16,6.30)	5.90(5.40,6.36)	0.33
Carboplatin/ Paclitaxel	41	6.17(5.15,6.67)	5.92(5.25,6.29)	0.48
Cisplatin	42	5.40(4.66,5.77)	5.38(4.67,5.68)	0.80
Docetaxel	42	5.26(4.74,5.75)	4.96(4.43,5.42)	0.14
Doxorubicin	49	5.17(4.20,5.58)	5.11(4.56,5.56)	0.82
Etoposide	39	5.49(4.66,6.00)	5.41(4.83,5.84)	0.85
Gemcitabine	48	5.27(4.46,5.55)	5.11(4.68,5.55)	0.64
Ifosfamide	30	5.58(5.32,5.80)	5.68(5.25,5.87)	0.90
Paclitaxel	47	5.59(4.99,6.21)	5.30(4.80,5.74)	0.08
Topotecan	52	5.39(4.65,5.74)	5.20(4.54,5.65)	0.99

Table 4 Chemoresponse assay results (expressed as a continuous variable corresponding to categorized results (R = 3, IR = 2, NR = 1)) for metachronous tumor pairs

	Number of pairs	Primary median (IQR) RI SCORE	Recurrent median (IQR) RI SCORE	p
Carboplatin	46	2(1–3)	1(1–2)	0.06
Carboplatin/ Gemcitabine	35	2(1–3)	2(2–3)	0.36
Carboplatin/ Paclitaxel	41	3(1–3)	2(1–3)	0.67
Cisplatin	42	2(1–2)	2(1–2)	1.00
Docetaxel	42	1(1–2)	1(1–2)	0.51
Doxorubicin	49	1(1–2)	1(1–2)	0.89
Etoposide	39	2(1–2)	2(1–2)	0.21
Gemcitabine	48	1(1–2)	1(1–2)	0.33
Ifosfamide	30	2(1–2)	2(1–2)	0.83
Paclitaxel	47	2(1–3)	1(1–2)	0.04
Topotecan	52	1.5(1–2)	1(1–2)	0.70

postulate that after initial debulking surgery, patients may harbor residual tumor in poorly vascularized areas. Such tumors would be shielded from systemic chemotherapy, retain their initial drug responsiveness, and contribute to tumor regrowth and recurrence. Because the length of time between end of treatment and subsequent recurrence plays an important role in the development of drug resistance, [19] it is possible that if we had examined patients with longer time to recurrence, we may have observed greater shifts toward increased resistance.

A study conducted by Zajchowski, et al. examined differences in biomarker expression via immunohistochemical analysis in primary and recurrent ovarian cancer specimens over a much longer time interval. In the majority of patients examined, the interval between treatments was >2 years, and as high as ≈ 8 year from the primary to last-received recurrent specimen. These patients received between 1–5 prior chemotherapies. Though differences were found in the expression of certain markers within each matched tumor pair, overall biomarker profiles for the matched patient specimens were very similar [20]. A study examining a larger patient population is needed to validate these findings.

A commonly held view is that chemoresponsiveness may change between primary diagnosis and recurrence of disease with intervening administration of chemotherapy. This may be due to the selection and clonal expansion of drug-resistant cells. Indeed, we observed a trend toward increased resistance to paclitaxel in our primary analysis, and a significant shift toward increased chemoresistance for paclitaxel, and a marginally significant shift toward increased chemoresistance for carboplatin, when examining change categorically. Although the treatment information was not included in the scope of this entire analysis, many of the patients in this study are assumed

to have received platinum/taxane-based treatment as first-line chemotherapy. This assumption is supported by the treatment information garnered from the subset of patients enrolled in the ChemoFx PRO study. Exposure to these particular drugs may, in part, explain the more evident shift towards resistance observed with carboplatin and paclitaxel from primary to recurrent tumor (i.e., acquired drug resistance). Notably, there was no evidence for the development of cross-resistance; we did not observe an increase in resistance at recurrence for common second-line treatment agents, such as doxorubicin, gemcitabine, and topotecan.

The theory of acquired drug resistance may explain our results and those of a previous study of metachronous pairs conducted by Matsuo et al.; paclitaxel resistance was higher upon recurrence in a sample of 29 epithelial ovarian cancer patients treated with adjuvant platinum/taxane therapy. In addition, in a sample of 65 patients, recurrent surgery after initial cytoreduction was significantly associated with increased resistance to paclitaxel [19]. Similar increases in paclitaxel resistance in recurrent disease have been reported in other series [20,21]. Additional studies have shown limited, albeit, significant increases in carboplatin [22] and more commonly, paclitaxel, [22,23] chemoresistance throughout the course of disease in primary epithelial ovarian cancer, with no changes in any other cytotoxic agents examined. Clinically, it has been shown that while taxanes have activity as later-line agents in ovarian cancer, resistance emerges over time and this increased resistance is very likely due to intervening therapies [24].

Heterogeneity of drug response is a serious clinical problem encountered when administering chemotherapy. Chemoresponse assays may help the physician avoid administering certain chemotherapeutic agents when a patient's tumor is found to be resistant to those agents. Our results suggest that the chemosensitivity profiles provided by ChemoFx in the primary setting may be valuable for use in both the primary and recurrent setting. Since very few patients undergo a secondary surgery, the opportunity to use results from tissue collected at initial cytoreduction underscores the importance of our current findings. The primary setting may be the physician's only chance to collect a specimen and thus chemoresponse results in the primary setting may be critical to that patient's future treatment.

The limitations of this study are those inherent to retrospective studies, including potential selection biases and lack of blinding and control groups. We were also limited in statistical power by a small sample size and short time to recurrence. Additionally, the use of assay results to guide chemotherapy treatment may be a potential confounder.

Conclusions

In summary, we observed a trend toward increased chemoresistance at recurrence for the common first-line gynecologic cancer treatment agent paclitaxel, and a marginally significant trend toward increased chemoresistance at recurrence for the first-line gynecologic cancer treatment agent carboplatin, but no change in chemoresponsiveness between primary diagnosis and recurrence of disease for other common chemotherapy drugs, including common second-line agents such as doxorubicin, gemcitabine, and topotecan. Our results are consistent with clinical observations and established biologic concepts, suggesting that an in vitro assay may be a useful tool in both research and clinical practice. Drug resistance remains a major obstacle in cancer therapy. Further research is needed to better elucidate the mechanisms by which tumors acquire drug resistance and to define the role of chemoresistance assays in the treatment of gynecologic cancers.

Competing interest
Candace K. McClure was an employee of Precision Therapeutics, Inc during the time of this trial. Additionally, during the time of this trial James Fiorica was on the speaker's bureau for Precision Therapeutics, Inc. All other authors report no competing interest.

Authors' Contributions
HJD and BJM had the concept and design for the manuscript. All authors carried out the study and assisted with the collection and assembly of data. All authors assisted with the writing of the manuscript. All authors read and approved the final manuscript.

Acknowledgement
The authors wish to thank Daniele A. Sumner, BA for her assistance in editing this manuscript. The authors are solely responsible for the content of this manuscript.

Author details
[1]The University of Texas MD Anderson Cancer Center, Houston, TX, USA. [2]Sarasota Memorial Hospital, Sarasota, FL, USA. [3]Precision Therapeutics, Inc, Pittsburgh, PA, USA. [4]University of South Alabama Mitchell Cancer Institute, Mobile, AL, USA. [5]South Florida Center for Gynecologic Oncology, Boca Raton, FL, USA. [6]North Shore LIJ Health System/Biomedical Research Alliance of New York, Manhassett, NY, USA. [7]Georgia Gynecologic Oncology, Atlanta, GA, USA. [8]University of Arizona Cancer Center, Creighton University School of Medicine at Dignity Health St. Joseph's Hospital and Medical Center, 500 W. Thomas Road, Suite 600, Phoenix, AZ 85013, USA.

References
1. Siegel R, Ma J, Zou Z, Jemal A: **Cancer statistics, 2014.** *CA Cancer J Clin* 2014, **64:**9–29.
2. du Bois A, Luck HJ, Meier W, Adams HP, Mobus V, Costa S, Bauknecht T, Richter B, Warm M, Schroder W, Olbricht S, Nitz U, Jackisch C, Emons G, Wagner U, Kuhn W, Pfisterer J, Arbeitsgemeinschaft gynäkologische Onkologie Ovarian Cancer Study Group: **A randomized clinical trial of cisplatin/paclitaxel versus carboplatin/paclitaxel as first-line treatment of ovarian cancer.** *J Natl Cancer Inst* 2003, **95:**1320–1329.
3. du Bois A, Weber B, Rochon J, Meier W, Goupil A, Olbricht S, Barats JC, Kuhn W, Orfeuvre H, Wagner U, Richter B, Lueck HJ, Pfisterer J, Costa S, Schroeder W, Kimmig R, Pujade-Lauraine E, Arbeitsgemeinschaft Gynaekologische Onkologie; Ovarian Cancer Study Group; Groupe d'Investigateurs Nationaux pour l'Etude des Cancers Ovariens: **Addition of epirubicin as a third drug to carboplatin-paclitaxel in first-line treatment of advanced ovarian cancer: a prospectively randomized gynecologic cancer intergroup trial by the Arbeitsgemeinschaft Gynaekologische Onkologie Ovarian Cancer Study Group and the Groupe d'Investigateurs Nationaux pour l'Etude des Cancers Ovariens.** *J Clin Oncol* 2006, **24:**1127–1135.
4. Fruehauf JP: **In vitro assay-assisted treatment selection for women with breast or ovarian cancer.** *Endocr Relat Cancer* 2002, **9:**171–182.
5. Neijt JP, Engelholm SA, Tuxen MK, Sorensen PG, Hansen M, Sessa C, de Swart CA, Hirsch FR, Lund B, van Houwelingen HC: **Exploratory phase III study of paclitaxel and cisplatin versus paclitaxel and carboplatin in advanced ovarian cancer.** *J Clin Oncol* 2000, **18:**3084–3092.
6. Ozols RF, Bundy BN, Greer BE, Fowler JM, Clarke-Pearson D, Burger RA, Mannel RS, DeGeest K, Hartenbach EM, Baergen R, Gynecologic Oncology Group: **Phase III trial of carboplatin and paclitaxel compared with cisplatin and paclitaxel in patients with optimally resected stage III ovarian cancer: a Gynecologic Oncology Group study.** *J Clin Oncol* 2003, **21:**3194–3200.
7. McGuire WP, Hoskins WJ, Brady MF, Kucera PR, Partridge EE, Look KY, Clarke-Pearson DL, Davidson M: **Cyclophosphamide and cisplatin compared with paclitaxel and cisplatin in patients with stage III and stage IV ovarian cancer.** *N Engl J Med* 1996, **334:**1–6.
8. Bookman MA: **Developmental chemotherapy and management of recurrent ovarian cancer.** *J Clin Oncol* 2003, **21:**149s–167s.
9. Cannistra SA: **Is there a "best" choice of second-line agent in the treatment of recurrent, potentially platinum-sensitive ovarian cancer?** *J Clin Oncol* 2002, **20:**1158–1160.
10. Ozols RF: **Recurrent ovarian cancer: evidence-based treatment.** *J Clin Oncol* 2002, **20:**1161–1163.
11. Markman M, Bookman MA: **Second-line treatment of ovarian cancer.** *Oncologist* 2000, **5:**26–35.
12. **Chemosensitivity/Resistance assay included as part of the NCCN principles of chemotherapy.** [http://www.medicalnewstoday.com/releases/180642.php]
13. **NCCN clinical guidelines in oncology: epithelial ovarian cancer/ fallopian tube cancer/primary peritoneal cancer, version 2.2011.** [http://www.nccn.org/professionals/physician_gls/pdf/ovarian.pdf]
14. Brower SL, Fensterer JE, Bush JE: **The ChemoFx assay: an ex vivo chemosensitivity and resistance assay for predicting patient response to cancer chemotherapy.** *Methods Mol Biol* 2008, **414:**57–78.
15. Gallion H, Christopherson WA, Coleman RL, DeMars L, Herzog T, Hosford S, Schellhas H, Wells A, Sevin BU: **Progression-free interval in ovarian cancer and predictive value of an ex vivo chemoresponse assay.** *Int J Gynecol Cancer* 2006, **16:**194–201.
16. Herzog TJ, Krivak TC, Fader AN, Coleman RL: **Chemosensitivity testing with ChemoFx and overall survival in primary ovarian cancer.** *Am J Obstet Gynecol* 2010, **203:**68.e1-6.
17. Tewari KS, Mehta RS, Burger RA, Yu IR, Kyshtoobayeva AS, Monk BJ, Manetta A, Berman ML, Disaia PJ, Fruehauf JP: **Conservation of in vitro drug resistance patterns in epithelial ovarian carcinoma.** *Gynecol Oncol* 2005, **98:**360–368.
18. Tewari KS, Kyshtoobayeva AS, Mehta RS, Yu IR, Burger RA, DiSaia PJ, Fruehauf JP: **Biomarker conservation in primary and metastatic epithelial ovarian cancer.** *Gynecol Oncol* 2000, **78:**130–136.
19. Matsuo K, Eno ML, Im DD, Rosenshein NB: **Chemotherapy time interval and development of platinum and taxane resistance in ovarian, fallopian, and peritoneal carcinomas.** *Arch Gynecol Obstet* 2010, **281:**325–328.
20. McAlpine JN, Eisenkop SM, Spirtos NM: **Tumor heterogeneity in ovarian cancer as demonstrated by in vitro chemoresistance assays.** *Gynecol Oncol* 2008, **110:**360–364.
21. Matsuo K, Im DD, Rosenshein NB: **Increased paclitaxel resistance in recurrent epithelial ovarian cancer: analysis of metachronous tumors.** *Int J Clin Oncol* 2010, **15:**325–327.
22. Pospiskova M, Spenerova M, Pilka R, Kudela M, Hajdúch M, Srámek V, Melichar B, Cwiertka K: **Repeated chemosensitivity testing in patients with epithelial ovarian carcinoma.** *Eur J Gynaecol Oncol* 2010, **31:**295–298.
23. Geisler JP, Linnemeier GC, Thomas AJ, Manahan KJ: **Extreme drug resistance is common after prior exposure to paclitaxel.** *Gynecol Oncol* 2007, **106:**538–540.
24. McCourt C, Dessie S, Bradley AM, Schwartz J, Brard L, Dizon DS: **Is there a taxane-free interval that predicts response to taxanes as a later-line treatment of recurrent ovarian or primary peritoneal cancer?** *Int J Gynecol Cancer* 2009, **19:**343–347.

15

Fertility-sparing management in cervical cancer: balancing oncologic outcomes with reproductive success

Karla Willows[1], Genevieve Lennox[1] and Allan Covens[1,2]*

Abstract

Background: Cervical cancer is the fourth most common cancer among women worldwide, many of who are still within their reproductive lifespan. Advances in screening and treatment have increased the 5-year survival for early stage disease to over 90 % in developed countries. The focus is now shifting to reducing morbidity and improving fertility outcomes for cervical cancer patients. Radical trachelectomy with lymph node assessment became the standard of care for selected women with lesions <2 cm who desire fertility preservation. However, several questions still remain regarding the degree of surgical radicality required for tumors <2 cm, and fertility-sparing options for women with early-stage disesase ≥2 cm, and those with more advanced disease. Here, we compile a narrative review of the evidence for oncologic and pregnancy outcomes following radical trachelectomy, non-radical fertility-sparing surgery, and the use of neoadjuvant chemotherapy prior to surgery for larger lesions. We also review the literature for assisted reproductive technologies in women with more advanced disease.

Findings: Available literature suggests that the crude recurrence and mortality rates after radical trachelectomy are <5 and <2 %, respectively (approx. 11 and 4 % for tumors ≥ 2 cm). Among 1238 patients who underwent fertility-sparing surgery for early cervical cancer there were 469 pregnancies with a 67 % live birth rate. Among 134 cases with lesions ≥ 2 cm, there were ten conceptions with a live birth rate of 70 %. Outcomes after non-radical surgery (simple trachelectomy or cervical conization) are similar, although only applicable among a highly selected patient population. For patients ineligible for fertility-preserving surgery or who require adjuvant radiation therapy, current options include ovarian transposition and cryopreservation of oocytes or embryos but other techniques are under investigation.

Conclusion: Today, many cervical cancer survivors have successful pregnancies. For those with early-stage disease, minimally invasive and fertility sparing techniques have resulted in improved obstetrical outcomes without compromising oncologic safety. Results from three ongoing trials on non-radical surgery for low-risk tumors <2 cm will further inform the need for radical surgery in such patients. For those in whom natural childbearing is unachievable, advances in assisted reproductive technologies provide reproductive options. Despite our advances, the effects of cervical cancer survivorship on quality of life are not fully elucidated.

Keywords: Fertility-sparing, Cervical cancer, Trachelectomy, Non-radical, Neoadjuvant chemotherapy, Assisted reproductive technologies, Quality of life,

* Correspondence: al.covens@sunnybrook.ca
[1]Division of Gynecologic Oncology, Department of Obstetrics and Gynecology, University of Toronto, M700-610 University Avenue, Toronto M5G 2 M9, ON, Canada
[2]Division of Gynecologic Oncology, T2051 Odette Cancer Centre, University of Toronto, 2075 Bayview Avenue, Toronto M4N 3 M5, ON, Canada

Background

Cervical cancer is the fourth most common cancer in women worldwide, with over half a million new cases diagnosed annually [1]. It affects women at a significantly younger age than most other malignancies. According to the Surveillance, Epidemiology, and End Results (SEER) database, between 2008 and 2012, 39 % of new cases diagnosed in the US were in women under the age of 45 [2]. Over the past several decades, most developed countries have seen a significant reduction in overall mortality with 5-year survival rates for localized disease surpassing 90 % [2]. Combined with a trend towards delayed childbearing, this has resulted in a cohort of cervical cancer survivors who are still well within their reproductive lifespan.

Loss of fertility, regardless of cause, is a source of significant psychological distress among women [3]. Several studies suggest that cervical cancer survivors have significantly more reproductive concerns, compared to age-matched controls, including grief about inability to bear children, and an inability to talk openly about fertility [3, 4]. In 2006 the American Society of Clinical Oncology highlighted the importance of addressing future fertility and potential fertility preservation options with patients prior to cancer therapy [5].

Radical trachelectomy (RT) was first described by Eugen Aburel for the treatment of early-stage cervical cancers in the 1950s [6]. This technique was all but forgotten until the 1990s when it was revitalized by Dargent et al. in 1994 [7], to preserve fertility in selected cases through a vaginal approach (VRT). This ushered in a new era of fertility-sparing options for women with early-stage cervical cancer. Over two decades of accumulated data show that for women with small volume disease, this procedure has acceptable surgical morbidity and oncological outcomes [8]. As a result, radical trachelectomy, with pelvic lymph node assessment, became the standard of care for selected women early-stage with disease <2 cm who desire to maintain their fertility [9].

However, several questions still remain about the degree of radicality required, as well as the optimal management of lesions greater than 2 cm. There continues to be a push towards less invasive procedures to reduce peri-operative morbidity, and reduce preterm delivery and perinatal morbidity without compromising oncologic safety. The purpose of this review is to examine the current state of fertility sparing management of cervical cancer, including management of ≥2 cm early stage disease and novel technologies in assisted reproduction for women with locally advanced disease.

Main text

Methods

We searched Ovid EMBASE (from 1974 to 2016 week 13) and Ovid MEDLINE in process & other non-indexed citations (from inception to March 2016) for relevant citations. We performed key-word searches combining various disease-specific terms (e.g. cervical cancer, uterine cervix carcinoma) with treatment specific terms (e.g. trachelectomy, conization, neoadjuvant chemotherapy). We limited our search to English language studies. To identify ongoing planned or unpublished trials, we searched the US National Institute of Health's clinical trial registry at ClinicalTrials.gov. All searches were supplemented by hand searching the reference lists of key papers for relevant citations. Articles were organized based on topics deemed to be relevant by the authors. Crude recurrence, mortality, and birth rates were calculated from large reports of radical trachelectomy overall, radical trachelectomy for lesions ≥2 cm, non-radical fertility sparing procedures, and fertility-sparing procedures after neoadjuvant chemotherapy. Where follow-up studies were available, we included only the most recent and complete series to avoid double counting patients. A narrative review of these topics is presented here.

Early-stage disease

Early-stage cervical cancer includes disease that is confined to the cervix, measuring ≤ 4 cm, with no apparent spread to adjacent structures or distant organs (International Federation of Gynecology and Obstetrics-FIGO- stages IA1-IB1) [10]. Given the low risk (≤1 %) of either pelvic lymph node or parametrial involvement in stage 1A1 squamous cell carcinoma of the cervix, standard treatment usually consists of cone biopsy or extrafascial hysterectomy, depending on the patient's desire for fertility preservation [10, 11]. Traditional thinking has dictated that beyond stage IA1 (or in the presence of other high risk features) the increased risk of local spread to the parametria and upper vagina necessitates a more radical surgical approach including lymph node assessment.

Excellent oncological outcomes have been obtained with radical hysterectomy accompanied by bilateral pelvic lymph node dissection for early-stage disease. Five-year overall survival rates range from 73 to 98 % [12–14]. However, this procedure carries a significant risk of surgical morbidity, including increased blood loss, transfusion, and injuries to the bladder, bowel, ureters, and obturator nerve [15–17]. Long-term bladder, anorectal, and sexual dysfunction have been described [18–20]. Over time, minimally invasive and nerve sparing approaches have been developed to reduce morbidity [10], and the degree of surgical radicality required has been challenged with favourable survival and recurrence rates [21, 22].

Eligibility for fertility sparing management

To be eligible for fertility sparing management of cervical cancer, two main criteria must be met; 1) the patient's desire for, and likelihood of, fertility must be sufficiently high, and 2) oncologic safety must be acceptable. A pre-operative fertility workup may be considered, particularly in those with a history of infertility [23]. The patient's age should be considered with respect to ovarian reserve and the increased risk of pregnancy complications with advanced maternal age [23, 24]. Eligibility for fertility-sparing surgery should reflect local jurisdictional age-related eligibility policies for assisted reproductive technologies.

Oncologic safety can be assessed in terms of clinicopathologic risk factors for recurrence. These include tumour size, depth of stromal invasion, presence of lymphovascular space invasion (LVSI), lymph node and parametrial involvement and the feasibility of achieving tumour-free margins [25–27].

Clinical stage, including vaginal and parametrial spread, should be assessed by an expert (e.g. Gynecologic Oncologist) [23]. Although tumours > 2 cm are at greater risk of lymph node metastasis and recurrence [28, 29], there is a general consensus that larger, expohytic tumours with minimal stromal invasion may be considered for fertility-sparing procedures [30, 31]. In a small prospective trial of 30 patients desiring fertility-preservation, magnetic resonance imaging was shown to have 100 % positive and negative predictive value in assessing suitability for radical trachelectomy [32].

For early stage disease, the difference in recurrence and mortality between squamous carcinomas and adenocarcinomas seems negligible, and both may be considered as candidates for fertility-preservation [33, 34]. A review at our centre found no significant difference in recurrence free survival between 74 patients with adenocarcinoma and 66 patients with squamous cell carcinoma treated with radical vaginal trachelectomy [35]. Although there have been reports of higher incidence of ovarian involvement in adenocarcinoma of the cervix, compared to squamous carcinomas, the overall risk remains low. A review by Touhami and Plante reported a 2 % incidence of ovarian metastasis among those with stage 1B adenocarcinomas of the cervix, among which 96.7 % had other clinical and pathologic features that would preclude fertility-sparing [36]. The authors argue that the risk of surgical menopause in the premenopausal population eligible for fertility-sparing outweighs the risk of ovarian involvement, and therefore advocate that ovarian preservation remains an option in the case of early adenocarcinomas of the cervix.

However, non-squamous, non-adenocarcinomas have significantly worse prognosis [37]. In a few early series that included neuroendocrine carcinomas for fertility-sparing, rapid recurrence was observed [28–30]. Many have thus questioned the inclusion of these aggressive histologies in fertility sparing procedures. LVSI alone should not preclude fertility-sparing management. A review by Beiner et al. found that among patients undergoing radical vaginal trachelectomy, 28 % had LVSI, and only 5 % had nodal metastases [38]. While exclusion on this basis is unmerited, extensive LVSI does put these patients at increased risk of nodal involvement [39].

Little prospective data exists as to the optimal surgical margin for trachelectomy specimen. A retrospective review by McCann et al. found that for patients with stage 1A2–2A cervical cancer undergoing radical hysterectomy, close surgical margins (defined as margins ≤5 mm), while not an independent risk factor for recurrence, were associated with other intermediate and high risk features, including lymph node positivity, parametrial involvement, increased size of primary lesion, increased depth of stromal invasion and LVSI [40]. Coincidently, most experts in the area had previously empirically adopted 5 mm as the minimum margin [41, 42]. Therefore, based on extrapolation of data on recurrence following radical hysterectomy and the above empiricism, we believe that optimal surgical margins after fertility-sparing management are at least 5 mm.

Lymph node assessment

Assessment for lymph node metastases is critical for any patient with greater than 3 mm depth of invasion (i.e. > stage IA1) or other high risk features (e.g. LVSI, high-risk histologies) on a biopsy specimen. Suspicious nodes should be sought on pre-operative CT or MRI but the sensitivity and specificity of these modalities in early cervical cancer is modest, given the low prevalence of enlarged nodes in this population [11]. Combined PET-CT may identify small metastases, however the utility and significance of these remains controversial, particularly in those receiving neoadjuvant chemotherapy prior to surgical management [43].

In the absence of grossly positive nodes on imaging, definitive nodal assessment must be made operatively. Frozen section may be utilized to assess for nodal metastases and positive surgical margins, in which case fertility-sparing surgery may be aborted, or the surgical procedure altered (eg. complete ipsilateral pelvic and para-aortic lymphadenectomy). However, frozen section is not universally practiced due to the concerns regarding false negatives, and loss of tissue for permanent pathological processing. A range of false negative rates for intra-operative frozen section in early cervical cancer has been reported. For stage 1A2–1B1, Panici et al. report a false negative rate of 4.2 % [44]; for stage 1B1–2B, Scholz et al. report a false negative rate of 19 % [45]. Since 2015, the National Comprehensive Cancer Network (NCCN) recommends the consideration of sentinel lymph node procedure (SLNP) for early-stage cervical cancer measuring less than 2 cm [9]. Gortzak examined the use of sentinel lymph node procedure among 81 women undergoing successful sentinel lymph node procedure for early cervical cancer (stage 1A–1B1). They reported a false negative rate of 21.4 % (3/14 negative sentinel nodes). Two of the three cases involved micrometastases <2 mm found only after ultrastaging, highlighting the importance of this element of the sentinel lymph node procedure [46]. Despite a high false negative rate, intraoperative frozen section remains useful in this setting, due to the low prevalence of nodal involvement in early cervical cancer. In this case, the finding of a negative node on frozen section has a negative predictive value of over 97 % [47, 48].

It is recommended that both intraoperative, and final pathology be reviewed by a pathologist specializing in gynecology and that ultrastaging be performed for sentinel lymph nodes. Ultimately, the clinician needs to evaluate all available information, and come to a decision regarding further surgery to define the extent of disease (staging), versus adjuvant therapy be it chemo, radiation, or both- the former not necessarily precluding fertility sparing.

Radical fertility-sparing surgical management

Radical vaginal trachelectomy (VRT) accompanied by laparoscopic pelvic lymph node dissection has become an accepted treatment modality for fertility preservation in early cervical cancer measuring <2 cm. In 2007, a review of 520 cases found a recurrence and mortality rate of 4.2 and 2.8 %, respectively [49].

Radical trachelectomy can also be performed abdominally (ART), laparoscopically (LRT), and robotically (RRT). An advantage to these alternative approaches is that they more closely resemble the radical hysterectomy familiar to gynecologic oncologists, and do not require special skills in vaginal surgery [34]. Additionally, an abdominal approach allows for potentially greater parametrial resection compared to the vaginal approach [50]. In 2013, Cao et al. performed a matched case-control study comparing surgical approaches in 126 patients undergoing radical trachelectomy [51]. They found no significant differences between VRT and ART for mean operating time, perioperative complications or postoperative complications. Although VRT resulted in higher pregnancy rates (35.5 v. 8.8 %) and live birth rates (23.3 v. 8.8 %), it also resulted in higher rates of recurrence (9.8 v. 0 %) and death from disease (2.8 v. 0 %) [51]. Our review of large case series' of radical trachelectomy identified oncologic outcomes in 1312 patients eligible for fertility sparing management of early cervical cancer (Table 1). After accounting for adjuvant treatments, 91 % successfully preserved their fertility. The crude recurrence and mortality rates in this group were 4.5 and 1.7 %, respectively. We identified 13 studies that

reported individual-level data on recurrences after radical trachelectomy. Fifty-six patients recurred at a median of 18 months after surgery (range 3–108 months). The majority (66 %) of recurrent cases had evidence of intermediate or high-risk features on surgical pathology, or a non-squamous, non-adenocarcinoma histology (Table 2).

Once tumour-free margins (>5 mm) have been achieved, many surgeons insert a cerclage suture around the lower uterine segment, in anticipation of future pregnancy [34]. In an attempt to prevent isthmic stenosis (which occurs in approximately 15 % of cases [52]) we suture a rubber catheter into the os of the lower uterine segment. In our center, this is removed 3 weeks post-operatively [34]. Alternatively, some advocate for the routine use of a temporary intrauterine device for this purpose [53]. If stenosis is suspected, cervical dilatation can be performed [52]. Our review of obstetrical outcomes among 1238 patients who had undergone successful fertility-sparing management for early cervical cancer identified 469 pregnancies, resulting in a 67 % crude live birth rate (Table 3).

Regardless of the approach, higher recurrence rates have been found in patients with larger tumours [51]. Our review of the literature identified 189 cases (for which individual-level data was extractable) of lesions >2 cm eligible for radical trachelectomy (Table 4). Among those who successfully underwent fertility sparing surgery, we identified an overall crude recurrence rate of 11 % and a crude disease-related mortality rate of 4 %. Many feel that lesions ≥2 cm should be triaged to the abdominal approach, where a wider parametrial resection is more attainable [50, 54]. The use of neoadjuvant chemotherapy in this population is discussed below. Furthermore, we identified 134 cases of lesions ≥2 cm where fertility sparing management was successful, resulting in ten conceptions, with a live birth rate of 70 % (Table 5). Ultimately, approximately 25–30 % of women who try to conceive post radical trachelectomy will be infertile [52]. Although three quarters of cases can be attributed to cervical factor, the remaining cases are due to other causes, highlighting the importance of a pre-operative fertility workup in some cases [52].

Non-radical surgical management

Parametrectomy is responsible for the majority of complications related to radical surgery [55]. Among a subgroup of patients with low-risk pathologic features (lesion <2 cm, depth of invasion <10 mm, and negative pelvic nodes), the risk of parametrial involvement is estimated to be as low as 0.6 % (90 % CI 0–1.1 %) [56]. Furthermore, after diagnostic LEEP/conization procedures, approximately 65 % of radical trachelectomy specimens have no residual disease [57–59]. Therefore, many patients with early cancers are over-treated at the

Table 1 Oncologic outcomes after radical trachelectomy (where $N > 100$ reported)

Study	Eligible for fertility sparing (N)	Stage (N)	Histology (N)	LVSI+ (N)	Approach	LN+ (N)	Required adjuvant therapy (N)	Successful fertility sparing (N)	Primary recurrences (N) (mos)	Dead of disease (N) (mos)	Median follow up months (range)
Shepherd 2006 [108]	123	IA2 = 2 IB1 = 121	83 SCC 33 AC 3 AS 4 other	39	VRT	7	11	112	5 (15, 19, 21, 31, 84)	4 (26, 26, 32, 32)	45[a] (1–120)
Marchiole 2007 [109]	118	IA1 = 10 IA2 = 19 IB1 = 83 IIA = 6	90 SCC 25 AC/AS 3 rare	43	LAVRT	5	8	97	7 (7, 11, 18, 19, 20, 21, 93)	5 (21, 24, 26, 27. 41)	95 (31–234)
Plante 2011 [57]	140	IA1 = 7 IA2 = 30 IB1 = 97 IB2 = 3 IIA = 3	78 SCC 52 AC 10 AS	40	VRT	5	15	110	6 (–)	2 (–)	95 (4–225)
Helpman 2011 [35]	140	All IA-IB	74 AC 66 SCC	55	VRT	8	9	140	8 (–)	0	60 (–)
Wethington 2012 [110]	101	IA1 = 3 IA2 = 8 IB1 = 88 IB2 = 1 IIA = 1	40 SCC 6 AS 54 AC 1 clear cell	47	ART	19	20	70	4 (–)	0	32 (1–124)
Cao 2013 [51]	150	18 IA1 19 IA2 113 IB1	135 SCC 15 AC	8	VRT ART	0	0	150	7 (–)	2 (–)	25 (6–91)
Mangler 2014 [111]	320[¥]	IA1 = 46 IA2 = 68 IB2 = 207	220 SCC 97 AC 5 AS	94	VRT	–	–	320	10 (mean 26.1 month, range 3–108)	5 (16, 19, 22, 29, 30)	48 (0–216)
Hauerberg 2015 [112]	120	CIS = 2 IA1 = 7 IA2 = 8 IB1 = 103	82 SCC 36 AC 2 AS	30	VRT	4	12	108	6 (–)	2 (–)	55.7 (5.5–147)
Vieira 2015 [113]	100	IA1 = 6 IA2 = 25 IB1 = 69	49 SCC 42 AC 7 AS 2 mixed	25	ART RRT LRT	2	9	83	0	0	51 (10–147)
Total	N = 1312							N = 1190	N = 53	N = 20	
Crude rates (%)									Recurrence rate = 4.5 %[#]	Mortality rate = 1.7 %[#]	

Abbreviations: LVSI+ presence of lymphovascular space invasion, *LN+* lymph node metastasis, *SCC* squamous cell carcinoma, *AC* adenocarcinoma, *AS* adenosquamous carcinoma, *LAVRT* laparoscopic-assisted vaginal radical trachelectomy, *ART* abdominal radical trachelectomy, *VRT* vaginal radical trachelectomy, *RRT* robotic radical trachelectomy

[a]Only mean follow up is reported

[#]Crude recurrence and mortality rates among those who successfully had fertility preservation

[¥]In the original study, the sum of the stages and histologies are 321 and 322, respectively, but the reported *N* is 320

Table 2 Histopathologic features among recurrences after radical trachelectomy (N = 56)

Intermediate/high risk features	N
Histology	
Squamous cell carcinoma	26
Adenocarcinoma	18
Adenosquamous	4
Clear cell	1
Neuroendocrine	2
Glassy cell	1
Not reported	4
Size	
≥ 2 cm	20
Lymphovascular space invasion	
positive	22
Lymph nodes	
positive	8
Margins	
positive	1
No intermediate/high risk features	19

risk of increased surgical morbidity without the benefit of improved oncologic outcomes. A review by Reade et al. identified 341 patients who had undergone simple hysterectomy or simple trachelectomy for the treatment of stage ≥ IA2 cervical cancer. They found a crude recurrence rate of 6.3 %, and a crude disease-related mortality

rate of 1.5 % [11], which are comparable to those achieved by radical trachelectomy [49, 51]. Given these findings, non-radical surgery (simple trachelectomy or conization) could be considered for fertility-sparing in the management of small lesions with favourable prognostic features [55, 56, 60].

Our review of the literature identified 203 cases of early-stage cervical cancer eligible for non-radical, fertility-sparing surgery (Table 6). All patients had lesions <2 cm. Sixty patients underwent simple trachelectomy, and 138 underwent conization. Among 185 cases where fertility-sparing was successful, the crude recurrence rate was 2.7 % and the crude mortality rate was 0.5 %. Among 124 women where fertility preservation was successful, we identified 71 pregnancies with a live birth rate of 68 % (Table 7). Both oncologic outcomes and pregnancy rates compare favourably to literature reports of those undergoing radical trachelectomy. However, it should be noted that the available data is from non-randomized studies of highly selected patient populations with more favourable prognostic factors compared to those undergoing radical surgery.

We identified three ongoing prospective trials designed to assess the efficacy of non-radical surgery in the treatment of low-risk early-stage cervical cancer. The SHAPE trial (NCT01658930) is a randomized trial comparing simple hysterectomy to radical hysterectomy (or cone biopsy to radical trachelectomy) in addition to pelvic lymph node assessment for cases of early-stage

Table 3 Obstetrical outcomes after radical trachelectomy (where N > 50 reported)

Study	Successful fertility sparing management[#]	Attempted to conceive	Conceptions	T1/T2 losses	Live births (ongoing pregnancy)	Median follow up months for entire series (range)
Bernardini 2003 [114]	80	39	22	4	18	–
Hertel 2006 [29]	106	–	18	3	12 (3)	29 (1–128)
Shepherd 2006 [108]	112	63	55	–	28 (3)	45[a] (1–120)
Li 2011 [53]	56	10	2	0	1 (1)	23 (1–78)
Plante 2011 [57]	110	–	106	29	77	95 (4–225)
Kim 2012 [115]	77	35	27	7	20	–
Wethington 2012 [110]	70	38	31	9	16 (6)	32 (1–124)
Cao 2013 [51]	150	77	20	9	14	25 (6–91)
Nishio 2013 [116]	114	69	31	5	21 (5)	33
Vieira 2015 [113]	83	34	19	5	10 (4)	51 (10–147)
Hauerberg 2015 [112]	108	72	77	21	53 (3)	55.7 (5.5–147)
Kasuga 2016 [117]	172	109	61	13	43 (5)	–
Total	1238	546	469	105	313 (30)	
Crude rates (%)				T1/T2 loss rate = 22.4 %	Live birth rate = 66.7 % &	

Abbreviations: *T1* first trimester, *T2* second trimester
[a]Only mean follow up is reported
[#]Excludes those who had completion hysterectomy, or received fertility-compromising adjuvant treatment
& Does not include ongoing pregnancies

Table 4 Oncologic outcomes of radical trachelectomy for lesions ≥ 2 cm (where N > 10 reported)

Study	N with lesions ≥ 2 cm who underwent fertility sparing surgery	Approach	N recurrences (mos)	N dead of disease (mos)	Median follow up months for entire series (range)
Marchiole 2007 [109]	21	LAVRT	6 (7, 11, 18, 20, 21, 93)	4 (21, 24, 27, 41)	95 (31–234)
Nishio 2009 [118]	13	ART	5 (4, 8, 14, 18, 23)	0	27 (1–67)
Cao 2013 [51]	48	VRT ART	5 (–)	2 (–)	34.3[a]
Li 2013 [119]	61	ART	0	0	30 (2–108)
Lintner 2013 [120]	31	ART	4 (5, 6, 10, 14)	2 (16, 22)	90 (60–148)
Wethington 2013 [121]	15	ART LAVRT VRT	1 (9)	0	44 (1–90)
Total	N = 189		N = 21	N = 8	
Crude rates (%)			Recurrence rate = 11.1 %[#]	Mortality rate = 4.2 %[#]	

Abbreviations: *LAVRT* laparoscopic-assisted vaginal radical trachelectomy, *ART* abdominal radical trachelectomy, *VRT* vaginal radical trachelectomy
[a]Only mean follow up is reported
[#]Crude recurrence and mortality rates among those who successfully underwent fertility sparing surgery, notwithstanding adjuvant treatment received

(IA2–IB1 < 2 cm), low-risk (stromal invasion <10 mm on LEEP/cone, or <50 % on MRI) cervical cancer [61]. The goal is to demonstrate that in selected cases, non-radical surgery (simple hysterectomy or cone biopsy) is non-inferior to the gold standard radical surgery (radical hysterectomy or radical trachelectomy) with respect to oncologic safety. Treatment-related morbidity, quality of life, and cost-effectiveness are also being evaluated. ConCerv (NCT01048853) is a prospective, international, multicenter cohort study. The goal is to assess the oncologic safety and feasibility of simple hysterectomy or cone biopsy for early-stage (IA2–IB1 < 2 cm) low-risk (negative LVSI, negative margins on cone specimen) cervical cancer [62]. GOG 278 (NCT01649089) is a large prospective cohort study [63]. This study's primary objectives are to examine the changes before and after non-radical surgical treatment (simple hysterectomy or cone biopsy for fertility preservation plus pelvic lymphadenectomy) on functional outcomes of bladder, bowel and sexual function for early stage cervical cancer. Women with stage IA1 (LVSI+) and IB1 (<2 cm)

carcinoma of the cervix with ≤ 10 mm of invasion on diagnostic pathology are eligible for entry. After a pre-operative survey on quality of life, women are stratified based on desire to preserve fertility. Those desiring fertility preservation undergo conization, whereas those not desiring future fertility undergo extrafascial hysterectomy. All patients undergo pelvic lymphadenectomy. Patients with high-risk features on final pathology are offered appropriate adjuvant treatment, and are followed for survival only. Otherwise, patients undergoing non-radical (simple hysterectomy) and fertility-sparing (conization) surgery are assessed at routine post-operative visit and every 6 months there-after for validated quality of life measures, including surgical morbidity, sexual function, fertility intentions, reproductive concerns and impact of therapeutic choice overall. Efficacy (recurrence) is an important secondary objective.

It is hoped that these trials will help to define a select group of patients for whom non-radical surgical management is oncologically safe.

Table 5 Obstetrical outcomes of radical trachelectomy for lesions ≥ 2 cm (where N > 10 reported)

Study	Successful fertility sparing management[#]	Attempted to conceive	Conceptions	T1/T2 loss	Live births (ongoing)	Median follow up months for entire series (range)
Cao 2013 [51]	48	24	3	0	3	34.3[a]
Li 2013 [119]	55	9	3	2	1	30.2 (2–108)
Lintner 2013 [120]	31	8	4	1	3	90 (60–148)
Total	134	41	10	3	7	
Crude rates (%)				T1/T2 loss rate = 30 %	Live birth rate = 70 %	

Abbreviations: *T1* first trimester, *T2* second trimester
[a]Only mean follow up is reported
[#]Excludes those who had completion hysterectomy, or received fertility-compromising adjuvant treatment

Table 6 Oncologic outcomes of non-radical fertility sparing procedures (where N > 10 reported)

Study	N eligible	Surgical procedure (includes pelvic LN assessment)	Successful fertility sparing surgery	N recurrences (mos)	N dead of disease (mos)	Median follow up months for entire series (range)
Bisseling 2007 [122]	18	18 cone	18	0	0	72[a]
Rob 2007 [123]	26	15 ST 7 cone	20	1 (14)	0	49 (18–84)
Landoni 2007 [124]	11	11 cone	11	0	0	20 (7–29)
Fagotti 2011 [125]	17	17 cone	13	0	0	16 (8–101)
Maneo 2011 [126]	36	36 cone	31	3 (20, 34, 36)	1 (72)	66 (18–168)
Raju 2012 [127]	15	15 ST	15	0	0	96 (12–120)
Palaia 2012 [128]	14	14 ST	14	0	0	38 (18–96)
Plante 2013 [129]	16	16 ST	16	0	0	27 (1–65)
Andikyan 2014 [130]	10	9 cone 1 cx bx	9	0	0	17 (1–83)
Bouchard-Fortier 2014 [55]	29	29 cone	29	0	0	21 (1–112)
Salihi 2015 [131]	11	11 cone	9	1 (40)	0	58 (13–122)
Total	203	138 Cone 60 ST	185	N = 5	N = 1	
Crude rates (%)				Recurrence rate = 2.7 %[#]	Mortality rate = 0.5 %[#]	

Abbreviations: *ST* simple trachelectomy, *cx bx* cervical biopsy
[a]Only mean follow up is reported
[#]Crude recurrence and mortality rates among those who successfully underwent fertility sparing surgery, notwithstanding adjuvant treatment received

Bulky (2–4 cm) early-stage disease and the use of neoadjuvant chemotherapy

For 2–4 cm FIGO stage IB1 and IIA disease, neoadjuvant chemotherapy (NACT) has been shown to reduce nodal metastases, parametrial infiltration, and overall tumour size, theoretically making otherwise unresectable (for fertility preserving purposes) disease amenable to surgical management [64–66]. Although meta-analysis of the available data has yet to show a survival advantage for the use of NACT in early cervical cancer, its use in the context of fertility preservation has been gaining attention [66].

Our literature review identified 80 cases of ≥2 cm stage IB1–IIA disease eligible for NACT prior to fertility-sparing surgery (Table 8). The crude recurrence rate is 6.3 % and one patient died from her recurrent disease. The use of NACT has resulted in at least 36 pregnancies with a 72.2 % live birth rate (Table 9).

The timing of nodal assessment with respect to NACT is not standardized. A study by Vercillino et al. in 2012

Table 7 Obstetrical outcomes of non-radical fertility sparing procedures (where N > 10 reported)

Study	Successful fertility sparing management[#]	Conceptions	T1/T2 losses	Live births (ongoing)	Median follow up months for entire series (range)
Bisseling 2007 [122]	18	18	5	13	72[a]
Rob 2007 [123]	20	15	6	8 (1)	49 (18–84)
Landoni 2007 [124]	11	3	0	3	20 (7–29)
Fagotti 2011 [125]	13	2	0	2	16 (8–101)
Maneo 2011 [126]	31	21	6	14 (1)	66 (18–168)
Raju 2012 [127]	15	4	0	4	96 (12–120)
Plante 2013 [129]	16	8	0	4 (4)	27 (1–65)
Total	124	71	17	48 (6)	
Crude rates (%)			T1/T2 loss rate = 23.9 %	Live birth rate = 67.6 % &	

Abbreviations: *T1* first trimester, *T2* second trimester
[a]Only mean follow up is reported
[#]Excludes those who had completion hysterectomy, or received fertility-compromising adjuvant treatment
& Does not include ongoing pregnancies

Table 8 Oncologic outcomes of fertility-sparing surgery after NACT (where N > 5 reported)

Study	N who received NACT	Timing of LN assessment (N positive LN)	NACT regimen	Surgical procedure	N recurrence (mos)	N dead of disease (mos)	Median follow up months for entire series (range)
Maneo 2008 [65]	21	After NACT (2)	TIP/TEP x 3	Cone	0[a]	0	69 (10–124)
Robova 2010 [132]	15	After NACT (1)	TI/TAx3	ST	3 (–)	1 (–)	76.5 (17–142)
Marchiole 2011 [64]	7	After NACT (0)	TIP/TEP x2-3	VRT	0	0	22 (5–49)
Vercecllino 2012 [133]	6	Before NACT (0)	1-TP 5-TIP	VRT	0	0	30.6 (8–70)
Lanowska 2014 [134]	20	Before NACT (0)	TIP/TP × 2-3	VRT	1 (20)	0	23 (1–88)
Salihi 2015 [131]	11	Before NACT (1)	2 TIP x3 4 ddCP x3 5 wCP x3	Cone	1 (40)	0	58 (13–122)
Total	N = 80				N = 5	N = 1	
Crude rates (%)					Recurrence rate = 6.3 %[#]	Mortality rate = 1.3 %[#]	

Abbreviations: *NACT* neoadjuvant chemotherapy, *LN* lymph node, *ST* simple trachelectomy, *VRT* vaginal radical trachelectomy, *TP* cisplatin + paclitaxel, *TI* cisplatin + ifosfamide, *TA* cisplatin + doxorubicin (for adenocarcinoma), *TIP* cisplatin + paclitaxel + ifosfamide, *TEP* cisplatin + paclitaxel + epirubicin (for adenocarcinoma), *ddCP* dose dense carboplatin + paclitaxel, *wCP* weekly carboplatin + paclitaxel
[#]Crude recurrence and mortality rates among those who successfully underwent fertility sparing surgery, notwithstanding adjuvant treatment received
[a]N = 3 patients developed CIN in the residual cervix

showed higher rates of recurrence among a subset of women with positive nodes, in whom fertility-sparing surgery was aborted, compared to women with negative nodes that went on to have NACT and VRT. They suggested that nodal assessment prior to NACT identifies a high-risk group in whom fertility preservation should be avoided [43]. Conversely, some contend that the use of NACT prior to lymph node assessment in these patients may result in fewer nodal metastases, and thus a higher number of patients eligible for fertility-sparing surgery [43]. Our review of the literature identified only 3 series where nodal assessment was carried out prior to NACT (Table 6). While nodal involvement is one of the most significant negative prognostic factors in early-stage cervical cancer, up-front lymph node assessment could theoretically be used to tailor NACT regimen, rather than to exclude potential candidates for fertility-sparing surgery [43].

Advanced-stage disease

For patients who require hysterectomy and/or pelvic radiotherapy, fertility preservation depends on assisted reproductive technologies. Recognized options include oocyte or embryo cryopreservation prior to cancer therapy and ovarian transposition [5, 67]. The American Society for Reproductive Medicine in 2013 argues that given similar fertilization and pregnancy rates to IVF/ICSI with fresh oocytes, oocyte cryopreservation should no longer be considered experimental [68]. Fertility preservation options that are still considered investigations include ovarian tissue cryopreservation/transplantation and uterine transplantation [5, 69, 70].

The estimated lethal radiation dose to destroy 50 % of oocytes is ≤2 Gy [71] and dependent on age, doses as low as 6 Gy can render a woman menopausal, [72, 73]. The uterus also undergoes irreversible damage after

Table 9 Obstetrical outcomes of fertility-sparing surgery after NACT (where N > 5 reported)

Study	Successful fertility sparing management[#]	Conceptions	T1/T2 losses	Live births (ongoing)	Median follow up months for entire series (range)
Maneo 2008 [65]	16	10	1	9	69 (10–124)
Robova 2010 [132]	12	7	0	6 (1)	76.5 (17–142)
Marchiole 2011 [64]	7	1	0	0 (1)	22 (5–49)
Lanowska 2014 [134]	18	7	2	4 (1)	23 (1–88)
Salihi 2015 [131]	9	11	4	7	58 (13–122)
Total	62	36	7	26 (3)	
Crude rates (%)			19.4 % T1/T2 loss rate	72.2 % live birth rate	

Abbreviations: *T1* first trimester, *T2* second trimester
[#]Excludes those who had completion hysterectomy, or received fertility-compromising adjuvant treatment
& Does not include ongoing pregnancies

doses from 14 to 30 Gy via reduced uterine volume, reduced elasticity of the uterine musculature and uterine vascular damage [71, 74].

Ovarian transposition was developed as a method to protect the ovaries from the effects of radiation. Due to the theoretical risk of remigration of the ovaries, the ASCO recommendations on fertility preservation suggest performing the transposition as close to the radiation treatment date as possible [5]. Even after the ovaries are transposed, short-term hormonal function is preserved in only approximately 50–93 %, with failure likely related to radiation scatter, remigration, and compromised ovarian blood supply [5, 75–80]. For all of the above reasons, we feel it is important that Gynecologic Oncologists familiar with the radiation borders perform such surgeries. Hwang et. al demonstrated that transposing the ovaries more than 1.5 cm above the iliac crest was significantly associated with successful preservation of ovarian function after treatment [81]. Despite increased success with higher fixation, the Royal College of Obstetricians and Gynecologists recommends that oocyte retrieval be considered for cervical cancer patients prior to the administration of radiation therapy due to the significant risk of ovarian failure after transposition [82]. New random-start ovarian hyperstimulation protocols decrease total time for the IVF cycle without compromising oocyte yield and maturity [83]. Apart from the risk of failure of ovarian transposition, there is also a concern about the risk of metastases in transposed ovaries [84–86]. Given that oophorectomy is not part of the standard treatment of cervical cancer, this risk is not considered prohibitive. Regardless, it seems that ovarian transposition is provided to only a small fraction of eligible patients [87]. A study Salih et. al. in 2015 also suggested that few cervical cancer patients who undergo ovarian transposition end up pursuing in vitro fertilization [88]. The reality is that patients who undergo ovarian transposition require a gestational carrier, which is fraught with ethical, financial and legal issues [89]. Although successful pregnancies have been reported for cervical cancer patients after oocyte retrieval from transposed ovaries and transfer to a gestational carrier, these reports are rare [90–92]. It seems that for most women, the main benefit of ovarian transposition is maintenance of hormonal function rather than preservation of fertility.

Experimental technique for fertility preservation

Ovarian tissue cryopreservation is an experimental technique for fertility preservation. It is sometimes offered to patients who require immediate gonadotoxic treatment of malignancies where there is insufficient time to offer ovulation induction and cryopreservation of oocytes or embryos. Ovarian tissue can be cryopreserved as cortical biopsies, cortical strips or as whole ovaries, but only cortical biopsies and strips have been successfully transplanted after cryopreservation [69]. The ovarian tissue can be transplanted into a pelvic (orthotopic) or extrapelvic (heterotopic) site. When cortical strips are transplanted orthotopically, they are transplanted either into the medulary portion of a remaining ovary or onto the peritoneum of the ovarian fossa [69]. Studies have reported normal menstrual cycles within 4–9 months after transplantation and graft survival from several months up to 7 years [69, 93–96]. There have been at least 24 births reported after orthotopic transplantation of cortical ovarian tissue, but many of these reports are confounded by the presence of native ovarian tissue [69, 95, 97–99]. Locations of heterotopic transplantation of ovarian tissue resulting in restoration of ovarian function include the forearm, abdominal wall and chest wall [69, 100–102]. Although oocyte retrieval and fertilization with IVF have been reported, there have been no reported live births with this technique. The risk of malignancy from autotransplanted ovarian tissue in cancer patients is not clear, but in a systematic review of 289 patients, metastases were common in patients with leukemia, but less common in most other cancers including cervical cancer [103].

Another experimental procedure that has had recent media attention is uterine transplantation. A 1-year follow-up report of the first uterine transplant trial was published in 2015 [104]. The trial involved uterine transplantation in 9 patients with normal ovarian function who had previously undergone IVF and had cryopreserved embryos. One patient had a history of hysterectomy for cervical cancer. Of the 9 transplanted uteri, 2 were removed within the first 6 months, one due to chronic infection and the other due to bilateral uterine vessel thrombosis. In addition to these grade III surgical complications in the recipients, one of the donors developed a ureterovaginal fistula. Participants were placed on an immunosuppressive protocol. After 1 year of follow-up, 5 of the 7 recipients who kept their transplanted uterus experienced rejection episodes which were all asymptomatic and managed with an intensification of the immunosuppressive regimen. Spontaneous menses occurred in all 7 women within 2 months of transplantation. The plan was to transfer embryos after 12–18 months post-transplant, and a 4–6 month rejection-free period, and to remove the uterus after 1–2 successful pregnancies. As of December, 2015 there were apparently 4 healthy babies born to this cohort [70].

Patient reported outcomes after fertility-sparing management

While we have made impressive technological advances in early cervical cancer management, the long-term effects of cancer survivorship on quality of life are still not fully understood [105]. Several prospective observational studies have assessed patient reported outcomes after fertility-sparing surgery in early cervical cancer. In 2010, Carter et al. conducted a 2-year prospective study assessing the emotional, sexual, and quality of life concerns of women undergoing radical trachelectomy versus radical hysterectomy for treatment of early-stage cervical cancer [105]. Pre-operatively, both groups reported increased depression, distress, and sexual dysfunction. Although these measurements improved over time, they did not differ significantly by surgery type. This highlights the challenges faced by young cancer survivors in general. After a few years of procedural experience with non-radical fertility-sparing surgery, Song et al., in 2013, examined the effects of surgical radicality on sexual functioning [106]. Women who had undergone non-radical surgery experienced less sexual dysfunction than those who had undergone radical surgery. There was no difference between those who had undergone radical trachelectomy versus radical hysterectomy [106]. While these non-randomized studies generate important hypotheses, they are limited by small sample sizes.

In addition to GOG 278, a prospective questionnaire-based study is currently assessing quality of life and sexual function in women who have undergone radical abdominal trachelectomy [107]. It is expected that these studies will shed light on the patient experience, both in terms of fertility-sparing and non-radical management of early-stage cervical cancer.

Conclusions

Today, many cervical cancer survivors have the option of becoming a parent. For those with early-stage disease, minimally invasive and fertility sparing techniques have resulted in improved obstetrical outcomes without compromising oncologic safety. For others, natural fertility and childbearing may be unachievable. However, advances in assisted reproductive technologies continue to make pregnancy and/or parenthood a possibility for those who desire it.

Several questions still remain. The safety of non-radical, fertility-sparing surgery has mainly been demonstrated in the context of small, non-randomized comparisons that are fraught with selection bias. The appropriate timing of NACT with respect to nodal assessment, in this context, has yet to be elucidated. The significance of nodal micrometastases remains unclear. For those fortunate enough to undergo fertility preservation and achieve pregnancy, management should be standardized. Centres of excellence should be established, involving gynecologic oncologists, reproductive endocrinologists, maternal fetal medicine specialists, and psychologists specializing in sexual and reproductive health. Ultimately, as we continue

to seek answers to our objective questions, the patient-centered purpose of this quest should not be forgotten.

Abbreviations

AC: Adenocarcinoma; ART: Abdominal radical trachelectomy; AS: Adenosquamous carcinoma; ASCO: American Society of Clinical Oncology; CT: Computed tomography; Cx bx: Cervical biopsy; FIGO: International Federation of Gynecology and Obstetrics; GOG: Gynecologic Oncology Group; Gy: Gray; ICSI: Intracytoplasmic sperm injection; IVF: In vitro fertilization; LARVT: Laparoscopic-assisted vaginal radical trachelectomy; LEEP: Loop electrical excision procedure; LN: Lymph node; LRT: Laparoscopic radical trachelectomy; LVSI: Lymphovascular space invasion; MRI: Magnetic resonance imaging; NACT: Neoadjuvant chemotherapy; NCCN: National Comprehensive Cancer Network; PET-CT: Positron emission tomography-computed tomography; RRT: Robotic radical trachelectoomy; RT: Radical trachelectomy; SCC: Squamous cell carcinoma; SEER: Surveillance, Epidemiology, and End Results database; SLNP: Sentinel lymph node procedure; ST: Simple trachelectomy; T1: First trimester; T2: Second trimester; VRT: Vaginal radical trachelectomy

Acknowledgments
None.

Funding
No funding was specifically obtained for this review.

Authors' contributions
KW was involved in data acquisition, analysis, and interpretation, and was responsible for drafting >80 % of the manuscript. GL was also involved in data acquisition, and interpretation, drafting parts of the review, and revisions of the final manuscript. AC was involved in conception and design of the review, revisions of the manuscript and provided content expertise throughout. All authors gave final approval for publication.

Competing interests
The authors declare that they have no competing interests.

References
1. Ferlay J, Soerjomataram I, Dikshit R, Eser S, Mathers C, Rebelo M, et al. Cancer incidence and mortality worldwide: sources, methods and major patterns in GLOBOCAN 2012. Int J Cancer. 2015;136(5):E359–86.
2. Howlader N NA, Krapcho M, Garshell J, Miller D, Altekruse SF, Kosary CL, Yu M, Ruhl J, Tatalovich Z,Mariotto A, Lewis DR, Chen HS, Feuer EJ, Cronin KA (eds). . SEER Cancer Statistics Review, 1975–2012. Bethesda, MD: National Cancer Institute., 2015.
3. Carter J, Rowland K, Chi D, Brown C, Abu-Rustum N, Castiel M, et al. Gynecologic cancer treatment and the impact of cancer-related infertility. Gynecol Oncol. 2005;97(1):90–5.
4. Wenzel L, Dealba I, Habbal R, Kluhsman BC, Fairclough D, Krebs LU, et al. Quality of life in long-term cervical cancer survivors. Gynecol Oncol. 2005;97(2):310–7.
5. Lee SJ, Schover LR, Partridge AH, Patrizio P, Wallace WH, Hagerty K, et al. American Society of Clinical Oncology recommendations on fertility preservation in cancer patients. J Clin Oncol Off J Am Soc Clin Oncol. 2006;24(18):2917–31.
6. Capilna ME, Ioanid N, Scripcariu V, Gavrilescu MM, Szabo B. Abdominal radical trachelectomy: a Romanian series. Int J Gynecol Cancer Off J Int Gynecol Cancer Soc. 2014;24(3):615–9.

7. Dargent DBJ, Roy M, et al. La trachelectomie elargie (TE) une alternative a l'hysterectomie radicale dans le traitement des cancers infiltrants developes sur la face externe du col uterin. J Obstet Gynaecol. 1994;2:285–92.

8. Sagae S, Monk BJ, Pujade-Lauraine E, Gaffney DK, Narayan K, Ryu SY, et al. Advances and Concepts in Cervical Cancer Trials: A Road Map for the Future. Int J Gynecol Cancer Off J Int Gynecol Cancer Soc. 2015;26:199–207.

9. Koh WJ, Greer BE, Abu-Rustum NR, Apte SM, Campos SM, Cho KR, et al. Cervical Cancer, Version 2.2015. Journal of the National Comprehensive Cancer Network : JNCCN. 2015;13:395–404; quiz

10. Salicru SR, de la Torre JF, Gil-Moreno A. The surgical management of early-stage cervical cancer. Curr Opin Obstet Gynecol. 2013;25(4):312–9.

11. Reade CJ, Eiriksson LR, Covens A. Surgery for early stage cervical cancer: how radical should it be? Gynecol Oncol. 2013;131(1):222–30.

12. Covens A, Rosen B, Murphy J, Laframboise S, Depetrillo AD, Lickrish G, et al. Changes in the demographics and perioperative care of stage IA (2)/IB (1) cervical cancer over the past 16 years. Gynecol Oncol. 2001;81(2):133–7.

13. Comerci G, Bolger BS, Flannelly G, Maini M, de Barros LA, Monaghan JM. Prognostic factors in surgically treated stage IB-IIB carcinoma of the cervix with negative lymph nodes. Int J Gynecol Cancer Off J Int Gynecol Cancer Soc. 1998;8(1):23–6.

14. Quinn MA, Benedet JL, Odicino F, Maisonneuve P, Beller U, Creasman WT, et al. Carcinoma of the cervix uteri. FIGO 26th Annual Report on the Results of Treatment in Gynecological Cancer. International journal of gynaecology and obstetrics: the official organ of the International Federation of Gynaecology and Obstetrics. 2006;95 Suppl 1:S43-103.

15. Pikaart DP, Holloway RW, Ahmad S, Finkler NJ, Bigsby GE, Ortiz BH, et al. Clinical-pathologic and morbidity analyses of Types 2 and 3 abdominal radical hysterectomy for cervical cancer. Gynecol Oncol. 2007;107(2):205–10.

16. Alexander-Sefre F, Chee N, Spencer C, Menon U, Shepherd JH. Surgical morbidity associated with radical trachelectomy and radical hysterectomy. Gynecol Oncol. 2006;101(3):450–4.

17. Covens A, Rosen B, Gibbons A, Osborne R, Murphy J, Depetrillo A, et al. Differences in the morbidity of radical hysterectomy between gynecological oncologists. Gynecol Oncol. 1993;51(1):39–45.

18. Pieterse QD, Maas CP, ter Kuile MM, Lowik M, van Eijkeren MA, Trimbos JB, et al. An observational longitudinal study to evaluate miction, defecation, and sexual function after radical hysterectomy with pelvic lymphadenectomy for early-stage cervical cancer. Int J Gynecol Cancer Off J Int Gynecol Cancer Soc. 2006;16(3):1119–29.

19. Bergmark K, Avall-Lundqvist E, Dickman PW, Henningsohn L, Steineck G. Vaginal changes and sexuality in women with a history of cervical cancer. N Engl J Med. 1999;340(18):1383–9.

20. Sood AK, Nygaard I, Shahin MS, Sorosky JI, Lutgendorf SK, Rao SS. Anorectal dysfunction after surgical treatment for cervical cancer. J Am Coll Surg. 2002;195(4):513–9.

21. Landoni F, Maneo A, Zapardiel I, Zanagnolo V, Mangioni C. Class I versus class III radical hysterectomy in stage IB1-IIA cervical cancer. A prospective randomized study. Eur J Surg Oncol J Eur Soc Surg Oncol Br Assoc Surg Oncol. 2012;38(3):203–9.

22. Landoni F, Maneo A, Cormio G, Perego P, Milani R, Caruso O, et al. Class II versus class III radical hysterectomy in stage IB-IIA cervical cancer: a prospective randomized study. Gynecol Oncol. 2001;80(1):3–12.

23. Ribeiro Cubal AF, Ferreira Carvalho JI, Costa MF, Branco AP. Fertility-sparing surgery for early-stage cervical cancer. International journal of surgical oncology. 2012;2012:936534.

24. Jacobsson B, Ladfors L, Milsom I. Advanced maternal age and adverse perinatal outcome. Obstet Gynecol. 2004;104(4):727–33.

25. Delgado G, Bundy BN, Fowler Jr WC, Stehman FB, Sevin B, Creasman WT, et al. A prospective surgical pathological study of stage I squamous carcinoma of the cervix: a Gynecologic Oncology Group Study. Gynecol Oncol. 1989;35(3):314–20.

26. Peters 3rd WA, Liu PY, Barrett 2nd RJ, Stock RJ, Monk BJ, Berek JS, et al. Concurrent chemotherapy and pelvic radiation therapy compared with pelvic radiation therapy alone as adjuvant therapy after radical surgery in high-risk early-stage cancer of the cervix. J Clin Oncol Off J Am Soc Clin Oncol. 2000;18(8):1606–13.

27. Sedlis A, Bundy BN, Rotman MZ, Lentz SS, Muderspach LI, Zaino RJ. A randomized trial of pelvic radiation therapy versus no further therapy in selected patients with stage IB carcinoma of the cervix after radical hysterectomy and pelvic lymphadenectomy: A Gynecologic Oncology Group Study. Gynecol Oncol. 1999;73(2):177–83.

28. Mathevet P, Laszlo de Kaszon E, Dargent D. Fertility preservation in early cervical cancer]. Gynecol Obstet Fertil. 2003;31(9):706–12.

29. Hertel H, Kohler C, Grund D, Hillemanns P, Possover M, Michels W, et al. Radical vaginal trachelectomy (RVT) combined with laparoscopic pelvic lymphadenectomy: prospective multicenter study of 100 patients with early cervical cancer. Gynecol Oncol. 2006;103(2):506–11.

30. Plante M, Renaud MC, Francois H, Roy M. Vaginal radical trachelectomy: an oncologically safe fertility-preserving surgery. An updated series of 72 cases and review of the literature. Gynecol Oncol. 2004;94(3):614–23.

31. Schlaerth JB, Spirtos NM, Schlaerth AC. Radical trachelectomy and pelvic lymphadenectomy with uterine preservation in the treatment of cervical cancer. Am J Obstet Gynecol. 2003;188(1):29–34.

32. Peppercorn PD, Jeyarajah AR, Woolas R, Shepherd JH, Oram DH, Jacobs IJ, et al. Role of MR imaging in the selection of patients with early cervical carcinoma for fertility-preserving surgery: initial experience. Radiology. 1999;212(2):395–9.

33. Gien LT, Beauchemin MC, Thomas G. Adenocarcinoma: a unique cervical cancer. Gynecol Oncol. 2010;116(1):140–6.

34. Gien LT, Covens A. Fertility-sparing options for early stage cervical cancer. Gynecol Oncol. 2010;117(2):350–7.

35. Helpman L, Grisaru D, Covens A. Early adenocarcinoma of the cervix: is radical vaginal trachelectomy safe? Gynecol Oncol. 2011;123(1):95–8.

36. Touhami O, Plante M. Should ovaries be removed or not in (early-stage) adenocarcinoma of the uterine cervix: a review. Gynecol Oncol. 2015;136(2):384–8.

37. Agarwal S, Schmeler KM, Ramirez PT, Sun CC, Nick A, Dos Reis R, et al. Outcomes of patients undergoing radical hysterectomy for cervical cancer of high-risk histological subtypes. Int J Gynecol Cancer Off J Int Gynecol Cancer Soc. 2011;21(1):123–7.

38. Beiner ME, Covens A. Surgery insight: radical vaginal trachelectomy as a method of fertility preservation for cervical cancer. Nat Clin Pract Oncol. 2007;4(6):353–61.

39. Marchiole P, Buenerd A, Benchaib M, Nezhat K, Dargent D, Mathevet P. Clinical significance of lympho vascular space involvement and lymph node micrometastases in early-stage cervical cancer: a retrospective case-control surgico-pathological study. Gynecol Oncol. 2005;97(3):727–32.

40. McCann GA, Taege SK, Boutsicaris CE, Phillips GS, Eisenhauer EL, Fowler JM, et al. The impact of close surgical margins after radical hysterectomy for early-stage cervical cancer. Gynecol Oncol. 2013;128(1):44–8.

41. Plante M, Roy M. New approaches in the surgical management of early stage cervical cancer. Curr Opin Obstet Gynecol. 2001;13(1):41–6.

42. Ismiil N, Ghorab Z, Covens A, Nofech-Mozes S, Saad R, Dube V, et al. Intraoperative margin assessment of the radical trachelectomy specimen. Gynecol Oncol. 2009;113(1):42–6.

43. Eiriksson L, Covens A. Advancing fertility-sparing treatments in cervical cancer: where is the limit? Gynecol Oncol. 2012;126(3):317–8.

44. Panici PB, Angioli R, Palaia I, Muzii L, Zullo MA, Manci N, et al. Tailoring the parametrectomy in stages IA2-IB1 cervical carcinoma: is it feasible and safe? Gynecol Oncol. 2005;96(3):792–8.

45. Scholz HS, Lax SF, Benedicic C, Tamussino K, Winter R. Accuracy of frozen section examination of pelvic lymph nodes in patients with FIGO stage IB1 to IIB cervical cancer. Gynecol Oncol. 2003;90(3):605–9.

46. Gortzak-Uzan L, Jimenez W, Nofech-Mozes S, Ismiil N, Khalifa MA, Dube V, et al. Sentinel lymph node biopsy vs. pelvic lymphadenectomy in early stage cervical cancer: is it time to change the gold standard? Gynecol Oncol. 2010;116(1):28–32.

47. Gubbala PK, Laios A, Wang Z, Dhar S, Pathiraja PJ, Haldar K, et al. Routine Intraoperative Frozen Section Examination to Minimize Bimodal Treatment in Early-Stage Cervical Cancer. Int J Gynecol Cancer Off J Int Gynecol Cancer Soc. 2016;26(6):1148–53.

48. Lv X, Chen L, Yu H, Zhang X, Yan D. Intra-operative frozen section analysis of common iliac lymph nodes in patients with stage IB1 and IIA1 cervical cancer. Arch Gynecol Obstet. 2012;285(3):811–6.

49. Dursun P, Leblanc E, Nogueira MC. Radical vaginal trachelectomy (Dargent's operation): a critical review of the literature. Eur J Surg Oncol J Eur Soc Surg Oncol Br Assoc Surg Oncol. 2007;33(8):933–41.

50. Einstein MH, Park KJ, Sonoda Y, Carter J, Chi DS, Barakat RR, et al. Radical vaginal versus abdominal trachelectomy for stage IB1 cervical cancer: a comparison of surgical and pathologic outcomes. Gynecol Oncol. 2009;112(1):73–7.

51. Cao DY, Yang JX, Wu XH, Chen YL, Li L, Liu KJ, et al. Comparisons of vaginal and abdominal radical trachelectomy for early-stage cervical cancer:

preliminary results of a multi-center research in China. Br J Cancer. 2013;109(11):2778–82.

52. Boss EA, van Golde RJ, Beerendonk CC, Massuger LF. Pregnancy after radical trachelectomy: a real option? Gynecol Oncol. 2005;99(3 Suppl 1):S152–6.

53. Li J, Li Z, Wang H, Zang R, Zhou Y, Ju X, et al. Radical abdominal trachelectomy for cervical malignancies: surgical, oncological and fertility outcomes in 62 patients. Gynecol Oncol. 2011;121(3):565–70.

54. Abu-Rustum NR, Neubauer N, Sonoda Y, Park KJ, Gemignani M, Alektiar KM, et al. Surgical and pathologic outcomes of fertility-sparing radical abdominal trachelectomy for FIGO stage IB1 cervical cancer. Gynecol Oncol. 2008;111(2):261–4.

55. Bouchard-Fortier G, Reade CJ, Covens A. Non-radical surgery for small early-stage cervical cancer. Is it time? Gynecol Oncol. 2014;132(3):624–7.

56. Covens A, Rosen B, Murphy J, Laframboise S, Depetrillo AD, Lickrish G, et al. How important is removal of the parametrium at surgery for carcinoma of the cervix? Gynecol Oncol. 2002;84(1):145–9.

57. Plante M, Gregoire J, Renaud MC, Roy M. The vaginal radical trachelectomy: an update of a series of 125 cases and 106 pregnancies. Gynecol Oncol. 2011;121(2):290–7.

58. Lanowska M, Mangler M, Spek A, Grittner U, Hasenbein K, Chiantera V, et al. Radical vaginal trachelectomy (RVT) combined with laparoscopic lymphadenectomy: prospective study of 225 patients with early-stage cervical cancer. Int J Gynecol Cancer Off J Int Gynecol Cancer Soc. 2011;21(8):1458–64.

59. Shepherd JH. Cervical cancer. Best practice & research Clinical obstetrics & gynaecology. 2012;26(3):293–309.

60. Ramirez PT, Pareja R, Rendon GJ, Millan C, Frumovitz M, Schmeler KM. Management of low-risk early-stage cervical cancer: should conization, simple trachelectomy, or simple hysterectomy replace radical surgery as the new standard of care? Gynecol Oncol. 2014;132(1):254–9.

61. Radical Versus Simple Hysterectomy and Pelvic Node Dissection in Patients With Low-risk Early Stage Cervical Cancer (SHAPE). ClinicalTrials.gov Identifier: NCT01658930. https://clinicaltrials.gov/ct2/show/NCT01658930. Accessed 26 May 2016.

62. Conservative Surgery for Women with Cervical Cancer. ClinicalTrials.gov Identifier: NCT01048853. https://clinicaltrials.gov/ct2/show/NCT01048853. Accessed 26 May 2016.

63. Studying the Physical Function and Quality of Life Before and After Surgery in Patients With Stage 1 Cervical Cancer. ClinicalTrials.gov Identifier: NCT01649089. https://clinicaltrials.gov/ct2/show/NCT01649089. Accessed 26 May 2016.

64. Marchiole P, Tigaud JD, Costantini S, Mammoliti S, Buenerd A, Moran E, et al. Neoadjuvant chemotherapy and vaginal radical trachelectomy for fertility-sparing treatment in women affected by cervical cancer (FIGO stage IB-IIA1). Gynecol Oncol. 2011;122(3):484–90.

65. Maneo A, Chiari S, Bonazzi C, Mangioni C. Neoadjuvant chemotherapy and conservative surgery for stage IB1 cervical cancer. Gynecol Oncol. 2008;111(3):438–43.

66. Kim HS, Sardi JE, Katsumata N, Ryu HS, Nam JH, Chung HH, et al. Efficacy of neoadjuvant chemotherapy in patients with FIGO stage IB1 to IIA cervical cancer: an international collaborative meta-analysis. Eur J Surg Oncol J Eur Soc Surg Oncol Br Assoc Surg Oncol. 2013;39(2):115–24.

67. ACOG. Committee Opinion No. 584: oocyte cryopreservation. Obstet Gynecol. 2014;123(1):221–2.

68. Pfeifer S, Goldberg J, McClure R, Lobo R, Thomas M, Widra E, Licht M, Collins J, Cedars M, Racowsky C, Vernon M, Davis O, Gracia C, Catherino W, Thornton K, Rebar R, La Barbera A. Mature oocyte cryopreservation: a guideline. Fertility and sterility. 2013;99(1):37–43.

69. Pfeifer S, Goldberg J, Lobo R, Pisarska M, Thomas M, Widra E, Sandlow J, Licht M, Rosen M, Vernon M, Catherino W, Davis O, Dumesic D, Gracia C, Odem R, Thornton K, Reindollar R, Rebar R, La Barbera A. Ovarian tissue cryopreservation: a committee opinion. Fertility and sterility. 2014;101(5):1237–43.

70. Brannstrom M. Uterus transplantation. Current opinion in organ transplantation. 2015;20(6):621–8.

71. Wallace WH, Thomson AB, Kelsey TW. The radiosensitivity of the human oocyte. Human reproduction (Oxford, England). 2003;18 (1):117–21.

72. Lushbaugh CC, Casarett GW. The effects of gonadal irradiation in clinical radiation therapy: a review. Cancer. 1976;37(2 Suppl):1111–25.

73. Ghadjar P, Budach V, Kohler C, Jantke A, Marnitz S. Modern radiation therapy and potential fertility preservation strategies in patients with cervical cancer undergoing chemoradiation. Radiation oncology (London, England). 2015;10:50.

74. Critchley HO, Wallace WH, Shalet SM, Mamtora H, Higginson J, Anderson DC. Abdominal irradiation in childhood; the potential for pregnancy. Br J Obstet Gynaecol. 1992;99(5):392–4.

75. Clough KB, Goffinet F, Labib A, Renolleau C, Campana F, de la Rochefordiere A, et al. Laparoscopic unilateral ovarian transposition prior to irradiation: prospective study of 20 cases. Cancer. 1996;77(12):2638–45.

76. Barahmeh S, Al Masri M, Badran O, Masarweh M, El-Ghanem M, Jaradat I, et al. Ovarian transposition before pelvic irradiation: indications and functional outcome. J Obstet Gynaecol Res. 2013;39(11):1533–7.

77. Olejek A, Wala D, Chimiczewski P, Rzempoluch J. Hormonal activity of transposed ovaries in young women treated for cervical cancer. Int J Gynecol Cancer Off J Int Gynecol Cancer Soc. 2001;15(1):5–13.

78. Huang KG, Lee CL, Tsai CS, Han CM, Hwang LL. A new approach for laparoscopic ovarian transposition before pelvic irradiation. Gynecol Oncol. 2007;105(1):234–7.

79. Ishii K, Aoki Y, Takakuwa K, Tanaka K. Ovarian function after radical hysterectomy with ovarian preservation for cervical cancer. J Reprod Med. 2001;46(4):347–52.

80. Pahisa J, Martinez-Roman S, Martinez-Zamora MA, Torne A, Caparros X, Sanjuan A, et al. Laparoscopic ovarian transposition in patients with early cervical cancer. Int J Gynecol Cancer Off J Int Gynecol Cancer Soc. 2008;18(3):584–9.

81. Hwang JH, Yoo HJ, Park SH, Lim MC, Seo SS, Kang S, et al. Association between the location of transposed ovary and ovarian function in patients with uterine cervical cancer treated with (postoperative or primary) pelvic radiotherapy. Fertility and sterility. 2012;97 (6):1387–93.e1-2.

82. Farthing AG-MS. Fertility Sparing Treatments in Gynaecological Cancers. RCOG Guidelines: Royal College of Obstetricians and Gynaecologists, 2013 February, 2013. Report No.: 35 Contract No.: 35.

83. Cakmak H, Rosen MP. Random-start ovarian stimulation in patients with cancer. Curr Opin Obstet Gynecol. 2015;27(3):215–21.

84. Delotte J, Ferron G, Kuei TL, Mery E, Gladieff L, Querleu D. Laparoscopic management of an isolated ovarian metastasis on a transposed ovary in a patient treated for stage IB1 adenocarcinoma of the cervix. J Minim Invasive Gynecol. 2009;16(1):106–8.

85. Shigematsu T, Ohishi Y, Fujita T, Higashihara J, Irie T, Hayashi T. Metastatic carcinoma in a transposed ovary after radical hysterectomy for a stage 1B cervical adenosquamous cell carcinoma. Case report. Eur J Gynaecol Oncol. 2000;21(4):383–6.

86. Morice P, Haie-Meder C, Pautier P, Lhomme C, Castaigne D. Ovarian metastasis on transposed ovary in patients treated for squamous cell carcinoma of the uterine cervix: report of two cases and surgical implications. Gynecol Oncol. 2001;83(3):605–7.

87. Han SS, Kim YH, Lee SH, Kim GJ, Kim HJ, Kim JW, et al. Underuse of ovarian transposition in reproductive-aged cancer patients treated by primary or adjuvant pelvic irradiation. J Obstet Gynaecol Res. 2011;37(7):825–9.

88. Salih SM, Albayrak S, Seo S, Stewart SL, Bradley K, Kushner DM. Diminished Utilization of in Vitro Fertilization Following Ovarian Transposition in Cervical Cancer Patients. J Reprod Med. 2015;60:345–53.

89. Brezina PR, Zhao Y. The ethical, legal, and social issues impacted by modern assisted reproductive technologies. Obstetrics and gynecology international. 2012;2012:686253.

90. Giacalone PL, Laffargue F, Benos P, Dechaud H, Hedon B. Successful in vitro fertilization-surrogate pregnancy in a patient with ovarian transposition who had undergone chemotherapy and pelvic irradiation. Fertil Steril. 2001;76(2):388–9.

91. Zinger M, Liu JH, Husseinzadeh N, Thomas MA. Successful surrogate pregnancy after ovarian transposition, pelvic irradiation and hysterectomy. J Reprod Med. 2004;49(7):573–4.

92. Agorastos T, Zafrakas M, Mastrominas M. Long-term follow-up after cervical cancer treatment and subsequent successful surrogate pregnancy. Reprod Biomed Online. 2009;19(2):250–1.

93. Donnez J, Dolmans MM, Demylle D, Jadoul P, Pirard C, Squifflet J, et al. Livebirth after orthotopic transplantation of cryopreserved ovarian tissue. Lancet (London, England). 2004;364 (9443):1405–10.

94. Radford JA, Lieberman BA, Brison DR, Smith AR, Critchlow JD, Russell SA, et al. Orthotopic reimplantation of cryopreserved ovarian cortical strips after

high-dose chemotherapy for Hodgkin's lymphoma. Lancet (London, England). 2001;357 (9263):1172–5.

95. Schmidt KL, Andersen CY, Loft A, Byskov AG, Ernst E, Andersen AN. Follow-up of ovarian function post-chemotherapy following ovarian cryopreservation and transplantation. Human reproduction (Oxford, England). 2005;20 (12):3539–46.

96. Callejo J, Salvador C, Miralles A, Vilaseca S, Lailla JM, Balasch J. Long-term ovarian function evaluation after autografting by implantation with fresh and frozen-thawed human ovarian tissue. J Clin Endocrinol Metab. 2001;86(9):4489–94.

97. Grynberg M, Poulain M, Sebag-Peyrelevade S, le Parco S, Fanchin R, Frydman N. Ovarian tissue and follicle transplantation as an option for fertility preservation. Fertil Steril. 2012;97(6):1260–8.

98. Meirow D, Levron J, Eldar-Geva T, Hardan I, Fridman E, Zalel Y, et al. Pregnancy after transplantation of cryopreserved ovarian tissue in a patient with ovarian failure after chemotherapy. N Engl J Med. 2005;353(3):318–21.

99. Demeestere I, Simon P, Buxant F, Robin V, Fernandez SA, Centner J, et al. Ovarian function and spontaneous pregnancy after combined heterotopic and orthotopic cryopreserved ovarian tissue transplantation in a patient previously treated with bone marrow transplantation: case report. Human reproduction (Oxford, England). 2006;21 (8):2010–4.

100. Kim SS, Lee WS, Chung MK, Lee HC, Lee HH, Hill D. Long-term ovarian function and fertility after heterotopic autotransplantation of cryobanked human ovarian tissue: 8-year experience in cancer patients. Fertil Steril. 2009;91(6):2349–54.

101. Oktay K, Buyuk E, Veeck L, Zaninovic N, Xu K, Takeuchi T, et al. Embryo development after heterotopic transplantation of cryopreserved ovarian tissue. Lancet (London, England). 2004;363 (9412):837–40.

102. Rosendahl M, Loft A, Byskov AG, Ziebe S, Schmidt KT, Andersen AN, et al. Biochemical pregnancy after fertilization of an oocyte aspirated from a heterotopic autotransplant of cryopreserved ovarian tissue: case report. Human reproduction (Oxford, England). 2006;21 (8):2006–9.

103. Bastings L, Beerendonk CC, Westphal JR, Massuger LF, Kaal SE, van Leeuwen FE, et al. Autotransplantation of cryopreserved ovarian tissue in cancer survivors and the risk of reintroducing malignancy: a systematic review. Hum Reprod Update. 2013;19(5):483–506.

104. Johannesson L, Kvarnstrom N, Molne J, Dahm-Kahler P, Enskog A, Diaz-Garcia C, et al. Uterus transplantation trial: 1-year outcome. Fertil Steril. 2015;103(1):199–204.

105. Carter J, Sonoda Y, Baser RE, Raviv L, Chi DS, Barakat RR, et al. A 2-year prospective study assessing the emotional, sexual, and quality of life concerns of women undergoing radical trachelectomy versus radical hysterectomy for treatment of early-stage cervical cancer. Gynecol Oncol. 2010;119(2):358–65.

106. Song T, Choi CH, Lee YY, Kim TJ, Lee JW, Kim BG, et al. Sexual function after surgery for early-stage cervical cancer: is there a difference in it according to the extent of surgical radicality? J Sex Med. 2012;9(6):1697–704.

107. Radical Trachelectomy for Cervical Cancer. ClinicalTrials.gov Identifier: NCT00813007. https://clinicaltrials.gov/ct2/show/NCT00813007. Accessed 26 May 2016.

108. Shepherd JH, Spencer C, Herod J, Ind TE. Radical vaginal trachelectomy as a fertility-sparing procedure in women with early-stage cervical cancer-cumulative pregnancy rate in a series of 123 women. BJOG. 2006;113(6):719–24.

109. Marchiole P, Benchaib M, Buenerd A, Lazlo E, Dargent D, Mathevet P. Oncological safety of laparoscopic-assisted vaginal radical trachelectomy (LARVT or Dargent's operation): a comparative study with laparoscopic-assisted vaginal radical hysterectomy (LARVH). Gynecol Oncol. 2007;106(1):132–41.

110. Wethington SL, Cibula D, Duska LR, Garrett L, Kim CH, Chi DS, et al. An international series on abdominal radical trachelectomy: 101 patients and 28 pregnancies. Int J Gynecol Cancer Off J Int Gynecol Cancer Soc. 2012;22(7):1251–7.

111. Mangler M, Lanowska M, Kohler C, Vercellino F, Schneider A, Speiser D. Pattern of cancer recurrence in 320 patients after radical vaginal trachelectomy. Int J Gynecol Cancer Off J Int Gynecol Cancer Soc. 2014;24(1):130–4.

112. Hauerberg L, Hogdall C, Loft A, Ottosen C, Bjoern SF, Mosgaard BJ, et al. Vaginal Radical Trachelectomy for early stage cervical cancer. Results of the Danish National Single Center Strategy. Gynecol Oncol. 2015;138:304–10.

113. Vieira MA, Rendon GJ, Munsell M, Echeverri L, Frumovitz M, Schmeler KM, et al. Radical trachelectomy in early-stage cervical cancer: A comparison of laparotomy and minimally invasive surgery. Gynecol Oncol. 2015;138:585–9.

114. Bernardini M, Barrett J, Seaward G, Covens A. Pregnancy outcomes in patients after radical trachelectomy. Am J Obstet Gynecol. 2003;189(5):1378–82.

115. Kim CH, Abu-Rustum NR, Chi DS, Gardner GJ, Leitao Jr MM, Carter J, et al. Reproductive outcomes of patients undergoing radical trachelectomy for early-stage cervical cancer. Gynecol Oncol. 2012;125(3):585–8.

116. Nishio H, Fujii T, Sugiyama J, Kuji N, Tanaka M, Hamatani T, et al. Reproductive and obstetric outcomes after radical abdominal trachelectomy for early-stage cervical cancer in a series of 31 pregnancies. Human reproduction (Oxford, England). 2013;28 (7):1793–8.

117. Kasuga Y, Nishio H, Miyakoshi K, Sato S, Sugiyama J, Matsumoto T, et al. Pregnancy Outcomes After Abdominal Radical Trachelectomy for Early-Stage Cervical Cancer: A 13-Year Experience in a Single Tertiary-Care Center. Int J Gynecol Cancer Off J Int Gynecol Cancer Soc. 2016;26(1):163–8.

118. Nishio H, Fujii T, Kameyama K, Susumu N, Nakamura M, Iwata T, et al. Abdominal radical trachelectomy as a fertility-sparing procedure in women with early-stage cervical cancer in a series of 61 women. Gynecol Oncol. 2009;115(1):51–5.

119. Li J, Wu X, Li X, Ju X. Abdominal radical trachelectomy: Is it safe for IB1 cervical cancer with tumors >/= 2 cm? Gynecol Oncol. 2013;131(1):87–92.

120. Lintner B, Saso S, Tarnai L, Novak Z, Palfalvi L, Del Priore G, et al. Use of abdominal radical trachelectomy to treat cervical cancer greater than 2 cm in diameter. Int J Gynecol Cancer Off J Int Gynecol Cancer Soc. 2013;23(6):1065–70.

121. Wethington SL, Sonoda Y, Park KJ, Alektiar KM, Tew WP, Chi DS, et al. Expanding the indications for radical trachelectomy: a report on 29 patients with stage IB1 tumors measuring 2 to 4 cm. Int J Gynecol Cancer Off J Int Gynecol Cancer Soc. 2013;23(6):1092–8.

122. Bisseling KC, Bekkers RL, Rome RM, Quinn MA. Treatment of microinvasive adenocarcinoma of the uterine cervix: a retrospective study and review of the literature. Gynecol Oncol. 2007;107(3):424–30.

123. Rob L, Charvat M, Robova H, Pluta M, Strnad P, Hrehorcak M, et al. Less radical fertility-sparing surgery than radical trachelectomy in early cervical cancer. Int J Gynecol Cancer Off J Int Gynecol Cancer Soc. 2007;17(1):304–10.

124. Landoni F, Parma G, Peiretti M, Zanagnolo V, Sideri M, Colombo N, et al. Chemo-conization in early cervical cancer. Gynecol Oncol. 2007;107(1 Suppl 1):S125–6.

125. Fagotti A, Gagliardi ML, Moruzzi C, Carone V, Scambia G, Fanfani F. Excisional cone as fertility-sparing treatment in early-stage cervical cancer. Fertil Steril. 2011;95(3):1109–12.

126. Maneo A, Sideri M, Scambia G, Boveri S, Dell'anna T, Villa M, et al. Simple conization and lymphadenectomy for the conservative treatment of stage IB1 cervical cancer. An Italian experience. Gynecol Oncol. 2011;123(3):557–60.

127. Raju SK, Papadopoulos AJ, Montalto SA, Coutts M, Culora G, Kodampur M, et al. Fertility-sparing surgery for early cervical cancer-approach to less radical surgery. Int J Gynecol Cancer Off J Int Gynecol Cancer Soc. 2012;22(2):311–7.

128. Palaia I, Musella A, Bellati F, Marchetti C, Di Donato V, Perniola G, et al. Simple extrafascial trachelectomy and pelvic bilateral lymphadenectomy in early stage cervical cancer. Gynecol Oncol. 2012;126(1):78–81.

129. Plante M, Gregoire J, Renaud MC, Sebastianelli A, Grondin K, Noel P, et al. Simple vaginal trachelectomy in early-stage low-risk cervical cancer: a pilot study of 16 cases and review of the literature. Int J Gynecol Cancer Off J Int Gynecol Cancer Soc. 2013;23(5):916–22.

130. Andikyan V, Khoury-Collado F, Denesopolis J, Park KJ, Hussein YR, Brown CL, et al. Cervical conization and sentinel lymph node mapping in the treatment of stage I cervical cancer: is less enough? Int J Gynecol Cancer Off J Int Gynecol Cancer Soc. 2014;24(1):113–7.

131. Salihi R, Leunen K, Van Limbergen E, Moerman P, Neven P, Vergote I. Neoadjuvant chemotherapy followed by large cone resection as fertility-sparing therapy in stage IB cervical cancer. Gynecol Oncol. 2015;139:447–51.

132. Robova H, Halaska M, Pluta M, Skapa P, Strnad P, Lisy J, et al. The role of neoadjuvant chemotherapy and surgery in cervical cancer. Int J Gynecol Cancer Off J Int Gynecol Cancer Soc. 2010;20(11 Suppl 2):S42–6.

133. Vercellino GF, Piek JM, Schneider A, Kohler C, Mangler M, Speiser D, et al. Laparoscopic lymph node dissection should be performed before fertility preserving treatment of patients with cervical cancer. Gynecol Oncol. 2012;126(3):325–9.

134. Lanowska M, Mangler M, Speiser D, Bockholdt C, Schneider A, Kohler C, et al. Radical vaginal trachelectomy after laparoscopic staging and neoadjuvant chemotherapy in women with early-stage cervical cancer over 2 cm: oncologic, fertility, and neonatal outcome in a series of 20 patients. Int J Gynecol Cancer Off J Int Gynecol Cancer Soc. 2014;24(3):586–93.

16

Very late recurrence of Diethylstilbestrol - related clear cell carcinoma of the cervix: case report

Ablavi Adani-Ifè[1,2*], Emma Goldschmidt[2], Pasquale Innominato[2], Ayhan Ulusakarya[2], Hassan Errihani[1], Philippe Bertheau[3] and Jean François Morère[2]

Abstract

Clear cell adenocarcinoma of the cervix is a rare tumor of the lower genital tract. It has been described in young women with a history of intra uterine exposure to diethylstilbestrol. This tumor is characterized by a greater tendency for late recurrences. In this article, we report the case of one exposed-patient who developed recurrence as liver metastases, 24 years after the initial treatment. This case demonstrates the need and the importance for continued follow-up in individuals prenatally exposed to diethylstilbestrol.

Keywords: Clear cell adenocarcinoma, Cervix, Diethylstilbestrol, Recurrence

Background

Clear cell adenocarcinoma of the cervix is an uncommon malignancy accounting for 4–9 % of cervical adenocarcinomas which represent about 5–10 % of all tumors of the cervix [1, 2]. It has been first described in young women exposed *in utero* to Diethylstilbestrol (DES) by Herbst et al. [3] and its incidence is in on the order of 1.0 per 1000 exposed persons [4, 5]. Clear cell adenocarcinomas of the lower genital tract have a greater tendency to recur late and develop metastases in distant sites more frequently than squamous cell carcinomas [6–8]. We report here the case of one patient who developed recurrence 24 years after the initial treatment.

Case presentation

In July 1990, a 20-year-old woman presented with abnormal vaginal bleeding. Her past medical history was only significant for *in utero* DES exposure. Physical examination revealed a budding tumor involving the anterior lip of the uterine cervix. The pelvic Computed Tomography (CT) scan showed an enlargement of the cervix which was deviated to the right. The mass came in contact with the rectal wall but did not invade the bladder or the parameters. Biopsy confirmed the diagnosis of clear

cell adenocarcinoma of the cervix. Disease extention evaluation including chest and abdominal scan was normal. A laparotomy with bilateral ovarian transposition and iliac lymphadenectomy was performed. The pathological examination of resected lymph nodes was negative. After the initial surgery, the patient was treated with brachytherapy (65 Grays). Because of an insufficient tumor response to the brachytherapy, the patient underwent two cervical conizations. After the second conization, surgical margins were negative for malignancy. The patient was then followed up regularly with colposcopic evaluation and annual Pap smear.

Despite the conservative treatment, the patient was unable to conceive. Fourteen years later in December 2004, she complained of metrorrhagia. Pelvic ultrasound revealed an abnormal uterine mass of 28 mm. The patient underwent radical hysterectomy and right annexectomy. The pathological analysis of the mass revealed a leiomyoma and the right annex was normal. The patient was followed up regularly and was considered to be free of disease until February 2014 when she developed abdominal pain and weight loss. Abdominal CT scan showed multiple hepatic masses and peritoneal carcinomatosis. A hepatic percutaneous biopsy revealed a tumor with tubular pattern consisting of large and polygonal cells with clear or eosinophilic cytoplasm CK7+, CK20-, TTF1-, ER-, PR-, HER2-, CDX2- and CK5/6- (Fig. 1). Based on these characteristics, the tumor was considered as metastatic diffusion of the previously treated clear cell

* Correspondence: solangeadaniife@yahoo.fr
[1]Department of Oncology, National Institute of Oncology, Avenue Allal El Fassi, BP 6542, Rabat 10100, Maroc
[2]Department of Oncology, Paul Brousse University Hospital AP-HP, 12-14 Avenue Paul Vaillant Couturier, 94800 Villejuif, France
Full list of author information is available at the end of the article

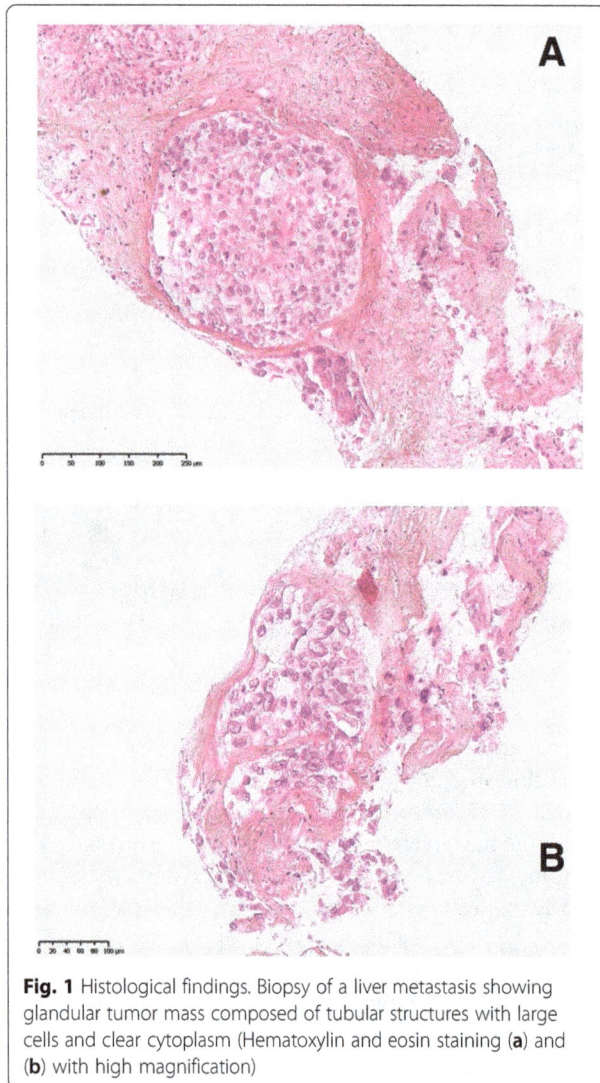

Fig. 1 Histological findings. Biopsy of a liver metastasis showing glandular tumor mass composed of tubular structures with large cells and clear cytoplasm (Hematoxylin and eosin staining (**a**) and (**b**) with high magnification)

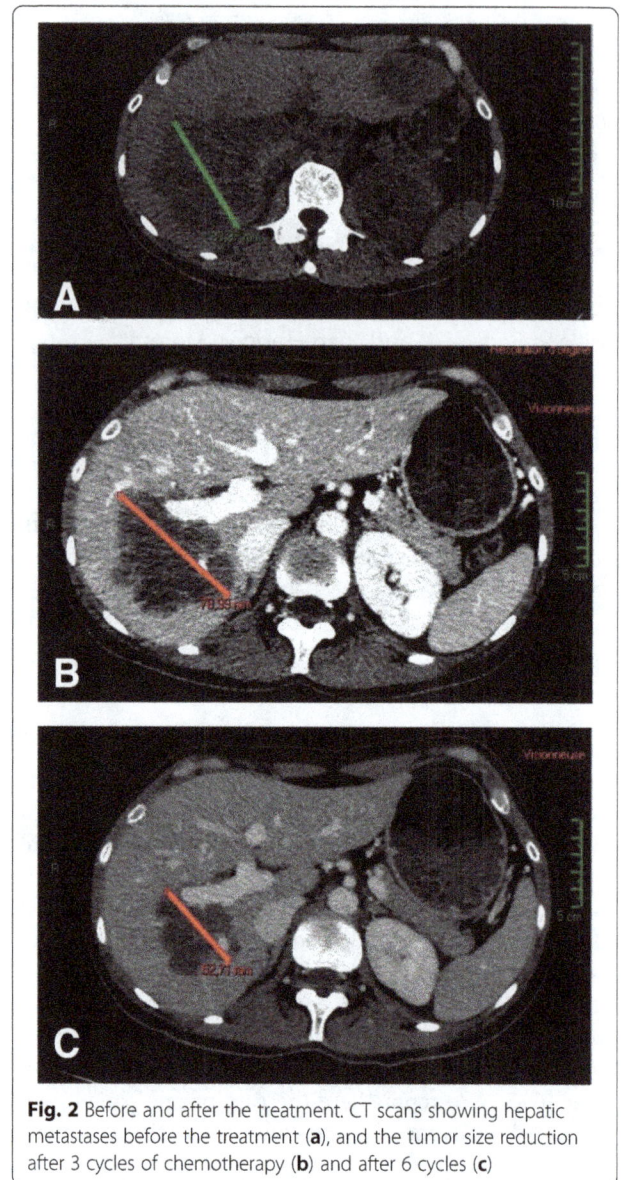

Fig. 2 Before and after the treatment. CT scans showing hepatic metastases before the treatment (**a**), and the tumor size reduction after 3 cycles of chemotherapy (**b**) and after 6 cycles (**c**)

adenocarcinoma. Imaging studies for the relapsed disease including a FDG-PET-scan confirmed hepatic and peritoneal lesions. The patient received combination chemotherapy regimen including weekly paclitaxel (80 mg/m^2), carboplatin (AUC = 5) and bevacizumab (7.5 mg/kg) both administered every three weeks. To date, she has received 7 cycles of this combination with excellent tolerance and the follow up CT scans have showed a partial response with reduction of tumor size after 3 and 6 cycles (Fig. 2).

Discussion

Diethylstilbestrol (DES) is an oral synthetic nonsteroidal estrogen that was used to prevent miscarriage, premature birth and other pregnancy complications between 1938 and 1971 in the United States [9] and until early 1980's in various European countries [9, 10]. Exposure to DES during a critical period of organogenesis disturbs the developing uterine muscle layers, causes abnormalities

of the uterotubal junction, and prevents stratification of the vaginal epithelium and resorption of vaginal glands, resulting in vaginal adenosis [10]. In female offspring, *in utero* exposure to DES has been associated with potential risks of cervicovaginal clear cell adenocarcinoma, congenital anomalies and epithelial changes of the reproductive tract, subfertility and adverse pregnancy outcomes, earlier age at menopause, breast cancer and cervical intra epithelial neoplasia [10].

DES related clear cell adenocarcinoma usually occurs between the age of 15 and 27 with a median of 19 years [4] and have a predilection for the ectocervix and upper third of the vagina [11]. Pathologically, the tumors can display solid, tubular, cystic and papillary patterns or mixed patterns [12, 13] with the tubular-cystic pattern being the most common presentation [13]. Survival rates approaching 90 % can be expected in patients with clear cell adenocarcinoma with papillary and tubulocystic features while tumors with more solid pattern have less favorable prognosis [14]. Most cases of clear cell carcinoma related to DES exposure have been diagnosed at stage one or two [5]. Patients with early stage are highly curable with surgery or radiotherapy or combination of both modalities [15–17]. However, clear cell adenocarcinoma can also be diagnosed in unexposed women. It can occur in older women [12, 18] and in about 25% of cases in young women, there is no history of maternal medication [19].

Most recurrences of clear cell adenocarcinoma of the vagina and cervix are diagnosed within the 3 years after primary tumor treatment [8] but late recurrences have been reported with few cases 8 years after initial diagnosis [7, 14, 20, 21]. To date the latest recurrence reported in DES exposed patients is 19 years after initial therapy [11]. Here, we present the case of a woman with intra uterine DES exposure who developed recurrence as distant metastases without local relapse, 24 years after initial curative treatment. In 1991, Goodman and coll reported a local recurrence of clear cell adenocarcinoma of the vaginal remnant presenting 20 years after initial surgery. Basing on the 20 years disease -free period, the absence of nodal, lymphatic or vascular involvements and the absence of distant spread in their case, they suggested a new primary tumor rather than a late recurrence [22]. In our patient, the absence of local relapse suggests the possibility that quiescent tumor cell may have been initially present in the liver and peritoneum and became activated after a prolonged interval and/or evolved slowly and finally became symptomatic.

In the cases reported by Herbst et al. [8], recurrences were more frequent in the pelvis (60 %), the lungs (36 %) and supraclavicular lymph nodes (12 %). One patient was reported with cerebellar metastases [20] but liver metastases from DES related clear cell adenocarcinoma of cervix have never been described. Because of a similar histological morphology, this diagnosis can be confused with that of primary clear cell carcinoma of liver, which is a particular and rare histological type of hepatocellular carcinoma [23, 24]. However, most of primary clear cell carcinoma of the liver occur in patients with liver cirrhosis [25] and the cases reported in patients with normal liver are uncommon [26]. Nevertheless, for the present case, immunostaining of biopsy samples excluded primary clear cell carcinoma of liver.

Local recurrences of clear cell adenocarcinoma of the cervix can be effectively treated with surgery, radiotherapy or combined modality [21]. Surgery or radiation therapy can be used to treat also limited metastatic recurrence. In disseminated recurrent disease, systemic chemotherapy including various cytotoxic drugs (alkylant agents, 5-fluorouracil, adriamycine, vinca-alcaloids, actinomycine D, cisplatin) or progestational agents has been used [8, 21] but no effective regimen is currently considered as the reference treatment [8, 21]. However paclitaxel has been administrated to one patient, and has permitted to obtain stable disease on CT scan and the decrease of the initially high CA 125 tumor marker [11]. Our patient is being treated with a combination of paclitaxel, carboplatin and bevacizumab which is an anti-angiogenic (anti Vascular Endothelial Growth Factor) monoclonal antibody. This regimen is active, inducing a clinical improvement (symptom disappearance) and a morphologic partial response.

Conclusions

To summarize, this case represents the longest reported disease-free interval till recurrence and the first description of metastatic liver disease of DES related clear cell adenocarcinoma of the cervix. It reemphasizes the necessity of long term surveillance of DES exposed women and confirms previous reports recommending the importance of frequent follow-up examination not only of the pelvis but also of all distant potential sites of metastasis. It also shows that treatment with paclitaxel, carboplatin and bevacizumab can be an effective and safe therapeutic option for treating recurrence of this rare tumor.

Competing interests

The authors declare that they have no competing interests

Authors' contributions

AA has contributed to the management and the follow up of the patient and drafted the manuscript. EG has contributed to the management and the follow up of the patient and helped to draft the manuscript. PI, AU helped to draft the manuscript. PB carried out histological and immunohistochemical studies of the biopsy. HE, JFM revised and helped to draft the manuscript. All authors read and approved the final manuscript.

Acknowledgements

We thank Fatiha Bouhidel for her contribution in providing the anatomopathological pictures

Author details

[1]Department of Oncology, National Institute of Oncology, Avenue Allal El Fassi, BP 6542, Rabat 10100, Maroc. [2]Department of Oncology, Paul Brousse University Hospital AP-HP, 12-14 Avenue Paul Vaillant Couturier, 94800 Villejuif, France. [3]Laboratory of Cytopathology, Saint Louis Hospital AP-HP, Avenue Claude Vellefaux, 75010 Paris, France.

References

1. Reich O, Tamussino K, Lahousen M, Pickel H, Haas J, Winter R. Clear cell carcinoma of the uterine cervix: pathology and prognosis in surgically treated stage IB-IIB disease in women not exposed in utero to diethylstilbestrol. Gynecol Oncol. 2000;76 Suppl 3:331–35.
2. Ding DC, Chang FW, Yu MH. Huge clear cell carcinoma of the cervix in teenager not associated with diethylstilbestrol: a brief case report. Eur J Obstet Gynecol Reprod Biol. 2004;117:115–16.
3. Herbst AL, Ulfelder H, Poskanzer DC. Adenocarcinoma of the vagina association of maternal stilbestrol therapy with tumor appearance in young women. N Engl J Med. 1971;284:878.
4. Melnick S, Cole P, Anderson D, Herbst A. Rates and risks of diethylstilbestrol-related clear cell adenocarcinoma of the vagina and cervix. An update. N Engl J Med. 1987;316:514–16.
5. Herbst AL, Anderson D. Clear cell adenocarcinoma of the vagina and cervix secondary to intrauterine exposure to diethylstilbestrol. Semin Surg Oncol. 1990;6 Suppl 6:343–46.
6. Robboy SJ, Herbst AL, Scully RE. Clear cell adenocarcinoma of the vagina and the cervix in young females: Analysis of 37 tumors that persisted or recurred after primary therapy. Cancer. 1974;34 Suppl 3:606–14.
7. Jones WB, Koulos JP, Saigo PE, Lewis Jr JL. Clear cell adenocarcinoma of the lower genital tract: Memorial Hospital 1974–1984. Obstet Gynecol. 1987;70 Suppl 4:573–77.
8. Herbst AL, Norusis MJ, Rosenow PJ, Welch WR, Scully RE. An analysis of 346 cases of clear cell adenocarcinoma of the vagina and cervix with emphasis on recurrence and survival. Gynecol Oncol. 1979;7:111–22.
9. Schrager S, Potter BE. Diethylstilbestrol Exposure. Am Fam Physician. 2004;69:2395–400.
10. Hatch E. Outcome and follow-up of diethylstilbestrol (DES) exposed individuals. 2014. http://www. Uptodate.com. Accessed 9 Aug 2014.
11. Fishman DA, Williams S, Small Jr W, Keh P, Gerbie MV, Schwartz PE, et al. Late recurrence of vaginal clear cell adenocarcinoma. Gynecol Oncol. 1996;62:128–32.
12. Kaminski PF, Maier RC. Clear Cell Adenocarcinoma of the cervix unrelated to diethylstilbestrol exposure. Obstet Gynecol. 1983;62:720–27.
13. Dickersin GR, Welch WR, Erlandson R, Robboy SJ. Ultrastructure of 16 cases of clear cell adenocarcinoma of the vagina and cervix in young women. Cancer. 1980;45:1615–24.
14. Herbst AL, Cole P, Norusis MJ, Welch WR, Scully RE. Epidemiologic aspects and factors related to survival in 384 Registry cases of clear cell adenocarcinoma of the vagina and cervix. Am J Obstet Gynecol. 1979;135:876–86.
15. Hill EC, Galante M. Radical surgery in the management of clear cell adenocarcinoma of the cervix and vagina in young women. Am J Obstet Gynecol. 1981;140:221–6.
16. Senekjian EK, Frey KW, Anderson D, Herbst AL. Local therapy in stage I clear cell adenocarcinoma of the vagina. Cancer. 1987;60:1319–24.
17. Wharton JT, Rutledge FN, Gallager HS, Fletcher G. Treatment of clear cell adenocarcinoma in young females. Obstet Gynecol. 1975;45:365–8.
18. Hanselaar A. Loosbroek, Schuurbiers O, Helmerhorst T, Bulten J, Bernheim J. Clear cell adenocarcinoma of the vagina and cervix. An update of the central Netherlands Registry showing Twin Age Incidence Peaks. Cancer. 1997;79:2229–36.
19. Herbst A. Clear cell adenocarcinoma and the current status of the DES-exposed females. Cancer. 1981;48:484–8.
20. Burks RT, Schwartz AM, Wheeler JE, Antonioli D. Late recurrence of clear cell adenocarcinoma oh the cervix: case report. Obstet Gynecol. 1990;76:525–7.
21. Jones WB, Tan LK, Lewis JL. Late recurrence of clear cell adenocarcinoma of the vagina and cervix: A report of three cases. Gynecol Oncol. 1993;54:266–71.
22. Goodman A, Sullinger JC, Rice LW, Fuller AF. Clear cell adenocarcinoma of the vagina: A second primary in a diethylstilbestrol-exposed woman? Gynecol Oncol. 1991;43:173–7.
23. Ji SP, Li Q, Dong H. Therapy and prognostic features of primary clear cell carcinoma of the liver. World J Gastroenterol. 2010;16(6):764–9.
24. Murakata LA, Ishak KG, Nzeako UC. Clear cell carcinoma of the liver: a comparative immunohistochemical study with renal clear cell carcinoma. Mod Pathol. 2000;13:874–81.
25. Liu Z, Ma W, Li H, Li Q. Clinicopathological and prognostic features of primary clear cell carcinoma of the liver. Hepatol Res. 2008;38:291–9.
26. Takahashi A, Saito H, Kanno Y, Abe K, Yokokawa J, Irisawa A, et al. Case of clear-cell hepatocellular carcinoma that developed in the normal liver of a middle-aged woman. World J Gastroenterol. 2008;14(1):129–31.

17

Preference of elderly patients' to oral or intravenous chemotherapy in heavily pre-treated recurrent ovarian cancer: final results of a prospective multicenter trial

Radoslav Chekerov[1]*[iD], Philipp Harter[2], Stefan Fuxius[3], Lars Christian Hanker[4], Linn Woelber[5], Lothar Müller[6], Peter Klare[7], Wolfgang Abenhardt[8], Yoana Nedkova[1], Isil Yalcinkaya[1], Georg Heinrich[9], Harald Sommer[10], Sven Mahner[10], Pauline Wimberger[11], Dominique Koensgen-Mustea[12], Rolf Richter[13], Gülten Oskay-Oezcelik[7,13], Jalid Sehouli[1,13] and On behalf of the Ovarian Cancer Study Group of the North-Eastern German Society of Gynaecological Oncology (NOGGO)

Abstract

Background: Palliative systemic treatment in elderly gynaecological cancer patients remains a major challenge. In recurrent ovarian cancer (ROC), treosulfan an active alkylating drug showed similar cytotoxicity whether as oral (p.o.) or intravenous (i.v.) application. The aim of this innovative trial was to evaluate the preference of elderly patients ($\geq$65 years) for p.o. or i.v. chemotherapy focusing compliance, outcome, toxicities, and geriatric aspects as secondary endpoints.

Methods: Patients with ROC had the free choice between treosulfan i.v. (7000 mg/m^2 d1, q29d) or p.o. (600 mg/m^2 daily d1-28, q57d). Only indecisive participants were randomized.

Results: Overall 123 patients with 2nd to 5th recurrence were registered and 119 received at least one cycle of chemotherapy. 85.7% preferred treosulfan i.v. and 14.3% oral, where only three patients were randomized. Main reasons for i.v. preference associated with individual expectations of lower rate of gastrointestinal disorders, higher activity and tolerability of treatment. Median of applied chemotherapies was three (range 1–12 cycles), with most common grade 3/4 toxicities thrombopenia (18.7%), leukopenia (15.7%), ascites (7.6%), bowel obstruction (6.7%), and abdominal pain (4.2%). Median time until progression/overall survival was 5.2/7.8 months (i.v.), and 5.6/10. 4 months (p.o.), respectively, without significant differences in efficacy.

Conclusions: Elderly patients with recurrent ovarian cancer asked and demonstrated active participation in the decision-making process of their oncological treatment and favoured predominantly the i.v. application. Treosulfan was generally well-tolerated despite comorbidities and heavy pre-treatment. Our study demonstrates that patients' preference did not influence prognosis negatively and remains important in gynaecologic oncology decision practice.

EudraCT Nr.: 2004-000719-25; NCT 00170690

Keywords: Recurrent ovarian cancer, Elderly, Patient preference, Treosulfan

* Correspondence: radoslav.chekerov@charite.de
[1]Department of Gynaecology, European Competence Centre for Ovarian Cancer, Charité Universitätsmedizin, Berlin, Germany
Full list of author information is available at the end of the article

Background

Treatment of elderly ovarian cancer patients remain a great challenge in the palliative situation, where innovative therapies conflicts with clinical routine [1–3]. In general some physicians consider critical surgical or systemic treatment [4, 5] while many observers reported inadequate treatment quality in elderly compared to younger patients [3, 6–8]. Otherwise age was one of the common exclusion criteria in clinical trials, so their results could not consequently be transferred to senior cancer cohorts. Additional, age-dependent limitations of functional reserves are not well understood, but complex and require elaborate assessment [9, 10]. In particular, individual preferences and knowledge of patient reported outcome measures are key aspects of palliative concepts [11]. Resent published data have confirmed opposing expectations and individual preferences by cancer patients and their physicians [11–13]. Today data focusing elderly ovarian cancer patients, their preferences and expectations for therapy are still limited, thus to change the primary perspective in a clinical trial is provoking but could generate a helpful insight to gynaecologic oncologists.

As factors of decision-making in oncology are poorly understood, there is an ongoing intensive discussion about new conceptual and scientific approaches [14]. Not only efficacy and toxicity, but also patient's acceptance of and compliance with treatment can significantly influence outcome [1, 3]. Inadequate therapy of elderly results quite often due to the erroneous belief that age alone determines lower tolerability to surgery and chemotherapy [15]. There is also controversial experience that, even in a palliation, elderly women can possibly tolerate debulking surgery and chemotherapy well, but still prediction of the individual aspects, benefits and risk is still not possible [8, 16]. Thus optimising strategies for increasing compliance and satisfaction with care should involve patients into the treatment decision-making process, above all respecting their expectations and preferences [13, 17, 18].

Treosulfan is a bifunctional alkylating prodrug showing activity for the i.v. formulation either as a single agent or in combination with other cytotoxic drugs such a cisplatin [19–21]. Furthermore, oral treosulfan demonstrated a high and constant bioavailability [22], which may lead to the same efficacy. Since both formulations show a similar efficacy and moderate toxicity, it seems attractive for evaluating individual therapy preferences. Treosulfan is approved in several European countries for the treatment of ovarian cancer and characterized by proven effectivity and mild toxicity (e.g. little hair loss and non-haematological side-effects), which makes it attractive for geriatric and multimorbid patients [23].

The innovative concept of this trial involved elderly patients with recurrent ovarian cancer to determine active their preference for therapy after detailed patient consultation on treatment aims and risks. Primary study objectives were the individual preference and free patient's choice to chemotherapy with either i.v. or p.o. treosulfan. Additionally, we evaluated the reasons for individual choice and analysed compliance, tolerability, and efficacy of the different application routes. Patients were free to participate on geriatric assessment measures.

Methods

Study design

This was an open-label, multicentre trial of treosulfan in elderly women with ROC. Patients were enrolled into the study after failure of platinum-containing treatment, irrespective of their treatment-free interval, following an innovative registration design: they were free to choose between oral and i.v. treosulfan treatment. Only indecisive participants were randomized.

Patients were enrolled at 27 German institutions (18 hospitals, nine outpatient facilities). Women ≥ 65 years with recurrent ovarian, peritoneal, or fallopian tube cancer were eligible. Key inclusion criteria were as follows (selection): ECOG ≤ 2, serum creatinine ≤ 1.25 × upper normal limit (UNL), bilirubin ≤ 1.25 × UNL (in the presence of liver metastases ≤ 5 × UNL), and adequate bone marrow function (leucocytes $\geq 2.0 \cdot \times 10^9$/l, and platelet count $\geq 100 \times 10^9$/l). Initially, only patients in the second line situation (first recurrence) were allowed to participate, but due to emerging trial results and improvement of national guidelines for the treatment of ovarian cancer, the subsequent change of inclusion criteria to patients with at least two previous therapies (≥3rd line situation) was amended.

The primary aim was to explore the preference and compliance of elderly participants for the palliative treatment with oral or i.v. medication. Secondary objectives included compliance, toxicity, progression-free and overall survival. Additional quality of life, functional and comorbidity measures and geriatric assessments were performed according to the preference of the participants.

This trial was planned by the North-Eastern German Society of Gynaecological Oncology (NOGGO) Ovarian Cancer Study Group. The study was performed according to ICH-GCP (International Conference on Harmonization - Good Clinical Practice) guidelines after obtaining central ethical committee's approval and trial registration (EudraCT Nr.: 2004-000719-25; NCT 00170690). Written informed consent was provided by each participant.

Treatment plan and toxicity evaluation

Patients received a standard dose of 7000 mg/m² treosulfan i.v. on day 1 of a 28-day cycle or 600 mg/m² p.o. on days 1–28 of a 56-day cycle for a maximum of

12 months or until disease-progression or development of unacceptable toxicity.

The screening started within 14 days prior to start of therapy included an evaluation of the medical history, a physical examination, and a tumour evaluation, staged by CA 125 and radiological imaging (chest x-ray, ultrasound, CT or MRI scan). Laboratory analyses comprised haematology (biweekly), serum chemistry, and urine analysis. Evaluation of response was performed every 12 weeks or in case of symptoms or signs of tumour progression.

Toxicity was classified according to the NCI- CTCAE version 2.0. Safety analyses were performed on all patients who received at least one therapy cycle. In order to account for the limited haematopoietic resources of elderly patients, chemotherapy was applied only if leukocyte was $\geq 3.5 \times 10^9/l$ and platelets $\geq 100 \times 10^9/l$.

In cases of dose reduction due to severe haematological toxicity, no re-escalation was allowed. Tumour progression, intolerable toxicity (grade 3/4), and/or a treatment delay > 2 weeks led to discontinuation of treatment.

Statistical analysis

The preference for oral or i.v. treosulfan was expected to result in a variable compliance. Description of compliance differences between the two treatment arms by 15% was defined as clinically significant. We used Fleiss statistical measurement to optimize the sample size [24]. Setting the test criteria to alpha = 5%, beta = 20% and a drop-out rate of 5%, 160 patients were initially intended to be recruited for this trial. Due to a slow recruitment we performed a prior evaluation with 123 patients identifying highly representative differences in preference and compliance, which were statistically significant to close early trial recruitment.

Results are presented as proportions, means, medians, and rates, and their adequate measures of distribution. We used a one-sample test of proportions to address the primary hypothesis. All other endpoints were evaluated in an exploratory fashion, and 95% confidence intervals (CI) were computed where appropriate.

Evaluation of response was performed by CA 125 monthly and by radiological assessment every 3 months. Response was measured according to UICC-criteria and CA-125 assessment criteria, established by Rustin et al. [25]. Progression-free survival and overall survival were defined as the interval between the first day of the study drug application and disease progression or death due to any cause. Both were calculated by the Kaplan-Meier method.

Results

Patient characteristics

Out of 123 registered patients, 119 received at least one cycle of chemotherapy and were eligible for the final analysis (Fig. 1). Generally, there were no significant differences in the global patient characteristics (Table 1). The median age at recruitment was 71 years (range of 65–87 years). Most women were diagnosed with advanced stage III/IV high-grade carcinomas of serouspapillary histology and were in good condition (ECOG 0–1). The majority had received three previous cytotoxic treatments (three in the i.v. and two in the oral preference arm). Most patients were treated in this study due to second or third recurrence (56.3%), but 32% had four or more recurrences in their medical history. Because the protocol allowed to register patients independently of their platinum-free interval, the rate of late recurrences with a treatment-free interval >12 months was between 35 and 52% (oral vs. i.v. group). Distant metastases were rare and typically localized to the liver or lung. The median number of concomitant diseases was 5 (range 1–9), mostly of cardiovascular, musculoskeletal or gastrointestinal character (Table 2).

Preference for chemotherapy

During the registration process patients were asked to realize their preference or to be randomized to treatment. Most them ($n = 116$, 97.5%) preferred to choose the application form of chemotherapy, thus only 3 indecisive women were randomized. A total of 85.7% or 102 patients realized their free choice to receive chemotherapy as i.v. application, where three were randomized to this arm. Seventeen patients (14.3%) preferred the oral therapy (no randomization to oral therapy). The main reasons for individual preference to i.v. or p.o. treosulfan are listed in Table 2.

Toxicity profile

In both treatment arms, most non-haematological and haematological toxicities were of grade 1 or 2. The most common grade 3/4 haematological side-effects were thrombocytopenia, leukopenia, and neutropenia. Severe non-haematological events were rare. Moreover, a remarkably low rate of alopecia was observed (13.7% with grade 1/2, no grade 3). No therapy-related death was observed (Table 3).

Treatment delay and discontinuation

In total, 421 cycles of treosulfan (median 3, range 1–12) were administered. Dose reductions were performed in 27 courses of treosulfan therapy (6.4%, 1 oral and 26 i.v. arm, see Table 3), whereas for 96 courses (22.8%), an interval prolongation was necessary. The main reason for dose reduction were haematological AEs and for treatment delay haematological toxicity and organisational reasons/preference.

Six Patients (35.3%) preferring oral application received three courses of therapy, but only three patients (17.6%) finished all planned 6 cycles (12 months). In the

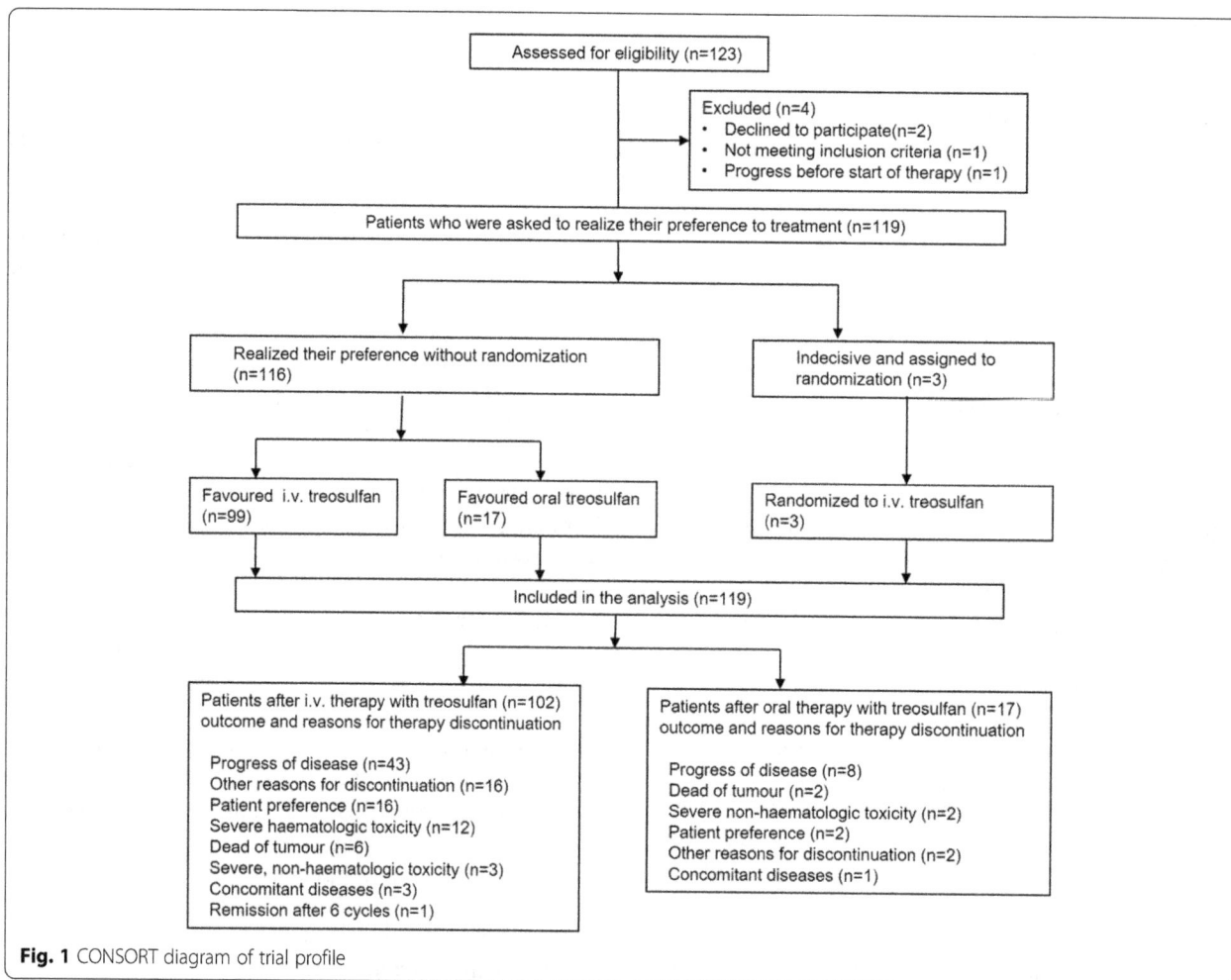

Fig. 1 CONSORT diagram of trial profile

i.v. group, 26 patients (25.4%) received six courses, but only one received the maximum of 12 chemotherapies. Disease progression and patient's choice were main reasons for discontinuing treatment. Subsequently 11.8% of the i.v. participants discontinued therapy due to haematological toxicities, whereas non-haematological events were twice as high in the oral group (Table 3).

Response, survival, and follow-up

Seventy-four patients (65 i.v./ 9 p.o.) were considered assessable for radiological response. One patient showed complete response (1/0), 13 (11/2) partial remission (PR), 15 (14/1) stable disease (SD), 45 (39/6) progressive disease (PD), and 45 were not assessable for response (lost of follow-up). During the study follow-up period, 105 patients (88.2%) died, mostly documented to disease progress.

Median follow-up was 11.4 months. Median progression-free survival in this study was 3.7 months (i.v. 3.5 months/p.o. 4.2 months). Median overall survival was 8.0 months, with 7.8 months (i.v.) and 10.4 months (p.o.),

respectively (Fig. 2). There was no statistically significant difference between the two arms regarding survival.

Geriatric aspects

The highest participation in the geriatric assessment with ADL and iADL questionnaires was achieved at the start of therapy (70%), but declined during the study period to less than 10%. Interestingly the proportion of patients which declared to need support or help in their activities of daily living (ADL) was significantly higher within the individuals with preference for oral treatment, but this effect was not demonstrated for the iADL-score. Geriatric measurements did not demonstrate specific differences in the patient preference profiles (Fig. 2).

Discussion

The key objectives in the treatment of recurrent ovarian cancer (ROC) are preventing disease-related symptoms, prolonging progression-free survival, and maintaining quality of life [2, 26]. However, as more patients achieve long-term survival, palliative care has evolved to include all aspects of cancer survivorship, which increase the

Table 1 Patients' characteristics and distribution of clinical parameters according to individual preference, n = 119

Parameter of disease (n, %)	Preference to treatment	
	i.v. (n = 102)	oral (n = 17)
Median age, in years (range)	72 (65–87)	70 (65–77)
ECOG		
0	22 (21.6)	4 (23.5)
1	68 (66.7)	10 (58.8)
2	12 (11.7)	3 (17.7)
FIGO stage at primary diagnosis		
I	2 (2)	1 (5.9)
II	7 (6.9)	1 (5.9)
III	62 (60.8)	13 (76.5)
IV	25 (24.5)	2 (11.7)
not documented	6 (5.9)	-
Histology		
Serous papillary	59 (57.8)	13 (76.5)
Mucinous	12 (11.7)	3 (17.7)
Endometrioid	8 (7.8)	1 (5.9)
Others or NOS	23 (22.6)	-
Grading at primary diagnosis		
G1	2 (2)	-
G2	29 (28.4)	5 (29.4)
G3	61 (59.8)	12 (70.6)
not documented	10 (9.8)	-
Type of treatment in the adjuvant situation or last recurrence		
Surgical tumordebulking	100 (98)	17 (100)
Chemotherapy	101 (99)	17 (100)
Previous hormonal treatment	8 (7.8)	2 (11.8)
Previous Radiotherapy	6 (5.9)	1 (5.9)
Relapse-free interval after primary platinum based therapy		
< 6 months	21 (20.6)	4 (23.5)
6–12 months	28 (27.5)	7 (41.2)
> 12 months	53 (51.9)	6 (35.3)
Type of previous chemotherapy regimens (n = 372)		
platinum/taxan based	182 (56.9)	22 (44.9)
anthracyclin	38 (11.9)	6 (12.2)
topotecan	45 (14)	9 (18.4)
taxan	12 (3.8)	1 (2.1)
others	43 (13.4)	11 (22.4)
No. of previous chemotherapies for all median (min. / max.)	3 (1–8)	
	3 (1–8)	2 (1–7)

Table 1 Patients' characteristics and distribution of clinical parameters according to individual preference, n = 119 (Continued)

Recurrent situation at time of registration		
1. Recurrence	13 (12.7)	1 (5.9)
2. Recurrence	25 (24.5)	8 (47)
3. Recurrence	30 (29.4)	4 (23.5)
4. Recurrence	15 (14.7)	2 (11.8)
> 4 Recurrencies	19 (18.6)	2 (11.8)

need of new and thoroughly considered approaches focusing individual expectations, preference and acceptance of treatment [13, 27, 28]. Demographic switch increase the expectations on clinicians and health care providers, since multimodal management and identification of subgroups with specific tumour characteristics is gaining key importance [3, 29]. In this prospective study, we evaluated the new strategy giving elderly patients the opportunity to choose free the application route of their chemotherapy and analysed prospectively their preferences. The great majority of 97% realized their preference, demonstrating clearly high motivation to participate to the decision making process. Unexpectedly most patients preferred the i.v. application of the drug, associating oral intake over long period with expected higher gastrointestinal risks for reflux, hyperacidemia, nausea, change of taste, loss of appetite or diarrhoea.

The monthly i.v. infusion seemed for many to be more comfortable, since regular hospital and physician contacts does not negatively influence patient's autonomy and compliance, as described by others [5, 18]. These findings are remarkable, as physicians tend often to inconsequent management of geriatric patients [3, 5, 26]. Multiple analyses demonstrated in the past, that elderly were treated suboptimal, commonly under-represented in clinical trials, which resulted in their unfavourable outcome [3, 7]. Although data do not support the suggestion that age – independently of any other factors – is a negative prognostic factor, we need new clinical instruments to evaluate additionally aspects of acceptance, preference and satisfaction with care, as well as social and psychological scopes of treatment [1, 5]. Our trial offers here unique aspects and insights to traditional management and can help for more individualisation of palliative ovarian cancer care.

Patient's preference is known to be complex, to base on individual experiences and reflecting on relevant life events and be difficult to assess [30, 31]. Acceptance of and compliance with oncological therapy plays a key role for improving efficacy and prolonging survival. Age is the strongest demographic factor affecting patients' preferences: younger and better-educated patients, and women

Table 2 Reasons for treatment preference and concomitant diseases (n = 119)

Characteristics	i.v., n = 102, (%)	Oral, n = 17, (%)
Preference to therapy regime	99 (83.2)	17 (14.3)
Randomization (for indecisive patients)	3 (2.5)	0
Main reasons for therapy preference		
Wish to avoid gastrointestinal disorders	20 (19.6)	0
Disfavour / poor toleration of oral drugs	12 (17.8)	0
Oblivion / daily oral intake is unsure	14 (13.7)	0
Believe i.v. application is saver over i.v. port	15 (14.7)	0
More effective / higher treatment pressure	13 (12.3)	1 (5.9)
Oral drug application not possible - short bowel/subileus	4 (3.9)	0
Pre-existing chronic diarrhoea / vomiting	4 (3.9)	0
Expect better tolerability	4 (3.9)	0
Wish no hospital treatment / more independence / privacy	0	6 (35.3)
The handling of the therapy is simple	0	4 (23.5)
Continuity of the drug administration / maintenance effect	0	2 (11.8)
Made bad experience with venous puncture	0	1 (5.9)
Reason for preference not documented	16 (17.6)	3 (17.7)
Concomitant diseases (multiple answers)		
Cardiovascular	92 (90.2)	17 (100)
Musculoskeletal	37 (36.3)	7 (41.2)
Pulmonary	28 (27.5)	2 (11.8)
Lower gastrointestinal tract	39 (38.2)	4 (23.5)
Upper gastrointestinal tract	27 (26.5)	4 (23.5)
Metabolic and hormonal	25 (24.5)	6 (35.3)
Hepatic	27 (26.5)	3 (17.7)
Renal	12 (11.8)	6 (35.3)
Urinary tract	21 (20.6)	2 (11.8)
Neurological	27 (26.5)	7 (41.2)
Psychiatric	6 (5.9)	4 (23.5)

Table 3 Toxicity, dose reduction and reasons for therapy discontinuation (n = 119)

Parameter	i.v., n = 102 (%)	Oral, n = 17 (%)
Toxicity (grade 3 or 4)	742 AE's [a]	14 AE's
Haematological (all grade)		
Thrombocytopenia	38.6	30
Leucopenia	27.3	50
Neutropenia	16.3	10
Anemia	11.6	10
Febrile Neutropenia	7	-
Non-haematological (all grade)		
Ascites	9.9	11
Subileus (severe constipation)	8.6	11
Constipation	6.2	-
Abdominal pain	4.9	11
Ileus (bowel obstruction)	4.9	-
Vomiting	4.9	-
Nausea	3.7	-
Diarrhoea	2.5	11
Rectal incontinence	2.5	-
Others (< 1%)	51.8	56
Dose reduction (27 of all 421 cycles)	6.4	
(26 of 376 i.v. cycles vs. 1 of 45 oral cycles)	6.9	2.2
Prolongation of treatment interval (> 14d)	25	4.4
Reasons for early therapy discontinuation		
Progressive disease	42	47.1
Patients preference	15.7	11.8
Other reasons	15.7	11.8
Haematological toxicity (grade 3/4)	11.8	-
Dead of tumour	5.9	11.8
Non-haematological toxicity (grade 3/4)	2.9	11.8
Concomitant disease	2.9	5.9
Complete remission	1	-
Main cause of death		
Tumour related	80.4	82.4
Others	7.8	5.9

[a]adverse events

in general, were reported to prefer more active role in decision-making [31]. Degner et al. identified a large variation in preferred and attained levels of involvement in the treatment decisions for breast cancer patients [32]. Our analysis identified that, even after extensive pre-treatment (median of 3 previous therapies) and in highly palliative situation elderly ovarian cancer patients prefer to realize their individual preference and accept the corresponding treatment. Therapy discontinuation remained low, mostly due to tumour progression or toxicity. The i.v. regimen seems to demonstrate a partly favourable toxicity compared to oral treosulfan. Interestingly, this corresponds

ADL

iADL

Fig. 2 Distribution of severe geriatric assessment inside patients with i.v. and oral preference. ADL = activities of daily living; iADL = instrumental activities of daily living

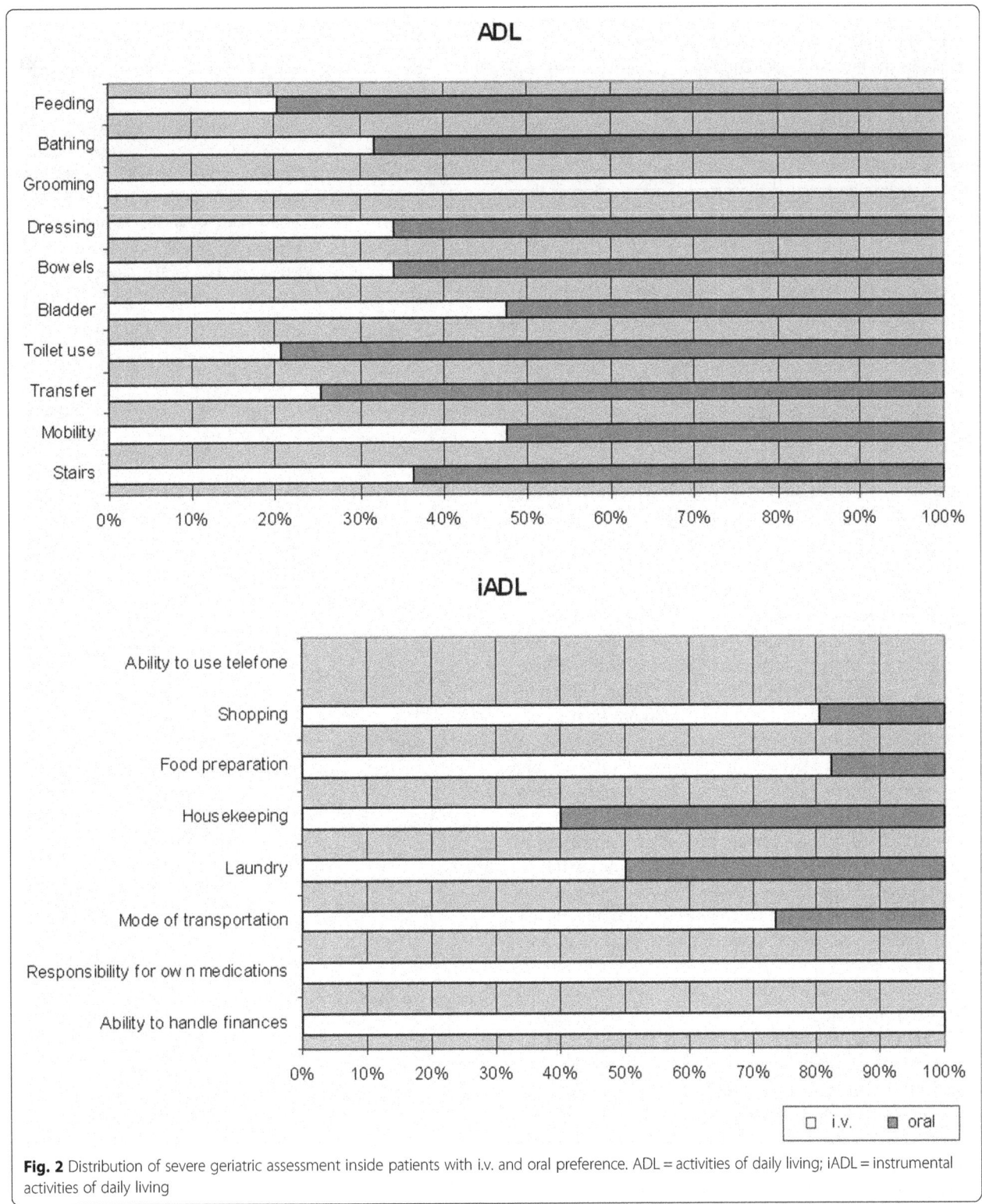

with the patients' expectation of a milder effect on the gastrointestinal tract, which, in turn, was declared to guarantee more safety. On the other hand, patients expected a better control over their treatment since the application takes place in a hospital/outpatient department and

associated the corresponding influence with expected positively affection on their outcome. This reflects report of close relationship of oncological patients to their treating physicians and palliative care teams as one of their most important representatives during the treatment [11, 13, 28].

Otherwise the possibility of realizing one's own preference evidently has the strongest psychological impact [33].

Despite all limitations of the small patient cohort and the non-mandatory evaluation of geriatric measures, this trial report interesting insight into a very complex palliative cohort of geriatric patients. Although the observed disease stabilisation was mostly brief, only a small number of participants interrupted their study participation at their own request, keeping their compliance and acceptance high. Despite methodical limitations due to the imbalance of patient distribution, our results are comparable with data by Pfeiffer et al, who reported preference for i.v. chemotherapy within colon cancer outpatients, probably due to expected lower toxicity [18].. In contrast, other groups reported preference for oral chemotherapy, within younger breast cancer patients associated with their better functional and physiological status, less comorbidities, and the wish for more individuality in their daily activities [1, 13].. A certain bias in the trial design consisted, perhaps, in the fact that, in most cases, in these trials an established i.v. drug was compared to an "innovative" oral formulation, which seemed more attractive [17, 18, 32, 34].

The frequency of concomitant diseases registered in our cohort was high, mostly of moderate severity, and, typically, resulted in more co-medication. It is well-known that multimorbidity may influence patient decisions, favouring tolerability while trying to balance risks and potential benefits [6]. Recently published data has not reported significant impact on early treatment discontinuation of chemotherapy in cohort of 1213 patients with relapsed ovarian cancer [35]. Although only some physical and emotional domains of quality of life were described most salient, there is no prospective evaluation in ovarian cancer patients and distinct domains are more than heterogeneous [36, 37]. Exemplarily patients after extensive tumour debulking with gross bowel resection, who are not able to resorb oral drugs due to consequently insufficient bowel metabolism, needs quite different treatment strategy as an elderly and frail patient with accumulated gastrointestinal toxicity [35, 38]. Thus, knowledge of late effects of cancer survivals and their individual preferences could help to modify possible ineffective treatment and increase satisfaction with care, but have to be studied systematic in a prospective approach [13, 38].

Summarising elderly ovarian cancer patients demonstrated a high motivation to realize their treatment preference, despite their comorbidity, co-medication and previous chemotherapy experience. The preference for i.v. chemotherapy in this palliative cohort could be described with subjective expectations and individual explanations to toxicity, safety and treatment potency which are difficult to be quantified objective. As expected there were no severe toxicities or differences in efficacy observed [39, 40]. Thus the concept of a patient's free choice following preference for the drug application form could be an attractive option in the treatment of ROC, especially in elderly and comorbid patients with heavily pre-treated recurrence.

Conclusions

Elderly patients with recurrent ovarian cancer have clear preferences and are motivated to participate to the treatment decision process. In the palliative situation they preferred the i.v. application of treosulfan, based on individual experience with toxicity, comorbidity and co-medication, which reflects their specific geriatric situation.

Abbreviations

ADL: Activities of daily living; AE: Adverse event/s; ECOG: Eastern Cooperative Oncology Group; iADL: Instrumental activities of daily living; ROC: Recurrent ovarian cancer

Acknowledgements

We would like to thank the Ovarian Cancer Study Group of the North-Eastern Society for Gynaecological Oncology (NOGGO) for concept, coordination, data management and follow-up acquisition.
The authors acknowledge Alcedis GmbH, Giessen, Germany for independent data monitoring and processing.
This study was presented in part at the 14th Biennial Meeting of the International Gynaecologic Cancer Society, Vancouver, Canada, October 13–16, 2012

Funding

This study was sponsored by
Medac Gesellschaft fuer klinische Spezialpraeparate mbH, Headquarters: Hamburg
Managing directors: Heiner Will, Dr. Rainer Dickhardt, Joerg Hans, Jens Denker, Nikolaus Graf Stolberg, Dr. Ulrich Kosciessa; Register court: Hamburg HRB 14 332
The design of the study, patient collection and registration, analysis and interpretation of data and the writing of this manuscript was organized and coordinated only by the authors and the Ovarian Cancer Study Group of the North-Eastern Society for Gynaecological Oncology (NOGGO).

Authors' contributions

RC, RR, GOO and JS participated in the design of the study and performed the statistical analysis. RC, PK, GH, HS, SM, DKM and JS conceived of the study, and participated in its design and coordination and helped to draft the manuscript. PH, SF, LRH, LW, LM, WA, YN, IY, PW, RR, GOO participated in the study and helped to draft the manuscript. All authors read and approved the final manuscript.

Competing interests

The authors declare that they have no competing interests.

Informed consent to participate

Informed consent was obtained from all individual participants included in the study.

Author details

[1]Department of Gynaecology, European Competence Centre for Ovarian Cancer, Charité Universitätsmedizin, Berlin, Germany. [2]Department of Gynaecology and Gynaecologic Oncology, Kliniken Essen Mitte, Essen, Germany. [3]Onkologische Schwerpunktpraxis Heidelberg, Heidelberg, Germany. [4]Department of Gynaecology and Obstetrics, Gynaecological Cancer Center of the University Schleswig-Holstein, Campus Lübeck, Lübeck, Germany. [5]Department of Gynaecology and Gynaecologic Oncology, University Medical Center Hamburg-Eppendorf, Hamburg, Germany. [6]Onkologische Schwerpunktpraxis Leer, Leer, Germany. [7]Praxisklinik Krebsheilkunde für Frauen, Berlin, Germany. [8]Onkologische Schwerpunktpraxis im Elisenhof, Munich, Germany. [9]Gynäkologisch-onkologische Schwerpunktpraxis, Fürstenwalde, Germany. [10]Department of Gynaecology and Obstetrics and Comprehensive Cancer Center, University of Munich, Munich, Germany. [11]Department of Gynecology and Obstetrics, Technische Universität Dresden, Dresden, Germany. [12]Department of Gynaecology and Obstetrics, University Medicine Greifswald, Greifswald, Germany. [13]North-Eastern German Society for Gynaecologic Oncology, Ovarian Cancer Study Group, Berlin, Germany.

References

1. Bonanni B, Lazzeroni M. Acceptability of chemoprevention trials in high-risk subjects. Ann Oncol. 2013;24 Suppl 8:viii42–6.

2. Hall M, Rustin G. Recurrent ovarian cancer: when and how to treat. Curr Oncol Rep. 2011;13:459–71.

3. Hilpert F, Wimberger P, du Bois A, Pfisterer J, Harter P. Treatment of elderly ovarian cancer patients in the context of controlled clinical trials: a joint analysis of the AGO Germany experience. Onkologie. 2012;35:76–81.

4. Colombo N, et al. Newly diagnosed and relapsed epithelial ovarian carcinoma: ESMO Clinical Practice Guidelines for diagnosis, treatment and follow-up. Ann Oncol. 2010;21 Suppl 5:v23–30.

5. Lambrou NC, Bristow RE. Ovarian cancer in elderly women. Oncology (Huntingt). 2003;17:1075–81. discussion 1081, 1085-1076, 1091.

6. Mahner S, et al. A prospective multicenter study of treosulfan in elderly patients with recurrent ovarian cancer: results of a planned safety analysis. J Cancer Res Clin Oncol. 2012;138:1413–9.

7. Petignat P, et al. Poorer survival of elderly patients with ovarian cancer: a population-based study. Surg Oncol. 2004;13:181–6.

8. Braicu EI, et al. Primary versus secondary cytoreduction for epithelial ovarian cancer: a paired analysis of tumour pattern and surgical outcome. Eur J Cancer. 2012;48:687–94.

9. Kolb GF, Weissbach L. Demographic change : changes in society and medicine and developmental trends in geriatrics. Urologe A. 2015;54:1701–9.

10. Clegg A, Young J, Iliffe S, Rikkert MO, Rockwood K. Frailty in elderly people. Lancet. 2013;381:752–62.

11. Nelson EC, et al. Patient reported outcome measures in practice. BMJ. 2015; 350:g7818.

12. De Cock L, Kieffer A, Kurtz JE, Joly F, Weber B. [Expectations of patients with ovarian cancer. Results of the European investigation EXPRESSION III in French patients from GINECO group]. Bull Cancer. 2015;102:217–25.

13. Oskay-Ozcelik G, et al. Breast cancer patients' expectations in respect of the physician-patient relationship and treatment management results of a survey of 617 patients. Ann Oncol. 2007;18:479–84.

14. Stuart GC, et al. 2010 Gynecologic Cancer InterGroup (GCIG) consensus statement on clinical trials in ovarian cancer: report from the Fourth Ovarian Cancer Consensus Conference. Int J Gynecol Cancer. 2011;21:750–5.

15. Petignat P, Vlastos G. Why do ovarian cancer patients not consult a gynecologic oncologist? Gynecol Oncol. 2002;87:157. author reply 158.

16. Fotopoulou C, et al. Clinical outcome of tertiary surgical cytoreduction in patients with recurrent epithelial ovarian cancer. Ann Surg Oncol. 2011;18:49–57.

17. Singh JA, et al. Preferred roles in treatment decision making among patients with cancer: a pooled analysis of studies using the Control Preferences Scale. Am J Manag Care. 2010;16:688–96.

18. Pfeiffer P, et al. Patient preference for oral or intravenous chemotherapy: a randomised cross-over trial comparing capecitabine and Nordic fluorouracil/ leucovorin in patients with colorectal cancer. Eur J Cancer. 2006;42:2738–43.

19. Gropp M, Meier W, Hepp H. Treosulfan as an effective second-line therapy in ovarian cancer. Gynecol Oncol. 1998;71:94–8.

20. Breitbach GP, et al. Treosulfan in the treatment of advanced ovarian cancer: a randomised co-operative multicentre phase III-study. Anticancer Res. 2002;22:2923–32.

21. Meier W, et al. Topotecan versus treosulfan, an alkylating agent, in patients with epithelial ovarian cancer and relapse within 12 months following 1st-line platinum/paclitaxel chemotherapy. A prospectively randomized phase III trial by the Arbeitsgemeinschaft Gynaekologische Onkologie Ovarian Cancer Study Group (AGO-OVAR). Gynecol Oncol. 2009;114:199–205.

22. Hilger RA, et al. Investigation of bioavailability and pharmacokinetics of treosulfan capsules in patients with relapsed ovarian cancer. Cancer Chemother Pharmacol. 2000;45:483–8.

23. Chekerov R, et al. Treosulfan in the treatment of advanced ovarian cancer - results of a german multicenter non-interventional study. Anticancer Res. 2015;35:6869–75.

24. Senn S. Review of Fleiss, statistical methods for rates and proportions. Res Synth Methods. 2011;2:221–2.

25. Rustin GJ. Follow-up with CA125 after primary therapy of advanced ovarian cancer has major implications for treatment outcome and trial performances and should not be routinely performed. Ann Oncol. 2011;22 Suppl 8:viii45–8.

26. Kurtz JE, et al. Ovarian cancer in elderly patients: carboplatin and pegylated liposomal doxorubicin versus carboplatin and paclitaxel in late relapse: a Gynecologic Cancer Intergroup (GCIG) CALYPSO sub-study. Ann Oncol. 2011;22:2417–23.

27. Rowland JH, Hewitt M, Ganz PA. Cancer survivorship: a new challenge in delivering quality cancer care. J Clin Oncol. 2006;24:5101–4.

28. Economou D. Palliative care needs of cancer survivors. Semin Oncol Nurs. 2014;30:262–7.

29. Barnholtz-Sloan JS, et al. Ovarian cancer: changes in patterns at diagnosis and relative survival over the last three decades. Am J Obstet Gynecol. 2003;189:1120–7.

30. Brennan PF, Strombom I. Improving health care by understanding patient preferences: the role of computer technology. J Am Med Inform Assoc. 1998;5:257–62.

31. Say R, Murtagh M, Thomson R. Patients' preference for involvement in medical decision making: a narrative review. Patient Educ Couns. 2006;60:102–14.

32. Degner LF, et al. Information needs and decisional preferences in women with breast cancer. JAMA. 1997;277:1485–92.

33. Hwang KH, Cho OH, Yoo YS. Symptom clusters of ovarian cancer patients undergoing chemotherapy, and their emotional status and quality of life. Eur J Oncol Nurs. 2016;21:215–22.

34. Mikhail SE, Sun JF, Marshall JL. Safety of capecitabine: a review. Expert Opin Drug Saf. 2010;9:831–41.

35. Woopen H, et al. The influence of comorbidity and comedication on grade III/IV toxicity and prior discontinuation of chemotherapy in recurrent ovarian cancer patients: An individual participant data meta-analysis of the North-Eastern German Society of Gynecological Oncology (NOGGO). Gynecol Oncol. 2015;138:735–40.

36. Donovan KA, et al. Recommended patient-reported core set of symptoms and quality-of-life domains to measure in ovarian cancer treatment trials. J Natl Cancer Inst. 2014;106(7):1–4.

37. King MT, et al. Development of the measure of ovarian symptoms and treatment concerns: aiming for optimal measurement of patient-reported symptom benefit with chemotherapy for symptomatic ovarian cancer. Int J Gynecol Cancer. 2014;24:865–73.

38. Tew WP, Fleming GF. Treatment of ovarian cancer in the older woman. Gynecol Oncol. 2015;136:136–42.

39. Sehouli J, et al. Nonplatinum topotecan combinations versus topotecan alone for recurrent ovarian cancer: results of a phase III study of the North-Eastern German Society of Gynecological Oncology Ovarian Cancer Study Group. J Clin Oncol. 2008;26:3176–82.

40. Edwards SJ, Barton S, Thurgar E, Trevor N. Topotecan, pegylated liposomal doxorubicin hydrochloride, paclitaxel, trabectedin and gemcitabine for advanced recurrent or refractory ovarian cancer: a systematic review and economic evaluation. Health Technol Assess. 2015;19:1–480.

18

Socio-demographic characteristics influencing cervical cancer screening intention of HIV-positive women in the central region of Ghana

Nancy Innocentia Ebu

Abstract

Background: The burden of HIV and cervical cancer is concentrated in sub-Saharan Africa. Women with HIV are more likely to have persistent HPV infection leading to cervical abnormalities and cancer. Cervical cancer screening seems to be the single most critical intervention in any efforts to prevent cervical cancer. The purpose of this study was to determine the socio-demographic factors influencing intention to seek cervical cancer screening by HIV-positive women in the Central Region of Ghana.

Methods: A descriptive cross-sectional study involving a convenience sample of 660 HIV-positive women aged 20 to 65 years receiving antiretroviral therapy in HIV care centres in the Central Region of Ghana was conducted using an interviewer-administered questionnaire. The data were summarised and analysed using frequencies, percentages and binary logistic regression.

Results: The study revealed that 82.0% of HIV-positive women intended to obtain cervical cancer screening. Level of education was a determinant of cervical cancer screening intention. HIV-positive women with low levels of education were 2.67 times (95% CI, 1.61–4.42) more likely to have intention to screen than those with no formal education. Those with high levels of education were 3.16 times (95% CI, 1.42–7.02) more likely to have intention to screen than those with no formal education. However, age, religion, marital status, employment status, and ability to afford the cost of cervical cancer screening were not determinants of intention to screen.

Conclusions: Education of women of all ages needs to be a priority, as it could enable them to adopt appropriate health behaviours and engage in cervical cancer screening. Additionally, interventions to improve understanding of cervical cancer screening among HIV-positive women are highly recommended. These include health education about the disease and availability of screening options in HIV/AIDS care centres.

Keywords: Cervical cancer screening, Cervical cancer, Socio-demographics, HIV-positive women, Intention, Ghana, Developing countries

Correspondence: nebu@ucc.edu.gh
Department of Public Health, School of Nursing and Midwifery, University of Cape Coast, Cape Coast, Ghana

Socio-demographic characteristics influencing cervical cancer screening intention of HIV positive women...

141

Background

Cancer of the cervix is an important concern in global health. Globally, cervical cancer is the second most prevalent cancer that impacts the health and mortality of women. It is estimated that 500,000 cases are diagnosed yearly, with over 250,000 deaths as a result of the condition [1]. Cervical cancer is a major cause of morbidity and mortality among women in poor resource settings, especially in Africa [1]. Significant proportions of cancers (over 80%) that occur in sub-Saharan Africa are discovered in late stages, mostly due to lack of information and limited access to preventive services [2, 3]. Late-stage disease is associated with low survival rates after surgery or radiotherapy. In addition, treatment options may not be available in developing economies, or they may be too costly and inaccessible to vulnerable women. Cervical cancer is potentially preventable, as effective screening programmes can lead to a significant reduction in the morbidity and mortality associated with this cancer [4]. The Global Health Group reports that more than 288,000 women die each year worldwide due to cervical cancer and the disease mostly affects vulnerable and disadvantaged women in society [5]. Most screening activities in developing countries do not reach vulnerable women, and consequently a high proportion of cervical cancer cases are diagnosed at an advanced stage [6].

The burden of HIV and cervical cancer is concentrated in sub-Saharan Africa. Women with HIV are more likely to have persistent HPV infection leading to cervical abnormalities and cancer [7, 8]. A systematic review reports that HIV infection could lead to a faster progression of cervical cancer due to a strong association between HIV infection and invasive cervical cancer [9]. This suggests that HIV-positive women need to screen early for an HIV-related cancer like cervical cancer to reduce risks of cancer. Previous studies conducted in sub-Saharan cultures have posited that socio-demographics, such as income, age and religion [10–15], level of education, marital status and age [16–18], influenced cervical cancer screening. However, the Health Belief Model (HBM) suggests that socio-demographic factors are modifiable variables which may influence an individual to engage in health behaviour [19]. Additionally, in Ghana, although cervical cancer may impact the health of HIV-positive women, few of the empirical works on cervical cancer screening focused on the attitudes and knowledge of women in general [20–22], and did not include HIV-positive women who are the most vulnerable group. This study therefore hypothesised that socio-demographic factors predict intention of HIV-positive women to seek cervical cancer screening.

Methods

A descriptive cross-sectional study was conducted in the Central Region of Ghana. The region is located in the southern part of Ghana. The region recorded an HIV prevalence of 1.8 in the 2016 HIV sentinel survey, which suggests the presence of HIV infection in the region [23]. The study population, comprised all HIV-positive women in the Central Region, was estimated to be 6019 [24]. However, the accessible population was HIV-positive women receiving care in the various antiretroviral care centres in the Central Region, and was estimated to be 3483 [24]. The study includes HIV-positive women who were between the ages of 20 to 65 years, and had been receiving regular care in health facilities that provide care to people living with HIV/AIDS (PLWHIV) in the Central Region.

However, terminally ill clients and those with dementia were excluded as they might not be in a position to provide valid responses. Using a power formula derived by Ogah [25], a sample size of 660 HIV-positive women was estimated for the study. Six health facilities that provide care for PLWHIV in the Central Region were randomly selected for the study. The study also employed the probability proportionate to size sampling in determining the number of HIV-positive women to participate in the study from the facilities selected for the study. Accidental quota sampling technique was used in selecting HIV-positive women from the various health facilities until the sample size was reached.

Data collection

A questionnaire was designed to identify the socio-demographic characteristics of HIV-positive women that influence intention to screen. It was guided by the HBM and Theory of Planned Behaviour. The questions were adopted from Ebu et al. [22] and Mupepi et al. [26]. The socio-demographic information considered included: age, marital status, religion, level of education, employment status and ability to afford the cost of cervical cancer screening. The independent variables for the study were; level of education, marital status, age, employment status, religion, and ability to afford the cost of cervical cancer screening. The dependent variable was intention to obtain cervical cancer screening. Data were collected from HIV-positive women who visited the health facilities during the period of data collection and volunteered to participate in the study. The data collectors were six HIV nurse prescribers (nurses who have been trained to provide antiretroviral therapy services to clients) who were trained for that purpose. The data was collected over a ten-week period. The Institutional Review Board of the University of Cape Coast and Ethical Review Committee of the Ghana Health Service gave ethical approval for the study to be conducted. Written informed consent was obtained from all participants.

Data analysis

Data were analysed using frequencies, percentages and binary logistic regression analysis. Independent variables were categorised. Levels of education were high level of education (tertiary school), low level of education (primary and secondary), and no formal education. Marital status was married (married or cohabiting) or unmarried (single, divorced, or widowed). Employment status was working or non-working (student, retired, or unemployed). Religion comprised Christians and Muslims. Age was classified by 30 years and above and under 30. The ability to afford cervical cancer screening was classified as very affordable, fairly affordable or not affordable. The independent variables were categorical and measured on the nominal scale. The dependent variable was intention to obtain cervical cancer screening and was measured as either "Yes" or "No".

Results

The descriptive statistics of the respondents showed that 79.2% ($n = 523$) were above 30 years old, and 20.8% ($n = 137$) were under 30. With regard to their marital status, 53.2% ($n = 351$) were married while 46.8% ($n = 309$) were not married. A high proportion of the respondents, 89.7% ($n = 592$), were Christians while 10.3% ($n = 68$) were Muslims. Again, 21.7% ($n = 143$) were not formally educated, 62.1% ($n = 410$) had low level of education and only 16.2% ($n = 107$) had high level of education. Additionally, 54.2% ($n = 358$) were working while 45.8% ($n = 302$) were not working. More than half of the respondents, 55.3%

($n = 365$) viewed the cost of screening as not affordable while 44.7% ($n = 295$) perceived it as affordable. In connection with the intention of the respondents, 82.0% ($n = 540$) of HIV-positive women had intention to obtain cervical cancer screening while 18.0% ($n = 120$) did not have any intention. The results in Table 1 show that low levels of education (primary and secondary) and high education (tertiary) statistically significantly contributed to intention to screen, with p-values of 0.001 and 0.005 respectively using respondents with no formal education as the reference category. Respondents with a low level of education were 2 times more likely to have intention to screen [OR] 2.67 (95%CI = 1.61–4.42). Comparatively, those with tertiary or a high level of education were approximately 3 times more likely to have intention to screen [OR] 3.16 (95% CI = 1.42–7.02). However, marital status ($p = 0.492$, OR = 1.17, [95% CI, 0.74–1.86]), religion ($p = 0.808$, OR = 1.09, [95% CI, 0.55–2.18]), age ($p = 0.704$, OR = 1.12, [95% CI, 0.63–2.00]), employment status ($p = 0.045$, OR = 1.63, [95% CI, 1.01–2.64]), and ability to afford the cost of cervical cancer screening ($p = 0.411$, OR = 1.25, [95% CI, 0.73–2.13]) did not contribute statistically significantly to the prediction of intention in the model.

Discussion

The findings suggest that respondents with low to high levels of education are likely to screen than those with no

Table 1 Binary Logistic Regression to Predict Intention to Seek Cervical Cancer Screening based on Socio-Demographic Characteristics

Variables	n (%)	β	Wald	p-value	OR	95% CI for OR	
						Lower	Upper
Level of Education							
High	93 (17)	1.15	7.97	0.005	3.16	1.42	7.02
Low	350 (65)	0.98	14.35	0.001	2.67	1.61	4.42
No education (Ref.)	97 (18)						
Marital Status							
Married	297 (55)	0.16	0.47	0.492	1.17	0.74	1.86
Not married (Ref.)	243 (45)						
Religion							
Christianity	486 (90)	0.09	0.06	0.808	1.09	0.55	2.18
Islam (Ref.)	54 (10)						
Age (in years)							
30 and above	427 (79)	0.11	0.15	0.704	1.12	0.63	2.00
Under 30 (Ref.)	113 (21)						
Employment Status							
Working	311 (58)	0.49	4.02	0.045	1.63	1.01	2.64
Not working (Ref.)	229 (42)						
Ability to Afford Cervical Cancer Screening							
Affordable	255 (47)	0.22	0.68	0.411	1.25	0.73	2.13
Not affordable (Ref.)	285 (53)						
Constant		2.16	35.35	0.001	8.70		

formal education. A possible explanation for this outcome is that women who are educated may have increased understanding of health care services. Education seems to be an enabling factor that can help women to have a better understanding about cervical cancer and the screening facilities available. Educated women may also be in a better position to evaluate their level of risk concerning the disease. The level of educational attainment could facilitate decisions in accessing health services including cervical screening. Several studies have affirmed education as an important predictor of intention to screen and cervical cancer screening behaviour [27–30].

The present finding is consistent with previous studies, which could be due to the similarity in how level of education was measured [16, 29]. Level of education is known to be a modifiable factor, as it is known to modify other constructs in the HBM. Education is an individual characteristic that can influence subjective perception of screening [19, 31]. It has commonly been assumed that women with some level of education have better chances of using maternal health care services compared to those without any formal education [12, 32]. Education has a high tendency of changing beliefs and unfavourable behaviours if interventions are designed and targeted to address specific notions in respect to health and illness [33].

The findings suggest that women with no formal education may not have intention to seek cervical screening. Women who are illiterate or have not had any form of education may have poor access to health services and experience low quality of life. Importantly, they may delay in seeking health care, even when symptoms of the disease are obvious, compared to better educated women, who may respond faster [33]. Other empirical works have demonstrated that illiterate women may be less likely to seek cervical cancer screening [32, 34, 35]. Despite the heterogeneity in the methodology and in the characteristics of the population employed in these studies, the findings suggest that women with no formal education may be at high risk of contracting cervical cancer. Education, therefore, allows women to have improved socio-economic status and decreased morbidity and mortality, as they become more empowered to control the determinants of their health [36].

Marital status was not a determinant of intention to screen. A possible explanation could be due to how this concept was measured in this study, as those who were cohabiting were regarded as being in marital relationship. Additionally, respondents who are divorced and widowed were added to single women and considered unmarried. This finding confirms previous studies in which no significant relationship was found between those who were married and the unmarried in relation to cervical cancer screening intention [17, 29, 32]. Although there was heterogeneity in the methodology

employed in these studies, the results were similar to the present study because the studies focused on women and the conceptual basis could be linked to the HBM. Ogunwale et al. explained that HIV-positive women who had not had cervical cancer screening were younger and had multiple sexual partners or had had sexual intercourse with a man with multiple sexual partners [37]. It is well documented that in Ghana, and other African societies, men tend to dominate affairs of women at the household level, including in decisions about seeking preventive healthcare [38]. In Nigeria, marital status was found not to be a predictor of cervical cancer screening uptake, as women had abysmally low knowledge and poor perception of the disease [39].

Similarly, respondents' religion did not statistically contribute significantly to the prediction of intention to screen. The result is consistent with that of Ezechi et al. [28] and Modibbo et al. [14], in which religion did not predict cervical cancer screening intention. Categorisation of respondents' religion in these previous studies was similar to that of the present study, and that may have influenced the outcome. Previous studies explained that, in the African context, religious and cultural beliefs of modesty, cervical cancer being viewed as a curse from God and a shameful disease associated with immorality [14], and male dominance over decisions about seeking health care may create barriers for many women [38].

Age also was not a determinant of cervical cancer screening intention. A possible explanation for this outcome could be that age was dichotomised into those under 30 and above 30 in this study. It could also be related to the fact that 79% of HIV-positive women with intention to screen were aged 30 years and above. This finding is consistent with previous studies in which age did not significantly predict willingness to have Pap test [17, 32]. This suggests that age is not an essential factor that may facilitate HIV-positive women's intention to seek screening. It seems regularly seeking preventive health services, specifically cervical cancer screening, is not well grounded in the culture of Ghanaians, which may suggest that women of all ages may not seek screening services. Perhaps in Ghana and some African cultures, utilisation of preventive health services and health-care-seeking behaviours are not well defined. Consequently, most women intend to seek or actually seek health care when symptoms of the disease are conspicuous [40].

Statistically, employment status did not contribute significantly to the prediction of intention to seek cervical cancer screening. A possible explanation for this outcome is that, although employment provides a sense of self-esteem and could result in personal fulfillment, HIV-positive women may have issues with stigma and entertain fears that other people may get to know of their HIV status. This could potentially deter those who work and could afford cervical cancer screening from engaging in such an important behaviour. In addition, some of these women may lack knowledge about cervical cancer and they may also have specific barriers regarding screening. In this study, 42% of HIV-positive women with intention to screen were not working. The fact that these women were not in any formal job could affect their perception of their intention to seek cervical cancer screening. The finding confirms previous studies in which employment status was not a determinant of screening [41, 42]. It seems employment may not guarantee intention to participate in a health promotion activity. This suggests that other important factors could influence intention. HIV-positive women encounter unique problems, including stigma, discrimination, and fear of obtaining a positive cervical cancer screening result [43–46], despite being in active employment and having the financial resources for health. It could be explained that the socialisation processes of young and mature women in the Ghanaian culture's strict traditions can deprive women of status, which can affect their pattern of health care seeking [47].

It is evident from the findings that ability to afford cervical cancer screening was not a determinant of intention to screen. A possible explanation for this outcome is that HIV-positive women have unique challenges regarding cervical cancer screening, as 53% of HIV-positive women with intention to screen perceived the cost as not being affordable. In previous studies conducted in developing settings, the ability to afford cervical cancer screening did not result in cervical cancer screening intention [28, 46, 48]. The ability to afford cervical cancer screening is a factor which has the potential of modifying perception constructs in the HBM [19]. However, HIV-positive women may have low socio-economic status and self-esteem that can impact utilisation of health services [49].

Previous studies found cost of cervical cancer screening to be a critical barrier to screening [50–53], if women perceived the cost to be high. One previous study reported that women may be willing to have cervical cancer screening if employers pay for the cost of screening [54]. This demonstrates an urgent need for women to be supported to act on their intention to screen [55]. For instance, in Ghana, although women play a critical role in nation building and form approximately 50% of the workforce, they are mostly involved in informal sector jobs such as trading and farming. Only 1% are in administrative positions in the public sector [56]. This suggests that it may be difficult for HIV-positive women to pay for cervical cancer screening which costs from 9.2 to 14.7 euros.

Conclusions

The findings imply that some level of education encourages women to have positive attitudes and intention toward cervical cancer screening. Cervical cancer screening education should be designed to target HIV-positive women, especially those who are not literate since they may be at increased risk of developing the disease. It is critical that education of both young and mature women be promoted, as it may form an integral part in ensuring positive health behaviours. These findings indicate that women who are not educated may not utilise health services, as misconceptions and personal beliefs about it could be a barrier [15, 25]. Therefore, the family, community, civil society and government should view female education as a priority. Education of women has a positive impact on them, their family and the entire society. Interventions that could improve HIV-positive women's understanding of cervical cancer screening, including health education about the disease and screening options in HIV/AIDS care centres, are highly recommended. Age, marital status, employment status, religion, and ability to afford cervical cancer screening, on the other hand, do not appear to influence intention to engage in cervical cancer screening. These factors may not be critical in designing interventions for HIV-positive women in the Central Region of Ghana.

Abbreviations

HBM: Health Belief Model; HIV: Human Immunodeficiency Virus; TPB: Theory of Planned Behaviour; WHO: World Health Organisation

Acknowledgements

The author wishes to acknowledge the support of all the HIV nurse prescribers who volunteered to collect the data for this study. She is grateful to the staff of the Antiretroviral units for their support during the data collection stage of the research at the following hospitals in Ghana: Saltpond, Swedru, Breman Assikuma, Abura Dunkwa, and Assin Foso. She also wishes to extend her gratitude to Mrs. Esther Nketsia and Mrs. Florence Offei of the Cape Coast Teaching Hospital for their support and encouragement. The author appreciates the kind contribution of Dianne Slager of Kirkhof College of Nursing, Grand Valley State University, Grand Rapids, MI, United States of America.

Funding

The study did not receive any funding or support in any form from any funding institution or organisation.

Authors' contributions

NIE conceptualised, designed and conducted the study. She analysed, interpreted the data and wrote the manuscript. She also revised the manuscript. The author read and approved the final manuscript.

Competing interests

The author does not have any personal or financial competing interests to declare in relation to this manuscript.

References

1. World Health Organisation. WHO guidance note on comprehensive cervical cancer prevention and control: a healthier future for girls and women. 2013. http://www.who.int/iris/bitstream/10665/78128/3/9789241505147_eng.pdf. Accessed 11 Jan 2016.

2. Kidanto HL, Kilewo CD, Moshiro C. Cancer of the cervix: knowledge and attitudes of female patients admitted at Muhimbili National Hospital, Dar-es-salaam. East Afr Med J. 2002;79(9):467–75.

3. Bingham A, Bishop A, Coffey P, Winkler J, Bradley J, Dzuba I, Agurto I. Factors affecting utilization of cervical cancer prevention services in low-resource settings. Salud Publica Mex. 2003;45:408–16.

4. Herdman C, Sherris J. Planning appropriate cervical cancer prevention programs. 2013. http://screening.iarc.fr/doc/cxca-planning-appro-prog-guide.pdf. Accessed 10 Jun 2013.

5. Global Health Group. Integrating cervical cancer screening into HIV services in sub-Saharan Africa: policy brief. 2012. http://www.globalhealthsciences.ucsf.edu. Accessed 21 Jan 2014.

6. Swaddiwudhipong W, Chaovakiratipong C, Nguntra P, Mahasakpan P, Lerdlukanavonge P, Koonchote S. Effect of a mobile unit on changes in knowledge and use of cervical cancer screening among rural Thai women. Int J Epidemiol. 1995;24(3):493–8.

7. Atashili J, Smith JS, Adimora AA, Eron J, Miller WC, Myers E. Potential impact of antiretroviral therapy and screening on cervical cancer mortality in HIV-positive women in sub-Saharan Africa: a simulation. PLoS One. 2011;6(4):e18527.

8. Ghebre RG, Grover S, Xu MJ, Chuang LT, Simonds H. Cervical cancer control in HIV-infected women: past, present and future. Gynecologic oncology reports. 2017;21:101–8.

9. Bonnet F, Lewden C, May T, Heripret L, Jougla E, Bevilacqua S, Costagliola D, Salmon D, Chêne G, Morlat P. Malignancy-related causes of death in human immunodeficiency virus–infected patients in the era of highly active antiretroviral therapy. Cancer. 2004;101(2):317–24.

10. Chen HY, Kessler CL, Mori N, Chauhan SP. Cervical cancer screening in the United States, 1993–2010: characteristics of women who are never screened. J Women's Health. 2012;21(11):1132–8.

11. Elit L, Krzyzanowska M, Saskin R, Barbera L, Razzaq A, Lofters A, Yeritsyan N, Bierman A. Sociodemographic factors associated with cervical cancer screening and follow-up of abnormal results. Can Fam Physician. 2012;58(1):e22–31.

12. Kahesa C, Kjaer S, Mwaiselage J, Ngoma T, Tersbol B, Dartell M, Rasch V. Determinants of acceptance of cervical cancer screening in Dar es salaam, Tanzania. BMC Public Health. 2012;12(1):1093.

13. Khan S, Woolhead G. Perspectives on cervical cancer screening among educated Muslim women in Dubai (the UAE): a qualitative study. BMC Womens Health. 2015;15(1):90.

14. Modibbo FI, Dareng E, Bamisaye P, Jedy-Agba E, Adewole A, Oyeneyin L, Olaniyan O, Adebamowo C. Qualitative study of barriers to cervical cancer screening among Nigerian women. BMJ Open. 2016;6(1):e008533.

15. Moser K, Patnick J, Beral V. Inequalities in reported use of breast and cervical screening in great Britain: analysis of cross sectional survey data. BMJ. 2009;338:b2025.

16. Nene B, Jayant K, Arrossi S, Shastri S, Budukh A, Hingmire S, Muwonge R, Malvi S, Dinshaw K, Sankaranarayanan R. Determinants of women s participation in cervical cancer screening trial, Maharashtra. India Bull World Health Organ. 2007;85(4):264–72.

17. Park MJ, Park EC, Choi KS, Jun JK, Lee HY. Sociodemographic gradients in breast and cervical cancer screening in Korea: the Korean National Cancer Screening Survey (KNCSS) 2005-2009. BMC Cancer. 2011;11(1):257.

18. William M, Kuffour G, Ekuadzi E, Yeboah M, ElDuah M, Tuffour P. Assessment of psychological barriers to cervical cancer screening among women in Kumasi, Ghana using a mixed methods approach. Afr Health Sci. 2013;13(4):1054–61.

19. Glanz K, Rimer BK, Viswanath K, eds. Health behavior and health education: theory, research, and practice. Wiley. 2008.

20. Abotchie PN, Shokar NK. Cervical cancer screening among college students in Ghana: knowledge and health beliefs. Int J Gynecol Cancer: official journal of the International Gynecological Cancer Society. 2009;19(3):412.

21. Adanu RM. Cervical cancer knowledge and screening in Accra, Ghana. J Womens Health Gend Based Med. 2002;11(6):487–8.

22. Ebu NI, Mupepi SC, Siakwa MP, Sampselle CM. Knowledge, practice, and barriers toward cervical cancer screening in Elmina, southern Ghana. Int J Womens Health. 2015;7:31.

23. National Aids Ccontrol Programme/Ghana Health Service/Ministry of Health. HIV sentinel survey report 2010. Accra: Author; 2017.

24. Ghana Health Service. Central regional health directorate: half year review report. Cape Coast: Author; 2015.

25. Ogah JK. Decision making in the research process: companion to students and beginning researchers. Accra: Adwinsa Publications (Gh) Limited; 2013.

26. Mupepi SC, Sampselle CM, Johnson TR. Knowledge, attitudes, and demographic factors influencing cervical cancer screening behavior of Zimbabwean women. J Women's Health. 2011;20(6):943–52.

27. Baskaran P, Subramanian P, Rahman RA, Ping WL, Taib NA, Rosli R. Perceived susceptibility, and cervical cancer screening benefits and barriers in Malaysian women visiting outpatient clinics. Asian Pac J Cancer Prev. 2013;14(12):7693–9.

28. Ezechi OC, Gab-Okafor CV, Ostergren PO, Pettersson KO. Willingness and acceptability of cervical cancer screening among HIV positive Nigerian women. BMC Public Health. 2013;13(1):46.

29. Sichanh C, Fabrice QU, Chanthavilay P, Diendere J, Latthaphasavang V, Longuet C, Buisson Y. Knowledge, awareness and attitudes about cervical cancer among women attending or not an HIV treatment center in Lao PDR. BMC Cancer. 2014;14(1):161.

30. Sudenga SL, Rositch AF, Otieno WA, Smith JS. Brief report: knowledge, attitudes, practices and perceived risk of cervical cancer among Kenyan women. Int J Gynecol Cancer: official journal of the International Gynecological Cancer Society. 2013;23(5):895.

31. Frank D, Swedmark J, Grubbs L. Colon Cancer screening in African American women. ABNF J. 2004;15(4):67.

32. Simou E, Maniadakis N, Pallis A, Foundoulakis E, Kourlaba G. Factors associated with the use of pap smear testing in Greece. J Women's Health. 2010;19(8):1577–85.

33. Gerald EI, Ogwuche CH. Educational level, sex and church affiliation on health seeking behaviour among parishioners in Makurdi metropolis of Benue state. Infect Dis Rep. 2014;1(2):311–6.

34. Lee M, Park EC, Chang HS, Kwon JA, Yoo KB, Kim TH. Socioeconomic disparity in cervical cancer screening among Korean women: 1998–2010. BMC Public Health. 2013;13(1):553.

35. Lyimo FS, Beran TN. Demographic, knowledge, attitudinal, and accessibility factors associated with uptake of cervical cancer screening among women in a rural district of Tanzania: three public policy implications. BMC Public Health. 2012;12(1):22.

36. Thomas D. How to reduce maternal deaths: rights and responsibilities. London: Department for International Development; 2005.

37. Ogunwale AN, Coleman MA, Sangi-Haghpeykar H, Valverde I, Montealegre J, Jibaja-Weiss M, Anderson ML. Assessment of factors impacting cervical cancer screening among low-income women living with HIV-AIDS. AIDS Care. 2016;28(4):491–4.

38. Abeliwine, E. Poverty means woman in Ghana. 2007. http://www.ibiswestafrica.com. Accessed 11 Jan 2016.

39. Abiodun OA, Olu-Abiodun OO, Sotunsa JO, Oluwole FA. Impact of health education intervention on knowledge and perception of cervical cancer and cervical screening uptake among adult women in rural communities in Nigeria. BMC Public Health. 2014;14(1):814.

40. Mandle E. Health promotion throughout the lifespan. 5th ed. New York: Mosby; 2002.

41. Matejic B, Vukovic D, Pekmezovic T, Kesic V, Markovic M. Determinants of preventive health behavior in relation to cervical cancer screening among the female population of Belgrade. Health Educ Res. 2011;26(2):201–11.

42. Hoque M, Hoque E, Kader SB. Evaluation of cervical cancer screening program at a rural community of South Africa. East Afr J Public Health. 2008;5(2):111–6.

43. Ezem BU. Awareness and uptake of cervical cancer screening in Owerri, south-eastern Nigeria. Ann Afr Med. 2007;6(3):94.

44. Ndikom CM, Ofi BA. Awareness, perception and factors affecting utilization of cervical cancer screening services among women in Ibadan, Nigeria: a qualitative study. Reprod Health. 2012;9(1):11.

45. Oche MO, Kaoje AU, Gana G, Ango JT. Cancer of the cervix and cervical screening: current knowledge, attitude and practices of female health workers in Sokoto, Nigeria. Niger Postgrad Med J. 2013;5(4):184–90.

46. Were E, Nyaberi Z, Buziba N. Perceptions of risk and barriers to cervical cancer screening at Moi teaching and referral hospital (MTRH), Eldoret, Kenya. Afr Health Sci. 2011;11(1):58–64.

47. Ardayfio-Schandorf E. Violence against women: the Ghanaian case. http://

citeseerx.ist.psu.edu/viewdoc/download? doi= 10.1.1.564.3095&re
=rep1&type=pdf. 2005. Accessed 18 Dec 2016.

48. Akinyemiju TF, McDonald JA, Lantz PM. Health care access dimensions and
     cervical cancer screening in South Africa: analysis of the world health
     survey. BMC Public Health. 2015;15(1):382.

49. Amu NJ. The role of women in Ghana's economy. Ghana: Friederich Ebert
     Foundation; 2005. http://library.fes.de/pdf-files/bueros/ghana/02990.pdf.
     Accessed 18 Dec 2016

50. Beining RM. Screening for cervical cancer—an exploratory study of urban
     women in Tamil Nadu. India: The University of Iowa; 2012.

51. Eze JN, Umeora OU, Obuna JA, Egwuatu VE, Ejikeme BN. Cervical cancer
     awareness and cervical screening uptake at the mater Misericordiae
     hospital, Afikpo, Southeast Nigeria. Ann Afr Med. 2012;11(4):238.

52. Sutton S, Rutherford C. Sociodemographic and attitudinal correlates of
     cervical screening uptake in a national sample of women in Britain. Soc Sci
     Med. 2005;61(11):2460–5.

53. Thippeveeranna C, Mohan SS, Singh I.R, Singh NN. Knowledge, attitude and
     practice of the pap smear as a screening procedure among nurses in a tertiary
     hospital in north eastern India. Asian Pac J Cancer Prev. 2013;14(2):849–52.

54. Kuroki H. Survey on the trends in uterine cervical cancer screening in
     Japanese women: the efficacy of free coupons in the screening. J Obstet
     Gynaecol Res. 2012;38(1):35–9.

55. Fort VK, Makin MS, Siegler AJ, Ault K, Rochat R. Barriers to cervical cancer
     screening in Mulanje, Malawi: a qualitative study. Patient Prefer Adherence.
     2011;5:125.

56. Ghana Statistical Service. Population and housing census: summary report
     of final results. 2012. http://www.statsghana.gov.gh/docfiles/2010phc/
     Census2010_Summary_report_of_final_results.pdf. Accessed 17 Jan 2016.

19

Therapeutic options for treatment of human papillomavirus-associated cancers -novel immunologic vaccines: ADXS11–001

Brett Miles[1], Howard P. Safran[2] and Bradley J. Monk[3*]

Abstract

Survival of patients with advanced, recurrent, or metastatic human papillomavirus (HPV)-associated cancer is suboptimal despite the availability of various treatment modalities. The recently developed bacterial vector *Listeria monocytogenes* (*Lm*) activates innate and adaptive immune responses and is expected to offer immunologic advantages. Axalimogene filolisbac (AXAL or ADXS11–001) is a novel immunotherapeutic based on the live, irreversibly attenuated *Lm* fused to the nonhemolytic fragment of listeriolysin O (*Lm*-LLO) and secretes the *Lm*-LLO-HPV E7 fusion protein targeting HPV-positive tumors. Herein are reported the development and recent results of various clinical trials in patients with HPV-associated cervical, head and neck, and anal cancers.

Keywords: ADXS11–001, AXAL, Human papillomavirus, HPV-positive cancers, Clinical trials

Introduction

Persistent human papillomavirus (HPV) infection is currently acknowledged as a direct cause of cervical, anogenital, and oropharyngeal cancers [1], and has been estimated to account for more than 5% of all cancers globally [2]. More than half of all cancers attributable to infection worldwide are caused by HPV (Table 1) [3]. Moreover, cervical cancer was the first type of cancer officially recognized by the World Health Organization to be attributable to a viral infection.

This review aims to describe current therapeutic options for HPV-associated cancers, with an emphasis on therapeutic cancer vaccines currently being tested in clinical trials, and a particular focus on describing the efficacy and safety of the novel immunogenic compound axalimogene filolisbac (AXAL or ADXS11–001) in patients with HPV-positive cervical, head and neck, and anal cancers.

Immunobiology of HPV

HPV belongs to a family of papillomaviruses that are composed of non-enveloped, double-stranded deoxyribonucleic acid (DNA) viruses able to infect the multilayer stratified tissue (eg, human epithelium). HPV is a sexually transmitted, circular virus encoding for 7 early (E1, E2, E4, E5, E6, E7, and E8) and 2 late, structural (L1 and L2) genes [4]. In cervical cancer, upon sexual transmission, HPV infects the basal epithelial cells of the cervical mucosa, leading to intracellular expression of low levels of viral proteins [5]. Viral DNA replicates following infection, and production of viral proteins is enhanced once HPV-infected cells leave the basal layer [6]. Chronic infection is maintained in approximately 10% of women because of the capacity of HPV to escape host immune surveillance [7]. The molecular mechanism accounting for persistent HPV infection and carcinogenesis involves the integration of viral DNA into the host genome, accompanied by deletion of both early and late HPV genes, namely E2, E4, E5, L1, and L2. The oncogenic potential of HPV is a result of two early viral proteins, E6 and E7. As a result of loss of the transcriptional regulator gene E2, these two oncoproteins are upregulated. The early viral protein E6 binds to the tumor suppressor gene p53, thereby inhibiting apoptosis of HPV-infected cells [8, 9]. The early viral protein E7 inhibits

* Correspondence: bradley.monk@usoncology.com
[3]Division of Gynecologic Oncology, Arizona Oncology (US Oncology Network), University of Arizona College of Medicine, Creighton University School of Medicine at St. Joseph's Hospital, 2222 E. Highland Ave, Suite 400, Phoenix, AZ 85016, USA
Full list of author information is available at the end of the article

Table 1 Estimated number of HPV-attributable new cancer cases, by anatomic site and gender

Cancer site	Number of new cases	Number of cases attributable to HPV	Attributable fraction, %	Number of cases attributable to HPV by gender	
				Male	Female
Cervix uteri	528,000	501,600	95	-	528,000
Anus	40,000	35,000	88	17,000	18,000
Vagina and vulva	49,000	20,000	41	-	20,000
Penis	26,000	13,000	51	13,000	-
Oropharynx	96,000	29,000	31	24,000	6000
Oral cavity and larynx	358,000	16,000	4.4	12,000	4000
Total	1 096000	641,000	58	66,000	575,000

HPV human papillomavirus

functionality of the tumor suppressor retinoblastoma product, thus allowing HPV to replicate in previously differentiated epithelial cells [9, 10]. Formation of complexes between these two viral proteins and the aforementioned tumor suppressor genes disturbs the normal cycle of cell regulation, causes genomic instability, and ultimately leads to neoplasia. A similar biomolecular process is the basis for development of other HPV-associated cancers.

HPV-associated cancers and current therapies
HPV-associated cancers and prevention of HPV infections
More than 100 HPV types have been identified to date [11]. Of these, the most frequently encountered high-risk HPV types, 16, 18, 31, and 45, are together responsible for approximately 80% of all cervical cancer cases [12–14]. HPV-16 and -18 have been identified as the two most prevalent high-risk HPV types and are accountable for approximately 62.6 and 15.7%, respectively, of cervical cancers [15]. Additionally, these two high-risk HPV types are responsible for 80–86% of vulvar and vaginal cancers, 89–95% of oropharyngeal cancers, 93% of anal cancers, and 63–80% of penile cancers [16].

Two prophylactic vaccines have been developed for prevention of HPV infection: Gardasil® (Merck and Co., Inc.), and Cervarix® (GlaxoSmithKline Biologicals). The quadrivalent vaccine Gardasil provides immunologic protection against infection with HPV-6, –11, –16, and –18 [17], whereas the bivalent vaccine Cervarix provides protection against infection with HPV-16 and -18 [18]. In addition, the nonavalent vaccine Gardasil 9 (Merck and Co., Inc.) has been demonstrated to protect against HPV-6, –11, –16, –18, –31, –33, –45, –52, and –58 [19]. However, despite recent advancements within the field of tumor immunology, no therapeutic vaccines for the treatment of HPV-associated cancers are currently available for general use in the clinical setting.

Current therapeutic options for HPV-associated cancers
Cervical and vulvar cancers
Pre-invasive genital tract neoplasia includes cervical intraepithelial neoplasia (CIN), vaginal neoplasia, and vulvar intraepithelial neoplasia (VIN). Current treatment strategies for CIN include minimally invasive therapies, such as loop electrosurgical excision procedure or cryotherapy [20]. These strategies focus on eliminating the HPV-positive precancerous cells, while maintaining cervical integrity and fertility [21].

The estimated number of new cervical cancer cases raises to 528,000 each year [3], with 95% cases attributable to HPV [22], while from the 49,000 new cases of vulvar and vaginal cancers estimated, 41% were attributable to HPV [3]. Chances of survival are high when cervical cancer is identified at early stages. (International Federation of Gynecology and Obstetrics [FIGO] stages IA2–IB1). Treatment consists of conization, radical hysterectomy (preferred), radical trachelectomy (for selected patients), or radiation therapy. Locally advanced tumors are generally treated with concomitant chemoradiotherapy that includes a cisplatin-based regimen [23]. Patients with persistent, recurrent, or metastatic cervical cancer have poor survival and increased morbidity caused by renal failure and clinical deterioration. For these patients, the standard of care consists of platinum-based chemotherapy doublets, such as cisplatin and paclitaxel [24, 25], usually administered in combination with the humanized monoclonal antibody directed against vascular endothelial growth factor (bevacizumab) [26]. The main treatment modalities of vulvar cancer consist of surgery, for localized disease, or a combination of surgery and radiation (with or without chemotherapy) when nodal metastases are present [27, 28]. For patients presenting with vaginal cancers, three types of standard treatment are generally used: surgery (e.g., laser surgery, wide local excision, vaginectomy, total hysterectomy), external or internal radiation therapy [29], and systemic or regional chemotherapy [30].

Head and neck cancers

High-risk oncogenic HPVs represent major risk factors for development of head and neck cancers [31]. These are primarily tumors of the oropharynx, specifically the tonsil and base of tongue. An estimated 96,000 new cases of cancer of the oropharynx was recently reported, out of which 29,000 were attributable to HPV [3]. In the United States it has recently been approximated that HPV-related head and neck cancers incidence is likely to surpass that of cervical cancers by the year 2020 [32]. The primary viral etiology of these cancers is HPV-16; however, up to 9% may be caused by additional serotypes (e.g., HPV-35, HPV-18) [33]. Despite increasing awareness and improved viral detection methods, identification of active disease remains problematic [34]. Patients with early stage disease can be treated with single-modality therapy. Minimally invasive transoral robotic surgery is also being investigated [35]. The most commonly employed therapies for locally advanced head and neck cancers include cisplatin and concurrent radiation. Concurrent epidermal growth factor receptor antibody and radiation is an alternative. More recent treatments for patients with head and neck cancers include targeted therapies, such as the anti-programmed death protein 1 (PD-1) monoclonal antibody nivolumab. In a phase II trial performed in patients with recurrent or metastatic squamous cell carcinoma of the head and neck, the overall survival (OS) of patients treated with nivolumab was higher than OS following standard platinum chemotherapy (7.5 vs 5.1 months). The 6-month progression-free survival (PFS) rate and the response rate of patients treated with nivolumab were also higher than in patients receiving standard therapy (19.7% vs 9.9% and 13.3% vs 5.8%), while the occurrence of grade 3 or 4 treatment-related adverse events (TRAEs) was lower following nivolumab treatment (13.1% vs 35.1%) [36]. This proof-of-concept phase II trial not only demonstrated the superior efficacy of nivolumab in patients with recurrent or metastatic squamous cell carcinoma of the head and neck, but also underlined the superior safety profile of nivolumab in this patient population.

Anal and penile cancers

Annually, 24,000 anal and 11,000 penile cancer cases are reported worldwide, with approximately 21,000 and 6500 cases, respectively, associated with HPV [1]. In 2012, these numbers increased to 40,000 for anal cancer and 26,000 for penile cancer, out of which 35,000 and 26,000 respectively, were reported as attributable to HPV [3]. Anal intraepithelial neoplasia (AIN) is generally treated with minimally invasive methods, such as laser ablation or infrared coagulation [37]; excision is reserved for high-grade AIN cases. The standard of treatment for localized anal cancer is concurrent chemoradiotherapy, consisting of concurrent radiation, mitomycin C, and 5-fluorouracil [38, 39]. Metastatic anal cancer is not curable. While there is no standard-of-care chemotherapy, options can include platinum analogues, taxanes, or antimetabolites. The best options for localized penile cancer consist of surgical treatments (e.g., excision, microsurgery, laser surgery, circumcision) and radiation, used as an adjuvant to surgery. Current treatment options for recurrent or metastatic penile cancer includes taxanes, platinum analogues, and ifosfamide. [40, 41].

Despite the various treatment modalities currently available, survival of patients presenting with one of the aforementioned advanced, recurrent, or metastatic HPV-associated cancers remains poor.

Therapeutic HPV vaccines

In patients with HPV-associated cancers, the standard functionality of the innate and adaptive immune systems is altered and tolerance or suppression mechanisms develop, capable of blocking or reversing antitumor immune responses [42, 43]. Tolerance mechanisms interfere with various steps of the antigen-presentation process as well as with the antitumoral activity of cluster of differentiation (CD)4-positive and CD8-positive T cells, thus rendering them nonfunctional. Immune suppression mechanisms include development of suppressive immune cell populations (e.g., regulatory T cells [Tregs], myeloid-derived suppressor cells [MDSCs], tumor-associated macrophages) with protumoral activity. Overall, HPV-induced diseases are associated with a lack of HPV-specific antitumoral immune responses and an excess of immune-suppressive cellular and humoral protumoral responses. Therefore, the main goal of therapeutic vaccines is to induce or greatly improve HPV-specific T-cell based immunity by making use of the constitutively expressed tumor-specific antigens E6 and E7.

Because of their reported efficacy, protein- and peptide-based vaccines are the most common forms of therapeutic HPV vaccines. Their mechanisms of action involve uptake of the peptide antigen and major histocompatibility complex molecules by dendritic cells, and cross-presentation to CD8-positive T cells (Fig. 1). A phase I study performed in patients with end-stage cervical cancer vaccinated with HPV-16 E6, alone or in combination with HPV-16 E7 overlapping long peptides, reported good vaccine tolerability and broad T-cell responses [44]. Several fusion protein-based vaccine formulations containing the oncogene E7 of the high-risk type HPV-16 have been tested in clinical trials in patients with high-grade AIN [45] or CIN [46, 47], as well as in patients with cervical cancer [48], and have demonstrated varying degrees of efficacy.

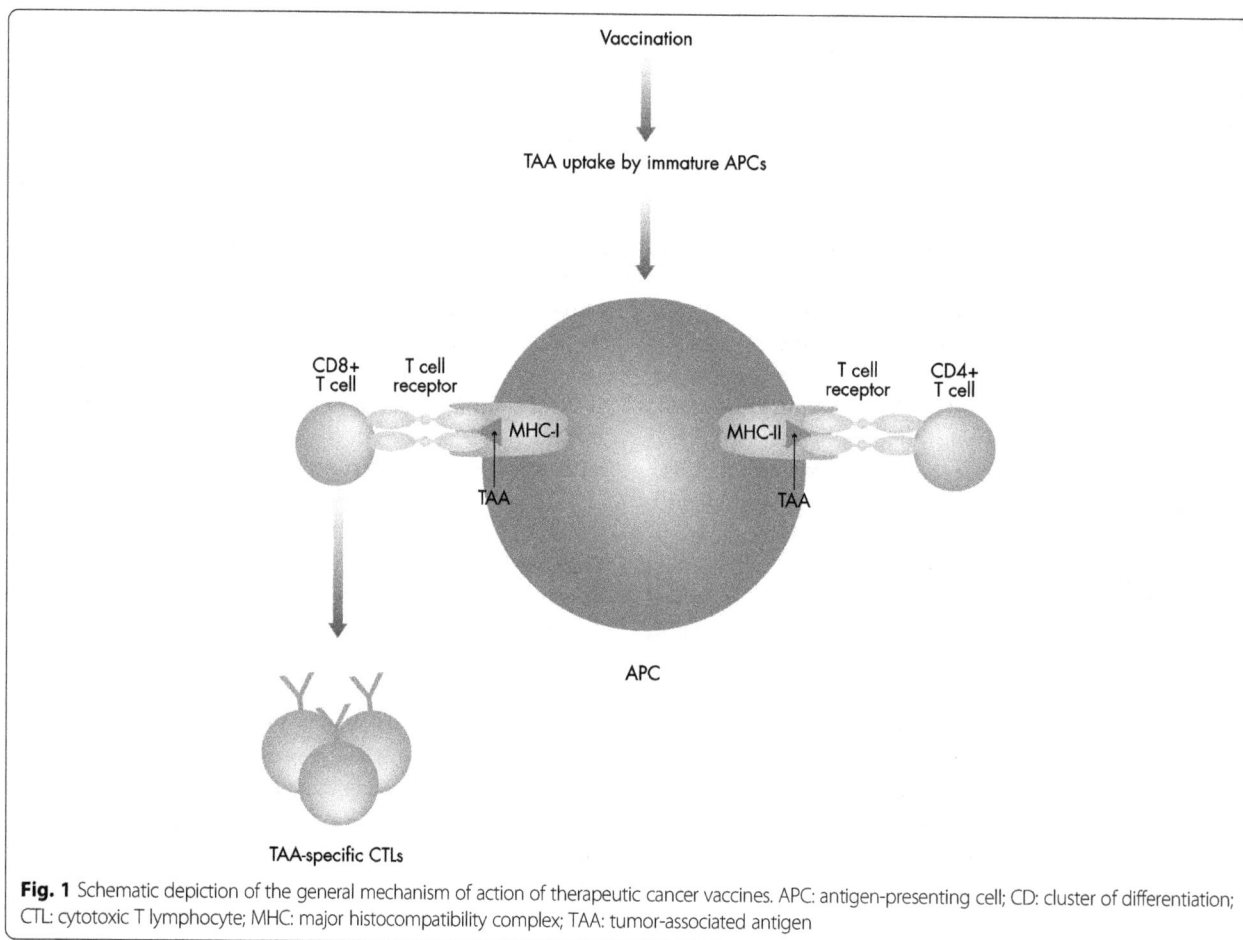

Fig. 1 Schematic depiction of the general mechanism of action of therapeutic cancer vaccines. APC: antigen-presenting cell; CD: cluster of differentiation; CTL: cytotoxic T lymphocyte; MHC: major histocompatibility complex; TAA: tumor-associated antigen

Nucleic acid and whole cell vaccines represent other potential immunotherapeutic strategies tested in clinical trials. A DNA vaccine containing E7 DNA fused with the heat shock protein 70 tested in patients with CIN grade 2/3 was reported to be safe, but induced only low-frequency E7-specific T-cell responses [49]. Similarly, autologous dendritic cells pulsed with HPV-16 or HPV-18 E7 recombinant proteins in patients with stage IB–IIA cervical cancer [50] or patients with late-stage disease [51] led to antigen-specific serologic responses of varying degrees; however, there was no sustained limitation on tumor burden. All of the aforementioned vaccine formulations were well tolerated and induced antigen-specific cell-mediated immunity to varying degrees. However, the rates of lesion regression observed within these studies were lower than 50%, with no direct correlation between clinical and immunologic responses reported. Recently, a phase II clinical trial was performed in patients with metastatic cervical cancer previously treated with chemotherapy or chemoradiotherapy. Following lymphocyte-depleting chemotherapy, patients received a single infusion of tumor-infiltrating T cells selected for HPV E6 and E7

reactivity. Objective tumor responses were observed in three of the nine patients enrolled: one patient presented with a three-month partial response, and two patients presented with complete responses that were ongoing at 22 and 15 months after treatment, respectively. This proof-of-concept study demonstrated durable, complete regression of metastatic cervical cancer following a single infusion of HPV-specific tumor-infiltrating T cells [52].

Another promising option for therapeutic vaccination is bacterial or viral vector-based vaccines (e.g., sindbis virus, equine encephalitis virus, or adenovirus). Thus far, the efficacy of some viral vector vaccines has been reported in preclinical models, while others have been tested in clinical trials. A recombinant vaccinia virus expressing the E2 protein of HPV-16 or HPV-18 led to complete lesion regression in CIN grade 2/3 patients [53], whereas a vaccine expressing a fusion protein of E6 and E7 caused therapeutic effects in patients with VIN in phase I/II clinical trials [54].

Nevertheless, survival outcomes of patients with HPV-associated cancers treated with the aforementioned vaccine combinations need to be greatly enhanced.

Axalimogene filolisbac (AXAL or ADXS11–001)

The bacterial vector most commonly used as an immunotherapeutic vaccine base is *Listeria monocytogenes* (*Lm*), because of its immunologic advantages. *Lm* is a gram-positive intracellular bacterium capable of escaping from the host cell phagosomes into the cytoplasm, thereby infecting host cells. Following infection of host cells, *Lm* has the ability to activate both the innate (neutrophils and macrophages) [55] and adaptive (CD4-positive and CD8-positive T cells) [56] immune responses. In cancer immunotherapy, *Lm* has been successfully used as a delivery vector for tumor-specific antigens.

Lm-listeriolysin O (LLO) immunotherapies have been reported to present with multiple simultaneous mechanisms of action that contribute to generation of a therapeutic response, enabled by their capacity to efficiently stimulate both innate and adaptive immune responses [57]. Upon administration, *Lm*-LLO immunotherapies have been shown to infect antigen-presenting cells, thereby initiating the process of antigen cross-presentation. This effect propagates to both arms of the adaptive immune system, leading to generation of activated CD4-positive and CD8-positive T cells. Additionally, *Lm*-LLO immunotherapies selectively reduce levels of intratumoral, but not splenic, Tregs and MDSCs, and present the capacity to induce maturation of immune cells to fully differentiated effector cells devoid of protumoral activity. Other advantages of *Lm*-LLO immunotherapies are their lack of induction of neutralizing antibodies and their capacity to facilitate chemotaxis of activated immune cells. Interestingly, *Lm*-LLO immunotherapies also stimulate robust immune memory responses; correlates of immune memory to *Lm* have been reported to develop just 5 h after exposure [58]. In various models, *Lm*-LLO immunotherapies have been shown to also induce therapeutic changes in the ratio of CD8-positive tumor-infiltrating lymphocytes to Tregs [59].

Because of the aforementioned promising results, one such *Lm*-LLO immunotherapy was used for development of AXAL, a novel immunotherapeutic agent for treatment of cervical cancer and other HPV-associated diseases. AXAL is based on the live, irreversibly attenuated *Lm* fused to the nonhemolytic fragment of LLO, and has been developed to secrete the *Lm*-LLO-E7 fusion protein targeting HPV-positive tumors [60]. AXAL is also bioengineered to be deficient of virulence-related transcription factors, such as peptide-chain release factor A [61, 62], induces antitumor T-cell immunity, and reduces tumor immune tolerance.

AXAL in clinical trials

Presently, AXAL is being evaluated in several clinical trials of patients with various HPV-associated tumors (Table 2) [61, 63–71]. Thus far, AXAL has most extensively been evaluated in cervical cancer, with various recently finalized or currently ongoing clinical trials having enrolled patients with cervical cancer at different stages.

AXAL in patients with cervical cancer

In 2009, Maciag et al. [61] published the first phase I clinical trial of AXAL, in which safety and efficacy were assessed in 15 patients with advanced cervical cancer whose disease presented no improvements following traditional therapies. Women with a history of listeriosis were excluded from this study. Doses of AXAL escalating from 1×10^9 colony-forming units (CFU) to 3.3×10^9 CFU and then 1×10^{10} CFU were administered to groups of five patients every 21 days for a total of two intravenous doses. Patients also received prophylactic antibiotics. Dose-limiting toxicity was achieved at the highest dose of 1×10^{10} CFU, with three of five patients developing hemodynamic instability and subsequently treated with medical interventions. All 15 patients reported at least one AE, as classified by the Common Terminology Criteria for Adverse Events version 3.0 [72]. The most common AEs reported by more than 50% of patients during the study were pyrexia (100%), vomiting (60%), musculoskeletal pain (57%), and chills, headache, and anemia (53%). Blood, urine, and feces analyses revealed the transient presence of *Lm*-LLO-E7 in only one patient receiving 1×10^9 CFU. Within the follow-up period of the study, two deaths were recorded. One death was caused by disease progression, while the second occurred in the setting of renal failure, followed by metabolic acidosis and cardiac arrest. Both were deemed unrelated to AXAL [61]. Overall, the results of this study showed an acceptable safety profile for AXAL at the dose of 1×10^9 CFU.

Considering the acceptable safety profile of AXAL observed in the study of Maciag et al., a single-arm, two-stage, phase II clinical trial is being conducted in patients with squamous or nonsquamous persistent, recurrent, metastatic cervical cancer that has progressed after systemic chemotherapy. In a Gynecologic Oncology Group (GOG) study, a total of 67 patients was estimated for enrolment at study initiation, with a target of 27 patients enrolled in the first study stage [63] (Table 2) [61, 63–71]. Eligible patients are 18 years of age or older, have a GOG performance status of 0 or 1, have measurable disease (Response Evaluation Criteria in Solid Tumors [RECIST] version 1.1), and have received one or more prior lines of systemic-dose chemotherapy (bevacizumab permitted) for squamous or non-squamous persistent or recurrent metastatic cervical cancer not amenable to curative therapy. In this study, AXAL safety and tolerability, as well as 12-month OS rates, were evaluated following administration of three doses of AXAL at

Table 2 Overview of AXAL in clinical studies (safety and efficacy)

Cancer type	Cancer stage	Investigator	Study phase (stage; NCT)	Mono–/Multi-therapy	Dosing regimen	Estimated enrollment	Efficacy	Safety (most frequent AEs)
Cervical cancer	Advanced	Maciag PC	I (60)	AXAL alone	Dose escalation: 1 × 10^9 CFU, 3.3 × 10^9 CFU, 1 × 10^{10} CFU	15	• Possible PR: 1 patient • SD: 7 patients • Progression of disease: 5 patients	• Pyrexia (100%) • Vomiting (60%) • Musculoskeletal pain (57%) • Chills; headache and anemia (53%) • Nausea and tachycardia (47%) DLT = 1 × 10^{10} CFU
	Persistent/recurrent/metastatic	GOG (Huh WK)	II (stage 1; NCT01266460) (62)	AXAL alone	1 × 10^9 CFU	67	• 12-month OS: 38.5% • Median PFS: 3.1 mo • Median OS: 7.7 mo • PR: 1 patient • SD: 9 patients	Drug-related AEs (38% of all AEs) • Vomiting • Chills • Fatigue • Fever
	Persistent/recurrent/metastatic	Ghamande SA	I–II (TiP; NCT02164461) (63)	AXAL alone	Dose escalation: 5 × 10^9 CFU, 1 × 10^{10} CFU	25	Pending	Treatment-related AEs (>3 patients) • Chills • Vomiting • Hypotension • Tachycardia • Fever • Nausea
	Recurrent/refractory	Petit R	II (CTRI/2010/091/001232) (64)	AXAL ± cisplatin	1 × 10^9 CFU + 40 mg/m^2	110	• 12-mo OS: 36% • 18-mo survival: 28% • Response rate: 11% (6 CRs; 6 PRs) • SD: 35 patients	• 79% of AEs: mild or moderate and unrelated to study drug
	High-risk locally advanced	GOG (Herzog TJ)	III (TiP; NCT02853604) (65)	AXAL alone	1 × 10^9 CFU	450	Pending	Pending
Head and neck cancer	Persistent/recurrent/metastatic	Cohen EW	I/II (TiP; NCT02291055) (66)	AXAL ± MEDI4736	Phase I: 1 × 10^9 CFU + 3 mg/kg (3 + 3 design for MEDI4736 dose escalation) Phase II: 1 × 10^9 CFU + 10 mg/kg	66	Pending	Pending
	Previously untreated, surgically resectable, stage II–IV patients (oropharyngeal cancer)	Miles B and Sikora A	II (NCT02002182) (67)	AXAL + transoral robotic surgery	1 × 10^9 CFU	30 (present time: 8/9 vaccinated patients; 10 observational group patients)	• Increased Ag-specific IFN-γ (5/8) or TNF-α (7/8) responses at 3/5 time points (other 2 time points pending) • Intratumoral expression of CD8 (4/8), PD-1 (6/8)	Pending

Table 2 Overview of AXAL in clinical studies (safety and efficacy) (Continued)

Oropharyngeal cancer	Jones TM	I (NCT01598792) (68)	AXAL alone	Dose escalation • 3.3 × 10^8 CFU • 1 × 10^9 CFU • 3.3 × 10^9 CFU	36	Pending	Pending	Pending
Anal cancer	Locally advanced	Safran H	I/II (TiP; NCT01671488) (69)	AXAL ± chemo-radiation (mitomycin, 5-fluorouracil, IMRT)	1 × 10^9 CFU	25	Pending	Pending
	Persistent/recurrent, locoregional/metastatic anorectal canal	Fakih M	II (stage 2 TiP; NCT02399813) (70)	AXAL alone	1 × 10^9 CFU	Stage 1 • 31 patients Stage 2 • 24 patients	Pending	Pending

Ag antigen, BID bi-daily, CR complete response, CTRI Clinical Trials Registry – India, DLT dose-limiting toxicity, IMRT intensity-modulated radiation therapy, NCT National Clinical Trial, PR partial response, SAE serious adverse event, TiP trial in progress

1×10^9 CFU every 28 days. Secondary endpoints were PFS, OS, and objective response (OR). To prevent development of the most common AEs reported in the study by Maciag et al., nonsteroidal anti-inflammatory agents were administered prophylactically. In total, 26 of the 29 patients who were enrolled in stage 1 received treatment. Safety analyses indicated that all treated patients experienced at least one AE: 91% were grade 1–2, and 38% were drug related, with nausea, vomiting, chills, fatigue, and fever the most common. The 38.5% (10 patients) 12-month OS rate observed in stage 1 of the study suggests that AXAL is an active agent with a net survival benefit for patients with squamous or nonsquamous persistent or recurrent metastatic cervical cancer. Median PFS was 3.1 months and median OS was 7.7 months. Preliminary evaluation of OR showed that one patient presented with unconfirmed partial response and nine patients presented with stable disease. Post-hoc efficacy analysis of the 18 patients who received all three per-protocol doses of AXAL showed a median OS longer than 1 year, and a 12-months OS rate of 55.6%, thus confirming the survival benefit offered by AXAL.

Another phase I, open-label, dose-escalation clinical trial being performed in patients with persistent, recurrent, or metastatic cervical squamous carcinoma or adenocarcinoma aims to evaluate the safety and tolerability of higher doses of AXAL, as well as tumor response, PFS, and correlative immunologic parameters [64] (Table 2) [61, 63–71]. Patients enrolled in this study had measurable disease (RECIST version 1.1) with documented disease progression on or intolerance to prior therapy, and had an Eastern Cooperative Oncology Group (ECOG) performance status of 0 or 1. Overall, 10 of 25 patients were enrolled, and nine of 10 patients were treated with AXAL every 3 weeks during a 12-week treatment cycle (six patients received 5×10^9 CFU and three patients received 1×10^{10} CFU). The primary endpoint of this study was AXAL safety and tolerability, with the recommended phase II dose (RP2D) selected based on a dose-limiting toxicity rate lower than 33%. Secondary objectives included evaluation of tumor response and PFS. All treated patients experienced at minimum one AE, of which 75% were TRAEs (eight of nine patients): 99% were grade 1–2, and the most common TRAEs occurring in three or more patients were chills, vomiting, hypotension, tachycardia, fever, and nausea. Only one grade 3 (hypotension) and no grade 4–5 TRAEs were reported. Analysis of tumor response and PFS, as well as correlative immunologic studies, is ongoing to assess if treatment intensity has an impact on the antitumor activity of AXAL. Lastly, another phase III clinical trial of AXAL (AIM2CERV) administered as adjuvant immunotherapy in patients with

high-risk, locally advanced cervical cancer following chemoradiation was opened for recruitment in September 2016 [65] (Table 2) [61, 63–71].

Given the observed safety and efficacy of AXAL when administered alone in patients with cervical cancer, combinatorial therapies containing AXAL were also assessed in clinical trials. The efficacy and safety of AXAL, administered with or without cisplatin, was evaluated in a phase II trial performed in India that enrolled 110 patients with recurrent or progressive invasive cervical cancer unresponsive to primary therapy [65] (Table 2) [61, 63–71]. Eligible patients were 18 years of age or older, had documented recurrent or progressing invasive cervical cancer, presented with measurable disease with at least one target lesion, and had ECOG performance status 2 or lower. Patients were randomized to AXAL alone (one cycle of three doses at 1×10^9 CFU administered every 4 weeks) or AXAL plus cisplatin (one preliminary AXAL dose followed by five weekly cisplatin treatments at the dose of 40 mg/m^2, followed by one AXAL cycle). The primary endpoint was OS; secondary endpoints were OR rates, PFS, and safety. Among the 109 patients who received treatment, AXAL was well tolerated; 79% of AEs were mild or moderate and unrelated to study drug. OS was found to be similar between the two treatment arms (median OS AXAL: 8.40 months; AXAL with cisplatin: 8.77 months). Furthermore, 22% of the treated patients alive at more than 18 months following AXAL therapy were deemed long-term survivors. No significant differences between the OR rates, disease control rates, duration of response, or PFS were observed between the two treatment groups.

AXAL in patients with head and neck cancer

In addition to the clinical trials performed in patients with cervical cancer, AXAL is also being investigated in other types of HPV-positive cancers, such as head and neck and anorectal cancer. Three phase I/II clinical trials in patients with head and neck cancer and two phase I/II clinical trials in patients with anorectal cancer are currently ongoing. The phase I/II randomized two-stage study by Cohen et al. is being performed in patients with recurrent, HPV-positive squamous cell carcinoma of the head and neck or cervix [67] (Table 2) [61, 63–71]. In phase I of this study, safety and efficacy of 1×10^9 CFU of AXAL administered every 4 weeks in combination with the PD-1 inhibitor durvalumab (MEDI-4736), used at escalating doses (dose level 1: 3 mg/kg; dose level 2: 10 mg/kg) administered every 2 weeks, will be assessed, and the RP2D of the combination therapy will be determined in up to 18 patients. In phase II of the study, 48 patients will be randomized to receive AXAL (1×10^9 CFU), durvalumab, or both, at the pre-established RP2D. The study allows patients to receive treatment for up to 1 year or, alternatively, discontinue treatment due to disease progression or unacceptable toxicity, and is currently ongoing.

Another clinical study of AXAL in patients with previously untreated, surgically resectable, stage II–IV oropharyngeal cancer is the "window of opportunity" phase II, two-stage trial that was initiated in 2014 [68] (Table 2) [61, 63–71]. Patients received AXAL at 1×10^9 CFU (two doses over 5 weeks, on the first and fifteenth days of treatment, respectively), prior to standard-of-care transoral robotic surgery. Of the eight of nine enrolled patients who completed study treatment, five patients presented with increased peripheral blood antigen-specific interferon gamma (IFN-γ) or tumor necrosis factor alpha (TNF-α) responses before treatment, on the day of surgery, and 5 weeks postsurgery. Additionally, intratumoral increases in posttreatment expression of CD8-positive T cells and PD-1 were recorded in four of eight and six of eight patients, respectively. These results are promising, as they indicate that effects of AXAL are not limited to the generation of robust antitumoral immune responses, but are also extended to the tumor microenvironment. Another phase I clinical trial evaluating the safety of escalating AXAL doses (from 3.3×10^8 to 3.3×10^9 CFU) in oropharyngeal cancer is also in progress [63] (Table 2) [61, 63–71].

AXAL in patients with anal cancer

In view of the reported efficacy of AXAL in cervical cancer and available immune response data in head and neck cancers, clinical trials aiming to evaluate this immunotherapeutic compound in HPV-positive anal cancers have recently been initiated. The phase I/II study by Safran et al. aims to assess safety and efficacy of AXAL when combined with intensity-modulated radiation therapy, mitomycin, and 5-fluorouracil for treatment of patients with anal cancer [70] (Table 2) [61, 63–71]. The phase II, two-stage study by Fakih et al. aims to assess the efficacy and safety of AXAL monotherapy (administered intravenously at a dose of 1×10^9 CFU every 3 weeks during nine-week treatment cycles) in patients with persistent, recurrent, locoregional, or metastatic squamous cell cancer of the anus. [71] (Table 2) [10, 63–71]. Both of these trials are ongoing, and results are expected to be made available in 2017.

Advantages of treatment with AXAL and future perspectives

AXAL seems to embody the main characteristics of a successful HPV therapeutic vaccine for patients with various HPV-associated cancers, both in terms of efficacy (i.e., capacity to engage both innate and adaptive immunity by promoting inflammation and inducing high numbers of antigen-specific cytotoxic T lymphocytes) and safety (i.e., reported tolerability). Additional benefits include the ability of AXAL to dampen intratumoral immune tolerance by reducing numbers and functionality of Tregs and MDSCs, as well as reducing secretion of immunosuppressive cytokines (e.g., interleukin-10 and transforming growth factor beta), both features of an immune response that would ordinarily contribute to a protumor microenvironment. Another advantage of AXAL immunotherapy is exemplified by its delivery vector, *Lm*, an attenuated bacterial vector characterized by lack of virulence yet retaining its adjuvant properties. Moreover, given the conserved nature of the E7 early gene in HPV, AXAL is expected to be effective irrespective of the HPV serotype associated with individual cases, which is particularly important in heterogeneous patient populations such as those with head and neck cancer. A further advantageous aspect of AXAL therapy is its potential to provide long-term immune modulation, an aspect of treatment that is currently lacking. In the case of HPV-associated oropharyngeal squamous cell carcinomas, which are known to involve longer survival and later recurrence compared to other head and neck cancers [72], the use of AXAL to bolster the antitumor response in conjunction with disease surveillance is an exciting yet currently unexplored option for preventing late recurrence in this setting. Potentially, treatment with AXAL could have an immediate impact improving patients' perception of care, which is often negatively affected by delays in scheduling surgery or radiotherapy. The effective and safe administration of AXAL in the weeks prior to definitive treatment has been indicated to be plausible in the window of opportunity study [68]. Another study that may have significant bearing on future strategies for AXAL use is AIM2CERV, the randomized phase III study of AXAL use following chemoradiation in patients with high-risk, locally advanced cervical cancer [66] (Fig. 2). In this setting, there is a clear unmet need, as patients have a 50% probability of disease recurrence or death following cisplatin-based chemoradiation plus brachytherapy. AIM2CERV will evaluate disease-free and OS as its endpoints; study enrollment is currently ongoing. Based on the studies described above and the windows of opportunity naturally occurring in different therapeutic scenarios, future directions of treatment with AXAL will most likely include administration in oropharyngeal squamous cell carcinomas and high-risk locally advanced cervical cancer, in combination with standard treatment options or alone.

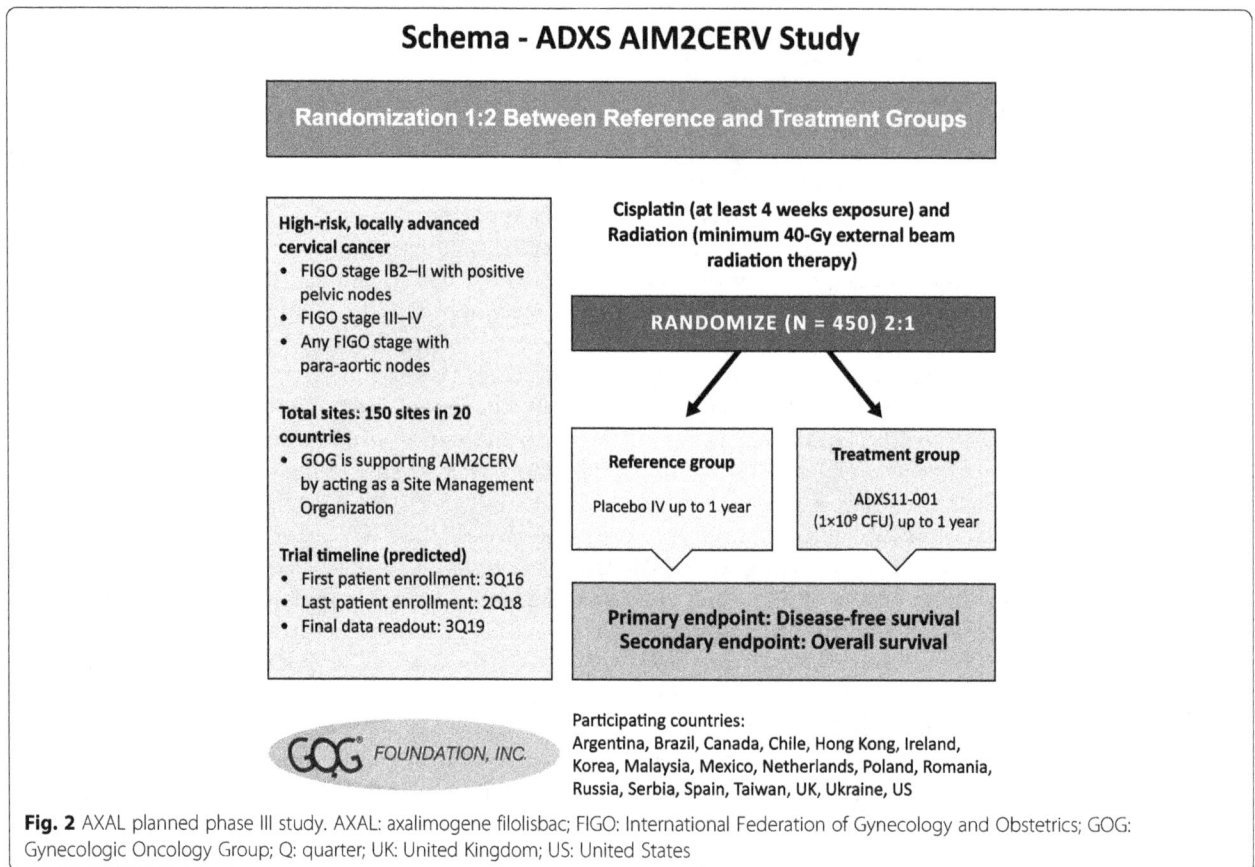

Schema - ADXS AIM2CERV Study

Randomization 1:2 Between Reference and Treatment Groups

High-risk, locally advanced cervical cancer
- FIGO stage IB2–II with positive pelvic nodes
- FIGO stage III–IV
- Any FIGO stage with para-aortic nodes

Total sites: 150 sites in 20 countries
- GOG is supporting AIM2CERV by acting as a Site Management Organization

Trial timeline (predicted)
- First patient enrollment: 3Q16
- Last patient enrollment: 2Q18
- Final data readout: 3Q19

Cisplatin (at least 4 weeks exposure) and Radiation (minimum 40-Gy external beam radiation therapy)

RANDOMIZE (N = 450) 2:1

Reference group
Placebo IV up to 1 year

Treatment group
ADXS11-001
(1×10^9 CFU) up to 1 year

Primary endpoint: Disease-free survival
Secondary endpoint: Overall survival

GOG® FOUNDATION, INC.

Participating countries:
Argentina, Brazil, Canada, Chile, Hong Kong, Ireland, Korea, Malaysia, Mexico, Netherlands, Poland, Romania, Russia, Serbia, Spain, Taiwan, UK, Ukraine, US

Fig. 2 AXAL planned phase III study. AXAL: axalimogene filolisbac; FIGO: International Federation of Gynecology and Obstetrics; GOG: Gynecologic Oncology Group; Q: quarter; UK: United Kingdom; US: United States

Conclusions

Considering the rising incidence of various HPV-associated cancers within the last years [73, 74], as well as HPV infection being more recently established as the principal cause of increased incidence in head and neck cancers [74], novel therapeutic options for HPV-associated cancers are stringently necessary. Novel therapeutic options for HPV-associated cancers include the use of vaccines based on DNA, peptides, or viral vectors. Delivery of HPV antigens using viral vectors, such as in the case of AXAL, has several advantages: in contrast to peptide immunization, CTL epitopes can be processed/presented naturally and delivered more effectively to target cells; in contrast to DNA immunization, the efficiency of introducing heterologous genes in target cells can be enhanced. While the exact costs for treatment with AXAL are not yet completely elucidated, given the long-term beneficial effects reported upon its administration to patients with HPV-positive tumors, it can be hypothesized that AXAL treatment will be cost-effective. Furthermore, considering the relatively straightforward method of AXAL production, the costs of a full course of AXAL are hypothesized to be far inferior to those of Sipuleucel-T treatment, for which a full course rises to $98,780 [75]. A more specific cost-estimate of the treatment will hopefully be possible in the near future, especially since treatment with AXAL is expected to be available within the next 5 years or earlier. In this regard, patients with high-risk locally advanced cervical cancer represent the ideal target patients for treatment with AXAL, also based on the promising results obtained so far in this patient population.

Although there is evidence in the literature demonstrating a growing incidence of decreased vaccine acceptance and hesitancy of usage [76], the various ongoing clinical trials with AXAL indicate its potential for widespread use across various types of HPV-associated cancers, thus placing AXAL among the promising immunotherapeutic tools of the future.

Abbreviations

Ag: Antigen; AIN: Anal intraepithelial neoplasia; AXAL: Axalimogene filolisbac; BID: bi-daily; CD: Cluster of differentiation; CFU: Colony-forming unit; CIN: Cervical intraepithelial neoplasia; CR: Complete response; CTRI: Clinical Trials Registry – India; DLT: Dose-limiting toxicity; DNA: Deoxyribonucleic acid; ECOG: Eastern Cooperative Oncology Group; FIGO: Federation of Gynecology and Obstetrics; GOG: Gynecologic Oncology Group; HPV: Human papillomavirus; IFN-γ: Interferon gamma; IMRT: Intensity-modulated radiation therapy; LLO: Listeriolysin O; *Lm*: *Listeria monocytogenes*; MDSCs: Myeloid-derived suppressor cells; NCT: National Clinical Trial; OR: Objective response; OS: Overall survival; PD-1: Programmed death protein 1; PFS: Progression-free survival; PR: Partial response; Q: Quarter; RECIST: Response Evaluation Criteria

Therapeutic options for treatment of human papillomavirus-associated cancers -novel immunologic...

157

In Solid Tumors; RP2D: Recommended phase II dose; TiP: Trial in progress; TNF-α: Tumor necrosis factor alpha; TRAEs: Treatment-related adverse events; Tregs: Regulatory T cells; UK: United Kingdom; US: United States; VIN: Vulvar intraepithelial neoplasia

Acknowledgements
The authors would like to thank Oana Draghiciu, PhD, from TRM Oncology, for medical writing assistance, funded by Advaxis, Inc. The authors are fully responsible for all content and editorial decisions for this review.

Funding
Medical writing assistance was funded by Advaxis, Inc.

Authors' contributions
BM, HPS, and BJM were integral in the writing, review, and revision of the manuscript. All authors read and approved the final manuscript.

Competing interests
BM has received research funding for the Window of Opportunity clinical trial (NCT02002182) from Advaxis Inc. BJM discloses that the St. Joseph's Hospital institution has received research grants from Amgen, Lilly, Genentech, Janssen/Johnson & Johnson, Array, TESARO, and Morphotek. BJM has received honoraria for speaker bureaus from Roche/Genentech, AstraZeneca, Myriad, and Janssen/Johnson & Johnson; and has been a consultant for Roche/Genentech, Merck, TESARO, AstraZeneca, Gradalis, Advaxis, Amgen, Pfizer, Bayer, Insys, Mateon (formerly OXiGENE), PPD, and Clovis. HPS has nothing to disclose.

Author details
[1]Department of Otolaryngology, Icahn School of Medicine at Mount Sinai, New York, NY, USA. [2]Brown University Oncology Research Group, Providence, RI, USA. [3]Division of Gynecologic Oncology, Arizona Oncology (US Oncology Network), University of Arizona College of Medicine, Creighton University School of Medicine at St. Joseph's Hospital, 2222 E. Highland Ave, Suite 400, Phoenix, AZ 85016, USA.

References
1. Forman D, de Martel C, Lacey CJ, Soerjomataram I, Lortet-Tieulent J, Bruni L, et al. Global burden of human papillomavirus and related diseases. Vaccine. 2012;30(suppl 5):F12–23.
2. de Martel C, Ferlay J, Franceschi S, Vignat J, Bray F, Forman D, et al. Global burden of cancers attributable to infections in 2008: a review and synthetic analysis. Lancet Oncol. 2012;13(6):607–15.
3. Plummer M, de Martel C, Vignat J, Ferlay J, Bray F, Franceschi S. Global burden of cancers attributable to infections in 2012: a synthetic analysis. Lancet Glob Health. 2016;4(9):e609–16.
4. Scheurer ME, Tortolero-Luna G, Adler-Storthz K. Human papillomavirus infection: biology, epidemiology, and prevention. Int J Gynecol Cancer. 2005;15(5):727–46.
5. Moody CA, Laimins LA. Human papillomavirus oncoproteins: pathways to transformation. Nat Rev Cancer. 2010;10(8):550–60.
6. Bodily J, Laimins LA. Persistence of human papillomavirus infection: keys to malignant progression. Trends Microbiol. 2011;19(1):33–9.
7. Grabowska AK, Riemer AB. The invisible enemy - how human papillomaviruses avoid recognition and clearance by the host immune system. Open Virol J. 2012;6:249–56.
8. Howie HL, Katzenellenbogen RA, Galloway DA. Papillomavirus E6 proteins. Virology. 2009;384(2):324–34.
9. Wise-Draper TM, Wells SI. Papillomavirus E6 and E7 proteins and their cellular targets. Front Biosci. 2008;13:1003–17.
10. Münger K, Basile JR, Duensing S, Eichten A, Gonzalez SL, Grace M, et al. Biological activities and molecular targets of the human papillomavirus E7 oncoprotein. Oncogene. 2001;20(54):7888–98.
11. Bernard HU, Burk RD, Chen Z, van Doorslaer K, Zur Hausen H, de Villiers EM. Classification of papillomaviruses (PVs) based on 189 PV types and proposal of taxonomic amendments. Virology. 2010;401(1):70–9.
12. Ling M, Kanayama M, Roden R, Wu TC. Preventive and therapeutic vaccines for human papillomavirus-associated cervical cancers. J Biomed Sci. 2000; 7(5):341–56.
13. Muñoz N, Bosch FX, de Sanjosé S, Herrero R, Castellsagué X, Shah KV, et al. Epidemiologic classification of human papillomavirus types associated with cervical cancer. N Engl J Med. 2003;348(6):518–27.
14. Schiffman M, Clifford G, Buonaguro FM. Classification of weakly carcinogenic human papillomavirus types: addressing the limits of epidemiology at the borderline. Infect Agent Cancer. 2009;4:8.
15. Guan P, Howell-Jones R, Li N, Bruni L, de Sanjosé S, Franceschi S, et al. Human papillomavirus types in 115,789 HPV-positive women: a meta-analysis from cervical infection to cancer. Int J Cancer. 2012;131(10):2349–59.
16. Chaturvedi AK. Beyond cervical cancer: burden of other HPV-related cancers among men and women. J Adolesc Health. 2010;46(4 suppl):S20–6.
17. FUTURE II Study Group. Quadrivalent vaccine against human papillomavirus to prevent high-grade cervical lesions. N Engl J Med. 2007;356(19):1915–27.
18. Centers for Disease Control and Prevention (CDC). FDA licensure of bivalent human papillomavirus vaccine (HPV2, Cervarix) for use in females and updated HPV vaccination recommendations from the Advisory Committee on Immunization Practices (ACIP). MMWR Morb Mortal Wkly Rep. 2010; 59(20):626–9.
19. Petrosky E, Bocchini JA Jr, Hariri S, Chesson H, Curtis CR, Saraiya M, et al. Use of 9-valent human papillomavirus (HPV) vaccine: updated HPV vaccination recommendations of the advisory committee on immunization practices. MMWR Morb Mortal Wkly Rep. 2015;64(11):300–4.
20. Stern PL, van der Burg SH, Hampson IN, Broker TR, Fiander A, Lacey CJ, et al. Therapy of human papillomavirus-related disease. Vaccine. 2012;30(suppl 5): F71–82.
21. Milinovic D, Kalafatic D, Babic D, Oreskovic LB, Grsic HL, Oreskovic S. Minimally invasive therapy of cervical intraepithelial neoplasia for fertility preservation. Pathol Oncol Res. 2009;15(3):521–5.
22. The Cancer Genome Atlas Research Network. Integrated genomic and molecular characterization of cervical cancer. Nature. 2017;541:169–75.
23. Rose PG. Combined-modality therapy of locally advanced cervical cancer. J Clin Oncol. 2003;21(10 suppl):211s–7s.
24. Moore DH, Blessing JA, McQuellon RP, Thaler HT, Cella D, Benda J, et al. Phase III study of cisplatin with or without paclitaxel in stage IVB, recurrent, or persistent squamous cell carcinoma of the cervix: a gynecologic oncology group study. J Clin Oncol. 2004;22(15):3113–9.
25. Monk BJ, Sill MW, McMeekin DS, Cohn DE, Ramondetta LM, Boardman CH, et al. Phase III trial of four cisplatin-containing doublet combinations in stage IVB, recurrent, or persistent cervical carcinoma: a Gynecologic Oncology Group study. J Clin Oncol. 2009;27(28):4649–55.
26. Tewari KS, Sill MW, Long HJ 3rd, Penson RT, Huang H, Ramondetta LM, et al. Improved survival with bevacizumab in advanced cervical cancer. N Engl J Med. 2014;370(8):734–43.
27. Gill BS, Bernard ME, Lin JF, Balasubramani GK, Rajagopalan MS, Sukumvanich P, et al. Impact of adjuvant chemotherapy with radiation for node-positive vulvar cancer: A National Cancer Data Base (NCDB) analysis. Gynecol Oncol. 2015;137(3):365–72.
28. National Comprehensive Cancer Network. NCCN Clinical Practice Guidelines in Oncology (NCCN Guidelines®). Vulvar cancer (squamous cell carcinoma). Version 1.2017. 2016. https://www.nccn.org/professionals/physician_gls/f_ guidelines.asp. Accessed 30 Nov 2016.
29. Eifel PJ, Berek JS, Markman MA. Cancer of the cervix, vagina, and vulva. In: DeVita Jr VT, Lawrence TS, Rosenberg SA, editors. DeVita, Hellman, and

Rosenberg's Cancer: Principles and Practice of Oncology. 9th ed. Philadelphia, Pa: Lippincott Williams & Wilkins; 2011. p. 1311–44.

30. Samant R, Lau B, Choan E, Le T, Tam T. Primary vaginal cancer treated with concurrent chemoradiation using Cis-platinum. Int J Radiat Oncol Biol Phys. 2007;69(3):746–50.

31. Olthof NC, Straetmans JM, Snoeck R, Ramaekers FC, Kremer B, Speel EJ. Next-generation treatment strategies for human papillomavirus-related head and neck squamous cell carcinoma: where do we go? Rev Med Virol. 2012;22(2):88–105.

32. Chaturvedi AK, Engels EA, Pfeiffer RM, Hernandez BY, Xiao W, Kim E, et al. Human papillomavirus and rising oropharyngeal cancer incidence in the United States. J Clin Oncol. 2011;29(32):4294–301.

33. Varier I, Keeley BR, Krupar R, Patsias A, Dong J, Gupta N, et al. Clinical characteristics and outcomes of oropharyngeal carcinoma related to high-risk non-human papillomavirus16 viral subtypes. Head Neck. 2016; 38(9):1330–7.

34. Truong Lam M, O'Sullivan B, Gullane P, Huang SH. Challenges in establishing the diagnosis of human papillomavirus-related oropharyngeal carcinoma. Laryngoscope. 2016;126(10):2270–5.

35. Cracchiolo JR, Baxi SS, Morris LG, Ganly I, Patel SG, Cohen MA, et al. Increase in primary surgical treatment of T1 and T2 oropharyngeal squamous cell carcinoma and rates of adverse pathologic features: National Cancer Data Base. Cancer. 2016;122(10):1523–32.

36. Ferris RL, Blumenschein G Jr, Fayette J, Guigay J, Colevas AD, Licitra L, et al. Nivolumab for recurrent squamous-cell carcinoma of the head and neck. N Engl J Med. 2016;375(19):1856–67.

37. Goldstone SE, Kawalek AZ, Huyett JW. Infrared coagulator: a useful tool for treating anal squamous intraepithelial lesions. Dis Colon rectum. 2005;48(5):1042–54.

38. Leon O, Guren MG, Radu C, Gunnlaugsson A, Johnsson A. Phase I study of cetuximab in combination with 5-fluorouracil, mitomycin C and radiotherapy in patients with locally advanced anal cancer. Eur J Cancer. 2015;51(17):2740–6.

39. National Comprehensive Cancer Network. NCCN Clinical Practice Guidelines in Oncology (NCCN Guidelines®). Anal carcinoma. Version 1.2017. 2016. https://www.nccn.org/professionals/physician_gls/f_guidelines.asp. Accessed 30 Nov 2016.

40. Di Lorenzo G, Buonerba C, Ferro M, Calderoni G, Bozza G, Federico P, et al. The epidermal growth factor receptors as biological targets in penile cancer. Expert Opin Biol Ther. 2015;15(4):473–6.

41. National Comprehensive Cancer Network. NCCN Clinical Practice Guidelines in Oncology (NCCN Guidelines®). Penile cancer. Version 2. 2016. 2016. https://www.nccn.org/professionals/physician_gls/f_guidelines.asp. Accessed 30 Nov 2016.

42. van Poelgeest MI, van Seters M, van Beurden M, Kwappenberg KM, Heijmans-Antonissen C, Drijfhout JW, et al. Detection of human papillomavirus (HPV) 16-specific CD4+ T-cell immunity in patients with persistent HPV16-induced vulvar intraepithelial neoplasia in relation to clinical impact of imiquimod treatment. Clin Cancer Res. 2005;11(14):5273–80.

43. Kobayashi A, Weinberg V, Darragh T, Smith-McCune K. Evolving immunosuppressive microenvironment during human cervical carcinogenesis. Mucosal Immunol. 2008;1(5):412–20.

44. Kenter GG, Welters MJ, Valentijn AR, Lowik MJ, Berends-van der Meer DM, Vloon AP, et al. Phase I immunotherapeutic trial with long peptides spanning the E6 and E7 sequences of high-risk human papillomavirus 16 in end-stage cervical cancer patients shows low toxicity and robust immunogenicity. Clin Cancer Res. 2008;14(1):169–77.

45. Palefsky JM, Berry JM, Jay N, Krogstad M, Da Costa M, Darragh TM, et al. A trial of SGN-00101 (HspE7) to treat high-grade anal intraepithelial neoplasia in HIV-positive individuals. AIDS. 2006;20(8):1151–5.

46. Frazer IH, Quinn M, Nicklin JL, Tan J, Perrin LC, Ng P, et al. Phase 1 study of HPV16-specific immunotherapy with E6E7 fusion protein and ISCOMATRIX adjuvant in women with cervical intraepithelial neoplasia. Vaccine. 2004; 23(2):172–81.

47. Roman LD, Wilczynski S, Muderspach LI, Burnett AF, O'Meara A, Brinkman JA, et al. A phase II study of Hsp-7 (SGN-00101) in women with high-grade cervical intraepithelial neoplasia. Gynecol Oncol. 2007;106(3):558–66.

48. Welters MJ, Kenter GG, Piersma SJ, Vloon AP, Löwik MJ, Berends-van der Meer DM, et al. Induction of tumor-specific CD4+ and CD8+ T-cell immunity in cervical cancer patients by a human papillomavirus type 16 E6 and E7 long peptides vaccine. Clin Cancer Res. 2008;14(1):178–87.

49. Trimble CL, Peng S, Kos F, Gravitt P, Viscidi R, Sugar E, et al. A phase I trial of a human papillomavirus DNA vaccine for HPV16+ cervical intraepithelial neoplasia 2/3. Clin Cancer Res. 2009;15(1):361–7.

50. Santin AD, Bellone S, Palmieri M, Zanolini A, Ravaggi A, Siegel ER, et al. Human papillomavirus type 16 and 18 E7-pulsed dendritic cell vaccination of stage IB or IIA cervical cancer patients: a phase I escalating-dose trial. J Virol. 2008;82(4):1968–79.

51. Ferrara A, Nonn M, Sehr P, Schreckenberger C, Pawlita M, Dürst M, et al. Dendritic cell-based tumor vaccine for cervical cancer II: results of a clinical pilot study in 15 individual patients. J Cancer Res Clin Oncol. 2003;129(9):521–30.

52. Stevanović S, Draper LM, Langhan MM, Campbell TE, Kwong ML, Wunderlich JR, et al. Complete regression of metastatic cervical cancer after treatment with human papillomavirus-targeted tumor-infiltrating T cells. J Clin Oncol. 2015;33(14):1543–50.

53. García-Hernández E, González-Sánchez JL, Andrade-Manzano A, Contreras ML, Padilla S, Guzmán CC, et al. Regression of papilloma high-grade lesions (CIN 2 and CIN 3) is stimulated by therapeutic vaccination with MVA E2 recombinant vaccine. Cancer Gene Ther. 2006;13(6):592–7.

54. Davidson EJ, Faulkner RL, Sehr P, Pawlita M, Smyth LJ, Burt DJ, et al. Effect of TA-CIN (HPV 16 L2E6E7) booster immunisation in vulval intraepithelial neoplasia patients previously vaccinated with TA-HPV (vaccinia virus encoding HPV 16/18 E6E7). Vaccine. 2004;22(21–22):2722–9.

55. Zenewicz LA, Shen H. Innate and adaptive immune responses to Listeria monocytogenes: a short overview. Microbes Infect. 2007;9(10):1208–15.

56. Pan ZK, Ikonomidis G, Lazenby A, Pardoll D, Paterson Y. A recombinant Listeria monocytogenes vaccine expressing a model tumour antigen protects mice against lethal tumour cell challenge and causes regression of established tumours. Nat Med. 1995;1(5):471–7.

57. Rothman J, Wallecha A, Maciag PC, Rivera S, Shahabi V, Paterson Y. The use of living Listeria monocytogenes as an active immunotherapy for the treatment of cancer. In: Fialho AM, Chakrabarty A, editors. Emerging cancer therapy: microbial approaches and biotechnological tools. New York: John Wiley & Sons, Inc.; 2010. p. 13–48.

58. Campisi L, Soudja SM, Cazareth J, Bassand D, Lazzari A, Brau F, et al. Splenic CD8α+ dendritic cells undergo rapid programming by cytosolic bacteria and inflammation to induce protective CD8+ T-cell memory. Eur J Immunol. 2011;41(6):1594–605.

59. Shahabi V, Reyes-Reyes M, Wallecha A, Rivera S, Paterson Y, Maciag P. Development of a Listeria monocytogenes based vaccine against prostate cancer. Cancer Immunol Immunother. 2008;57(9):1301–13.

60. Wallecha A, French C, Petit R, Singh R, Amin A, Rothman J. Lm-LLO-based immunotherapies and HPV-associated disease. J Oncol. 2012;2012:542851.

61. Maciag PC, Radulovic S, Rothman J. The first clinical use of a live-attenuated Listeria monocytogenes vaccine: a Phase I safety study of Lm-LLO-E7 in patients with advanced carcinoma of the cervix. Vaccine. 2009;27(30):3975–83.

62. de las Heras A, Cain RJ, Bielecka MK, Vázquez-Boland JA. Regulation of Listeria virulence: PrfA master and commander. Curr Opin Microbiol. 2011;14(2):118–27.

63. Huh WK, Brady WE, Moore KN, Lankes HA, Monk BJ, Aghajanian C, et al. A phase 2 study of live-attenuated Listeria monocytogenes cancer immunotherapy (ADXS11-001) in the treatment of persistent or recurrent cancer of the cervix (GOG-0265). J Clin Oncol. 2014;32(suppl): abstract TPS5617.

64. Ghamande SA, Dobbins R, Marshall L, Wheatley D, Price C, Mauro DJ, et al. Phase I study evaluating high dose ADXS11-001 treatment in women with carcinoma of the cervix. J Clin Oncol. 2015;33(suppl): abstract TPS3096.

65. Petit RG, Mehta A, Jain M, Gupta S, Nagarkar R, Kumar V, et al. ADXS11-001 immunotherapy targeting HPV-E7: final results from a Phase II study in Indian women with recurrent cervical cancer. J Immunother Cancer. 2014; 2(suppl 3): abstract P92.

66. Herzog T, Backes FJ, Copeland L, Estevez Diz MD, Hare TW, Huh W, et al. AIM2CERV: a randomized phase 3 study of adjuvant AXAL immunotherapy following chemoradiation in patients who have high-risk locally advanced cervical cancer (HRLACC). J Immunother Cancer. 2016;4(suppl 1): abstract P140.

67. Cohen EE, Moore KN, Slomovitz BM, Chung CH, Anderson ML, Morris SR, et al. Phase I/II study of ADXS11-001 or MEDI4736 immunotherapies alone and in combination, in patients with recurrent/metastatic cervical or human papillomavirus (HPV)-positive head and neck cancer. J Immunother Cancer. 2015;3(suppl 2): abstract P147.

68. Krupar R, Imai N, Miles B, Genden E, Misiukiewicz K, Saegner Y, et al. HPV E7 antigen-expressing Listeria-based immunotherapy (ADXS11-001) prior to

robotic surgery for HPV-positive oropharyngeal cancer enhances HPV-specific T cell immunity. Cancer Res. 2016;76(14 suppl): abstract LB-095.

69. U.S. National Institutes of Health. ClinicalTrials.gov. Safety study of recombinant *Listeria monocytogenes* (Lm) based vaccine virus vaccine to treat oropharyngeal cancer (REALISTIC). https://clinicaltrials.gov/ct2/show/NCT01598792. Accessed 30 Nov 2016.

70. U.S. National Institutes of Health. ClinicalTrials.gov. A phase I/II evaluation of ADXS11–001, mitomycin, 5-fluorouracil (5-FU) and IMRT for anal cancer (276). https://clinicaltrials.gov/ct2/show/NCT01671488. Accessed 30 Nov 2016.

71. Fakih M, O'Neil BH, Chiorean EG, Hochster HS, Chan E, Mauro D, et al. Phase II study of ADXS11–001 in patients with persistent/recurrent, locoregional or metastatic squamous cell carcinoma of the anorectal canal. J Clin Oncol. 2016;34(4 suppl): abstract TPS786.

72. Guo T, Rettig E, Fakhry C. Understanding the impact of survival and human papillomavirus tumor status on timing of recurrence in oropharyngeal squamous cell carcinoma. Oral Oncol. 2016;52:97–103.

73. Chaturvedi AK, Engels EA, Pfeiffer RM, Hernandez BY, Xiao W, Kim E, et al. Human papillomavirus and rising oropharyngeal cancer incidence in the United States. J Clin Oncol. 2011;29:4294–301.

74. Gillison ML, Chaturvedi AK, Anderson WF, Fakhry C. Epidemiology of human papillomavirus-positive head and neck squamous cell carcinoma. J Clin Oncol. 2015;33:3235–42.

75. Geynisman DM, Chien CR, Smieliauskas F, Shen C, Tina Shih YC. Economic evaluation of therapeutic cancer vaccines and immunotherapy: A systematic review. Hum Vaccin Immunother. 2014;10(11):3415–24.

76. Darden PM, Thompson DM, Roberts JR, Hale JJ, Pope C, Naifeh M, et al. Reasons for not vaccinating adolescents: National Immunization Survey of Teens, 2008-2010. Pediatrics. 2013;131(4):645–51.

20

Assessment of drug therapy problems among patients with cervical cancer at Kenyatta National Hospital, Kenya

Amsalu Degu[1*], Peter Njogu[2], Irene Weru[3] and Peter Karimi[1]

Abstract

Background: Although cervical cancer is preventable, it is still the second leading cause of cancer deaths among women in the world. Further, it is estimated that around 5–10% of hospital admissions are due to drug related problems (DRPs), of which 50% are avoidable. In cancer therapy, there is an immense potential for DRPs due to the high toxicity of most chemotherapeutic regimens. Hence, this study sought to assess DRPs among patients with cervical cancer at Kenyatta National Hospital (KNH).

Methods: A cross-sectional study was conducted at the oncology units of KNH. A total of 81 study participants were recruited through simple random sampling. Data were collected from medical records and interviewing patients. The appropriateness of medical therapy was evaluated by comparing with National Compressive Cancer Network and European Society for Medical Oncology practice guideline of cervical cancer treatment protocol. The degree of adherence was determined using eight-item Morisky medication adherence scale. The likelihood of drug interaction was assessed using Medscape, Micromedex and Epocrates drug interaction checkers. The data were entered in Microsoft Excel and analysed using statistical software STATA version 13.0. Descriptive statistics such as mean, percent and frequency were used to summarise patients' characteristics. Univariable and multivariable binary logistic regression were used to investigate the potential predictors of DRPs.

Result: A total of 215 DRPs were identified from 76 patients, translating to a prevalence of 93.8% and a mean of 2. 65 ± 1.22 DRPs. The predominant proportion of DRPs (48.2%) was identified in patients who had been treated with chemoradiation regimens. Adverse drug reactions 56(69.1%) and drug interactions 38(46.9%) were the most prevalent DRPs. Majority (67.9%) of the study population were adherent to their treatment regimens. Forgetfulness 18(69.2%), expensive medications 4(15.4%) and side effects of medications 4(15.4%) were the main reasons for medication non-adherence. Patients with advanced stage cervical cancer were 15.4 times (AOR = 15.4, 95% CI = 1. 3–185.87, $p = 0.031$) more likely to have DRPs as compared to patients with early stage disease.

Conclusion: Adverse drug reactions, drug interactions, and need of additional drug therapy were the most common DRPs identified among cervical cancer patients. Advanced stage cervical cancer was the only predictor of DRPs.

Keywords: Drug related problems, Cervical cancer, Kenyatta national hospital

* Correspondence: amsaludegu@yahoo.com
[1]Department of Pharmaceutics and Pharmacy Practice, University of Nairobi, College of Health Sciences, School of Pharmacy, P.O. Box 19676-00202, Nairobi, Kenya
Full list of author information is available at the end of the article

Background

In the past few decades, medicines have had a substantial positive effect on health by reducing mortality and disease burden. Interestingly, there is ample evidence that potential problems exists since the right medicine does not always reach the right patient and around 50% of all patients fail to take their medication correctly [1]. Moreover, irrational use of drugs is a major global problem, and World Health Organization (WHO) estimates that above 50% of all drugs are prescribed and dispensed inappropriately with consequent wastage of scarce resources and widespread health hazards [2].

A drug-related problem (DRP) is defined as an event involving drug therapy that has a potential to interfere with the desired health outcomes [3]. Alternatively, a drug therapy problem is any detrimental event experienced by a patient which impedes attainment of the desired goals of treatment. In the absence of appropriate intervention, medication problems have considerable negative impact on the health of the patients [4].

Drug-related problems are categorised into different classes, namely need for additional drug therapy, medication use without indication, improper drug selection, overdosage, sub-therapeutic dosage, adverse drug reactions (ADRs), drug interactions, inappropriate laboratory monitoring and non-adherence [4].

In cancer therapy, there is a tremendous potential for DRPs due to the high toxicity and the complexity of most chemotherapeutic regimens [5]. Cancer patients have a high incidence of coexisting chronic diseases and the treatment of cancer carry an inherent risk of DRPs [6]. Moreover, problems arising due to drugs are more common in cancer patients, and commonly present a major hurdle to health care providers [7].

Drug-related problems due to cancer chemotherapy can have severe consequences arising from the high toxicity and narrow therapeutic range of anticancer drugs [5]. Anticancer agents are differentiated from other class of drugs due to the frequency and severity of side effects at therapeutic doses [8]. Chemoradiation with cisplatin is associated with increased acute haematological and gastrointestinal toxicity in cervical cancer patients [9]. Since cancer patients receive multiple drug therapy, they are at a higher risk to develop DRPs. Accordingly, a substantial clinical need is required to address this problem by identifying cancer therapy-induced problems. Moreover, the prevalence of DRPs in patients with cervical cancer is not known in Kenya though the chemotherapeutic agents are expected to produce serious adverse outcomes to the patients. Thus, it was imperative that assessment was carried out to identify DRPs in cervical cancer patients to overcome these hurdles.

An extensive study of DRPs would render valuable perspicacity for the healthcare providers to lessen the incidence of DRPs [10]. However, there is a paucity of data on comprehensive DRPs among cervical cancer patients. Therefore, this study investigated the prevalence, types and predictors of DRPs in cervical cancer patients admitted at the oncology units of Kenyatta National Hospital.

Methods

Study design and setting

A cross-sectional study design was conducted from April to June 2017 at the oncology units of Kenyatta National Hospital (KNH), the biggest tertiary hospital in Kenya. Single population proportion formula was used to calculate the sample size [11].

$$n = \frac{Z_{\frac{\alpha}{2}}^2 \times P(1-P)}{d^2}$$

where: n is the minimum sample size required for large population ($\geq$10,000).

$Z_{\alpha/2}$ is the critical value for a 95% confidence interval (= 1.96 from Z- table).

P is the proportion of drug-related problems in cervical cancer patients. Since there were no previous studies in Kenya, P was assumed to be 50% (0.5).

d is the margin of error (5%)

Hence, estimated minimum sample size

$$(n) = \frac{(1.96)^2 \times 0.5(1-0.5)}{(0.05)^2} = 384$$

However, since study population was less than 10,000, we estimated the sample size using the following reduction formula.

Corrected sample size $= \frac{n \times N}{n+N}$ Where N = source population and n = estimated sample size for $N \geq 10,000$ population. According to KNH Health Information Department report, an average of 90 cervical cancer patients was on treatment in both inpatient and outpatient oncology units of KNH in the preceding three months period (September–November, 2016). The study was carried out for three months period, and hence the approximate size of the source population was 90 cervical cancer patients. Then, corrected sample size = $\frac{384 \times 90}{384+90} = 73$. Therefore, the corrected sample size with a 10% contingency for incomplete medical records of the patient and non-response provided a final sample size of 81 cervical cancer patients.

Eligibility criteria

Patients aged 18 years and above with documented diagnosis of cancer and, treatment regimens were targeted. However, only those who signed the informed consent were included in the study.

Data collection techniques

Two qualified nurses from the oncology units of KNH were trained to assist in data collection. Relevant information about each patient such as socio-demographic characteristics, histological types of cervical cancer, stage of cancer, types of co-morbidity, treatment regimen, ADR, the rate of adherence and reasons for non-adherence, were recorded by reviewing medical records and interviewing the patients. A pilot study was done in 10% of the sample size to ensure the validity of the data collection instruments. After pre-testing, all necessary adjustments were executed on the data collection instruments before implementing in the main study. The adequacy of medical therapy was evaluated using National Guidelines for Cancer Management in Kenya [12], National Compressive Cancer Network (NCCN) practice guideline of cervical cancer treatment [13], European Society for Medical Oncology (ESMO) practice guideline of cervical cancer [14] and WHO cancer pain management protocols [15]. The probability of drug interaction was assessed using Medscape, Micromedex, Web MD and Epocrates drug interaction checkers. The degree of adherence was determined using Eight-Item Morisky Medication Adherence Scale [16]. The Modification of Diet in Renal Disease (MDRD) Study eq. [17], Du Bois method [18] and Calvert formula [19] were used to determine estimated Glomerular filtration rate (eGFR), body surface area and carboplatin dosing, respectively. DRPs were categorised as the need of additional drug therapy, medication use without indication, improper drug selection, overdosage, sub-therapeutic dosage, adverse drug reactions, drug interactions, inappropriate laboratory monitoring and patient's non-adherence by the Cipolle et al. classification system [4].

Analysis

The data were entered into the Microsoft Excel worksheet and analysed using statistical software STATA version 13.0. Descriptive statistics such as percent and frequency were used to summarise categorical variables of patients' characteristics. Mean and standard deviation were used to compile continuous variables. The univariable and multivariable binary logistic regression analyses were employed to investigate the potential predictors of DRPs. A p-value of ≤0.05 was considered statistically significant.

Results

Sociodemographic characteristics of study participants

The study was conducted among 81 cervical cancer patients. The mean age of the study population was 53.3 ± 11.6 years, and the predominant portion of the study subjects 47(58.0%) were aged 50 years and above. Among the 81 study participants, 61(75.3%) were married, 44(54.3%) had a primary level of education, while only 2(2.5%) had attained tertiary level of education. Twenty four participants (29.6%) were housewives. The monthly income level of majority of the population 59(72.8%) was less than USD 100, and most of the patients 40(49.4%) were on treatment with 5–9 drugs (Table 1).

Clinical characteristics of the study participants

As illustrated in Fig. 1, three histological types of cervical cancer were identified among the study subjects. Squamous cell carcinoma (91.4%) was the most common type, followed by adenocarcinoma (7.4%) while invasive anaplastic carcinoma (1.2%) was the least common histological type.

The study showed that 44.4% and 35.8% of study population had stage II and III cervical cancer, respectively, with stages IIB (33.3%) and IIIB (28.4%) being the most prevalent. However, stages I and IV had low prevalence rates (Fig. 2).

Table 1 Sociodemographic characteristics of the study participants

Variables	Frequency	Percent
Age (years)		
29–39	10	12.3
40–50	24	29.6
≥ 51	47	58.0
Marital status		
Single	20	24.7
Married	61	75.3
Level of education		
Illiterate	10	12.3
Primary	44	54.3
Secondary	25	30.9
Tertiary	2	2.5
Occupation		
Housewife	24	29.6
Retired	9	11.1
Merchant	5	6.2
Unemployed	19	23.5
Farmer	16	19.8
Daily labourer	4	4.9
Private employee	3	3.7
Other	1	1.2
Monthly family income (USD)		
Very low (<100)	59	72.8
Low (100–200)	18	22.2
Average (200–500)	4	4.9
Number of drugs per patient		
< 5	31	38.3
5–9	40	49.4
> =10	10	12.3

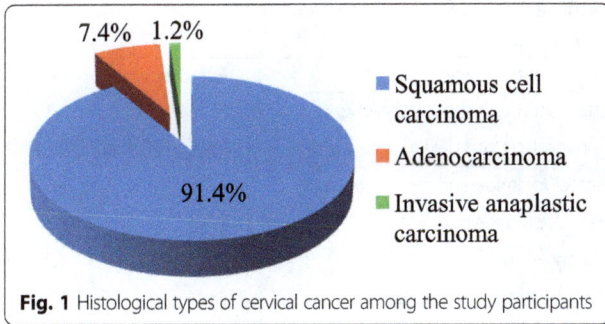

Fig. 1 Histological types of cervical cancer among the study participants

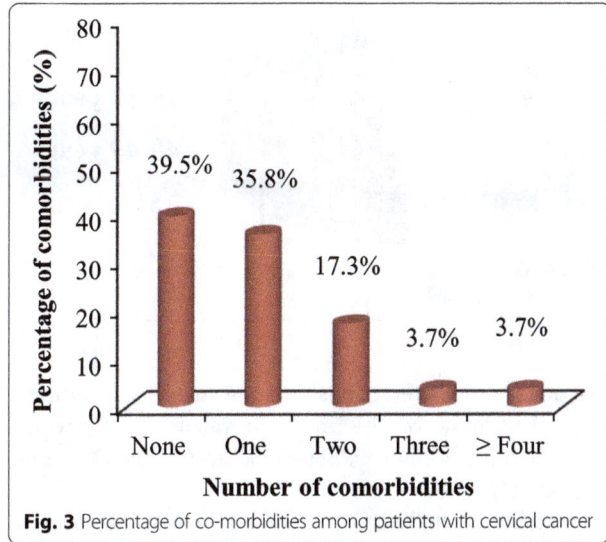

Fig. 3 Percentage of co-morbidities among patients with cervical cancer

Among the study population, 39.5% patients did not have co-existing co-morbidities. Nonetheless, 35.8%, 17.3%, and 3.7% patients had been diagnosed with one, two, three, and four and above co-morbidities, respectively (Fig. 3). Anaemia 21(25.9%), retroviral disease 15(18.3%) and hypertension 13(16.1%) were the most common types of co-morbidities. Conversely, pulmonary embolism, sepsis, acute kidney injury, goitre and gastric ulcer were the least frequent co-morbidities among the study participants (Table 2). When age was taken into consideration, most of the study participants (29.6%) who had co-existing co-morbidities were aged 51 years and above (Fig. 4).

Types of regimen used in the management of cervical cancer
Chemoradiation 41(50.6%) comprising of weekly cisplatin and daily radiotherapy was the most widely used treatment regimen in the management of cervical cancer in our setting. Further, hysterectomy and brachytherapy had been used in the management of 15(18.5%) and 11(13.6%) of the patients, respectively. Cisplatin and paclitaxel 9(11.1%) were the most commonly used combination anticancer agents in the treatment of cervical cancer (Table 3).

Granisetron and dexamethasone combination 32(39.5%) was the most commonly used prophylactic antiemetic regimen followed by a combination of ondansetron and dexamethasone 18(22.2%). Conversely, metoclopramide and ondansetron monotherapy were less frequently used in management of chemotherapy-induced emesis among the study subjects (Table 4).

The finding of the study showed that paracetamol, morphine, tramadol and codeine were the most commonly used analgesics among the study participants. Nonetheless, significant proportion (37.4%) of cervical cancer patients did not receive any form of pain medication (Table 5).

Prevalence of drug-related problems
A total of 215 DRPs were identified from 76 cervical cancer patients, translating to a prevalence of 93.8% and a mean of 2.65 ± 1.22 DRPs per patient. Adverse drug

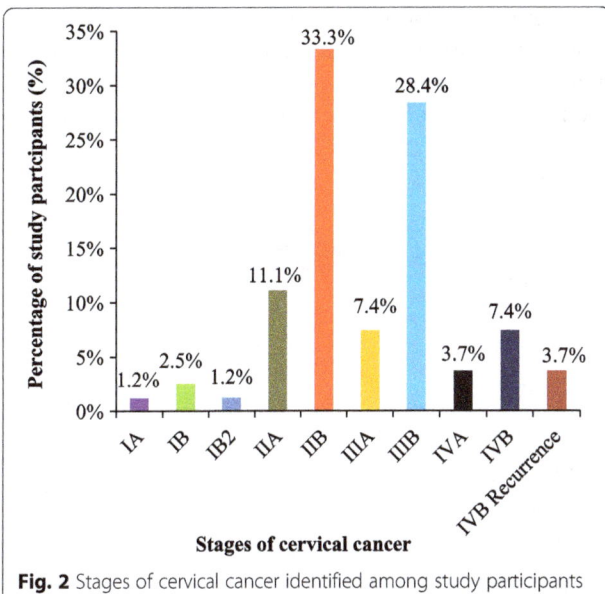

Fig. 2 Stages of cervical cancer identified among study participants

Table 2 Types of co-morbidities among patients with cervical cancer

Co-morbidity	Frequency	Percent
Anaemia	21	25.9
Retroviral disease	15	18.5
Hypertension	13	16.1
Hydronephrosis	13	16.1
Deep vein thrombosis	3	3.7
Rheumatoid arthritis	3	3.7
Chronic kidney disease	3	3.7
Type II diabetes mellitus	2	2.5
Acute kidney injury	1	1.2
Pulmonary embolism	1	1.2
Sepsis	1	1.2
Gastric ulcer	1	1.2
Goitre	1	1.2

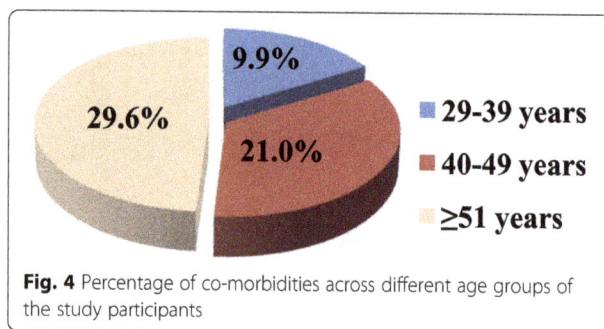

Fig. 4 Percentage of co-morbidities across different age groups of the study participants

Table 4 Types of prophylactic antiemetic regimens used in cervical cancer

Type of antiemetic	Frequency	Percent
Granisetron and dexamethasone	32	39.5
Ondansetron and dexamethasone	18	22.2
Metoclopramide and dexamethasone	4	4.9
Metoclopramide	2	2.5
Ondansetron	1	1.2
No-antiemetics given	24	29.6
Total	81	100.0

reactions, drug interactions and the need for additional drug therapy were the most prevalent DRPs, which accounted for 56(69.1%), 38(46.9%) and 32(39.5%) cases, respectively.

In addition, 26(32.1%) patients were non-adherent to their medications, and 16(19.8%) patients received a sub-therapeutic dose of their treatment regimens. Nevertheless, overdosage, improper drug selection, medication use without indication and inappropriate laboratory monitoring accounted for relatively low proportion of drug therapy problems (Table 6).

As illustrated in Fig. 5, most (54.3%) DRPs were found in the 51 years and above age group while the 40–50 years age group accounted for 28.4%. The least proportion of drug-related problems occurred in the 29–39 years age group.

As shown in Fig. 6, the predominant proportion of DRPs (48.2%) was identified in patients treated with chemoradiation regimens while 16.1% and 13.6% drug therapy problems were identified in patients who had been managed with radical hysterectomy and brachytherapy, respectively. An equivalent proportion (11.1%) of drug therapy problems were detected in patients treated with radiotherapy and combination of cisplatin and paclitaxel regimens. In contrast, the least proportion of drug therapy problems were identified in patients treated with the combination of carboplatin and paclitaxel and cisplatin and vinorelbine regimens.

According to the eight-item Morisky medication adherence scale, 67.9% of cervical cancer patients were highly adherent, 18.5% of patients had an average level of medication adherence, while 13.6% of patients were poorly adherent to their treatment regimens (Fig. 7).

Forgetfulness 18(69.2%), expensive medications 4(15.4%) and side effects of medications 4(15.4%) were the main reasons for non-adherence to medications in the participants. Long duration of therapy and complicated regimens accounted for equal contribution for medication non-adherence while lack of trust on the efficacy of medications was the least common reason for non-adherence in cervical cancer patients (Table 7).

As indicated in Tables 8, 45 drug-drug interactions were identified among the study participants. Ondansetron and dexamethasone were the most common interacting drugs accounting for 12(26.7%) of the total drug interactions. The other frequently encountered drug interactions were dexamethasone and paclitaxel 4(8.9%), and codeine and morphine 2(4.4%). Each of the other pairs of interacting drugs encountered in this study accounted for approximately 2.2% of the total drug interactions.

In terms of severity, 68.9% of the drug interactions were significant which required modification or close monitoring of the outcome of the drug interactions. Furthermore, 26.7% of drug interactions were considered as

Table 3 Types of regimen used in the management of cervical cancer

Regimen	Frequency	Percent
Chemoradiation (Cisplatin weekly + Radiotherapy)	41	50.6
Hysterectomy	15	18.5
Brachytherapy	11	13.6
Radiotherapy	10	12.3
Cisplatin + Paclitaxel	9	11.1
Carboplatin + Paclitaxel	5	6.2
Cisplatin +Vinorelbine	1	1.2

Table 5 Analgesics regimens used in cervical cancer at Kenyatta National Hospital

Type of analgesic	Frequency	Percent
Paracetamol	21	25.9
Morphine	12	14.8
Tramadol	12	14.8
Codeine	11	13.6
Diclofenac	6	7.4
Ibuprofen	5	6.2
meloxicam	3	3.7
Etoricoxib	1	1.2
Analgesic not given	30	37.4

Table 6 Categories of drug related problems

Type of drug related problem	Frequency	Percent
Adverse drug reaction	56	69.1
Drug interaction	38	46.9
Need for additional drug therapy	32	39.5
Non-adherence	26	32.1
Sub-therapeutic dose	16	19.8
Overdosage	15	18.5
Improper drug selection	13	16.1
Medication use without indication	10	12.4
Inappropriate laboratory monitoring	9	11.1

minor interactions. However, 4.4% of drug interactions were serious which necessitate the use of alternative medications in the treatment regimen (Fig. 8).

Of the 166 ADRs identified in this study, the most common were vomiting, nausea, and leucopenia which accounted for 40(49.4%), 24(29.6%), and 18(22.2%) ADRs, respectively. On the other hand, constipation, and thrombocytopenia were the least prevailing ADRs (Table 9).

Predictors of drug related problems

In the univariable and multivariable binary logistic regression analysis, patients whose cervical cancer was at an advanced stage were 15.4 times (AOR = 15.4, 95% CI = 1.3–185.87, p = 0.031) more likely to have DRPs compared to patients with early stage cervical cancer. Hence, stage of cervical cancer was the only predictor of DRPs in cervical cancer patients (Table 10).

Patients who had been treated with more than five drugs were 2.9 times (COR = 2.9, 95% CI = 1.10–7.78, p = 0.032) more likely to have ADRs as compared to patients treated with less than five medications. In addition, patients with advanced stage disease were 5.9 times (AOR = 5.9, 95% CI = 1.43–24.61, p = 0.017) more likely to have ADRs as compared to patients with early stage of cervical cancer. Nonetheless, patients between 40 and 50 years old were 0.1 times (AOR = 0.1, 95% CI = 0.02–0.6, p = 0.013) less likely to have ADRs compared to patients with less than 40 years of age (Table 11).

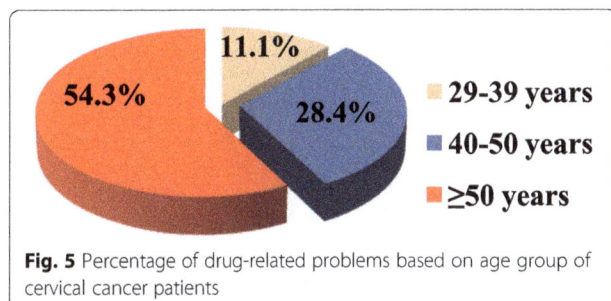

Fig. 6 Percentage of drug-related problems across different treatment regimens

The study revealed that patients with cervical cancer and retroviral disease were 8.8 times (AOR = 8.8, 95% CI = 1.22–68.23, p = 0.037) more likely to have drug interactions as compared to cervical cancer patients without concurrent retroviral disease. The other patient

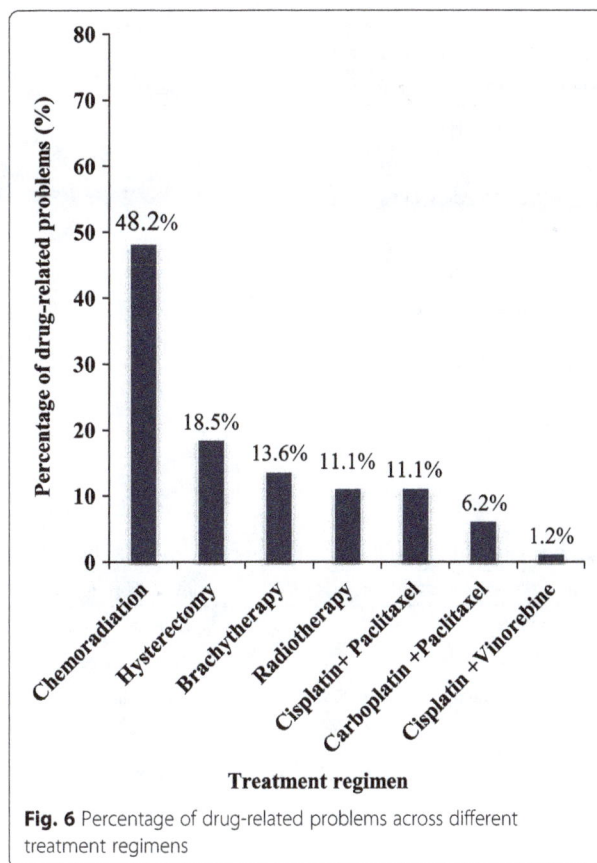

Fig. 5 Percentage of drug-related problems based on age group of cervical cancer patients

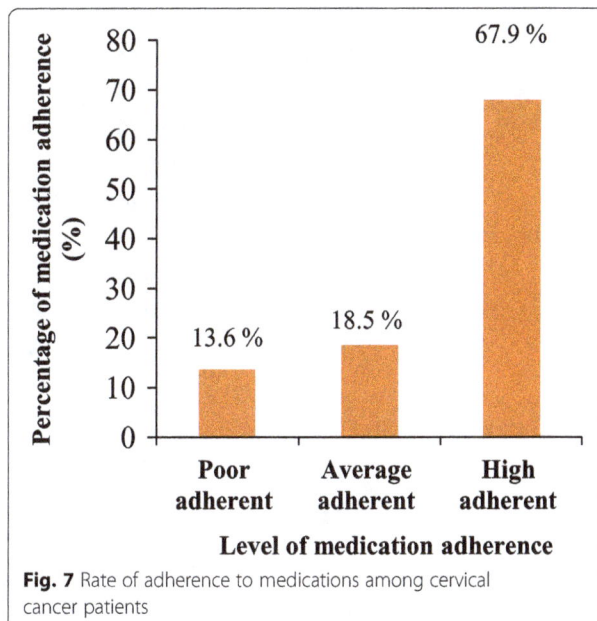

Fig. 7 Rate of adherence to medications among cervical cancer patients

Table 7 Reasons for medications non-adherence among cervical cancer patients (*n* = 26)

Reasons for medications non-adherence	Frequency	Percent
Forgetfulness	18	69.2
Expensive medications	4	15.4
side effects of medications	4	15.4
Long duration of therapy	2	7.7
Complicated regimens	2	7.7
Lack of trust on the efficacy of medications	1	3.8
Others	2	7.7

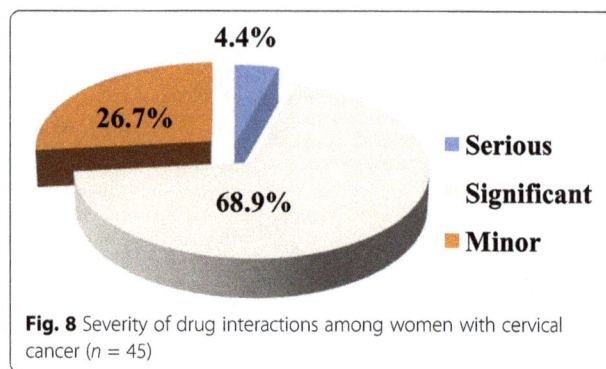

Fig. 8 Severity of drug interactions among women with cervical cancer (*n* = 45)

Table 8 Interacting drugs identified among cervical cancer patients (n = 45)

Severity of the interaction	Interacting drugs	Frequency	Percent
Serious interaction	Codeine + Tramadol	1	2.2
	Metronidazole + Erythromycin	1	2.2
Significant interaction	Amoxicillin +Hydrochlorothiazide	1	2.2
	Zidovudine +cisplatin	1	2.2
	Zidovudine +Cotrimoxazole	1	2.2
	Ceftriaxone + Enoxaparin	1	2.2
	Cisplatin + Gentamicin	1	2.2
	Codeine + Amitryptyline	1	2.2
	Codeine + Morphine	2	4.4
	Dexamethasone + Metronidazole	1	2.2
	Dexamethasone + Tramadol	1	2.2
	Dexamethasone + Paclitaxel	4	8.9
	Diclofenac + Dexamethasone	1	2.2
	Furosemide +Cisplatin	1	2.2
	Nifedipine + Atorvastatin	1	2.2
	Omeprazole + Ranferon	1	2.2
	Ondansetron + Dexamethasone	12	26.7
	Cotrimoxazole +Azithromycin	1	2.2
	Tenofovir + Cisplatin	1	2.2
Minor interaction	Dexamethasone + Amlodipine	1	2.2
	Diclofenac + Enoxaparin	1	2.2
	Eefavirenz + Paclitaxel	1	2.2
	Efavirenz +Tramadol	1	2.2
	Gabapentin + Paracetamol	1	2.2
	Metronidazole + Diclofenac	1	2.2
	Metronidazole + Gentamicin	1	2.2
	Metronidazole + Ibuprofen	1	2.2
	Metronidzole + Paclitaxel	1	2.2
	Nifedipine + Etoricoxib	1	2.2
	Omeprazole + Diazepam	1	2.2

Table 9 Types of adverse drug reactions in cervical cancer patients ($n = 81$)

Types of adverse drug reaction	Frequency	Percent
Vomiting	40	49.4
Nausea	24	29.6
Leucopoenia	18	22.2
Dizziness	13	16.0
Diarrhoea	10	12.3
Abdominal cramp & bloating	8	9.9
Neutropenia	8	9.9
Tinnitus	5	6.2
Low haemoglobin	4	4.9
constipation	3	3.7
thrombocytopenia	1	1.2
Others[a]	15	18.5

[a]Others include hypokalemia, skin rash, oesophageal irritation, bleeding, fatigue, loss of appetite

factors did not have statistically significant association with drug interactions (Table 12).

It was noted that patients treated with more than five drugs were 3.6 times (AOR = 3.6, 95% CI = 1.24–11.23, $p = 0.026$) more likely to have dosing problems as compared to patients treated with less than five medications. Besides, patients who had been managed with cisplatin and paclitaxel regimen were 9.8 times (AOR = 9.8, 95% CI = 1.25–77.81, $p = 0.030$) more likely to have dosing problems than patients who were not using this regimen (Table 13).

Discussion

The present study revealed that the mean age of the study participants was 53.3 ± 11.6 years, and the predominant portion of the study subjects 47(58.0%) were 51 years and above. This study is fairly comparable with similar studies conducted in India and Tanzania [20, 21].

Table 10 Univariable and multivariable binary logistic regression analysis of predictors of drug related problems

Variable	Univariable analysis		Multivariable analysis	
	COR (95% CI)	P value	AOR (95% CI)	P value
Age (years)				
29–39	1		1	
40–50	2.6(0.14–46.21)	0.525	3.4(0.13–241)	0.263
≥ 51	1.6(0.15–17.76)	0.689	2.3(0.14–59.22)	0.489
Education				
Illiterate	1		1	
Literate	1.9(0.18–18.81)	0.599	2.5(0.12–48.81)	0.541
Income (USD)				
< 100	1		1	
100–200	0.9(0.09–9.47)	0.938	1.2(0.12–13.52)	0.855
200–500	0.2(0.01–2.08)	0.162	0.1(0.00–1.13)	0.061
Marital status				
Single	1		1	
Married	0.8(0.08–7.23)	0.803	0.9(0.14–5.80)	0.927
Occupation				
Unemployed	1		1	
Employed	0.1(0.01–1.48)	0.096	0.1(0.01–1.41)	1.423
Co-morbidity				
No	1		1	
Yes	1.0(0.16–6.56)	0.982	0.8(0.11–5.11)	0.767
Number of medications				
< 5	1		1	
≥ 5	2.6(0.41–16.53)	0.321	2.5(0.32–21.61)	0.399
Stage of cervical cancer				
Early stage	1		1	
Advanced stage	9.9 (1.45–67.58)	0.019[*]	15.4 (1.3–185.87)	0.031[*]

COR Crude odds ratio, AOR Adjusted odds ratio, 95% CI 95% confidence interval, [*]Statistically significant: P value ≤0.05

Table 11 Univariable and multivariable binary logistic regression analysis of predictors of adverse drug reactions

Variable	Univariable analysis COR (95% CI)	P value	Multivariable analysis AOR (95% CI)	P value
Age (years)				
29–39	1		1	
40–50	0.2(0.02–1.45)	0.102	0.1(0.02–0.61)	0.013*
≥ 51	0.3(0.03–2.29)	0.227	0.2(0.03–1.2)	0.123
Education				
Illiterate	1		1	
Literate	1.59(0.41–6.26)	0.509	2.4(0.62–9.63)	0.231
Marital status				
Single	1		1	
Married	1.7(0.59–4.99)	0.314	1.7(0.52–5.93)	0.392
Occupation				
Unemployed	1		1	
Employed	0.9(0.08–10.44)	0.925	0.8(0.11–9.04)	0.845
Co-morbidity				
No	1		1	
Yes	0.8(0.30–2.15)	0.668	0.7(0.23–2.31)	0.582
Number of medications				
< 5	1		1	
≥ 5	2.9(1.12–7.78)	0.032*	2.9(0.91–9.0)	0.071
Type of cancer				
Adenocarcinoma & Invasive anaplastic carcinoma	1		1	
Squamous cell carcinoma	0.4(0.04–3.09)	0.343	0.1 (0.00–5.42)	0.271
Stage of cervical cancer				
Early stage	1		1	
Advanced stage	4.8(1.37–16.79)	0.014*	5.8(1.43–24.61)	0.017*

COR Crude odds ratio, *AOR* Adjusted odds ratio, *95% CI* 95% confidence interval, *Statistically significant: P value ≤0.05

Late incidence of cervical cancer in the older age may be due to the insidious transformation of the cervical epithelium into cancerous cells by the combined effects of high-risk strains of human papillomavirus (HPV) and other risk factors [22].

Most of the study population had stages IIB (33.3%) and IIIB (28.4%) cervical cancer while stages IA and IB2 were the least prevalent. Likewise, a similar study in India showed that stage IIIB (38%) and stage IIB (35%) were the most common clinical stages found in cervical cancer patients [21]. The high prevalence of locally advanced stage of cervical cancer patients in our setting may be due to inadequate understanding of the early symptoms of cervical cancer and poor habit of early screening. Moreover, since the majority of the patients had a maximum of primary level education, they might have inadequate understanding of the importance for early Pap smear screening leading to the predominance of advanced stage cervical cancer at the time of diagnosis. Most of the patients in stage I were managed using

surgical intervention. According to our eligibility criteria, the patients must be on drug or chemotherapy to be included in the study since we are as assessing drug related problems. Hence, majority of the patients in stage I were not eligible to be included in the study. Moreover, advanced radiological imaging techniques such as PET scan were not available in our facility to screen early stage of precancerous lesion in the cervix. That is why cervical cancer patients with stage I were least prevalent in our setting.

The mortality rate after stage IIIB was very high in our setting due to the progression of the disease. Besides, the rate of transfer to more advanced treatment facilities in advanced stage of the disease was very high. Those are the main reasons why cervical cancer patients with stage IV were very limited in our setting.

Most of the study participants (39.5%) did not have co-existing co-morbidities. Nonetheless, 35.8%, 17.3%, and 3.7% patients were diagnosed with one, two, three, and four and above co-morbidities, respectively. In contrast, a

Table 12 Univariable and multivariable binary logistic regression analysis of predictors of drug interactions

Variable	Univariable analysis COR (95% CI)	P value	Multivariable analysis AOR (95% CI	P value
Age (years)				
29–39	1		1	
40–50	1.1(0.22–6.73)	0.957	1.9(0.21–19.11)	0.558
≥ 51	0.2(0.02–1.54)	0.109	0.5 (0.04–6.11)	0.591
Education				
Illiterate	1		1	
Literate	1.1(0.13–10.38)	0.906	0.3(0.04–3.02)	0.318
Marital status				
Single	1		1	
Married	0.6(0.14–2.77)	0.529	1.2 (0.23–6.11)	0.851
Co-morbidity				
No	1		1	
Yes	6.1(0.71–51.61)	0.101	1.2(0.11–16.32)	0.882
Retroviral disease	14.0(2.93–66.72)	0.001[*]	8.8(1.22–68.23)	0.037[*]
Number of medications				
< 5	1		1	
≥ 5	0.45(0.11–1.85)	0.269	0.2(0.03–1.24)	0.081
Type of cancer				
Adenocarcinoma & Invasive anaplastic carcinoma	1		1	
Squamous cell carcinoma	0.3(0.42–1.62)	0.150	0.4(0.02–6.41)	0.723
Stage of cervical cancer				
Early stage	1		1	
Advanced stage	0.6(0.11–3.48)	0.597	1.5(0.21–11.72)	0.651

COR Crude odds ratio, AOR Adjusted odds ratio, 95% CI 95% confidence interval, [*]Statistically significant: P value ≤0.05

similar study in Zimbabwe indicated that majority of the study participants (79.4%) had concurrent co-morbidities [23]. In the present study, the most common co-morbidity was anaemia (25.9%) probably arising from tumour-induced bleeding and iron deficiency secondary to malignancy [24]. This finding is in agreement with an Iranian study in which anaemia was the most common (59.0%) complication among cervical cancer patients [25]. Contrastingly, a study done in Nigeria identified hypertension (29.8%) and diabetes mellitus (27.4%) as the most common co-morbidities in cervical cancer patients [26].

Retroviral disease (18.3%) was the second leading type of co-morbidity in cervical cancer patients. Correspondingly, a cross-sectional study in Zimbabwe showed that 25.6% of the study participants had a retroviral disease [27]. In addition, some studies have shown that a strong association exists between human immunodeficiency virus (HIV) infection and cervical cancer with a high prevalence of high-risk HPV DNA in women with HIV infection [28, 29]. This could probably be due to a weakened immune system secondary to retrovirus infection which puts them at higher risk of HPV infections.

Moreover, the retrovirus may augment the oncogenic activities of HPV which predispose the patients to develop cervical cancer [30]. Although thromboembolic disorders are among the top ranked co-morbidities in cervical cancer patients [31], they had relatively low occurrence among the study participants.

Chemoradiation was the most widely used treatment regimen in the management of cervical cancer at KNH accounting for 50.6% of treatment modalities which is higher than in a similar study conducted in Ethiopia (37.6%) [32]. In the present study, cisplatin and paclitaxel (11.1%) were the most commonly used combination anticancer agents in the treatment of cervical cancer. Contrastingly, cisplatin and 5-fluorouracil combination regimen was widely used in a Nigerian study [26].

The study showed that granisetron and dexamethasone combination was the most commonly used prophylactic antiemetic in our setting with a usage frequency of 39.5%, followed by a combination of ondansetron and dexamethasone (22.2%). Serotonin receptor type 3 (5-HT$_3$) antagonists such as ondansetron and granisetron are the gold standard treatment protocol for chemotherapy-induced nausea and

Table 13 Univariable and multivariable binary logistic regression analysis of predictors of dosing problems

Variable	Univariable analysis COR (95% CI)	P-Value	Multivariable analysis AOR (95% CI)	P-value
Age (years)				
29–39	1		1	
40–50	1.7(0.34–8.15)	0.529	2.4(0.32–17.61)	0.412
≥ 51	1.5(0.32–6.39)	0.625	1.7(0.24–11.52)	
Education				
Illiterate	1		1	
Literate	2.8(0.54–14.11)	0.221	4.2(0.60–30.01)	0.161
Marital status				
Single	1		1	
Married	1.6(0.54–4.82)	0.386	1.2(0.42–3.71)	0.761
Co-morbidity				
No	1		1	
Yes	0.4(0.17–1.11)	0.084	0.4(0.11–1.32)	0.125
Number of medications				
< 5	1		1	
≥ 5	3.2(1.15–8.73)	0.026[*]	3.6(1.24–11.23)	0.026[*]
Type of cancer				
Adenocarcinoma & Invasive anaplastic carcinoma	1		1	
Squamous cell carcinoma	1.6(0.29–8.96)	0.586	1.5(0.32–7.43)	0.614
Stage of cervical cancer				
Early stage	1		1	
Advanced stage	2.3(0.58–9.33)	0.231	3.2(0.72–13.62)	0.121
Treatment Regimen				
Cisplatin + Paclitaxel	3.7(0.9–16.5)	0.079	9.8(1.25–77.81)	0.030[*]

COR Crude odds ratio, AOR Adjusted odds ratio, 95% CI 95% confidence interval, *Statistically significant: P value ≤0.05

vomiting due to superior efficacy and better tolerability of side effects as compared to conventional antiemetics [33]. The 5-HT$_3$ receptor antagonists are also preferred over dopamine receptor antagonists since they are devoid of extrapyramidal side effects [34]. Previous studies reported that the efficacy of 5-HT$_3$-receptor antagonists was augmented with the addition of dexamethasone [35]. Although equivalent doses of different 5-HT$_3$-receptor antagonists had comparable efficacy [34], a combination of ondansetron and dexamethasone use was not common in our setting due to drug-drug interaction. This finding corroborated the frequent use of granisetron and dexamethasone combination in our setting which is in line with the standard protocol [35].

The finding of 93.8% prevalence of DRPs in our setting is fairly higher than in a similar Norwegian study (73%) [36]. However, the finding of this study is comparable with a similar study done in Nigeria which showed that the prevalence of DRPs in cervical cancer patients was 89.2% [26]. Besides, a mean of 2.65 ± 1.22 drug therapy problems were identified in the study population which

is relatively higher than 2.1 DRPs detected per patient in a study done in Norway [36]. The higher prevalence DRPs in our setting may be due to inadequate understanding of the disease and medications among the patients and absence of local standard treatment protocols for cervical cancer patients.

There was a high preponderance of DRPs in the 51 years and above age group that accounted for 54.3% of the cases. This could probably be due to the high prevalence of co-morbidities in patients 51 years and above (29.6%) and the ageing of the metabolising organs which predispose the patient to DRPs.

Adverse drug reactions (69.1%) and drug interactions (46.9%) were the most prevalent DRPs, a finding that is in agreement with a similar study done in Nigeria [26] but higher than a finding reported by a Singaporean study [37]. The high incidence of ADRs may be attributed to the complexity and immunosuppressive effects of cancer treatment regimens.

Nausea and vomiting were among the top ranking ADRs. These findings are in line with a study done in

India in which nausea and vomiting were prevalent among cancer patients treated with anticancer agents [38, 39]. This could probably be linked to the emetogenic potential of cisplatin and paclitaxel and the cytotoxic effects of anticancer agents in the highly proliferating cells of the gastrointestinal tract. Additionally, the higher incidence of nausea and vomiting could be due to poor management of delayed nausea and vomiting secondary to the anticancer agents.

Although morphine, tramadol and codeine were the most commonly used pain medications, only 3.7% of the population had constipation as ADR. In our facility, these pain medications were usually given along with stool softeners and this clinical practice could probably be the main reason why constipation due to these opioids-based pain medications was not a major issue in our setting. Pain control was in line with WHO guideline for pain control in cancer patients and hence we didn't notice any discrepancies except drug interactions due to the combined use of two opioid analgesics (i.e. codeine and morphine) among 4.4% of the study participants. Pain medications were considered as essential drugs for palliative care treatment in cancer patients in Kenya [40]. Hence, almost all public healthcare facilities offering cancer treatment were universally accessible to these essential drugs. However, controlled pain medications such as opioid analgesics were accessed to cancer patients under supervised prescription by the palliative care specialists. In addition, being controlled drugs those medicines may not be available at the lower level of healthcare facilities.

When age was taken into consideration, elderly patients (age ≥ 51 years) had encountered most (40.7%) of the ADRs. This finding is similar to that reported by Poddar et al. [41] where the incidence of ADRs among geriatric patients was significantly higher than other age groups. This may be due to diminished metabolising capacity and excretory functions in the elderly patients leading to accumulation of drugs in the body and thus increasing the risk of ADRs [42].

Chemoradiation was the most commonly used treatment modality and was also associated with the majority of the ADRs in our setting which is comparable with other studies [43, 44]. Furthermore, the present study revealed that 33.3% and 28.4% patients had stage IIB and IIIB cervical cancer, respectively which were categorised as locally advanced cervical cancer. It has been shown that chemoradiation is the standard treatment of choice in the management of locally advanced cervical cancer due to the overall tolerability of side effects and enhancement of survival [45, 46]. This could probably be the reason why this regimen was widely used in our setting and was therefore associated with the majority of the ADRs.

Due to the complexity of the chemotherapeutic regimens, cancer patients are susceptible to potential drug interactions. Not surprisingly, this study unveiled that 46.9% of cervical cancer patients had potential drug interactions in the treatment regimens. A similar study in Dutch reported 46% prevalence of potential drug interactions among cancer patients [47]. This high prevalence of drug interactions may step up the adverse effects of anticancer agents or lessen the therapeutic outcomes of the treatment regimen. With regard to severity, 68.9% significant drug interactions were detected from the treatment regimens of cervical cancer patients which is slightly higher than a study done in Tehran that reported a prevalence of 59.7% [48]. However, only 4.4% of the drug interactions were identified as serious drug interaction which necessitates use of alternative drug regimens.

Ondansetron and dexamethasone were the most common interacting drugs accounting for 26.7% of the total drug interactions. Previous studies reported that premedication of dexamethasone diminished the efficacy of paclitaxel in breast cancer and ovarian carcinoma [49, 50]. According to the findings of the present study, dexamethasone and paclitaxel accounted for 8.9% of the drug interactions. Thus, it is plausible to assume that the prophylactic use of dexamethasone antiemetic in paclitaxel-based regimens might reduce the antitumor activity of paclitaxel in cervical cancer patients.

A cross-sectional descriptive study conducted in Ethiopia revealed that 69.7% of cervical cancer patients were adherent to their treatment regimens while 30.3% of patients were non-adherent [32]. Similarly, 67.9% of cervical cancer patients were adherent to their treatment regimens in our setting. However, the rate of medication adherence (61.1%) among cervical cancer patients in India was slightly lower than our setting [51]. This could probably be due to the availability of better facilities to strengthen the awareness of the patients about their medications adherence at the Oncology Units of KNH.

Among 26 non-adherent cervical cancer patients, forgetfulness (69.2%), expensive medications (15.4%) and side effects of medications (15.4%) were the main reasons for non-adherence while long duration of therapy and complicated regimens contributed equivalently (7.7%) to medication non-adherence. On the other hand, lack of trust on the efficacy of medicines was the least common reason for non-adherence in cervical cancer patients at KNH. Comparatively, a study from Ethiopia revealed that long duration of therapy, side effects of the medication and expensive medication were among the top-ranking reasons for medication non-adherence in cervical cancer patients [32].

The present study revealed that patients with advanced stage cervical cancer were 15.4 times (AOR = 15.4, 95%

CI = 1.3–185.87, p = 0.031) more likely to have DRPs as compared to patients with early stage cervical cancer. In addition, patients with advanced stage cervical cancer were 5.9 times (AOR = 5.9, 95% CI = 1.4–24.6, p = 0.017) more likely to experience ADRs as compared to patients with early stage disease.

Koh et al. [52] reported that multiple uses of drugs were a significant predictor of the incidence of DRPs. Hence, the higher likelihood of DRPs in the advanced stage cervical cancer may be due to multiple medications secondary to the complexity of the conditions which predispose the patients to DRPs. Likewise, stage of cervical cancer was the only predictor of DRPs in cervical cancer patients. Previous studies in Sweden [53], Malaysia [54], Nigeria [26] and Ethiopia [55] reported that polypharmacy and presence of co-morbidities were positively associated with DRPs. Conversely, our study revealed that number of medications and presence of co-morbidities were not statistically significant predictors of drug related problems.

Patients who had been treated with more than five drugs were more likely to have ADRs and dosing problems and less likely to have inappropriate laboratory monitoring as compared to patients treated with less than five medications. Similarly, previous study in Pakistan showed that polypharmacy was positively associated with ADRs [56]. Moreover, a similar study in Singapore showed that chronic use of five or more drugs was associated with the presence of DRPs [37]. The higher likelihood of having ADRs may plausibly be due to the enhanced pharmacological effects of the drugs secondary to the undesired drug interaction at the level of metabolism and excretion.

In the univariable logistic regression analysis, patients who had been managed with cisplatin and paclitaxel regimen were 9.8 times more likely to have dosing problems. Additionally, cervical cancer patients with the retroviral disease were 8.8 times (AOR = 8.8, 95% CI = 1.2–68, p = 0.037) more likely to have drug interactions as compared to patients without concurrent retroviral disease. Conversely, the other sociodemographic factors did not have statistically significant association with drug interactions. The higher likelihood of having drug interactions may plausibly be due to the complexity of drug regimens in the management of both conditions. Previous studies showed that an increased risk of nephrotoxicity due to the combination tenofovir and platinum analogues such as cisplatin particularly in patients with renal insufficiency. Moreover, there was a mounting report of haematological toxicity with a combination of taxane class of anticancer agents such as paclitaxel and zidovudine [57]. Since the majority of cervical cancer patients with retroviral disease were treated with tenofovir and cisplatin-based regimens in our setting, they were a higher risk of having nephrotoxicity due to drug-drug interaction between the anticancer and anti retroviral agents. Hence, having a retroviral disease as co-morbidity in cervical patients might be an important predictor for drug interaction.

Conclusion
Adverse drug reactions, drug interactions, and need of additional drug therapy were the most common DRPs identified among cervical cancer patients. Nausea and vomiting were the most prevalent ADRs among the study participants. In the multivariable binary logistic regression analysis, advanced stage of cervical cancer and treatment with more than five drugs were significant predictors of ADRs. Likewise, coexisting retroviral disease and treatment with more than five medications were predictors of drug interactions and dosing problems, respectively.

Abbreviations
ADRs: Adverse Drug Reactions; AOR: Adjusted Odds Ratio; CI: Confidence Interval; COR: Crude Odds Ratio; DRPs: Drug Related Problems; ESMO: European Society for Medical Oncology; GFR: Glomerular Filtration Rate.; NCCN: National Compressive Cancer Network.; USD: United States Dollar.; WHO: World Health Organization

Acknowledgments
The authors would like to acknowledge AFIMEGQ Programme for financial support towards this project.

Funding
The study was conducted under the financial support of Africa for Innovation, Mobility, Exchange, Globalization and Quality (AFIMEGQ) Programme.

Author's contribution
AD conducted the actual study and the statistical analysis. AD, PN, IW and PK were involved in developing the idea, designing of the study and the write up of the manuscript. All authors approved the submitted version of the manuscript.

Competing interests
The authors declare that they have no competing interest.

Author details
¹Department of Pharmaceutics and Pharmacy Practice, University of Nairobi, College of Health Sciences, School of Pharmacy, P.O. Box 19676-00202, Nairobi, Kenya. ²Department of Pharmaceutical Chemistry, University of Nairobi, College of Health Sciences, School of Pharmacy, Nairobi 19676-00202, Kenya. ³Kenyatta National Hospital, Division of Pharmacy, Nairobi 20723-00202, Kenya.

References

1. World Health Organization. The Pursuit of responsible use of medicines: sharing and learning from Country experiences [Internet]. Amsterdam; 2012. Available from: http://apps.who.int/iris/bitstream/10665/75828/1/WHO_EMP_MAR_2012.3_eng.pdf?ua=1

2. World Health Organization. Essential medicines and health products [Internet]. 2015 [cited 2016 Oct 28]. Available from: http://www.who.int/medicines/areas/rational_use/en/

3. Ruths S, Viktil KK, Blix HS. Classification of drug-related problems. Tidsskr Nor Laegeforen. 2007;127(23):3073–6.

4. Cipolle R, Strand L, Morley P. Pharmaceutical care practice: the patient-centered approach to medication management services. 3rd ed. USA: McGraw-hill Education; 2012.

5. Jaehde U, Liekweg A, Simons S, Westfeld M. Minimising treatment-associated risks in systemic cancer therapy. Pharm World Sci. 2008;30(2):161–8.

6. Cehajic I, Bergan S, Bjordal K. Pharmacist assessment of drug-related problems on an oncology ward. Eur J Hosp Pharm. 2015;22(4):194–7.

7. Iftikhar A, Jehanzeb K, Ullah A. Clinical pharmacy services in medical oncology unit, Peshawar, Pakistan. Pharmacologyonline. 2015;1:10–2.

8. Ambili R. Toxicities of anticancer drugs and its management. Int J Basic Clin Pharmacol. 2012;1(1):2–12.

9. Ikushima H, Osaki K, Furutani S, Yamashita K, Kawanaka T, Kishida Y, et al. Chemoradiation therapy for cervical cancer: toxicity of concurrent weekly cisplatin. Radiat Med. 2006;24(2):115–21.

10. Koh Y, Kutty FB, Li SC. Drug-related problems in hospitalized patients on polypharmacy: the influence of age and gender. Ther Clin Risk Manag. 2005;1(1):39–48.

11. Kasiulevicius V, Sapoka V, Filipaviciute R. Sample size calculation in epidemiological studies. Gerontologija. 2006;7(4):225–31.

12. Ministry of Health. National Guidelines for Cancer Management Kenya [Internet]. 2013 [cited 2017 Jun 15]. Available from: http://kehpca.org/wp-content/uploads/National-Cancer-Treatment-Guidelines2.pdf

13. National Compressive Cancer Network. NCCN Clinical Practice Guidelines in Oncology: Cervical Cancer. [Internet]. 2016 [cited 2017 Jun 15]. Available from: https://www.nccn.org/professionals/physician_gls/pdf/cervical.pdf

14. Marth C, Landoni F, Mahner S, McCormack M, Gonzalez-Martin A, Colombo N. Cervical cancer: ESMO Clinical Practice Guidelines for diagnosis, treatment and follow-up. Ann Oncol. 2017;28(Supplement 4):iv72–83.

15. World Health Organization. Cancer pain relief: with a guide to opioid availability [Internet]. 1996 [cited 2016 Nov 30]. Available from: http://apps.who.int/iris/bitstream/10665/37896/1/9241544821.pdf

16. Oliveira-Filho AD, Barreto-Filho JA, Neves SJ, Lyra Junior DP. Association between the 8-item Morisky medication adherence scale (MMAS-8) and blood pressure control. Arq Bras Cardiol. 2012;99(1):649–58.

17. Levey AS, Coresh J, Greene T, Marsh J, Stevens LA, Kusek JW, et al. Expressing the modification of diet in renal disease study equation for estimating glomerular filtration rate with standardized serum creatinine values. Clin Chem. 2007;53(4):766–2.

18. Du Bois D, Du Bois EFA. Formula to estimate the approximate surface area if height and weight be known. 1916. Nutrition. 1989;5(5):303–11.

19. van Warmerdam LJ, Rodenhuis S, ten Bokkel Huinink WW, Maes RA, Beijnen JH. The use of the Calvert formula to determine the optimal carboplatin dosage. J Cancer Res Clin Oncol. 1995;121(8):478–86.

20. Majinge PM. Treatment outcome of cervical cancer patients at ocean road cancer institute, Dar es salaam [internet]. Muhimbili University of Health and Allied. Sciences. 2011; Available from: http://ihi.eprints.org/966/

21. Chauhan R, Trivedi V, Rani R, Singh U. A hospital based study of clinical profile of cervical cancer catients of Bihar, an eastern state of India. Womens Heal Gynecol. 2016;2(2):1–4.

22. Burd EM. Human papillomavirus and cervical cancer. Clin Microbiol Rev. 2003;16(1):1–17.

23. Kagura Y. A study to determine the relationship between prevalence of late stage diagnosis of cervical cancer and number of comorbid illnesses in women aged 65 years and above in Zimbabwe [internet]. University of Zimbabwe; 2015. Available from: http://ir.uz.ac.zw/jspui/bitstream/10646/2901/1/Kagura_A-Study_to_Determine_The_Relationship_Between_Prevalence_Of_Late_Stage_Diagnosis_Of_Cervical_Cancer_.pdf

24. Candelaria M, Cetina L, Duenas-Gonzalez A. Anemia in cervical cancer patients: implications for iron supplementation therapy. Med Oncol. 2005;22(2):161–8.

25. Shahbazian H, Marrefi MS, Arvandi S, Shahbazian N. Investigating the prevalence of anemia and its relation with disease stage and patients ' age with cervical cancer referred to Department of Radiotherapy and Oncology of Ahvaz Golestan hospital during 2004-2008. Int J Pharm Res Allied Sci. 2016;5(2):190–3.

26. Mustapha S. Drug related problems in cervical cancer patients on chemotherapy in Ahmadu Bello University teaching hospital, Nigeria [internet]. Near East University; 2016. Available from: http://docs.neu.edu.tr/library/6405400533.pdf

27. Chirenje ZM, Loeb L, Mwale M, Nyamapfeni P, Kamba M, Padian N. Association of cervical SIL and HIV-1 infection among Zimbabwean women in an HIV/STI prevention study. Int J STD AIDS. 2002;13(11):765–8.

28. Holmes RS, Hawes SE, Toure P, Dem A, Feng Q, Weiss NS, et al. HIV infection as a risk factor for cervical cancer and cervical intraepithelial neoplasia in Senegal. Cancer Epidemiol Biomark Prev. 2009;18(9):2442–6.

29. Adjorlolo-Johnson G, Unger ER, Boni-Ouattara E, Touré-Coulibaly K, Maurice C, Vernon SD, et al. Assessing the relationship between HIV infection and cervical cancer in Côte d'Ivoire: a case-control study. BMC Infect Dis. 2010;10:242.

30. Mandelblatt JS, Kanetsky P, Eggert L, Gold KIHIV. Infection a cofactor for cervical squamous cell neoplasia? Cancer Epidemiol Biomark Prev. 1999;8(1):97–106.

31. Barbera L, Thomas G. Venous thromboembolism in cervical cancer. Lancet Oncol. 2008;9(1):54–60.

32. Gebre Y, Zemene A, Fantahun A, Aga F. Assessment of treatment compliance and associated factors among cervical cancer patients in Tikur Anbessa specialized hospital, oncology unit, Ethiopia 2012. Int J Cancer Stud Res. 2015;4:67–74.

33. Hesketh PJ. Comparative review of 5-HT3 receptor antagonists in the treatment of acute chemotherapy-induced nausea and vomiting. Cancer Investig. 2000;18:163–73.

34. Goodin S, Cunningham R. 5-HT(3)-receptor antagonists for the treatment of nausea and vomiting: a reappraisal of their side-effect profile. Oncologist. 2002;7(5):424–36.

35. National Compressive Cancer Network. NCCN Clinical Practice Guideline in Oncology:Antiemsis version1 [Internet]. 2015 [cited 2017 Jul 23]. Available from: http://www.prolekare.cz/dokumenty/Antiemetikum_guidelines.pdf

36. Cehajic I, Bergan S, Bjorda K. Pharmacist assessment of drug-related problems on an oncology ward. Eur J Hosp Pharm. 2015;22(4):1–4.

37. Yeoh TT, Tay XY, Si P, Chew L. Drug-related problems in elderly patients with cancer receiving outpatient chemotherapy. J Geriatr Oncol. 2015;6(4):280–7.

38. Wahlang JB, Laishram PD, Brahma DK, Sarkar C, Lahon J, Nongkynrih BS. Adverse drug reactions due to cancer chemotherapy in a tertiary care teaching hospital. Ther Adv Drug Saf. 2017;8(2):61–6.

39. Sharma A, Kumari KM, Manohar HD, Bairy KL, Thomas J. Pattern of adverse drug reactions due to cancer chemotherapy in a tertiary care hospital in South India. Perspect Clin Res. 2015;6(2):109–15.

40. Ministry of Health. Kenya Essential Medicines List [Internet]. 2016 [cited 2017 Sep 21]. Available from: http://apps.who.int/medicinedocs/documents/s23035en/s23035en.pdf

41. Poddar S, Sultana R, Sultana R, Akbor MM, Azad MAK, Hasnat A. Pattern of adverse drug reactions due to cancer chemotherapy in tertiary care teaching Hospital in Bangladesh. Dhaka Univ. J Pharm Sci. 2009;8(1):11–6.

42. Klotz U. Pharmacokinetics and drug metabolism in the elderly. Drug Metab Rev. 2009;41(2):67–76.

43. Duenas-Gonzalez A, Cetina L, Coronel J, Gonzalez-Fierro A. The safety of drug treatments for cervical cancer. Expert Opin Drug Saf. 2016;15(2):169–80.

44. Surendiran A, Balamurugan N, Gunaseelan K, Akhtar S, Reddy KS, Adithan C. Adverse drug reaction profile of cisplatin-based chemotherapy regimen in a tertiary care hospital in India: an evaluative study. Indian J Pharmacol. 2010;42(1):40–3.

45. Todo Y, Watari H. Concurrent chemoradiotherapy for cervical cancer: background including evidence-based data, pitfalls of the data, limitation of treatment in certain groups. Chin J Cancer Res. 2016;28(2):221–7.

46. Lukka H, Hirte H, Fyles A, Thomas G, Elit L, Johnston M, et al. Concurrent cisplatin-based chemotherapy plus radiotherapy for cervical cancer–a meta-analysis. Clin Oncol. 2002;14(3):203–12.

47. van Leeuwen RW, Brundel DH, Neef C, van Gelder T, Mathijssen RH, Burger DM, et al. Prevalence of potential drug-drug interactions in cancer patients treated with oral anticancer drugs. Br J Cancer. 2013;108(5):1071–8.

48. Tavakoli-Ardakani M, Kazemian K, Salamzadeh J, Mehdizadeh M. Potential of drug interactions among hospitalized cancer patients in a developing country. Iran J Pharm Res. 2013;12:175–82.

49. Sui M, Chen F, Chen Z, Fan W. Glucocorticoids interfere with therapeutic efficacy of paclitaxel against human breast and ovarian xenograft tumors. Int J Cancer. 2006;119:712–7.

50. Hou WJ, Guan JH, Dong Q, Han YH, Zhang R. Dexamethasone inhibits the effect of paclitaxel on human ovarian carcinoma xenografts in nude mice. Eur Rev Med Pharmacol Sci. 2013;17(21):2902–8.

51. Dutta S, Biswas N, Muhkherjee G. Evaluation of socio-demographic factors for non-compliance to treatment in locally advanced cases of cancer cervix in a rural medical College Hospital in India. Indian J Palliat Care. 2013;19(3):158–65.

52. Koh Y, Kutty FB, Li SC. Drug-related problems in hospitalized patients on polypharmacy: the influence of age and gender. Ther Clin Risk Manag. 2005; 1(1):39–40.

53. Peterson C, Gustafsson M. Characterisation of drug-related problems and associated factors at a clinical pharmacist service-naive Hospital in Northern Sweden. Drugs Real World Outcomes. 2017;4(2):97–107.

54. Zaman Huri H, Hui Xin C, Sulaiman CZ. Drug-related problems in patients with benign prostatic hyperplasia: a cross sectional retrospective study. PLoS One. 2014;9(1):e86215.

55. Sisay EA, Engidawork E, Yesuf TA, Ketema EB. Drug related problems in chemotherapy of cancer patients. J Cancer Sci Ther. 2015;7(2):55–9.

56. Ahmed B, Nanji K, Mujeeb R, Patel MJ. Effects of polypharmacy on adverse drug reactions among geriatric outpatients at a tertiary care hospital in Karachi: a prospective cohort study. PLoS One. 2014;9(11):e112133.

57. Makinson A, Pujol JL, Le Moing V, Peyriere H, Reynes J. Interactions between cytotoxic chemotherapy and antiretroviral treatment in human immunodeficiency virus-infected patients with lung cancer. J Thorac Oncol. 2010;5(4):562–71.

21

Improving attendance to genetic counselling services for gynaecological oncology patients

Hanoon P. Pokharel[1,2,3*], Neville F. Hacker[1,2] and Lesley Andrews[4,5]

Abstract

Background: Gynaecological cancers may be the sentinel malignancy in women who carry a mutation in BRCA1 or 2, a mis-match repair gene causing Lynch Syndrome or other genes. Despite published guidelines for referral to a genetics service, a substantial number of women do not attend for the recommended genetic assessment. The study aims to determine the outcomes of systematic follow-up of patients diagnosed with ovarian or endometrial cancer from Gynaecologic-oncology multidisciplinary meetings who were deemed appropriate for genetics assessment.

Methods: Women newly diagnosed with gynaecological cancer at the Royal Hospital for Women between 2010 and 2014 (cohort1) and 2015–2016 (cohort 2) who were identified as suitable for genetics assessment were checked against the New South Wales/Australian Capital Territory genetic database. The doctors of non-attenders were contacted regarding suitability for re-referral, and patients who were still suitable for genetics assessment were contacted by mail. Attendance was again checked against the genetics database.

Results: Among 462 patients in cohort 1, flagged for genetic assessment, 167 had not consulted a genetic service at initial audit conducted in 2014. 86 (18.6%) women whose referral was pending clarification of family history and/or immunohistochemistry did not require further genetic assessment. Letters were sent to 40 women. 7 women (1.5%) attended hereditary cancer clinic in the following 6 months.

The audit conducted in 2016 identified 148 patients (cohort 2) appropriate for genetic assessment at diagnosis. 66 (44.6%) had been seen by a genetics service, 51 (34.5%) whose referral was pending additional information did not require further genetic assessment. Letters were sent to 15 women, of whom 9 (6.1%) attended genetics within 6 months.

Conclusions: To improve the effectiveness of guidelines for the genetic referral of women newly diagnosed with ovarian cancer, clinicians need to obtain a thorough family history at diagnosis; arrange for reflex MMR IHC according to guidelines; offer BRCA or panel testing to all women with non-mucinous ovarian cancer prior to discharge and systematically follow up all women referred to genetics at the post-op visit.

Keywords: BRCA1, BRCA2, Genetic testing, Mainstreaming, Hereditary cancer clinic, Efficacy, Effectiveness

Background

Gynaecological cancers have been recognised as the sentinel cancer in Lynch Syndrome, as well as Hereditary Breast Ovarian Cancer and site specific hereditary ovarian cancer, and provide an opportunity to identify families with mutations in MMR, BRCA1/2 or other gynaecological cancer predisposition genes according to

established guidelines [1]. Referral of women newly diagnosed with gynaecological cancer for genetic assessment is based on their personal and family history, their histopathology (high grade serous ovarian cancer in suspected BRCA1/2 mutation carriers or endometrioid, mucinous, clear cell or mixed endometrial or ovarian cancer in suspected Lynch Syndrome) or abnormal mismatch repair immunohistochemistry [2]. As BRCA1/2 mutation carriers can experience meaningful disease control from platinum based chemotherapy and poly ADP-ribose polymerase (PARP) inhibitor treatment

* Correspondence: hanoon.pokharel@gmail.com
[1]Gynaecologic Cancer Centre, Royal Hospital for Women, Sydney, Australia
[2]School of Women's and Children's Health, University of New South Wales, Sydney, Australia
Full list of author information is available at the end of the article

upon tumor relapse, there is an increasing clinical need to offer genetic testing to these women [3, 4]. Identification of a BRCA1 or BRCA2 mutation also alerts the woman to her increased risks of breast cancer. Women identified with Lynch Syndrome following a diagnosis of endometrial or ovarian cancer face a lifetime risk of colorectal cancer of around 30%, which is similar to the risk of endometrial cancer for an unaffected woman with a mis-match repair mutation, while the risk of ovarian cancer for an unaffected woman with Lynch Syndrome is around 9%.

With the advent next generation sequencing, panel testing has shown to increase the detection of germline mutations that lead to increased risk of breast, ovarian, and other cancers and can better guide individualized screening measures compared to limited BRCA testing alone. At the same time, multi-gene panel testing is more time-and cost-efficient [5].

Furthermore, predictive testing for family members of women with a pathogenic variant in genes such as the MMR genes, BRCA1/2, RAD51C, RAD51D and BRIP1 provides options for reducing their cancer risk, with screening, surgery or chemoprevention.

Despite the proven benefits for affected women and their relatives, ensuring all potential cases have genetics assessment is challenging. The normal workflow for genetic referral is shown in fig. 1 [6].

A previous audit of women diagnosed with a gynaecological cancer at the Royal Hospital for Women found that 167 of 462 women who were recommended for further genetics assessment between 2010 and 2014, had not been seen by a genetics service in New South Wales or Australian Capital Territory (NSW/ACT) by February 2016 [7]. This indicates that there is a gap between the efficacy and effectiveness of guidelines to identify gynaecological cancer mutation carriers.

A recent paper described the difference between efficacy and effectiveness with regard to the identification of BRCA1/2 mutation carriers amongst women diagnosed with breast cancer. Efficacy refers to the performance of an intervention under ideal and controlled circumstances. Effectiveness can be defined as the performance of an intervention under "real world" circumstances [8]. It was found that effectiveness of BRCA testing criteria was much lower than efficacy. Hence, the current testing criteria and procedures accompanying BRCA ½ testing are insufficient, and there is room for improving efficacy and effectiveness [8].

Irrespective of family history, 17% of women aged 70 years or younger with newly diagnosed high grade serous ovarian cancer (HGSOC) harbor a germline BRCA1/2 pathologic variant [9]. Despite International guidelines recommending testing for patients with high grade serous ovarian cancer (HGSOC) for germline BRCA1 and BRCA2 pathological variants, the uptake of genetic testing in this patient group remains low, with 19.6% of eligible patients with ovarian cancer declining test [10, 11]. The low rate of genetic testing in eligible patients is likely multifactorial. A lack of awareness or misunderstanding of referral guidelines are likely to contribute to non-referral [11].

Additionally the barriers to genetic counselling and testing have been identified in gynaecological oncology patients, including insufficient family history collection, lack of referral, insufficient insurance/cost of the appointment, anxiety for the results, lack of interest, patient/family not wanting to know information regarding cancer risks, and lack of understanding regarding benefits of genetic testing and available preventive measures [12–14].

At the time of our previous audit no formal follow- up recommendation was in place. We sought to determine if delayed (more than one year) or short-term (less than one year) follow- up improved adherence to multidisciplinary meeting recommendations regarding genetic assessment and patient attendance at hereditary cancer clinics.

Methods

All patients undergoing surgery at the Royal Hospital for Women Gynaecologic Cancer Unit are reviewed at the weekly multidisciplinary team (MDT) meeting which is attended by a genetic consultant or a genetic counsellor. Women diagnosed with ovarian, peritoneal, fallopian tube or endometrial cancer warranting further genetic assessment or genetic testing are then referred to the Hereditary Cancer Clinic.

Our previous study identified two cohorts of women. The first cohort included all cases of new or recurrent gynaecological cancer diagnosed between 2010 and 2014 who were recommended for genetics assessment at the weekly multidisciplinary review [7]. The statewide genetics database (Kintrak/Trakgene) identified those who had been assessed by a genetics service in New South Wales or Australian Capital Territory, allowing us to determine those who had not had appropriate genetics follow-up at a public genetics service. The second cohort was those women discussed at the review meeting between July 1, 2015 and June 30, 2016 who were recommended but had not had genetics assessment.

The treating gynaecologist of each woman was contacted and advised that genetics assessment was not recorded. They were asked to reply if further information had indicated if further information indicated genetics assessment was not indicated (clarification of family history, MMR IHC), if the woman was deceased, or if genetics assessment had been completed

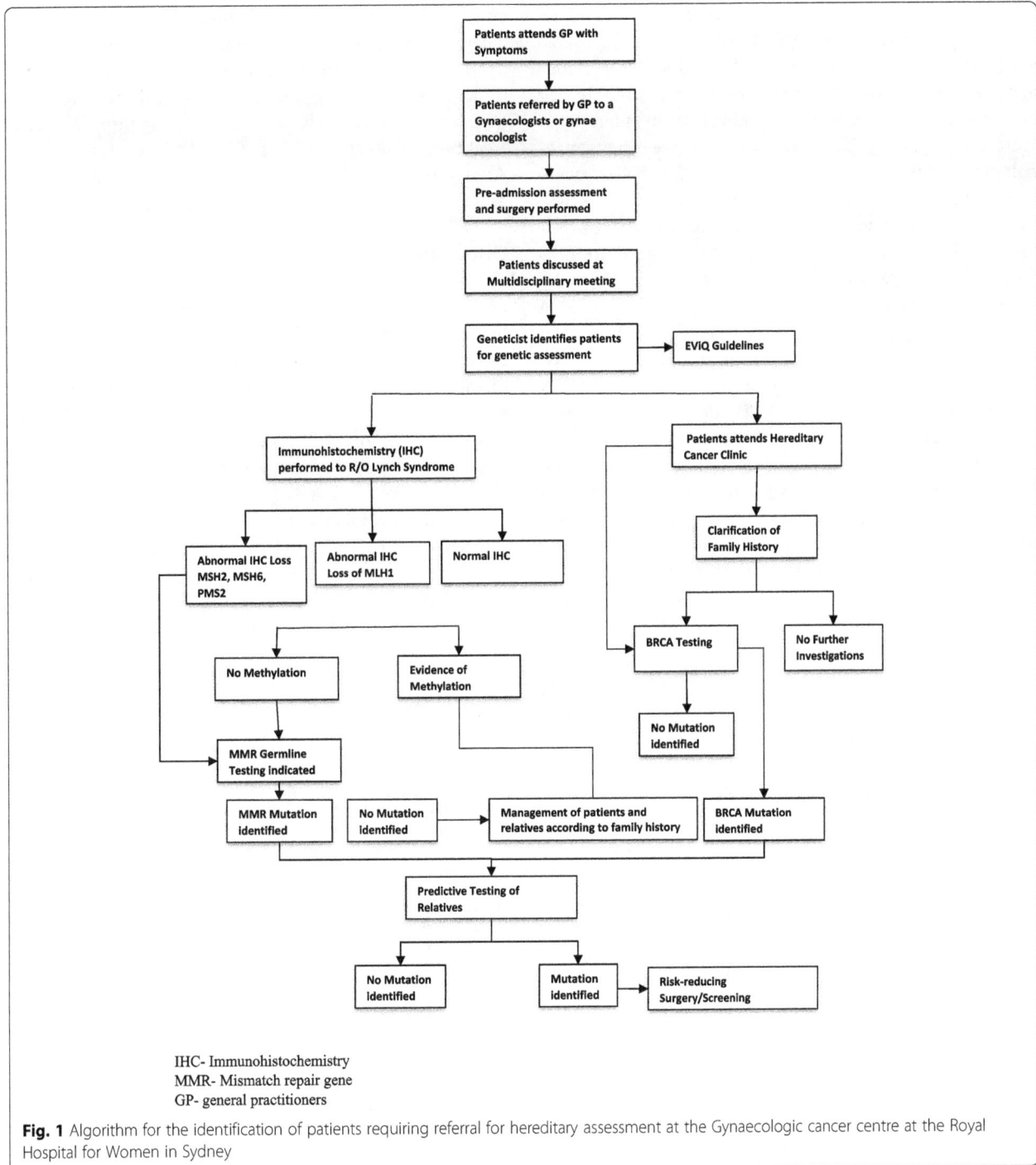

IHC- Immunohistochemistry
MMR- Mismatch repair gene
GP- general practitioners

Fig. 1 Algorithm for the identification of patients requiring referral for hereditary assessment at the Gynaecologic cancer centre at the Royal Hospital for Women in Sydney

outside of the New South Wales/Australian Capital Territory's genetics service. Those patients still requiring genetics assessment were sent a letter by the gynaecologist asking them to contact a hereditary cancer clinic from the included list of state-wide services.

Ethics approval was obtained from the Southern Eastern Sydney LDH Human Research Ethics Committee. HREC ref. no: 14/170(LNR/15/POWH/229).

Results

Of the 462 patients in cohort 1, 295 (63.9%) attended the Hereditary Cancer Clinic and 86 (18.6%) were deemed by a genetic counsellor to not require formal referral following clarification of family history or mismatch repair gene immunohistochemistry (MMR IHC) status. This left 81 patients (17.5%) who had not attended as recommended. 17 (3.7%) of these consulted a hereditary cancer service between initial ascertainment and this review. Review of the medical records of the remaining 64 patients (13.9%) indicated that 16 (3.5%) were deceased, and 5 (1%) had declined a genetics appointment leaving 43 patients (9.3%) suitable for genetics assessment who had never been seen by a Hereditary Cancer Clinic service. The treating gynaecologic oncologist was contacted; 2 (0.4%) were considered too unwell to attend and 1 (0.2%) had moved out of New South Wales (Fig. 2). Formal letters were sent to 40 patients (8.7%). After 6 months follow up, there were still 33 patients (7.1%) who failed to present to a Hereditary Cancer Clinic in New South Wales or Australian Capital Territory.

The audit of the 503 gynaecological cancer cases discussed at the multidisciplinary meetings in the year July 1 2015–June 30 2016 (cohort 2) identified 148 (29%) who were appropriate for genetics assessment. Of these, 66 (44.6%) had been seen by a genetics service by March 1, 2017, and 51 (34.5%) did not require further assessment after clarification of family history or immunohistochemistry status. Thirty-one patients (20.9%) had not attended a Hereditary Cancer Clinic by March 1, 2017. Of these, 7 (4.7%) declined genetic referral, and 1 (0.7%) was deceased. Treating gynaecological oncologists were

contacted regarding the remaining 23 women (15.5%). They reported 6 patients (4%) had declined genetic assessment and 2 patients (1.4%), who were currently undergoing active treatment, intended to attend a hereditary cancer clinic after completion of their treatment. Fifteen patients (10.1%) were sent letters. After 6 months follow-up, 6 patients (4.1%) had still not attended the hereditary cancer clinic (Fig. 3).

Discussion

Our audits of two retrospective cohorts of women diagnosed with gynaecological cancer has shown that despite having a member of a hereditary cancer team at multidisciplinary review meetings to identify women needing further assessment, approximately 10–15% of women do not receive that assessment. Further, we have demonstrated that information essential for determination of suitability for genetics assessment is frequently not available at the weekly meeting, such as detailed family history or MMR IHC status.

In an effort to optimise uptake, we have trialled a joint initiative between the gynaecological team and the hereditary cancer service to identify and contact nonattenders. Follow up of our original cohort with a letter

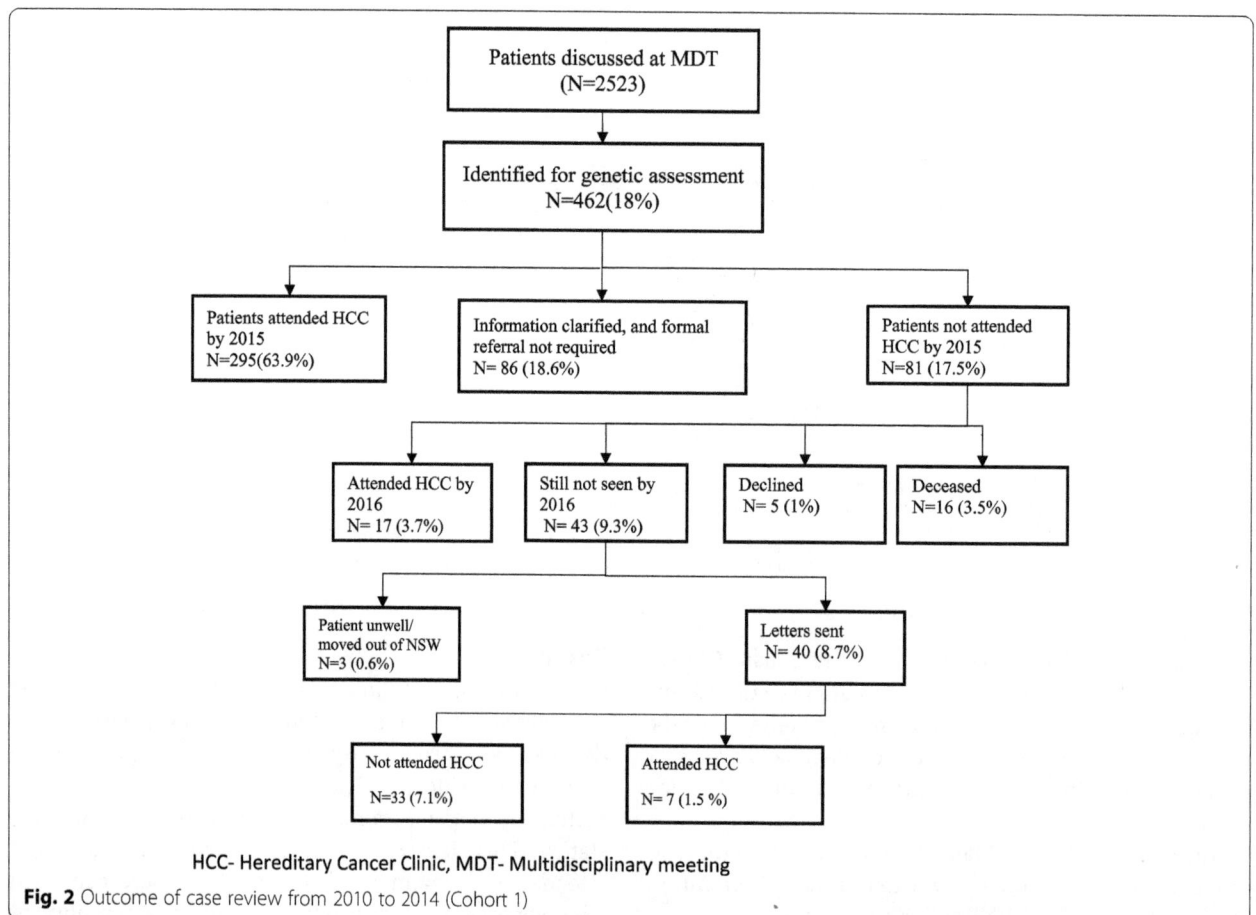

HCC- Hereditary Cancer Clinic, MDT- Multidisciplinary meeting

Fig. 2 Outcome of case review from 2010 to 2014 (Cohort 1)

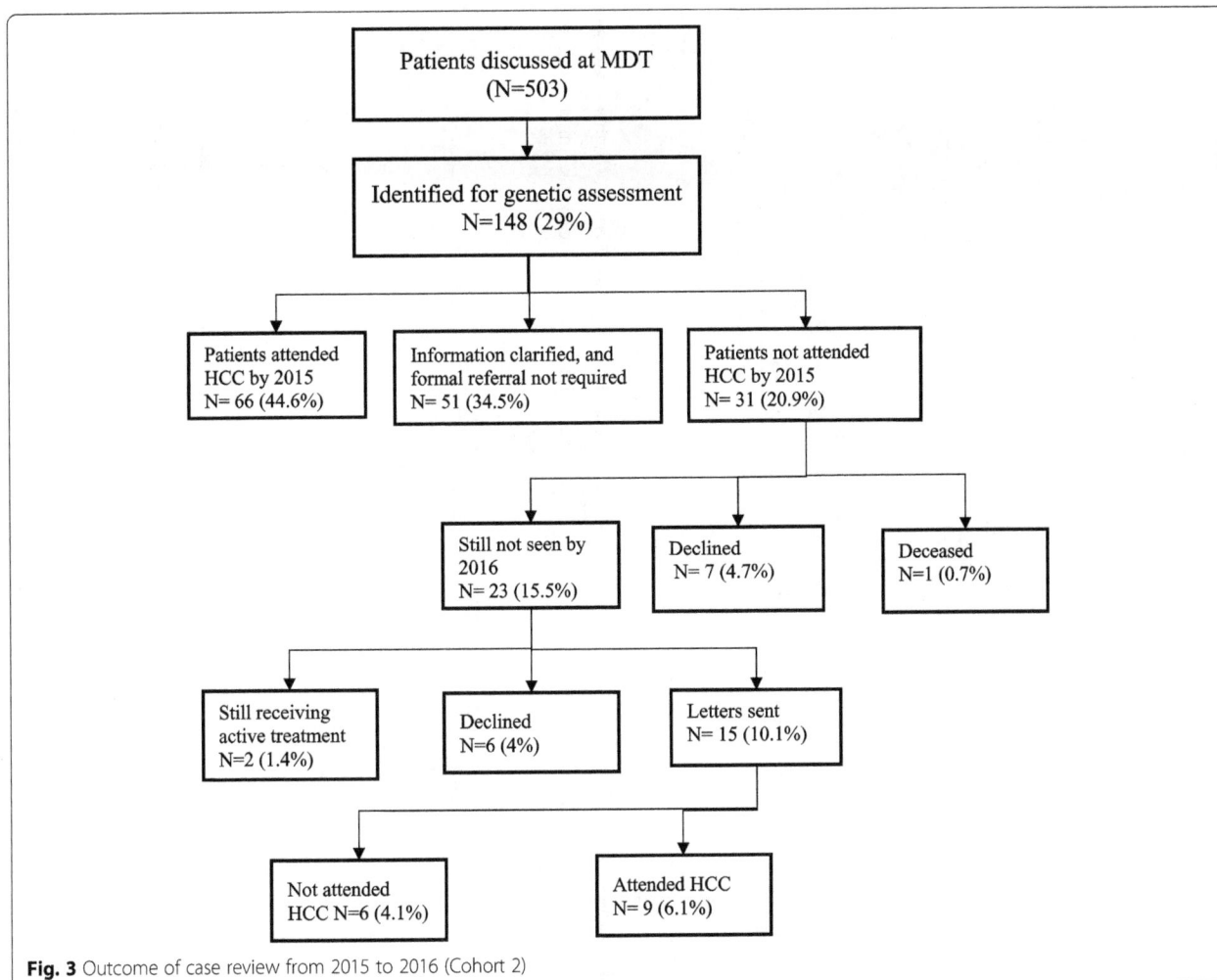

Fig. 3 Outcome of case review from 2015 to 2016 (Cohort 2)

indicated that late follow up improved attendance by only 1.5% (7/462). Short term follow- up of the second cohort (diagnosed 2015–2016) improved attendance by 6.1% (9/148). Hence, we recommend following up with patients in the short term, rather than the long term.

This process would optimise genetic assessment of gynaecological oncology patients, but requires ongoing interaction between both oncology and genetics services.

As an alternative to referral to a genetic service for women diagnosed with ovarian cancer, the introduction of "mainstreaming," whereby genetic testing of BRCA1/2 or panel of genes is done by the treating gynaecological or medical oncologist at diagnosis of primary or recurrent disease, has the potential to improve appropriate genetic assessment [15]. As a hybrid of mainstreaming, a genetic counsellor with specialized training and experience in familial cancer genetics, directly deployed into a gynaecologic oncology outpatient clinic and during chemotherapy sessions [15] has been reported to improve the uptake rate.

Our audit also identified that 18.6% and 34.5% patients in cohort 1 and 2 respectively who were identified as needing clarification of family history or immunohistochemistry when discussed at the meeting less than two weeks after surgery, were later found not to have indications for further genetic assessment. In most cases this was because family history information was incomplete or inaccurate, especially with confusion between ovarian, uterine and cervical cancers. With time, many women can gather information which is not available at the time of surgery (Figs. 2 and 3). Family history has been the foundation for genetic assessment and the basis for identifying patients at increased risk. Even when not providing full genetic assessment and testing services, oncologists are in a position to identify patients who may be at increased risk of cancer by recognizing the signs of an inherited syndrome. The general recommendation is to get a three-generational family history from all patients [16, 17]. Ideally, this history should include information on first-, second- and third- degree relatives, including the type of each primary cancer, age at

Table 1 Four steps to appropriate genetic assessment in gynaecological oncology for the first routine oncology follow-up visit (3-6 months)

1. Non-mucinous ovarian, fallopian tube or primary peritoneal cancer		BRCA testing alone or included in a panel
2. Histopathology	Mucinous ovarian cancer	MMR IHC
	Endometrioid or clear cell ovarian cancer	MMR IHC
	Endometrial cancer	MMR IHC
3. Family History	Ovarian cancer <50	Refer to hereditary cancer clinic for further assessment
	Breast cancer <50	Refer to hereditary cancer clinic for further assessment
	Endometrial or GIT cancer	MMR IHC
4. Post-operative follow up visit	Are investigations completed?	
	Has patient attended hereditary cancer clinic if referred?	

diagnosis, age at death, cause of death, and environmental exposures of all relatives with cancer. Many patients may not know these details on all family members at their first visit, so it is important to regularly update the history [18]. This is particularly important for the gynaecological oncologist, as ovarian and endometrial cancers are the sentinel cancer for many women with either a BRCA1 or 2 mutations or Lynch Syndrome, and can be facilitated by a family history questionnaire.

In a number of cases, routine MMR immunohistochemistry had not been done, prompting further assessment, however this could be accomplished if it was integral to histopathological examination for all endometrial cancer, with or without an upper age limit of age of 60 [19], and was included in the request by the gynaecological surgeon (Table 1).

By the time the patient is discharged, the gynaecological oncologist should have clear indications for the genetic management of the patient. This is particularly important for tertiary referral centres, because the patient may live remotely and have difficulty accessing a local genetic service (Table 1).

Our study shows that 16 patients (3.5%) in cohort 1 had deceased at the time of writing, which emphasizes the importance of early follow-up and intervention. In our opinion, the best way not to lose the patients recommended from the multidisciplinary meeting would be for patients to consult oncologists and the genetic counsellors on the same day at the post-operative visit.

A model of including a genetic counsellor in gynaecological cancer care [16, 20] has been shown to enable accurate family history assessment and appropriate IHC to be done, as well as concurrent genetic testing where indicated. This avoids patients being lost to follow up or becoming too ill or passing away before genetics assessment can be completed. Embedding a genetic counsellor in the cancer clinic proved effective, increasing uptake of genetic testing in eligible patients to over 90%.The median time from referral to delivery of genetic testing results was less than five months [16].

Conclusion

We have demonstrated in our recent cohort that 91.7% of eligible women had received genetic assessment, which seems effective and shows the small gap between the efficacy and effectiveness of guidelines for women diagnosed with gynaecological cancer. Even though, family history is often not helpful in determining genetic risk, effort taking a detail family history will not harm in selecting high risk patients for genetic testing. It is important to note that almost half of patients with a BRCA1/2 mutation and ovarian cancer have no family history of breast or ovarian cancer. For women with high-grade serous tubo-ovarian carcinomas, should be referred for genetic testing irrespective of their family history. A brief 4 step (Table 1) process for gynaecological oncologists is proposed to improve the effectiveness of guidelines for the genetic assessment of women with gynaecological cancer.

While mainstreaming is being adopted by some treating specialists, there will remain a cohort of women for whom hereditary cancer clinic referral is indicated, such as those with gynaecological cancers other than serous histology who have indications for genetic assessment.

Additionally, this model of improving the effectiveness of referral guidelines can be used for patients identified at other multidisciplinary meetings e.g.-breast or colorectal.

Acknowledgements

We would like to thank the treating gynaecologic oncologists at Royal hospital for Women, Sydney, Dr. Greg Robertson, Dr. Rhonda Farrell, and Dr. Archana Rao for following up their patients and giving us the required feedback.

Funding

None.

Authors' contributions

LA, HPP and NH contributed to the conceptualization and design of the study. LA, HPP and NH edited the manuscript. All authors read and approved the final manuscript.

Competing interests

The authors declare that they have no competing interests.

Author details

[1]Gynaecologic Cancer Centre, Royal Hospital for Women, Sydney, Australia. [2]School of Women's and Children's Health, University of New South Wales, Sydney, Australia. [3]Department of Obstetrics and Gynaecology, B P Koirala Institute of Health Sciences, Dharan, Nepal. [4]Hereditary Cancer Clinic, Prince of Wales Hospital, Sydney, Australia. [5]School of Medicine, University of New South Wales, Sydney, Australia.

References

1. https://www.eviq.org.au. Risk management for a female BRCA1 mutation carrier.
2. Hall MJ, Obeid EI, Schwartz SC, Mantia-Smaldone G, Forman AD, Daly MB. Genetic testing for hereditary cancer predisposition: BRCA1/2, lynch syndrome, and beyond. Gynecol Oncol. 2016;140(3):565–74.
3. Ledermann J, Harter P, Gourley C, Friedlander M, Vergote I, Rustin G, et al. Olaparib maintenance therapy in platinum-sensitive relapsed ovarian cancer. N Engl J Med. 2012;366(15):1382–92.
4. Scott CL, Swisher EM, Kaufmann SH. Poly (ADP-ribose) polymerase inhibitors: recent advances and future development. J Clin Oncol : Official J Am Soc Clin Oncol. 2015;33(12):1397–406.
5. Nimmi S, Kapoor KCB. Should multi-gene panel testing replace limited BRCA1/2 testing? A review of genetic testing for hereditary breast and ovarian cancers. World J of Surg Proced. 2016;6(1):13–8.
6. Pokharel HP, Hacker NF, Andrews L. Hereditary gynaecologic cancers in Nepal: a proposed model of care to serve high risk populations in developing countries. Hereditary Cancer Clinical Practice. 2017;15:12.
7. Pokharel HP, Hacker NF, Andrews L. Changing patterns of referrals and outcomes of genetic participation in gynaecological-oncology multidisciplinary care. Aust N Z J Obstet Gynaecol. 2016;56(6):633–8.

8.   Nilsson MP, Winter C, Kristoffersson U, Rehn M, Larsson C, Saal LH, et al. Efficacy versus effectiveness of clinical genetic testing criteria for BRCA1 and BRCA2 hereditary mutations in incident breast cancer. Familial Cancer. 2017;16(2):187–93.

9.   Alsop K, Fereday S, Meldrum C, deFazio A, Emmanuel C, George J, et al. BRCA mutation frequency and patterns of treatment response in BRCA mutation-positive women with ovarian cancer: a report from the Australian ovarian cancer study group. J Clin Oncol : Official J Am Soc Clin Oncol. 2012;30(21):2654–63.

10. Cohen PA, Nichols CB, Schofield L, Van Der Werf S, Pachter N. Impact of clinical genetics attendance at a gynecologic oncology tumor board on referrals for genetic counseling and BRCA mutation testing. Int J Gynecological Cancer : Official J Int Gynecological Cancer Soc. 2016;26(5):892–7.

11. Integrating genetic risk assessment into practice. J Oncol Pract. 2008;4(5):214–9.

12. Backes FJ, Mitchell E, Hampel H, Cohn DE. Endometrial cancer patients and compliance with genetic counseling: room for improvement. Gynecol Oncol. 2011;123(3):532–6.

13. Cross DS, Rahm AK, Kauffman TL, Webster J, Le AQ, Spencer Feigelson H, et al. Underutilization of lynch syndrome screening in a multisite study of patients with colorectal cancer. Genetics Med : Official J Am College Med Genet. 2013;15(12):933–40.

14. Batte BA, Bruegl AS, Daniels MS, Ring KL, Dempsey KM, Djordjevic B, et al. Consequences of universal MSI/IHC in screening ENDOMETRIAL cancer patients for lynch syndrome. Gynecol Oncol. 2014;134(2):319–25.

15. Kentwell M, Dow E, Antill Y, Wrede CD, McNally O, Higgs E, et al. Mainstreaming cancer genetics: a model integrating germline BRCA testing into routine ovarian cancer clinics. Gynecol Oncol. 2017;145(1):130–6.

16. George A, Riddell D, Seal S, Talukdar S, Mahamdallie S, Ruark E, et al. Implementing rapid, robust, cost-effective, patient-centred, routine genetic testing in ovarian cancer patients. Sci Rep. 2016;6:29506.

17. Levine DA, Karlan BY, Strauss JF, 3rd. Evolving approaches in research and Care for Ovarian Cancers: a report from the National Academies of sciences, engineering, and medicine. JAMA 2016;315(18):1943–1944.

18. van Altena AM, van Aarle S, Kiemeney LA, Hoogerbrugge N, Massuger LF, de Hullu JA. Adequacy of family history taking in ovarian cancer patients: a population-based study. Familial Cancer. 2012;11(3):343–9.

19. Buchanan DD, Tan YY, Walsh MD, Clendenning M, Metcalf AM, Ferguson K, et al. Tumor mismatch repair immunohistochemistry and DNA MLH1 methylation testing of patients with endometrial cancer diagnosed at age younger than 60 years optimizes triage for population-level germline mismatch repair gene mutation testing. J Clin Oncol Off J Am Soc Clin Oncol. 2014;32(2):90–100.

20. Randall LM, Pothuri B, Swisher EM, Diaz JP, Buchanan A, Witkop CT, et al. Multi-disciplinary summit on genetics services for women with gynecologic cancers: a Society of Gynecologic Oncology White Paper. Gynecol Oncol. 2017;146(2):217–24.

22

Mechanistic insights into ADXS11-001 human papillomavirus-associated cancer immunotherapy

Brett A. Miles[1*], Bradley J. Monk[2] and Howard P. Safran[3]

Abstract

Immune responses to the facultative intracellular bacterium *Listeria monocytogenes* (*Lm*) are robust and well characterized. Utilized for decades as a model of host-disease immunology, *Lm* is well suited for use as an immunotherapeutic bacterial vector for the delivery of foreign antigen. Genetic modification of *Lm* has been undertaken to create an attenuated organism that is deficient in its master transcriptional regulator, protein-related factor A, and incorporates a truncated, nonhemolytic version of the listeriolysin O (LLO) molecule to ensure its adjuvant properties while also preventing escape of the live organism from the phagolysosome. Delivery of a vaccine construct (*Lm*-LLO-E7; axalimogene filolisbac [AXAL] or ADXS11-001) in which the modified LLO molecule is fused with the E7 oncoprotein of human papillomavirus type 16 (HPV-16) consistently stimulates strong innate and E7 antigen-specific adaptive immune responses, resulting in reduction of tumor burden in animal cancer models. In the clinical setting, AXAL has shown early promise in phase I/II trials of women with cervical cancer, and several more trials are currently underway to assess the efficacy and safety of this antitumor vaccine in patients with HPV-positive head and neck and anal cancers.

Keywords: AXAL, ADXS11-001, Axalimogene filolisbac, Cancer immunotherapy, Mechanism of action, Human papillomavirus, Vaccine therapy

Introduction

Human papillomavirus: Prevalence, molecular structure, and biology

Several infectious agents are considered to be necessary causal agents of human cancers. Among these, persistent infections involving the human papillomaviruses (HPV) are estimated to be responsible for 5.2% of all cancers worldwide, with the majority of cases occurring in developing countries [1]. Infection with high-risk, oncogenic HPV subtypes is directly attributable to all cases of cervical cancer, approximately 90% of anal cancers, approximately 40% of penile, vulvar, and vaginal cancers, and around 12% of head and neck cancers, mainly of the oropharynx [1]. HPV subtypes 16, 18, 31, and 45 are the most frequently encountered high-risk HPV types; subtypes 16 and 18 alone are the causative agents of more than 70% of cervical cancer cases [2].

HPV is a circular, double-stranded, non-enveloped, icosahedral DNA virus. The HPV genome contains six or seven early genes, denoted E1, E2, E4, E5, E6, E7, and E8, which are required for maintenance of the viral genome, DNA replication, regulation of transcription, stimulation of cell growth, and inhibition of tumor suppressor genes [3]. E6 and E7 are the major oncogenes of HPV, and are used by the virus to evade the host immune system and access cell replication machinery [4]. In addition, the HPV genome contains two late genes, L1 and L2, which encode the major and minor capsid proteins, respectively [3].

When the integrity of the host cutaneous or mucosal epithelium has been compromised (e.g., microabrasions or other trauma), HPV infects the basal epithelial cells and establishes an episome. As the infected cells differentiate, early and late viral proteins are expressed, leading to viral assembly and eventual viral shed. In high-risk, oncogenic HPV subtypes, the E6 protein targets the p53 tumor suppressor protein, whereas E7 binds to the active form of

* Correspondence: Brett.Miles@mountsinai.org
[1]Division of Head and Neck Cancer Surgery, Department of Otolaryngology, Icahn School of Medicine at Mount Sinai, One Gustave L. Levy Place, New York, NY 10029, USA
Full list of author information is available at the end of the article

the retinoblastoma protein, thereby disrupting normal cell cycle regulation and providing the means to cause cellular alterations that potentially lead to neoplasia [3]. Cancer develops after a long latency period in which viral DNA persists, with ongoing viral integration into the host cell DNA, and continuous overexpression of the E6 and E7 early proteins, with consequent aberrant proliferation of the host cells [4, 5].

Review

Listeria monocytogenes: Versatile delivery vector for immunotherapy

Listeria monocytogenes (Lm) is an anaerobic, Gram-positive, facultative intracellular bacterium that is associated with opportunistic foodborne disease in susceptible hosts [6]. During active infection by Lm, the organism may disseminate via the bloodstream from the principal site of infection in the gastrointestinal tract and invade organs such as the spleen and liver, where it is phagocytosed by splenic and hepatic macrophages [7]. Following cellular invasion, Lm escapes the phagosome by secreting the pore-forming toxin listeriolysin O (LLO), a virulence factor that destroys the phagosomal membrane, and which allows the organism to undergo rapid cytosolic growth and actin nucleator A (ActA)-dependent cell-to-cell spread [8]. The entire Lm life cycle is dependent on the virulence gene and master transcriptional regulator protein-related factor A (prfA). ActA, an abundant surface protein that is upregulated more than 200-fold during intracellular growth in order for the bacterium to move toward the cell surface and spread to other cells [9], is activated in the host cytosol following allosteric activation of prfA, and subsequently mediates host actin polymerization. Once at the cell membrane, Lm forms a protrusion that is subsequently internalized by an adjacent macrophage, thereby disseminating the infection. Appropriate regulation of LLO and ActA by prfA is critical for Lm pathogenesis [8].

Lm has the ability to activate both the innate and adaptive immune responses (Fig. 1) [7, 10]. Following infection with Lm, innate immune responses are rapidly triggered in a stepwise manner, with the hallmarks of early resistance to infection being the production of interferon-gamma (IFN-γ) by natural killer cells and the subsequent activation of macrophages. At the cell surface, Toll-like receptors (TLRs) are an important link between the pathogen and subsequent immune activation, with TLR2 and TLR5 involved in the recognition of Lm pathogen-associated molecular patterns, such as peptidoglycan, lipoteichoic acid, lipoproteins, and bacterial flagellins [7, 11]. Myeloid differentiation primary response protein 88 is important in the innate immune defense against Lm, where its role in transmitting TLR-mediated signals is a required element for the full activation of immune responses [12].

Whereas TLRs are extracellular pattern recognition receptors involved in the activation of the inflammasome and production of pro-inflammatory cytokines, the nucleotide-binding oligomerization domain-like receptors (NLRs) are involved in the detection of cytosolic pathogens [13]. In particular, NLRC4 and NLRP3 detect cytosolic Lm with consequent activation of the inflammasome, while a further NLR, AIM2, specifically senses the bacterial DNA of Lm. The ensuing inflammatory response ensures the infiltration of large numbers of neutrophils and then macrophages to the site of infection, where they help to limit bacterial growth and, in the case of macrophages, drive the subsequent adaptive immune response [14].

During phagocytosis by infiltrating macrophages, any Lm bacteria that have not escaped the phagosome are phagocytosed and their processed antigen fragments are presented on the cell surface via major histocompatibility complex (MHC) class II. This interaction between the bacterial peptide/MHC class II complex and T cells that are able to recognize the antigen via their own receptors subsequently leads to the activation of cluster of differentiation 4-positive (CD4+) T cells [14]. In addition, bacteria that have escaped the phagosome into the cytosol may release antigenic fragments that are presented by MHC class I molecules to CD8+ cytotoxic T cells, with both CD4+ and CD8+ T cells involved in final clearance of the infection and generation of protective immunity [14, 15]. Lm is a strong stimulator of CD8+ T-cell responses in particular, with CD8+ T cells undergoing rapid programming to become long-lived CD8+ memory T cells, which provide protection against subsequent Lm infections [16]. Dendritic cells are an important link between the innate and adaptive immune responses, with their activation in response to the TLR signaling cascade required for co-stimulation of T cells and the effective activation of cell-mediated immunity [14, 16]. The CD8α subset of conventional dendritic cells is most effective in supporting this CD8+ T-cell memory formation [15].

Because of its well-established and robust immunologic effects, as well as decades-long use as a model of host-disease immunology, strains of Lm have been deployed as a therapeutic bacterial vector for the delivery of foreign antigens in both the preclinical and clinical settings [15]. The utility of the Lm vector is achieved through its genetic recombination with a truncated, nonhemolytic form of LLO, which eliminates the cytolytic activity of Lm and associated cell toxicity while preserving the significant immunogenic and adjuvant properties of the organism. For example, ADXS31-164 is an Lm-based vaccine that expresses a chimeric human HER2/neu gene fused to a nonhemolytic LLO fragment, which is expressed in the highly attenuated Lm vector LmddA. The vector lacks antibiotic selection markers and has the ability to spread from cell to cell. Despite this level of attenuation, ADXS31-164 was able to

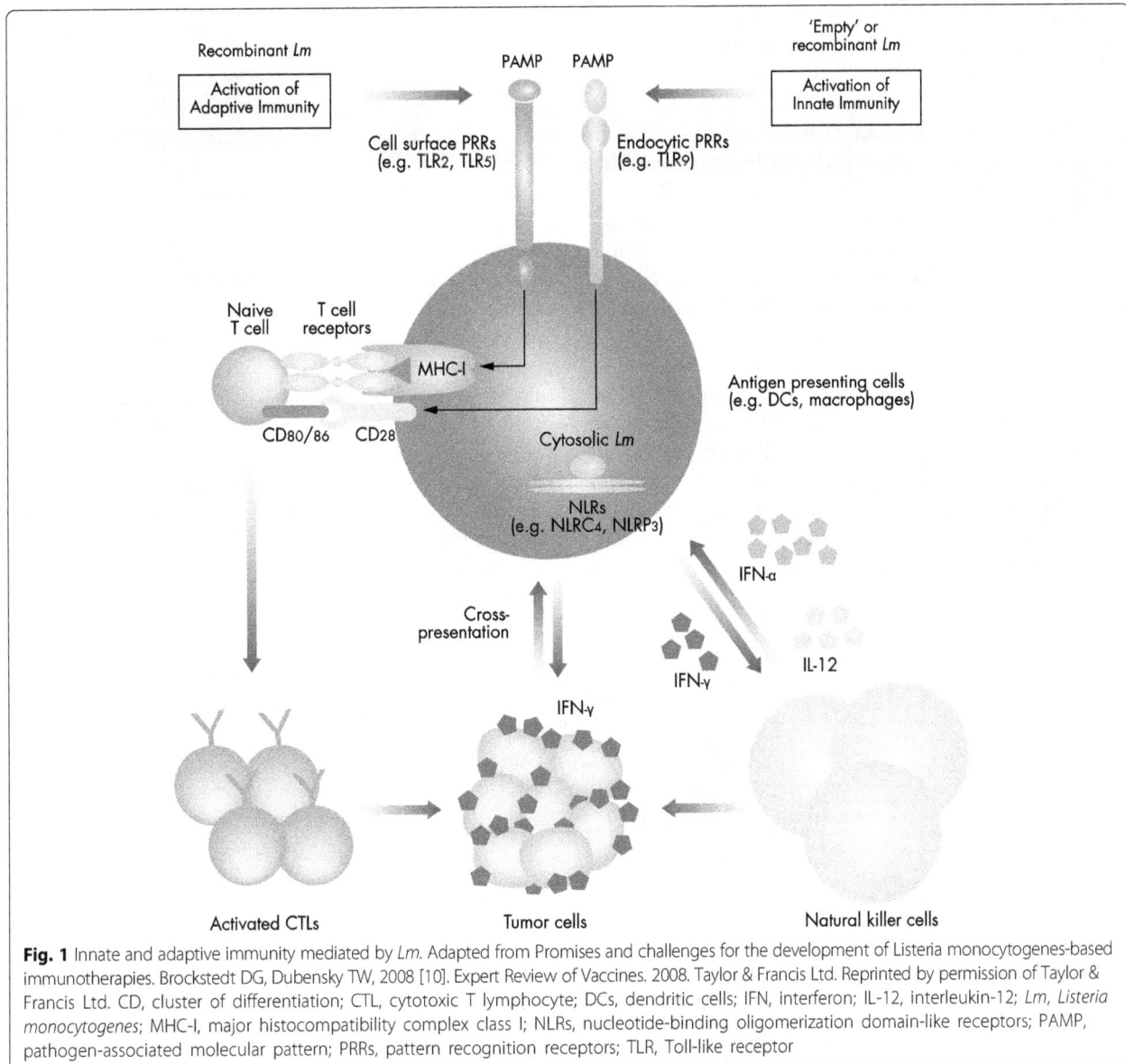

Fig. 1 Innate and adaptive immunity mediated by *Lm*. Adapted from Promises and challenges for the development of Listeria monocytogenes-based immunotherapies. Brockstedt DG, Dubensky TW, 2008 [10]. Expert Review of Vaccines. 2008. Taylor & Francis Ltd. Reprinted by permission of Taylor & Francis Ltd. CD, cluster of differentiation; CTL, cytotoxic T lymphocyte; DCs, dendritic cells; IFN, interferon; IL-12, interleukin-12; *Lm*, *Listeria monocytogenes*; MHC-I, major histocompatibility complex class I; NLRs, nucleotide-binding oligomerization domain-like receptors; PAMP, pathogen-associated molecular pattern; PRRs, pattern recognition receptors; TLR, Toll-like receptor

disrupt immune tolerance toward the HER2/neu self-antigen, eliciting strong T-cell responses in experimental animal tumor models that resulted in a reduction in regulatory T cells (Tregs), an increase in the CD8+/Treg ratio, and a reduction in tumor growth [17].

In the preclinical setting, *Lm*-based vaccine strategies were shown to potentiate CD8+ T-cell responses and inhibit neoangiogenesis in mouse models of breast, cervical, and head and neck cancers [17–22]. Singh et al. [18] demonstrated that five unique HER2/neu fragments secreted as a fusion protein with a truncated, nonhemolytic form of LLO and expressed in recombinant *Lm* controlled the growth of established NT2 mammary tumors, with the antitumor effect driven by a population of anti-HER2/neu CD8+ cytotoxic T cells [18]. In a syngeneic 4 T1 mouse tumor model, vaccination with a melanoma-associated

antigen b-*Lm*-LLO–based vaccine significantly reduced the number of metastases by 96% when compared to saline, and by 88% when compared to the vector control group (i.e., *Lm*-LLO alone) [19]. Administration of a vascular endothelial growth factor-targeted recombinant *Lm*-LLO–based vaccine in a mouse model of breast cancer led to eradication of some of the established tumors, reduction of microvascular density in the remaining tumors, and protection against tumor rechallenge and experimental metastases [20]. In an autochthonous mouse model for human epidermal growth factor receptor 2 (HER2)/neu + breast cancer, a novel human HER2/neu chimera *Lm*-based vaccine combining selected portions of individual fragments of the HER2/neu protein that contained most of the human leukocyte antigen epitopes prevented spontaneous tumor outgrowth, induced tumor regression in transplantable models, and prevented seeding of experimental lung metastases [21]. In a mouse model of HER2/neu-driven breast cancer, the *Lm*-LLO-CD105A and *Lm*-LLO-CD105B *Lm* recombinant vaccines that target endoglin (CD105) expressed in tumor vasculature were able to prevent neovascularization, thereby leading to therapeutic responses against primary and metastatic tumors [22].

In addition to breast tumor models, the antitumor activity of *Lm*-based vaccines has also been demonstrated in preclinical models of cervical and head and neck cancers [23–25]. A recombinant *Lm* construct that encoded the HPV-16 E7 gene was used to evaluate the potential potency of recombinant *Lm*-E7 as a therapeutic vaccine for cervical cancer in a syngeneic mouse model. When orally administered, the *Lm*-based vaccine induced an E7-specific cytotoxic T-cell response that could prevent and eradicate tumor growth in vaccinated mice because of enhancement of antigen-specific T-cell immunity [23]. These effects were confirmed by another study, which reported that an *Lm*-based HPV-16 E7 vaccine limited

autochthonous tumor growth in a transgenic mouse model of HPV-16–transformed tumors [25]. In a mouse model of head and neck cancer, the administration of an *Lm*-based ActA vaccine expressing the E7 protein of HPV-16 caused complete regression of HPV+ tumors in six of eight tested mice [24]. Consistent with other tumor models, the antitumor response was driven by the activation of cytotoxic T cells.

Listeriolysin O: Potent adjuvant for immunotherapy

LLO is a 529-amino acid hemolytic pore-forming protein crucial for the intracellular escape of *Lm* from the phagolysosome of infected cells [26]. In the context of tumor immunology, LLO is a very useful adjuvant because of its immunologic properties. Fusion of tumor antigens to the first 420-amino acid sequence of LLO, which excludes the hemolytic domain, helps to facilitate secretion of the antigen, increase antigen presentation, and stimulate maturation of dendritic cells (Fig. 2) [25, 27]. Details of this bioengineered version of the LLO

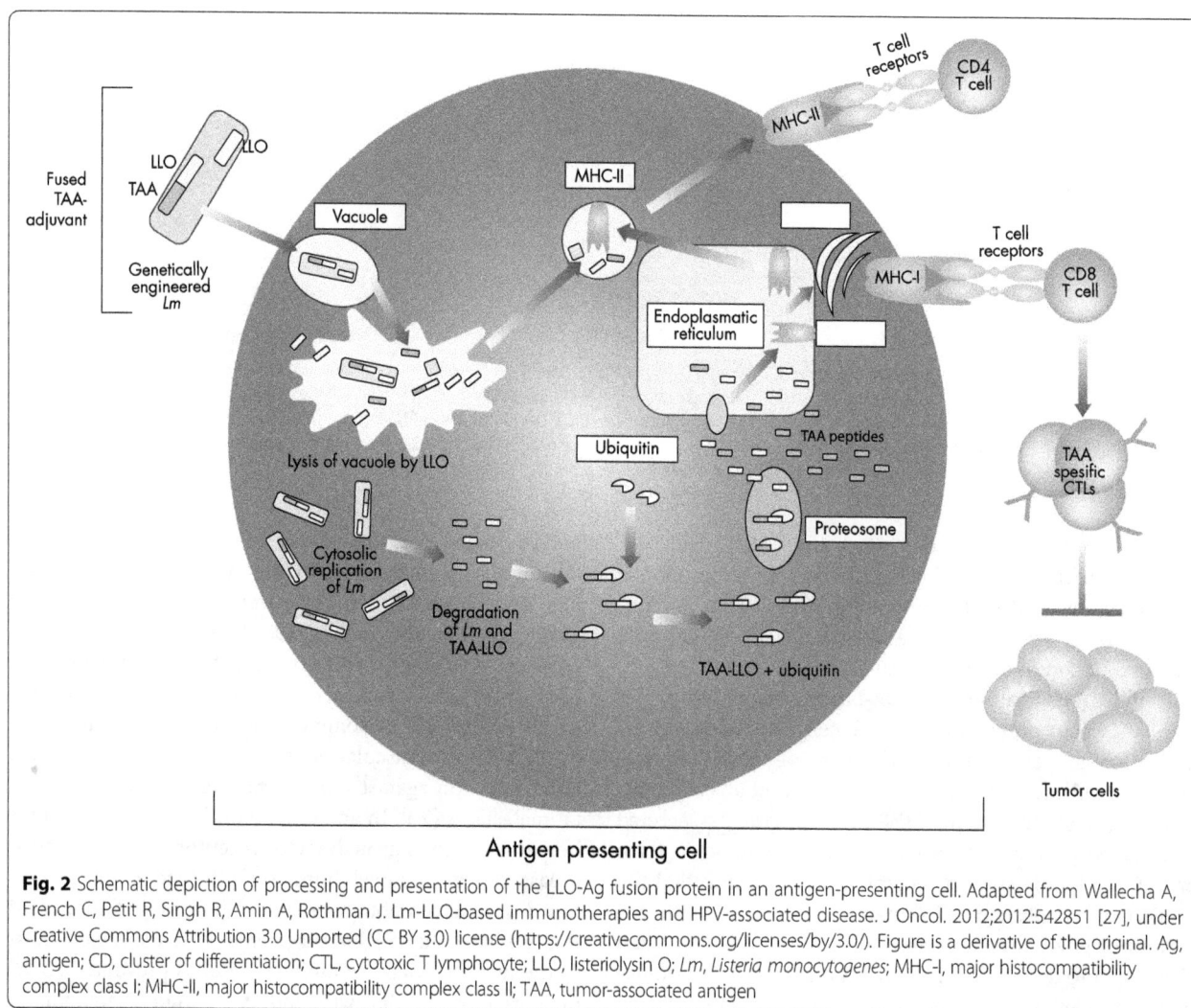

Fig. 2 Schematic depiction of processing and presentation of the LLO-Ag fusion protein in an antigen-presenting cell. Adapted from Wallecha A, French C, Petit R, Singh R, Amin A, Rothman J. Lm-LLO-based immunotherapies and HPV-associated disease. J Oncol. 2012;2012:542851 [27], under Creative Commons Attribution 3.0 Unported (CC BY 3.0) license (https://creativecommons.org/licenses/by/3.0/). Figure is a derivative of the original. Ag, antigen; CD, cluster of differentiation; CTL, cytotoxic T lymphocyte; LLO, listeriolysin O; *Lm, Listeria monocytogenes*; MHC-I, major histocompatibility complex class I; MHC-II, major histocompatibility complex class II; TAA, tumor-associated antigen

molecule were first published by Gunn et al., who prepared two recombinant *Lm* strains, one expressing the E7 protein of HPV-16 with no attempt to modify the LLO molecule (*Lm*-E7), and the second expressing E7 as a fusion protein joined to nonhemolytic LLO (*Lm*-LLO-E7) [28]. The two strains induced qualitatively different T-cell immune responses that correlated with their ability to induce regression of established HPV+ tumors in mice. *Lm*-LLO-E7, but not *Lm*-E7, induced the regression of E7-expressing tumors in a syngeneic mouse model with tumor regression dependent on a CD8+ T-cell response. The antitumor response to *Lm*-LLO-E7, but not *Lm*-E7, was reduced considerably with the depletion of CD4+ T cells, indicating the potency of the nonhemolytic LLO molecule as an immunologic adjuvant compared to the native LLO molecule. In contrast, *Lm*-E7 was shown to be an effective tumor immunotherapy in mice depleted of CD4+ T cells. Furthermore, antibody-mediated depletion of CD25+ cells improved the efficacy of *Lm*-E7 treatment [28]. In the years since, preclinical studies have shown that *Lm*-LLO-E7 is able to stimulate the expression of a wide range of pro-inflammatory cytokines by dendritic cells, such as interleukin-2 (IL-2), IL-12, tumor necrosis factor-α, and IFN-γ, as well as promote dendritic cell maturation, activate CD4+ T-cell–mediated adaptive immune responses, induce tumor antigen-specific CD8+ cytotoxic T cells, break immunologic tolerance, maintain protective immunity, and block tumor reoccurrence [29, 30]. Additionally,

LLO is capable of inducing chemokines and co-stimulatory molecules crucial for the development of potent innate and adaptive immune responses.

Axalimogene filolisbac (ADXS-HPV)
Molecular mechanism of action and immunotherapeutic effects

Axalimogene filolisbac (AXAL, or ADXS11-001) is a live, irreversibly attenuated *Lm*-LLO-E7 immunotherapy specifically developed for the treatment of HPV-associated cancers [31] (Fig. 3). As in earlier editions of *Lm*-LLO-E7, AXAL secretes an antigen-adjuvant fusion protein consisting of a truncated, nonhemolytic fragment of LLO fused to HPV-16 E7. AXAL was bioengineered from the prfA-deficient XFL-7 *Lm* strain, which renders the organism nonvirulent and also unable to escape the phagolysosome of the infected cell [32]. The strain was transformed using the pGG55 multicopy plasmid, which contains an expression cassette with the E7 gene fused to a truncated *hly* gene that encodes the first 441 amino acid residues of LLO and additionally contains a mutated copy of the prfA gene to partially restore XFL-7 virulence needed for plasmid retention in vivo.

AXAL targets tumors through a mechanism of action that results in activation of innate and adaptive immune responses. Briefly, the attenuated *Lm* expressing the HPV antigen fused to LLO is taken up by antigen-presenting cells via phagocytosis [33, 34]. Through its induction of pro-inflammatory cytokines from natural

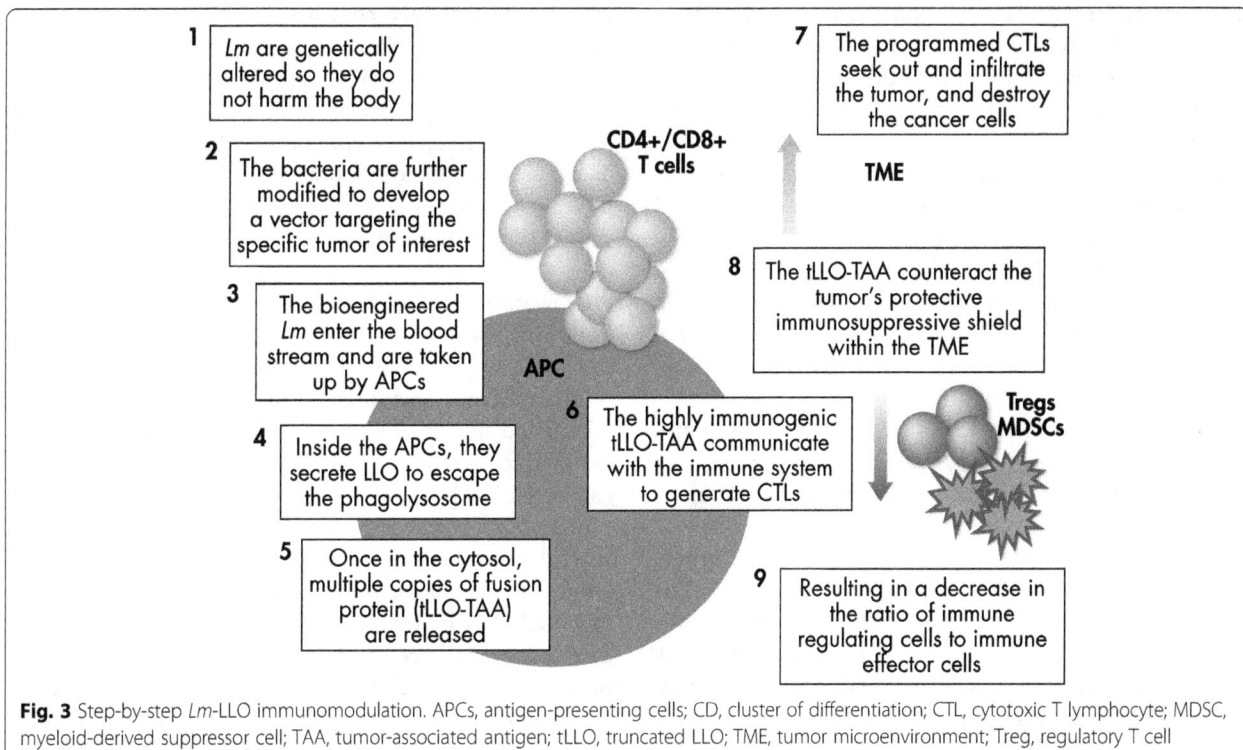

Fig. 3 Step-by-step *Lm*-LLO immunomodulation. APCs, antigen-presenting cells; CD, cluster of differentiation; CTL, cytotoxic T lymphocyte; MDSC, myeloid-derived suppressor cell; TAA, tumor-associated antigen; tLLO, truncated LLO; TME, tumor microenvironment; Treg, regulatory T cell

killer cells, recruitment of monocytes from the peripheral blood to the site of inflammation, and maturation of local dendritic cells, LLO helps to mediate a number of immunostimulatory effects that are an essential bridge between the innate and adaptive immune responses [33]. Antigenic peptides that result from the phagocytosis and breakdown of *Lm* are presented via MHC class II to antigen-specific CD4+ T cells. The immunogenic nature of LLO is further associated with a peptide sequence rich in proline, glutamic acid, serine, and threonine, which likely targets the protein for rapid ubiquitin-mediated proteasomal degradation, with antigenic fragments processed via this cytosolic pathway and subsequently presented via MHC class I to antigen-specific CD8+ T cells. Thus, both arms of the adaptive immune system are stimulated, resulting in the generation of strong T-cell–mediated effector immune responses and protective immunity [33, 34].

AXAL responses in mouse tumor models

Because of its capacity to effectively stimulate innate immunity and both arms of the adaptive immune response, AXAL presents attractive immunotherapeutic effects, which have been reported in both preclinical and clinical (Table 1 [25, 28, 32, 35–49]) studies. A study by Hussain and Paterson [35] shed light on the findings of Gunn et al. [28], who showed that antibody-mediated depletion of CD25+ cells improved the antitumor efficacy of *Lm*-E7 in a mouse cancer model. Hussain and Paterson showed in tumor-bearing mice that CD4 + CD25+ Tregs secreting transforming growth factor-β and the anti-inflammatory cytokine IL-10 are preferentially induced in mice vaccinated with *Lm*-E7, emphasizing the complexity of *Lm*-based immunotherapy. In a separate study, Peng et al. [36] reported that the ability of *Lm*-E7 and *Lm*-LLO-E7 vaccines to induce an antitumor response is correlated with myeloid dendritic cell maturation, as only *Lm*-LLO-E7 was able to induce IL-2 production by dendritic cells while also stimulating significantly higher levels of MHC class II molecules and co-stimulatory molecules necessary for stimulation of naive T cells [36]. This effect was independent of the E7 antigen, again indicating the adjuvant properties of LLO.

Loss of responsiveness to IFN-γ provides an immune escape mechanism for many human tumors, yet tumor sensitivity to IFN-γ was not required for inhibition of tumor angiogenesis or infiltration of CD4+ and CD8+ T cells to the tumor site in response to *Lm*-LLO-E7 in preclinical models [37]. Dominiecki et al. used the TC1 tumor cell line, which is immortalized with HPV E6 and E7 proteins and rendered unresponsive to IFN-γ. Although *Lm*-LLO-E7 was unable to induce tumor regression in the IFN-γ–insensitive model possibly because of an inability of the infiltrating T cells to penetrate the tumor mass, the capability of *Lm*-LLO-E7 to inhibit tumor angiogenesis in this model is nevertheless an encouraging finding. Using a similar model, a more recent preclinical study reported that administration of *Lm*-LLO-E7 increases the secretion of chemokine (C-X-C motif) ligand 9 (CXCL9) by TC1 tumor cells and mediated the intratumoral infiltration of CD8+ T cells [39]. This effect was IFN-γ dependent, since anti–IFN-γ antibody treatment resulted in a reduction in CXCL9 expression and a resultant decrease in the proportion of CD8+ T cells. In a transgenic mouse model of HPV-transformed cancer, *Lm*-LLO-E7 was shown to overcome tumor-induced central tolerance by expanding low-avidity and low-frequency E7-specific CD8+ T cells, which eradicate E7-expressing thyroid mouse tumors [38]. In an effort to evaluate the systemic immunologic effects that differentiate *Lm*-LLO-E7 vaccination from its control vector lacking E7 protein expression, Sewell et al. [25] showed that mice treated with *Lm*-LLO-E7 had significantly smaller tumors than control mice and possessed higher numbers of antigen-specific CD8+ T cells in the spleens, tumors, and peripheral blood [25].

Another tumor immune escape mechanism and therefore barrier for successful immunotherapy is tumor-mediated inhibitory responses that are effected via programmed cell death protein 1 (PD-1) interactions with its ligands, PD-L1 and PD-L2. A recent study conducted in a TC1 mouse tumor model showed that the combination of *Lm*-LLO-E7 with an anti–PD-1 antibody that blocks the PD-1/PD-L1 interaction significantly improved the immunotherapeutic efficacy of treatment compared with *Lm*-LLO-E7 alone [40]. In particular, the combination treatment led to a significant reduction in Tregs and myeloid-derived suppressor cells (MDSCs) in the spleen and tumor microenvironment, and significantly enhanced antigen-specific CD8+ T-cell peripheral and tumoral immune responses, thereby prolonging survival and promoting the complete regression of tumors in mice.

Brief overview of AXAL in clinical studies

Following the positive results obtained in the preclinical setting, assessment of the efficacy and safety of AXAL immunotherapy was initiated in phase I/II clinical trials conducted in patients with HPV-associated cancers, including cervical cancer, head and neck cancer, and anal cancer (Table 1 [25, 28, 32, 35–49]).

In patients with cervical cancer, AXAL was assessed in several phase I/II trials either as monotherapy or in combination with other anticancer therapies. The safety of AXAL was first assessed in 2009 in a phase I trial in 15 patients with previously treated metastatic, refractory, or recurrent cervical cancer. Single-agent AXAL was administered at dose levels of 1×10^9, 3.3×10^9, or 1×10^{10} colony-forming units (CFU) as an intravenous infusion

Table 1 Overview of AXAL in preclinical and clinical studies

AXAL IN PRECLINICAL MOUSE TUMOR MODELS	
Study (chronologic order)	**Results**
Gunn et al. [28]	Lm-LLO-E7 (but not Lm-E7) led to tumor regression
Hussain et al. [35]	Confirmation of above results Explanation: Lm-E7 induces Tregs (suppressive through production of IL-10 and TGF-β)
Peng et al. [36]	Lm-LLO-E7 infection of bone marrow DCs: DC maturation, IL-2 production, and expansion of E7-specific CTLs
Dominiecki et al. [37]	Sensitivity to IFN-γ is required for Lm-LLO-E7 therapeutic efficacy, but not for inhibition of tumor angiogenesis
Souders et al. [38]	Lm-LLO-E7 overcomes central tolerance by expanding low-avidity E7-specific CD8+ T cells that are not deleted during thymopoiesis and can eliminate solid tumors
Sewell et al. [25]	Lm-LLO-E7 led to higher numbers of antigen-specific CD8+ T cells than controls and inhibited autochthonous tumor growth
Guirnalda et al. [39]	Following Lm-LLO-E7, CXCL9 (produced as a result of IFN-γ stimulation of TC1 tumor cells) mediates intratumoral infiltration of CD8+ T cells
Mkrtichyan et al. [40]	Bone marrow DCs infected with Lm-LLO-E7 were found to upregulate expression of the PD-1 ligand, PD-L1 Anti–PD-1 antibody significantly enhances Lm-LLO-E7 immunotherapy efficacy

AXAL IN CLINICAL TRIALS					
Trial by investigator/ NCT identifier	**Indication**	**Mono/multi-therapy**	**Phase I**	**Phase II**	**Phase III**
Maciag et al. [32]	Advanced cervical cancer	AXAL alone			
Ghamande et al. [41] (NCT02164461)	Persistent/recurrent/metastatic cervical cancer	AXAL alone	→		
US National Institutes of Health [42] (NCT01598792)	Oropharyngeal cancer	AXAL alone			
US National Institutes of Health [43] (NCT01671488)	Anal cancer	AXAL ± chemoradiation (mitomycin, 5-fluorouracil, IMRT)			
Cohen et al. [44] (NCT02291055)	Recurrent/metastatic head and neck cancer	AXAL ± MEDI4736 (durvalumab)	→→		
Huh et al. [45] (NCT01266460)	Persistent/recurrent/metastatic cervical cancer	AXAL alone			
Basu et al. [46] (CTRI/2010/091/001232)	Recurrent/refractory cervical cancer	AXAL ± cisplatin			
Miles et al. [47] (NCT02002182)	Previously untreated, surgically resectable stage II–IV oropharyngeal cancer	AXAL + transoral robotic surgery		→→	
Fakih et al. [48] (NCT02399813)	Persistent/recurrent, locoregional/metastatic cancer of the anal canal	AXAL alone			
Herzog TJ [49] (NCT02853604)	High-risk locally advanced cervical cancer	AXAL alone			→→→

Abbreviations: *CTRI* Clinical Trials Registry – India, *DC* dendritic cell, *IMRT* intensity-modulated radiation therapy, *NCT* National Clinical Trial

followed by a second dose 3 weeks later [32]. The investigators reported an acceptable safety profile, with all patients experiencing a flu-like syndrome that responded to symptomatic treatment. At the highest dose, some patients had severe fever and dose-limiting hypotension, but no grade 4 adverse events were reported. Two patients died during the study; the deaths were considered unrelated to the administration of AXAL. Of 13 evaluable patients, five had disease progression, seven had stable disease, and one patient had an unconfirmed partial tumor response with a 32% reduction in tumor load. In a preliminary report of another phase I trial conducted in a similar population of previously treated women with advanced cervical cancer, AXAL was administered at a dose of 5×10^9 or 1×10^{10} CFU every 3 weeks for 12 weeks [41]. At the lower dose level, one patient of three experienced grade 3 hypotension as a dose-limiting toxicity. A total of 16 doses were safely administered, and accrual for the second dose level had not started at the time of preparation of this manuscript. Updated data are anticipated.

Two phase II studies of AXAL in women with persistent, recurrent and/or refractory cervical cancer have also been initiated [45, 46]. The first of these evaluates the activity of AXAL in patients with persistent or recurrent cervical cancer, with secondary objectives of evaluating progression-free survival, overall survival, and objective tumor response [45]. Patients will receive AXAL at a dose of 1×10^9 CFU on day 1 with a repeat dose every 28 days for three total doses in the absence of disease progression or unacceptable toxicity. Preliminary data from stage 1 of this trial show that treatment with AXAL led to a 38.5% 12-month overall survival rate in 26 patients. When evaluating safety data, grade 1 or 2 adverse events were reported in 19 of 26 patients (73%), with fatigue, chills, and fever the most common. Only 4 patients (15%) experienced a grade 3 adverse event (e.g., hypotension and cytokine release syndrome) and one patient (4%) experienced a grade 4 adverse event (lung infection and sepsis) [49]. Preliminary data are also available from a second phase II trial of AXAL being conducted in women from India with recurrent/refractory cervical cancer [46]. The primary endpoint of this open-label, randomized phase II study was to determine efficacy and safety of AXAL alone or in combination with cisplatin. In this study, 110 patients were randomized to either one cycle (three doses) of AXAL at 1×10^9 CFU or four doses of AXAL at 1×10^9 CFU together with cisplatin chemotherapy. Following treatment, when analyzing the treatment efficacy in these patients, an 11% response rate was observed, with an average response duration of 10.5 months in both treatment groups. Objective tumor responses included six patients with complete responses and six patients with a partial

response; tumor responses were observed in both treatment arms. Another 35 patients had stable disease for more than 3 months, for a disease control rate of 43%. Activity was observed against all high-risk HPV strains detected. The percentage of patients alive at 12 months was 36%, with an 18-month survival rate of 28%. When analyzing treatment safety, two grade 3 serious adverse events were reported, with nonserious adverse events predominantly of transient, noncumulative flu-like symptoms that either spontaneously resolved or responded to symptom-based treatment. The investigators concluded that AXAL can be safely administered in combination with chemotherapy, and is well tolerated with a predictable and manageable safety profile. Moreover, the 36% 12-month survival rate and 11% response rate in this disease setting were encouraging and support the activity of AXAL in recurrent cervical cancer [46].

More recently, a randomized phase III clinical trial (AIM2CERV) enrolling patients with high-risk locally advanced cervical cancer following chemoradiation who will receive AXAL as adjuvant immunotherapy was opened for recruitment in September 2016 [50] (Fig. 4). As patients with high-risk locally advanced cervical cancer present with a 50% probability of recurrence or death following chemoradiation and brachytherapy, there is a clear need for treatment modalities that will lead to improved outcomes. The AIM2CERV trial will evaluate overall survival and disease-free survival of these patients.

The efficacy and safety of AXAL has also been assessed in phase I/II clinical trials that enrolled patients with head and neck cancer, as well as cancer of the anal canal. Although a phase I dose-escalation trial conducted in patients with HPV-16+ oropharyngeal carcinoma was terminated early when two patients suffered dose-limiting toxicities postvaccination [42], a phase I/II trial is currently investigating AXAL and the fully humanized anti–PD-L1 antibody durvalumab alone or in combination in previously treated patients with recurrent/metastatic HPV + head and neck cancer [44]. The primary objective of the phase I study is to evaluate safety and tolerability of the combination regimen and to select a recommended phase II dose. Preliminary phase I results reported that 10 of the 11 enrolled patients (91%) had treatment-related adverse events, with the majority being grade 1 (7/11; 64%) or 2 (6/11; 55%), such as chills and/or rigors, fever, nausea, hypotension, diarrhea, fatigue, tachycardia, or headache [51]. The primary objective of phase II is to evaluate tumor response, progression-free survival, and safety of AXAL and durvalumab as monotherapy and in combination. A phase II trial in this setting is currently evaluating AXAL in patients with stage II–IV HPV+ oropharyngeal cancer prior to robotic surgery [47]. The primary objective is to determine the immunogenicity of AXAL. Preliminary data have yet to be reported.

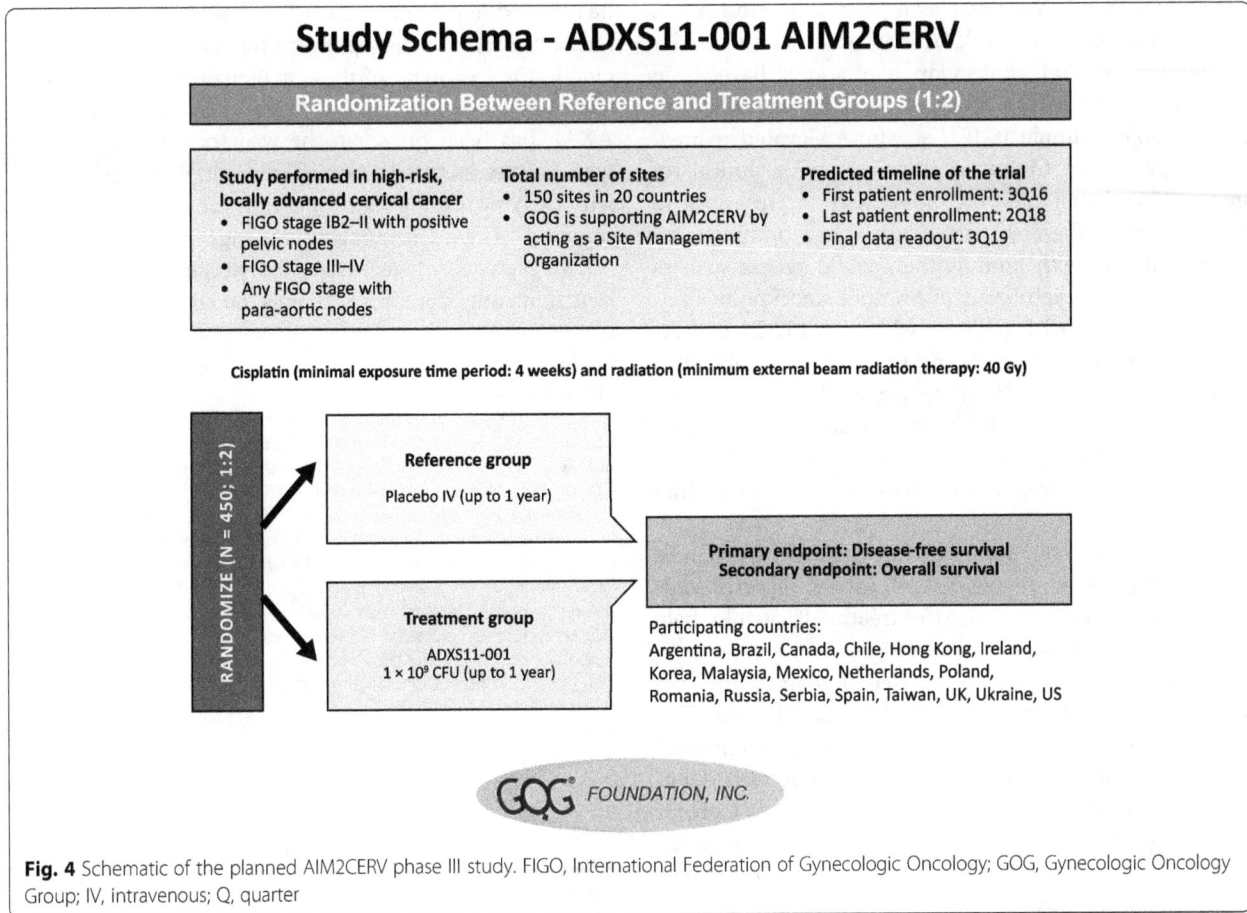

Fig. 4 Schematic of the planned AIM2CERV phase III study. FIGO, International Federation of Gynecologic Oncology; GOG, Gynecologic Oncology Group; IV, intravenous; Q, quarter

In anal cancer, a phase II trial is currently evaluating AXAL as single-agent therapy in patients with persistent/recurrent, locoregional or metastatic anal cancer [48]. Finally, a phase I/II trial is evaluating the combination of AXAL, mitomycin, 5-fluorouracil, and intensity-modulated radiation therapy in patients with anal cancer [43]. The first efficacy and safety data from these trials are expected to be available in 2017.

A topic of interest when evaluating AXAL in the clinical setting is its safety profile, particularly when administered in patients with persistent, recurrent, or metastatic disease who would benefit from co-administration of other immunotherapies. Preliminary evaluation of safety data from phase I/II trials with AXAL, administered alone or combined with other immunotherapeutic agents in patients with HPV+ cervical or head and neck cancers, reported that most adverse events were grade 1 or 2 and included fatigue, chills, fever, and nausea as the most common [46, 51]. Combined administration of AXAL with the anti–PD-L1 antibody durvalumab led to a similar range of adverse events as did AXAL monotherapy. In view of these preliminary results, it can be hypothesized that anticipated toxicities upon combination of AXAL with other immunotherapeutic agents would mainly consist of grade

1–2 adverse events similar to those already reported. Additionally, mild adverse events associated with infusion of AXAL could potentially be observed on the day of dosing; nevertheless, as previously described, these are transient and either self-resolve or respond readily to symptomatic treatment [46].

Another relevant aspect of immunotherapy with AXAL is the identification of predictive and prognostic biomarkers that might be evaluated upon treatment of HPV+ cancer patients, along with expected translational endpoints. In recent years, a relatively wide array of both cellular and molecular biomarkers predictive or prognostic for response to immunotherapy have been identified. Cellular biomarkers relevant for response to AXAL immunotherapy could potentially be of both anti- and protumoral effect. T-cell infiltration of various types of human tumors has been previously reported to be associated with improved clinical outcome [52, 53], whereas high numbers of circulating protumoral immune cell populations, such as MDSCs or Tregs, have been associated with worse overall survival [54, 55]. Considering that AXAL administration results in a decrease in the ratio of Tregs and MDSCs to antitumoral immune effector cells (Fig. 1) [10], these immunosuppressive cell populations might serve as useful prognostic biomarkers for immune response to AXAL. In addition to cellular biomarkers, several molecular biomarkers have been identified as predictors of response to immunotherapy. One notable example is IFN-γ, whose elevated expression in pretreated tumors is associated with clinical response [56]. Other relevant biomarkers for response to AXAL immunotherapy, particularly when administered in combination with immunotherapeutic agents such as durvalumab, are high levels of immune checkpoint molecules such as PD-L1; patients with high PD-L1 expression have been shown to be more likely to benefit from immunotherapy [57]. These cellular and molecular biomarkers could potentially predict response to AXAL, used as monotherapy or in combination with other immunotherapeutic agents, and therefore warrant further investigation.

In view of the often-severe disease burden experienced by cancer patients, acquisition of patient-reported outcomes, along with response to treatment, would help provide comprehensive clinical insights. Systematic measurements of these patient-reported outcomes are possible today with the use of existing validated tools. Two of the most commonly used measurement systems are the Functional Assessment of Anorexia/Cachexia Therapy (FAACT) and the Functional Assessment of Chronic Illness Therapy – Fatigue (FACIT-F) questionnaires, developed for assessment of anorexia/cachexia and fatigue experienced by cancer patients undergoing various treatments [58, 59]. Taking into consideration the preponderance of fatigue and nausea associated with the adverse events observed to date in clinical trials with AXAL immunotherapy, the patient-reported outcomes mentioned above bear relevance and could potentially be investigated in future clinical trials of AXAL.

Conclusions

Lm-based immunotherapy has progressed considerably since the completion of the first preclinical studies. Genetic engineering, utilized to obtain a recombinant, attenuated form of *Lm* as a bacterial vector, has enhanced the safety of *Lm*-based vaccines such that they have now been utilized successfully in clinical trials in humans. Moreover, the fusion of tumor antigens to LLO has greatly enhanced the immunologic and antitumor properties of these vaccines. As several studies have indicated, one major challenge for *Lm*-based vaccines is their capacity to induce CD25+ Treg cells with a propensity for immunosuppression along with the CD4+ and CD8+ effector T cells that are needed for protective immunity [28, 35]. However, this effect can be overcome by combining *Lm*-based vaccines with other targeted antitumoral therapies, such as monoclonal antibodies [40]. The current clinical status of AXAL, which continues to

be assessed in patients with HPV-associated cancers at different stages, provides optimism for the future of the vaccine in the treatment of these malignancies. Administered alone or in combination with various cancer therapies, AXAL has been proven to be well tolerated by patients with HPV-associated cancers in multiple investigations, with early promising signs of antitumor activity also being reported. These encouraging findings pave the way for AXAL phase III clinical trials and, at later stages, the potential introduction of AXAL into the clinical setting.

Abbreviations

ActA: Actin nucleator A; APC: Antigen-presenting cell; AXAL: Axalimogene filolisbac or ADXS11-001; CD: Cluster of differentiation; CFU: Colony-forming unit; CTL: Cytotoxic T lymphocyte; CTRI: Clinical Trials Registry – India; CXCL9: Chemokine (C-X-C motif) ligand 9; DC: Dendritic cell; FAACT: Functional Assessment of Anorexia/Cachexia Therapy; FACIT-F: Functional Assessment of Chronic Illness Therapy – Fatigue; FIGO: International Federation of Gynecologic Oncology; GOG: Gynecologic Oncology Group; HER2: Human epidermal growth factor receptor 2; HPV: Human papillomavirus; IFN-γ: Interferon gamma; IL: Interleukin; IMRT: Intensity-modulated radiation therapy; IV: Intravenous; LLO: Listeriolysin O; *Lm*: *Listeria monocytogenes*; MDSC: Myeloid-derived suppressor cell; MHC: Major histocompatibility complex; NCT: National Clinical Trial; NLR: Nucleotide-binding oligomerization domain-like receptor; PD-1: Programmed cell death protein 1; PD-L1: Programmed cell death protein 1 ligand 1; PD-L2: Programmed cell death protein 1 ligand 2; prfA: Protein-related factor A; Q: Quarter; TAA: Tumor-associated antigen; tLLO: Truncated listeriolysin O; TLR: Toll-like receptor; TME: Tumor microenvironment; Treg: Regulatory T cell

Acknowledgments

The authors would like to thank Oana Draghiciu, PhD, from TRM Oncology, for medical writing assistance, funded by Advaxis, Inc. The authors are fully responsible for all content and editorial decisions for this review.

Funding

Funding for medical writing assistance was provided by Advaxis, Inc.

Authors' contributions

BM, HPS, and BJM were integral in the writing, review, and revision of the manuscript. All authors read and approved the final manuscript.

Competing interests

BAM has received funding (institutional) from Advaxis for the clinical trial of ADXS11-001 vaccination prior to robotic surgery, HPV-positive oropharyngeal cancer (NCT02002182). BJM discloses that St. Joseph's Hospital institution has received research grants from Amgen, Lilly, Genentech, Janssen/Johnson & Johnson, Array, TESARO, and Morphotek. BJM has received honoraria for speaker bureaus from Roche/Genentech, AstraZeneca, Myriad, and Janssen/Johnson & Johnson, and has been a consultant for Roche/Genentech, Merck, TESARO, AstraZeneca, Gradalis, Advaxis, Amgen, Pfizer, Bayer, Insys, Mateon, PPD, and Clovis. HPS has nothing to disclose.

Author details

[1]Division of Head and Neck Cancer Surgery, Department of Otolaryngology, Icahn School of Medicine at Mount Sinai, One Gustave L. Levy Place, New York, NY 10029, USA. [2]Division of Gynecologic Oncology, University of Arizona College of Medicine, Creighton University School of Medicine at Dignity Health St. Joseph's Hospital and Medical Center, Phoenix, AZ, USA. [3]Brown University Oncology Research Group, Providence, RI, USA.

References

1. Parkin DM. The global burden of infection-associated cancers in the year 2002. Int J Cancer. 2006;118(12):3030–44.
2. Galani E, Christodoulou C. Human papilloma viruses and cancer in the post-vaccine era. Clin Microbiol Infect. 2009;15(11):977–81.
3. Scheurer ME, Tortolero-Luna G, Adler-Storthz K. Human papillomanvirus infection: biology, epidemiology, and prevention. Int J Gynecol Cancer. 2005;15(5):727–46.
4. zur Hausen H. Papillomaviruses and cancer: from basic studies to clinical application. Nat Rev Cancer. 2002;2(5):342–50.
5. Jabbar SF, Abrams L, Glick A, Lambert PF. Persistence of high-grade cervical dysplasia and cervical cancer requires the continuous expression of the human papillomavirus type 16 E7 oncogene. Cancer Res. 2009;69(10):4407–14.
6. Renier S, Hébraud M, Desvaux M. Molecular biology of surface colonization by Listeria monocytogenes: an additional facet of an opportunistic Gram-positive foodborne pathogen. Environ Microbiol. 2011;13(4):835–50.
7. Pamer EG. Immune responses to Listeria monocytogenes. Nat Rev Immunol. 2004;4(10):812–23.
8. Reniere ML, Whiteley AT, Portnoy DA. An in vivo selection identifies Listeria monocytogenes genes required to sense the intracellular environment and activate virulence factor expression. PLoS Pathog. 2016;12(7):e1005741.
9. Tilney LG, Portnoy DA. Actin filaments and the growth, movement, and spread of the intracellular bacterial parasite, Listeria monocytogenes. J Cell Biol. 1989;109(4 Pt 1):1597–608.
10. Brockstedt DG, Dubensky TW. Promises and challenges for the development of Listeria monocytogenes-based immunotherapies. Expert Rev Vaccines. 2008;7(7):1069–84.
11. Machata S, Tchatalbachev S, Mohamed W, Jänsch L, Hain T, Chakraborty T. Lipoproteins of Listeria monocytogenes are critical for virulence and TLR2-mediated immune activation. J Immunol. 2008;181(3):2028–35.
12. Edelson BT, Unanue ER. MyD88-dependent but Toll-like receptor 2-independent innate immunity to Listeria: no role for either in macrophage listericidal activity. J Immunol. 2002;169(7):3869–75.
13. Warren SE, Armstrong A, Hamilton MK, Mao DP, Leaf IA, Miao EA, et al. Cutting edge: cytosolic bacterial DNA activates the inflammasome via Aim2. J Immunol. 2010;185(2):818–21.
14. Zenewicz LA, Shen H. Innate and adaptive immune responses to Listeria monocytogenes: a short overview. Microbes Infect. 2007;9(10):1208–15.
15. Rothman J, Paterson Y. Live-attenuated Listeria-based immunotherapy. Expert Rev Vaccines. 2013;12(5):493–504.
16. Campisi L, Soudja SM, Cazareth J, Bassand D, Lazzari A, Brau F, et al. Splenic CD8α$^+$ dendritic cells undergo rapid programming by cytosolic bacteria and inflammation to induce protective CD8$^+$ T-cell memory. Eur J Immunol. 2011;41(6):1594–605.
17. Shahabi V, Seavey MM, Maciag PC, Rivera S, Wallecha A. Development of a live and highly attenuated Listeria monocytogenes-based vaccine for the treatment of Her2/neu-overexpressing cancers in human. Cancer Gene Ther. 2011;18(1):53–62.
18. Singh R, Dominiecki ME, Jaffee EM, Paterson Y. Fusion to Listeriolysin O and delivery by Listeria monocytogenes enhances the immunogenicity of HER-2/neu and reveals subdominant epitopes in the FVB/N mouse. J Immunol. 2005;175(6):3663–73.
19. Kim SH, Castro F, Gonzalez D, Maciag PC, Paterson Y, Gravekamp C. Mage-b vaccine delivered by recombinant Listeria monocytogenes is highly effective against breast cancer metastases. Br J Cancer. 2008;99(5):741–9.
20. Seavey MM, Maciag PC, Al-Rawi N, Sewell D, Paterson Y. An anti-vascular endothelial growth factor receptor 2/fetal liver kinase-1 Listeria monocytogenes anti-angiogenesis cancer vaccine for the treatment of primary and metastatic Her-2/neu + breast tumors in a mouse model. J Immunol. 2009;182(9):5537–46.
21. Seavey MM, Pan ZK, Maciag PC, Wallecha A, Rivera S, Paterson Y, et al. A novel human Her-2/neu chimeric molecule expressed by Listeria monocytogenes can elicit potent HLA-A2 restricted CD8-positive T cell responses and impact the growth and spread of Her-2/neu-positive breast tumors. Clin Cancer Res. 2009;15(3):924–32.
22. Wood LM, Pan ZK, Guirnalda P, Tsai P, Seavey M, Paterson Y. Targeting tumor vasculature with novel Listeria-based vaccines directed against CD105. Cancer Immunol Immunother. 2011;60(7):931–42.
23. Lin CW, Lee JY, Tsao YP, Shen CP, Lai HC, Chen SL. Oral vaccination with recombinant Listeria monocytogenes expressing human papillomavirus type 16 E7 can cause tumor growth in mice to regress. Int J Cancer. 2002;102(6):629–37.
24. Sewell DA, Douven D, Pan ZK, Rodriguez A, Paterson Y. Regression of HPV-positive tumors treated with a new Listeria monocytogenes vaccine. Arch Otolaryngol Head Neck Surg. 2004;130(1):92–7.
25. Sewell DA, Pan ZK, Paterson Y. Listeria-based HPV-16 E7 vaccines limit autochthonous tumor growth in a transgenic mouse model for HPV-16 transformed tumors. Vaccine. 2008;26(41):5315–20.
26. Guirnalda P, Wood L, Paterson Y. Listeria monocytogenes and its products as agents for cancer immunotherapy. Adv Immunol. 2012;113:81–118.
27. Wallecha A, Wood L, Pan ZK, Maciag PC, Shahabi V, Paterson Y. Listeria monocytogenes-derived listeriolysin O has pathogen-associated molecular pattern-like properties independent of its haemolytic ability. Clin Vaccine Immunol. 2013;20:177–84.
28. Gunn GR, Zubair A, Peters C, Pan ZK, Wu TC, Paterson Y. Two Listeria monocytogenes vaccine vectors that express different molecular forms of human papillomavirus-16 (HPV-16) E7 induce qualitatively different T cell immunity that correlates with their ability to induce regression of established tumors immortalized by HPV-16. J Immunol. 2001;167(11):6471–9.
29. Freeman MM, Ziegler HK. Simultaneous Th1-type cytokine expression is a signature of peritoneal CD4+ lymphocytes responding to infection with Listeria monocytogenes. J Immunol. 2005;175(1):394–403.
30. Sun R, Liu Y. Listeriolysin O as a strong immunogenic molecule for the development of new anti-tumor vaccines. Hum Vaccin Immunother. 2013; 9(5):1058–68.
31. Wallecha A, French C, Petit R, Singh R, Amin A, Rothman J. Lm-LLO-based immunotherapies and HPV-associated disease. J Oncol. 2012;2012:542851.
32. Maciag PC, Radulovic S, Rothman J. The first clinical use of a live-attenuated Listeria monocytogenes vaccine: a Phase I safety study of Lm-LLO-E7 in patients with advanced carcinoma of the cervix. Vaccine. 2009;27(30):3975–83.
33. Shahabi V, Maciag PC, Rivera S, Wallecha A. Live, attenuated strains of Listeria and Salmonella as vaccine vectors in cancer treatment. Bioeng Bugs. 2010;1(4):235–43.
34. Singh R, Wallecha A. Cancer immunotherapy using recombinant Listeria monocytogenes: transition from bench to clinic. Hum Vaccin. 2011;7(5):497–505.
35. Hussain SF, Paterson Y. CD4+CD25+ regulatory T cells that secrete TGFbeta and IL-10 are preferentially induced by a vaccine vector. J Immunother. 2004;2(5):339–46.
36. Peng X, Hussain SF, Paterson Y. The ability of two Listeria monocytogenes vaccines targeting human papillomavirus-16 E7 to induce an antitumor response correlates with myeloid dendritic cell function. J Immunol. 2004; 172(10):6030–8.
37. Dominiecki ME, Beatty GL, Pan ZK, Neeson P, Paterson Y. Tumor sensitivity to IFN-gamma is required for successful antigen-specific immunotherapy of a transplantable mouse tumor model for HPV-transformed tumors. Cancer Immunol Immunother. 2005;54(5):477–88.
38. Souders NC, Sewell DA, Pan ZK, Hussain SF, Rodriguez A, Wallecha A, et al. Listeria-based vaccines can overcome tolerance by expanding low avidity CD8+ T cells capable of eradicating a solid tumor in a transgenic mouse model of cancer. Cancer Immun. 2007;7:2.
39. Guirnalda P, Wood L, Goenka R, Crespo J, Paterson Y. Interferon γ-induced intratumoral expression of CXCL9 alters the local distribution of T cells following immunotherapy with Listeria monocytogenes. Oncoimmunology. 2013;2(8):e25752.
40. Mkrtichyan M, Chong N, Abu Eid R, Wallecha A, Singh R, Rothman J, et al. Anti-PD-1 antibody significantly increases therapeutic efficacy of Listeria monocytogenes (Lm)-LLO immunotherapy. J Immunother Cancer. 2013;1:15.
41. Ghamande SA, Dobbins R, Marshall L, Wheatley D, Prince C, Mauro DJ, et al. Phase I study evaluating high dose ADXS11-001 treatment in women with carcinoma of the cervix. J Clin Oncol. 2015;33(Suppl): abstract TPS3096.
42. US National Institutes of Health. ClinicalTrials.gov. Safety study of recombinant Listeria monocytogenes (Lm) based vaccine virus to treat

oropharyngeal cancer (REALISTIC). 2016. https://clinicaltrials.gov/ct2/show/NCT01598792. Accessed 3 Jan 2017.

43. US National Institutes of Health. ClinicalTrials.gov. A phase I/II evaluation of ADXS-001, mitomycin, 5-fluorouracil (5-FU) and IMRT for anal cancer (276). 2016. https://clinicaltrials.gov/ct2/show/NCT01671488. Accessed 3 Jan 2017.

44. Cohen EE, Moore KN, Slomovitz BM, Chung CH, Anderson ML, Morris SR, et al. Phase I/II study of ADXS11-001 or MEDI4736 immunotherapies alone and in combination, in patients with recurrent/metastatic cervical or human papillomavirus (HPV)-positive head and neck cancer. J Immunother Cancer. 2015;3(Suppl 2): poster P147.

45. Huh WK, Brady WE, Moore KN, Lankes HA, Monk BJ, Aghajanian C, et al. A phase 2 study of live-attenuated listeria monocytogenes cancer immunotherapy (ADXS11-001) in the treatment of persistent or recurrent cancer of the cervix (GOG-0265). J Clin Oncol. 2014;32(Suppl): abstract TPS5617.

46. Basu P, Mehta AO, Jain MM, Gupta S, Nagarkar RV, Kumar V, et al. ADXS11-001 immunotherapy targeting HPV-E7: Final results from a phase 2 study in Indian women with recurrent cervical cancer. J Clin Oncol. 2014;32(Suppl): abstract 5610.

47. Miles B, Gnjatic S, Donovan M, Genden EM, Misiukiewicz K, Krupar R, et al. Window of opportunity trial of HPV E7 antigen-expressing *Listeria*-based therapeutic vaccination prior to robotic surgery for HPV-positive oropharyngeal cancer. J Clin Oncol. 2015;33(Suppl): abstract TPS6088.

48. Fakih M, O'Neil BH, Chiorean EG, Hochster HS, Chan E, Mauro DJ, et al. Phase II study of ADXS11-001 in patients with persistent/recurrent, locoregional or metastatic squamous cell carcinoma of the anorectal canal. J Clin Oncol. 2016; 4(Suppl): abstract TPS786.

49. Herzog T. HPV – therapeutic strategies. Presented at the 34th Annual Meeting of the American Gynecological and Obstetrical Society; September 17–19, 2015; Half Moon Bay, CA.

50. Herzog T, Backes FJ, Copeland L, Estevez Diz MD, Hare TW, Huh W, et al. AIM2CERV: a randomized phase III study of adjuvant AXAL immunotherapy following chemoradiation in patients who have high-risk locally advanced cervical cancer (HRLACC). J Immunother Cancer. 2016;4(Suppl 1): abstract P140.

51. Slomovitz BM, Moore KM, Youssoufian H, Posner M. A phase I/II study of durvalumab alone or in combination with AXAL in recurrent/persistent or metastatic cervical or human papillomavirus (HPV) + squamous cell cancer of the head and neck (SCCHN): preliminary phase I results. J Immunother Cancer. 2016;4(Suppl 1): abstract P241.

52. Galon J, Pagès F, Marincola FM, Thurin M, Trinchieri G, Fox BA, et al. The immune score as a new possible approach for the classification of cancer. J Transl Med. 2012;10:1.

53. Galon J, Costes A, Sanchez-Cabo F, Kirilovsky A, Mlecnik B, Lagorce-Pagès C, et al. Type, density, and location of immune cells within human colorectal tumors predict clinical outcome. Science. 2006;313(5795):1960–4.

54. Funt S, Mu Z, Cipolla CK, Kania BE, Zheng J, Boyd ME, et al. Evaluation of monocytic myeloid-derived suppressor cell (M-MDSC) frequency in patients with metastatic urothelial carcinoma (mUC). J Clin Oncol. 2017;35(Suppl 6S): abstract 356.

55. Shou J, Zhang Z, Lai Y, Chen Z, Huang J. Worse outcome in breast cancer with higher tumor-infiltrating FOXP3+ Tregs: a systematic review and meta-analysis. BMC Cancer. 2016;16:687.

56. Herbst RS, Soria JC, Kowanetz M, Fine GD, Hamid O, Gordon MS, et al. Predictive correlates of response to the anti-PD-L1 antibody MPDL3280A in cancer patients. Nature. 2014;515(7528):563–7.

57. Masucci GV, Cesano A, Hawtin R, Janetzki S, Zhang J, Kirsch I, et al. Validation of biomarkers to predict response to immunotherapy in cancer: Volume 1 – pre-analytical and analytical validation. J Immunother Cancer. 2016;4:76.

58. Ribaudo JM, Cella D, Hahn EA, Lloyd SR, Tchekmedyian NS, Von Roenn J, et al. Re-validation and shortening of the Functional Assessment of Anorexia/Cachexia Therapy (FAACT) questionnaire. Qual Life Res. 2000;9(10):1137–46.

59. Webster K, Cella D, Yost K. The Functional Assessment of Chronic Illness Therapy (FACIT) Measurement System: properties, applications, and interpretation. Health Qual Life Outcomes. 2003;1:79.

23

Meeting report, "First Indian national conference on cervical cancer management -expert recommendations and identification of barriers to implementation"

K. S. Tewari[1*] (ID), A. Agarwal[2], A. Pathak[3], A. Ramesh[4], B. Parikh[5], M. Singhal[6], G. Saini[7], P. V. Sushma[8], N. Huilgol[9], S. Gundeti[10], S. Gupta[11], S. Nangia[12], S. Rawat[13], S. Alurkar[14], V. Goswami[15], B. Swarup[16], B. Ugile[16], S. Jain[16] and A. Kukreja[16]

Abstract

Objective: In India, cervical cancer accounts for almost 14% of all female cancer cases. Although poverty continues to cast a wide net over the Indian subcontinent, the preceding three decades have borne witness to improvements in nutrition and sanitation for many citizens. However, due to an absence of a national immunization program to cover human papillomavirus (HPV) vaccination and lack of accessible cervical cancer screening, the disease is characterized by late detection, lack of access to affordable and quality health care, and high mortality rates. Treatment of cervical cancer is stage-specific and depends on the patient's age, desire to preserve fertility, overall health, the clinician's expertise, and accessibility to resources. There is a paucity of uniform treatment protocols for various stages of cervical cancer in India. Considering all these parameters, a need to optimize treatment paradigms for the Indian population emerged.

Methods/materials: Three expert panel meetings were held in different regions of India from 2016 to 2017. They were comprised of 15 experts from across the country, and included surgical oncologists, radiation oncologists, and medical oncologists. The panel members reviewed the literature from both national and global sources, discussed their clinical experience and local practices and evaluated current therapeutic options and management gaps for women diagnosed with cervical cancer.

Results: This article summarizes the expert opinion from these meetings. It discusses the available resources and highlights the current therapeutic options available for different cervical cancer stages: early stage disease, locally advanced tumors, recurrent/persistent/metastatic cancer. An Indian consensus governing treatment options emerged, including guidelines for use of the only approved targeted therapy in this disease, the anti-angiogenesis drug, bevacizumab.

Conclusions: The panel concluded that given the availability of state-of-the-art imaging modalities, surgical devices, radiotherapeutics, and novel agents in several population-dense urban centers, a uniform, multi-disciplinary treatment approach across patient care centers is ideal but not realistic due to cost and a paucity of third party payors for most Indian citizens. Preventative strategies including visual inspection with acetic acid to screen for precursor lesions (i.e., cervical intraepithelial neoplasia) with immediate referral for cervical cryotherapy and possible large-scale roll-out of the HPV vaccine in the near future can be expected to reduce mortality rates significantly in this country.

Keywords: Cervical cancer, Cancer management, India, Expert opinion

* Correspondence: ktewari@uci.edu
[1]Division of Gynecologic Oncology, Department of Obstetrics & Gynecology, University of California, Irvine, The City Tower, 333 City Blvd, West - Suite 1400, Orange, CA, USA
Full list of author information is available at the end of the article

Introduction

As per GLOBOCAN, cervical cancer is the fourth most common cancer in women with an estimated 528,000 new cases (Fig. 1a) and 266,000 deaths in 2012 (Fig. 1b) [1].

In India, cervical cancer is the second most common cancer in women (aged 15–44 years) after breast cancer accounting for almost 14% of all female cancer cases [2, 3]. The age-adjusted incidence rate (AAIR) is 27.0 per 100,000 female population (Fig. 2) and age-adjusted mortality rate (AAMR) per 10,000 population is reported to be 12.4 [4, 5]. The higher mortality rate can be attributed largely to the lack of appropriate healthcare infrastructure in India [5, 6]. Cervical cancer in its advanced stage has a dismal outcome in terms of both prognosis and quality of life, registering approximately 67,477 deaths (23.3% of all cancer-related deaths) each year in Indian women [3, 7].

Screening and immunization programs availability in India

Several screening (visual inspection with acetic acid [VIA], magnified VIA [VIAM], visual inspection with Lugol's iodine [VILI], human papilloma virus [HPV] DNA testing and the Papanicolaou test) and diagnostic tests (cystoscopy, proctoscopy, examination under anesthesia) and imaging (computed tomography; CT; magnetic resonance imaging; MRI; positron emission tomography; PET scan; chest x-ray, and intravenous urography) are available for cervical cancer. However, their availability, specifically to patients residing in rural areas is limited [8–11].

Sankaranarayanan et al. (2009), in a cluster-randomized trial, assigned 131,746 healthy women aged 30 to 59 years to four groups (HPV testing, cytologic testing, visual inspection of the cervix with acetic acid [VIA], or standard care [control]). After 8 years of follow-up, the incidence rates of stage II or higher cervical cancer and death rates from cervical cancer were lowest in the HPV testing group. The hazard ratio (HR) for the detection of advanced cancer was 0.47 (95% confidence interval [CI]: 0.32–0.69) and for death was 0.52 (95% CI: 0.33–0.83) in the HPV-testing group when compared to the control group. In the other two experimental groups, significant reductions in the numbers of advanced cancers or deaths were not observed [12]. Further, Shastri et al., examined the feasibility and efficacy of VIA in reducing cervical cancer mortality by conducting a cluster-randomized study that included 151,538 women aged 35 to 64 years. After 12 years of follow-up, the VIA screening group showed 31% reduction in cervical cancer mortality when compared to the control group (rate ratios [RR]: 0.69; 95% CI: 0.54–0.88; $p = 0.003$) [13].

For cervical cancer, three types of vaccinations are already approved by the United States Food and Drug Administration which immunizes against various HPV types. They are HPV 2 (protects against subtype 16 and

18), HPV4 (6, 11, 16 and 18); and HPV9 (6, 11, 16, 18, 31, 33, 45, 52, and 58) [14]. With the exception of HPV immunization program in only two districts (Bathinda and Mansa) in the state of Punjab, currently there are no national HPV/cervical cancer immunization programs in India. The program has been launched with technical support from the World Health Organization (WHO) Country Office for India. First phase of the program has vaccinated approximately 10,000 girls of sixth standard in government schools of the above mentioned two districts, and is planned to be expanded to the other parts of the state with time [15].

Treatment options for cervical cancer

The International Federation of Gynecology and Obstetrics (FIGO) stratifies cervical cancer in four stages and the treatment depends on the cancer stage. Certain other factors can also impact the treatment decision such as location and type of cancer (squamous cell cancer or adenocarcinoma), age, overall health, and the patient's desire to have children [16]. Generally, early cancers are treated surgically, locally advanced cancers are treated with chemoradiation, and recurrent/metastatic cancers of the cervix may be salvaged with pelvic exenteration or palliated with systemic chemotherapy plus bevacizumab [16]. Apart from these, palliative care can be offered to patients to improve their quality of life and that of their respective families [17]. In India, cervical cancer is characterized by high incidence, late detection, lack of access to affordable and quality health care, and high mortality rates. Although, 360 million (30%) Indian population has taken up health insurance policies in the year 2015–2016, but there still remains a need to improve the awareness about health insurance policies among the rural communities where majority of the India's population resides [18, 19]. This expert opinion aims to highlight the treatment paradigm of cervical cancer from an Indian perspective and aims to help in the effective management of these patients.

Materials and methods

Three expert panel meetings were held at different regions in India. First two expert meetings were held at regional level in Delhi (Aug 6) and Hyderabad (June 18) in 2016, followed by a national level meeting in Mumbai in January 2017. Fifteen (15) members comprising of radiation oncologists, medical oncologists, surgical oncologists, and gynecologic oncologists were involved in this process (panel members listed in the Appendix). Although the meetings were supported by Roche, there were no Roche employees included among the expert panels physician roster. The expert opinion report was developed based on:

- Discussion by panel members who were convened to review the current therapeutic options and management gaps in cervical cancer patients

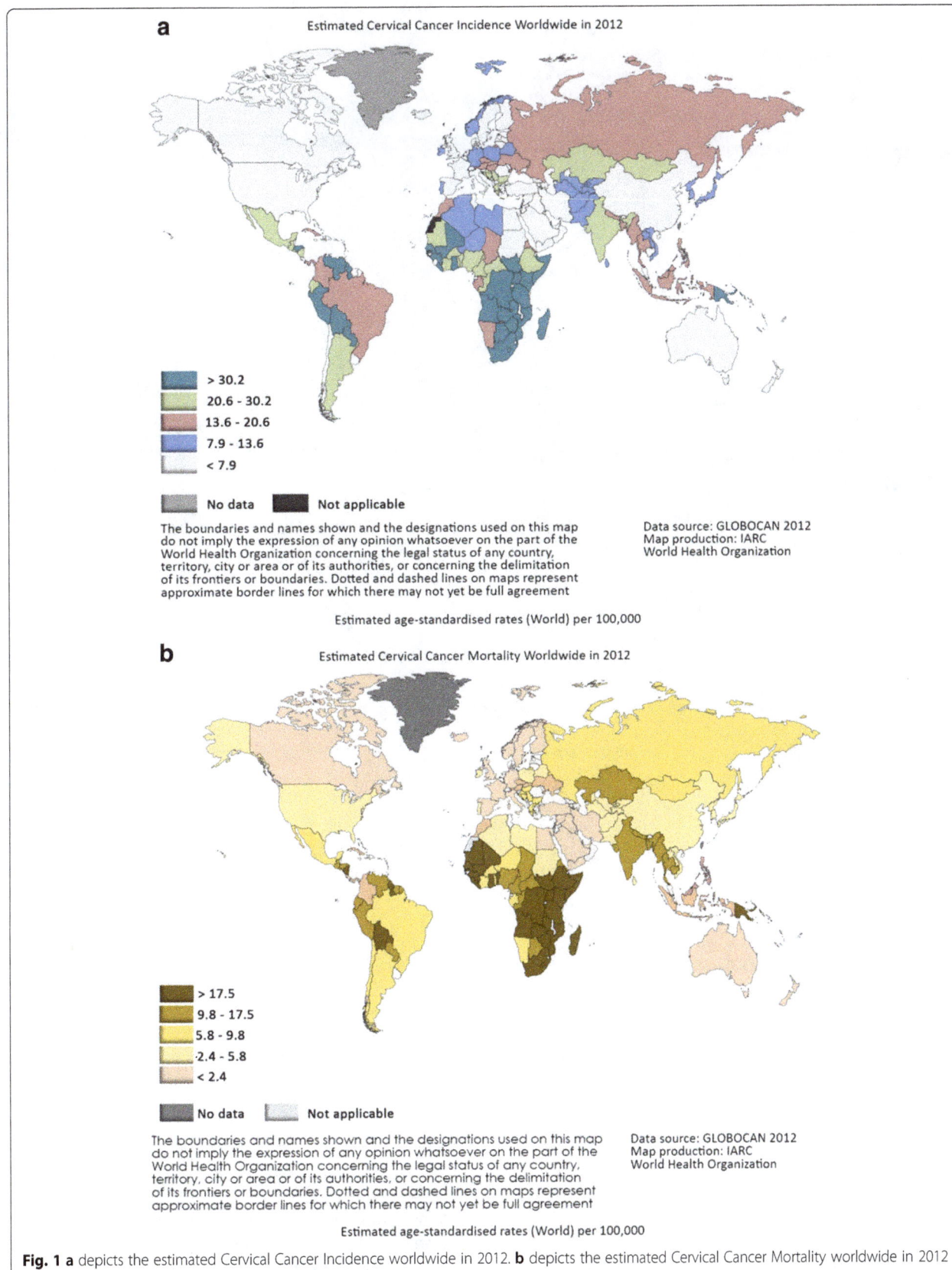

a Estimated Cervical Cancer Incidence Worldwide in 2012

Legend:
> 30.2
20.6 - 30.2
13.6 - 20.6
7.9 - 13.6
< 7.9
No data   Not applicable

The boundaries and names shown and the designations used on this map do not imply the expression of any opinion whatsoever on the part of the World Health Organization concerning the legal status of any country, territory, city or area or of its authorities, or concerning the delimitation of its frontiers or boundaries. Dotted and dashed lines on maps represent approximate border lines for which there may not yet be full agreement

Data source: GLOBOCAN 2012
Map production: IARC
World Health Organization

Estimated age-standardised rates (World) per 100,000

b Estimated Cervical Cancer Mortality Worldwide in 2012

Legend:
> 17.5
9.8 - 17.5
5.8 - 9.8
2.4 - 5.8
< 2.4
No data   Not applicable

The boundaries and names shown and the designations used on this map do not imply the expression of any opinion whatsoever on the part of the World Health Organization concerning the legal status of any country, territory, city or area or of its authorities, or concerning the delimitation of its frontiers or boundaries. Dotted and dashed lines on maps represent approximate border lines for which there may not yet be full agreement

Data source: GLOBOCAN 2012
Map production: IARC
World Health Organization

Estimated age-standardised rates (World) per 100,000

Fig. 1 a depicts the estimated Cervical Cancer Incidence worldwide in 2012. **b** depicts the estimated Cervical Cancer Mortality worldwide in 2012

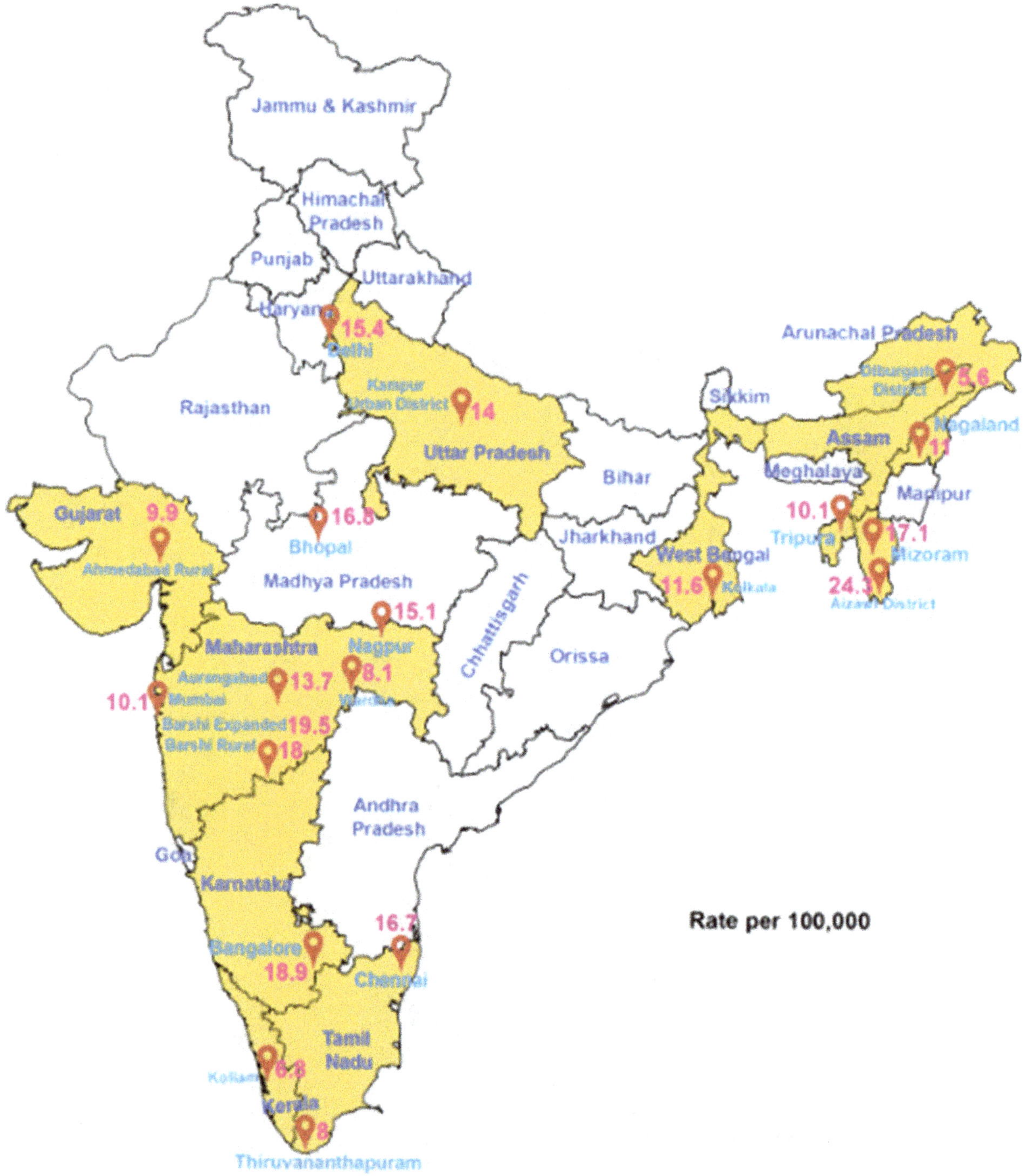

Fig. 2 Age adjusted Incidence of Cervical Cancer in India (rate per 100,000) as per the Different Population Based Cancer Registries are depicted in a political map of India

- A targeted review of literature from both national and global sources

This article highlights stage-specific cervical cancer treatment options, the Indian consensus and resource accessibility for the same.

Results
Treatment options, rationale for management, and recommendations specific to India
Early stage (FIGO stage IA-IB1 < 2 cm) desires fertility
For preservation of fertility, the National Comprehensive Cancer Network (NCCN) and the American Society of

Clinical Oncology (ASCO) guidelines recommends cone biopsy with negative margins for stage IA cervical cancer without lymphovascular space invasion (LVSI). Whereas, for stage IA cancer with LVSI and stage IA2, cone biopsy with negative margins with pelvic lymph node dissection (PLND) or radical trachelectomy with PLND is recommended. Radical trachelectomy with PLND is also recommended for stage IB1 [20, 21]. As per ASCO guidelines, women's with stage IB1 desiring fertility may also require adjuvant therapy if tumor is > 2 cm [21].

Patient survival with conization for stage IA cancer is similar to that with hysterectomy [22]. A Romanian study showed that radical vaginal trachelectomy and laparoscopic pelvic lymphadenectomy presents a safe therapeutic option in early stage cervical cancer with negligible recurrence rate and thus, promises to be a suitable option for young patients who want to retain their fertility [23]. Further, a Swedish study demonstrated that robotics-assisted laparoscopic radical trachelectomy in early stage cervical cancer patients is associated with high fertility rates (81%), low premature deliveries (6%), and an acceptable rate of tumor recurrence (4%) [24]. Studies have also shown that fertility sparing surgical management in the form of radical trachelectomy for early cervical cancer have a low rate of recurrence, few complications, and encouraging rates of conception and uneventful pregnancies although fertility treatment may be required [25, 26].

Indian consensus The panelists unanimously agreed that early stage cervical cancer can be effectively managed by cone biopsy and radical trachelectomy. Cone biopsy with removal of pelvic lymph nodes and radical trachelectomy with PLND are the best treatment options for fertility preservation. Pelvic lymphadenectomy for fertility preservation can be successfully carried out with laparoscopy.

Early stage IA2 to IB1

When preservation of fertility is not desired, the NCCN and ASCO guidelines recommends performing extrafascial or modified radical hysterectomy with PLND or pelvic external beam radiation therapy (EBRT) plus brachytherapy [20].

Indian consensus The panelists agreed that radical hysterectomy with PLND and tailored adjuvant radiotherapy/chemoradiation and/or brachytherapy should be recommended for women who do not desire fertility.

Early stage IA2 and IB1 (fertility not desired)

Guidelines recommend modified radical hysterectomy with PLND or pelvic EBRT plus brachytherapy for early stages IA2 and IB1, if fertility is not desired [20]. If surgery is chosen, it can be performed as an open

procedure or using minimally invasive techniques (eg. laparoscopy, robotic-assisted laparoscopy). In addition, patients with IB1 stage are also suggested to be treated with adjuvant radiotherapy or concomitant chemo-radiotherapy (CCRT), if required [21]. Presence of intermediate risk factors (vascular and lymphatic permeation, tumor size > 2 cm, and deep cervical stroma invasion) or high-risk factors (positive pelvic lymph nodes, parametrial infiltration, and positive surgical margins) in surgically treated early-stage cervical cancer patients can dictate the use of adjuvant radiation or chemoradiation [27]. Adjuvant pelvic radiotherapy in intermediate-risk stage IB cervical cancer patients who underwent radical hysterectomy and pelvic lymphadenectomy showed 15% recurrence rate compared to 28% in the patient group who had no further treatment ($p = 0.008$) [28]. Similarly, high risk cervical cancer patients who received CCRT and pelvic radiation therapy after radical surgery showed improved progression free survival (PFS) and overall survival (OS) when compared to patients treated with adjuvant pelvic radiation therapy and surgery (PFS: 80% vs. 63%; $p = 0.003$ and Overall Survival (OS): 81% vs. 71%; $p = 0.007$) [29]. Adjuvant treatment with pelvic EBRT is indicated in case of large tumor size, more than one-third stromal invasion and/or LVSI (Sedlis Criteria) [20, 28]. It has been suggested that intensity-modulated radiation therapy (IMRT) may reduce the radiation dose to bowel and other vital structures by virtue of its ability to intensify dose to cancerous tissues while sparing the surrounding healthy tissue. IMRT can be used in patients post hysterectomy and also in the treatment of para-aortic nodes [30].

Indian consensus Experts recommended adjuvant radiotherapy and cisplatin-based CCRT for cervical cancer patients with intermediate and high-risk factors for tumor recurrence. In cases where surgical expertise is unavailable, or the patient is unsuitable for surgery, radiation therapy with either intracavitary brachytherapy alone or along with external beam radiation therapy remains a viable treatment of choice.

Locally advanced disease IB2 to IVA

Treatment of locally advanced disease consists of pelvic EBRT with concurrent cisplatin-based chemotherapy and brachytherapy [20]. Table 1 present clinical studies assessing the efficacy and safety of chemotherapy and radiotherapy.

Lymphatic metastases are known to be higher in patients with locally advanced cervical cancer than in those at early stage. In spite of improved local control and OS with CCRT, almost 10–15% of the patients develop para-aortic lymph node (PALN) metastasis. Extended field irradiation combined with CCRT has shown better results in such cases. (Table 1) [38].

Table 1 Clinical Trials Assessing Efficacy and Safety of Chemotherapy and Radiotherapy in Locally advanced disease IB2 to IVA

Trials	Patient population	Treatment Arms	Results	Conclusions/Discussions
Morris et al. 1999 [31]	Cervical cancer confined to the pelvis (stages IIB through IVA or stage IB or IIA with a tumor diameter of at least 5 cm or involvement of pelvic lymph nodes)	Radiotherapy + chemotherapy (fluorouracil + cisplatin) vs. radiotherapy alone in high risk cervical cancer	5-year survival rate: 73% vs. 58%; $p = 0.004$	Addition of chemotherapy with fluorouracil and cisplatin to radiotherapy significantly improves survival rate
Kang et al. 2015 [32]	Patients will all tumor stages	Temporal treatment patterns for cervical cancer per guideline recommendations	Factors affecting likelihood of treatment per guidelines: age ($p < 0.0001$); tumor stage at diagnosis ($p = 0.002$) Reduction in all-cause mortality: 56%; cancer related mortality: 49%	Treatment per guideline recommendations reduced mortality rates and OS
Au-Yeung et al. 2013 [33]	Patients with Locally advanced cervix cancer patients	Carboplatin + radiation for locally advanced cervical cancer	No significant benefit in OS or DFS	Concurrent use of carboplatin along with radiation therapy does not impact survival rate
Sebastiao et al. 2016 [34]	Patients with cervical cancer stage IIB-IVA	Cisplatin + radiotherapy vs. carboplatin + radiotherapy in advanced cervical cancer	3-year PFS: 59% vs. 40% 3-year OS: 70% vs. 68%	Overall, both cisplatin and carboplatin were similar with respect to 3-years OS, PFS, ORR, and toxic effects
Hashemi et al. 2013 [35]	Patients with cervical cancer stage IIB to stage IVA	Gemcitabine + cisplatin + radiotherapy	ORR: 97.3% 3-year DFS: 67% OS: 72%	Inconclusive regarding the benefit with gemcitabine. Further phase III studies required to validate the results
Narayan et al. 2016 [36]	Patients with stage I(IB2) and locally advanced (stages II-IVA) cervical cancer	NACT followed by CCRT vs. CCRT	DFS: 58.3% vs. 41.8%; $p=0.001$	Combination NACT with paclitaxel and cisplatin may improve long-term survival of patients with cervical cancer
Gill et al. 2015 [37]	Patients with stage IB1 to IVA cervical cancer	MRI-guided high-dose-rate intracavitary brachytherapy for cervical cancer	2-year local control: 91.6%; DFS: 81.8%; cancer-specific survival rate: 87.6%	Excellent local control and considerable morbidity was observed
Li et al. 2014 [38]	Patients with stage IIb-IVa cervical squamous cell carcinoma, adenocarcinoma, or adenosquamous carcinoma; seven patients had lymph node metastasis	Raltitrexed/cisplatin with concurrent radiotherapy; additional radiation was administered to the lymph node metastases	OS: 90.7%	Favorable efficacy and acceptable adverse events

Legend: OS Overall survival, PFS Progression free survival, ORR Overall response rate, DFS Disease free survival, NACT Neoadjuvant chemotherapy, CCRT Concurrent chemoradiation therapy, MRI Magnetic resonance imaging

Extended-field CCRT is also an effective and a reasonable option for stage IIB-IVA cervical cancer patients with positive pelvic lymph nodes and radiologic negative PALN [39]. Internal radiation therapy/ intracavitary radiotherapy/ brachytherapy when combined with EBRT demonstrates good tolerance and is safe with acceptable morbidity [40, 41]. Brachytherapy is preferred after EBRT for radical treatment which delivers huge proportional radiation dose to the residual tumor while sparing the adjacent local organs (bladder and rectum) [42]. As per the International Commission on Radiation Units and Measurements (ICRU) report 38, brachytherapy can be administered at low-, medium-, and high-dose rate [43]. Higher dose is mandatory to achieve local control and poor tumor geometric conditions may require interstitial brachytherapy [44, 45].

Brachytherapy can be high dose rate (HDR) or low dose rate (LDR). In LDR brachytherapy, cesium-137 isotope is used, and a point A dose rate of < 0.4 Gray/hour is delivered. HDR brachytherapy uses iridium-192 isotope and a point A dose rate of > 12 Gray/hour. Although HDR is gaining more popularity in the recent years, the overall results and toxicity with HDR and LDR are considered to be comparable [46].

Main indications for interstitial brachytherapy include large tumors, lower vaginal involvement, lateral extension of disease, and ill-fitting intracavitary applicators [46]. Younger women can be offered the option for laparoscopic ovarian transposition to move ovaries out of radiation field. This helps in reducing the exposure to radiations by 90% [47].

Indian consensus The panel members jointly agreed that locally advanced cancers are best treated with CCRT. Adjuvant chemotherapy may be considered as per the clinician's perspective. Chemotherapy is for the systemic management while radiotherapy limits local disease. The choice of therapeutic regimen is as follows: cisplatin+ paclitaxel > > carboplatin + paclitaxel > cisplatin alone > > cisplatin + gemcitabine. The experts had a detailed discussion regarding the sequence of the two management options: radiotherapy and chemotherapy and finally it was concluded that the sequence of administering the modalities depends on the patient's condition, availability of radiotherapeutic units and the clinician's perspective. It was also agreed that the choice of treatment for a PALN negative stage IIB-IVA cervical cancer patient would include CCRT to the pelvis plus brachytherapy, and for a PALN positive patient, CCRT to pelvis with extended field radiotherapy plus brachytherapy.

Metastatic (stage IVB) disease
The prognosis of metastatic cervical cancer is usually poor and the main objectives of treatment include slowing the cancer growth and relieving the symptoms. The

management of stage IVB will be addressed together with the management of persistent and recurrent disease later in the paper.

Indian consensus The panel members unanimously agreed that systemic chemotherapy is mandatory for advanced stage cervical cancer patients while radiotherapy is essential for improvement of their symptoms including vaginal bleeding, pelvic pain, pain due to bone metastases etc. Cisplatin, carboplatin (chemotherapeutic agents), and bevacizumab (targeted therapy) are the available treatment choices. Considering increased toxicity, topotecan is not recommended for the management of advanced stage cervical cancer and the preferred therapeutic choice is cisplatin + paclitaxel + bevacizumab.

Persistent disease
The management of persistent disease along with metastatic and recurrent disease will be addressed later.

Indian consensus Adding bevacizumab to chemotherapy for persistent cervical cancer improves OS, progression free survival (PFS) and overall response rate (ORR). Combination therapy with cisplatin, paclitaxel and bevacizumab is superior than topotecan, paclitaxel, and bevacizumab regimen similar to that for metastatic (stage IV B) disease.

Recurrent disease-isolated central recurrence
Pelvic recurrence of cervical cancer is categorized into three categories; they are central pelvic, lateral pelvic and extra-pelvic. The management of central pelvic recurrence varies with the previous treatment received by the patient i.e. radical hysterectomy without adjuvant irradiation or only irradiation. Women's treated with irradiation in the past are only left with pelvic exenteration as a surgical therapeutic option [48]. NCCN also states that cancers recurring centrally (in the pelvis only) might see a better response with pelvic exenteration while in patients with recurrence at distant locations (such as lungs or bone), radiation and chemotherapy may be used [20].

A Korean study showed that with pelvic exenteration, the 5-year OS and 5-year DFS were 56 and 49% for metastatic cases [49]. Similarly, an Indian study reported a good 5-year OS (> 55%) in patients who underwent pelvic exenteration [50]. However, both the studies reported high morbidity rates associated with pelvic exenteration (44 and 62.50%, respectively) [49, 50].

Further, it is recommended that these patients should then undergo a pelvic reconstructive procedure which include bowel reconstruction, urinary reconstruction, and vagina reconstruction [51]. The reconstructive procedures are reported to lower morbidity rates. Continent diversions are preferred as they have been found to improve quality of life [52]. However, they too are associated with complications such as ureteral stricture/obstruction, difficult catheterization and pyelonephritis [53]. These patients require to be given post-operative care in intensive care units (ICUs). A patient is estimated to spend two to three days on an average in Intensive Care Unit post-surgery where regular care by the team involving intensive care team, colorectal surgeons for primary care, surgical specialty review, stoma therapy, nursing, and other health staff is required [54].

Indian consensus The panelists stated that pelvic exenteration may provide the opportunity of long-term survival in carefully selected cervical cancer patients. They also highlighted that pelvic exenteration is a morbid procedure creating a huge financial and psychological burden.

Recurrent disease non-exenteration candidate, first-line therapy

Although cisplatin administered intravenously (50 mg/m^2) every 3 weeks is considered the most effective single agent in the treatment of metastatic cervical cancer, patients who have already received cisplatin as a radio sensitizer, may not respond to the single drug regimen. Therefore, cisplatin-based combination therapies are used in these patients [55–57]. According to Pfaendler and Tewari (2016), the standard treatment for recurrent cancer patients is cisplatin plus paclitaxel [58].

Now-a-days studies are being conducted to assess the effectiveness of adding bevacizumab (vascular endothelial growth factor-specific angiogenesis) inhibitor to chemotherapeutic regimen in patients with recurrent, persistent, or metastatic cervical cancer. Recurrence after prior chemotherapy results in very poor prognosis of cervical cancer patients can be better dealt by incorporating bevacizumab in the treatment regime.

NCCN guidelines gives class 1 recommendation for bevacizumab to be given as first line treatment (in following combinations: cisplatin/paclitaxel/bevacizumab; topotecan/paclitaxel/bevacizumab; carboplatin/paclitaxel/bevacizumab) in patients with metastatic or recurrent cervical cancer [20].

Patients with metastatic disease may experience symptoms of vaginal bleeding, pelvic pain, pain due to bone metastases etc. Palliative radiotherapy must be used based on the site of metastases, patient's performance status and life expectancy, and potential treatment toxicity. Evidence suggests that longer duration of radiotherapy may not be required as short courses are as effective [59, 60].

Indian consensus

Experts agreed that without evidence of inferiority, carboplatin and paclitaxel are an alternative for patients with recurrent disease, unless they have not received prior chemoradiation therapy. In patients with renal dysfunction, carboplatin is better tolerated owing to its milder toxic profile. Adding bevacizumab to chemotherapy for recurrent cervical cancer improves OS, PFS and ORR as in patients with persistent disease. The combination therapy with cisplatin, paclitaxel and bevacizumab appears to be clinically more feasible than topotecan, paclitaxel and bevacizumab regimen.

Recurrent disease, second-line therapy

Kamura et al. (2013) in his review concluded that chemotherapy can be considered as a second line treatment for patients with recurrent cervical cancer, but is less effective due to drug resistance. A phase II trial has assessed the efficacy and tolerability of bevacizumab in patients with recurrent or persistent cervical cancer. The study results showed median PFS and OS times to be 3.40 months (95% CI: 2.53–4.53 months) and 7.29 months (95% CI: 6.11–10.41 months), respectively. Further, phase III clinical trials are warranted. It has suggested bevacizumab to be used as second or third line drug in patients with recurrent cervical cancer [61]. NCCN guidelines also recommend bevacizumab for second line treatment of recurrent cervical cancer in addition to other drugs (category 2B unless otherwise indicated) including docetaxel, 5-FU, gemcitabine, ifosfamide, mitomycin, irinotecan, albumin bound paclitaxel (i.e., nab-paclitaxel), topotecan, pemetrexed, and vinorelbine [20]. Chemotherapy is the only choice for a palliative therapy in patients with recurrent non-central cervical cancer who had previously been treated with surgery plus adjuvant irradiation and chemo (radiation) [48]. NCCN guidelines states that patients who had recurrence even after second line treatment (surgery or radiation therapy) can be given "chemotherapy or best supportive care, or can be enrolled in a clinical trial." [20]. It should be noted that in June 2018, the anti-PD-1 checkpoint inhibitor, pembrolizumab, was granted accelerated approved in the United States by the U.S. Food and Drug Administration for second-line therapy in women with recurrent cervical cancer. It is too early to determine the likelihood of availabilty of this drug and other immuno-oncology agents for this indication in India.

Indian consensus The panel agreed that palliative chemotherapy should be given to patients with recurrent cervical cancer as second line treatment. The need of best supportive care for these patients was also suggested.

Resources and feasibility

Availability of resources for management of cervical cancer in India is presented in Table 2.

Discussion

Treatment of cervical cancer is stage-specific and depends on patient's age, desire to preserve fertility, overall health, clinician's expertise, and accessibility to resources. This expert opinion highlights the current therapeutic options available for different cancer stages (early-, advanced, and recurrent) and Indian consensus on their treatment options.

Majority of the early-stage cancers are treated with surgery which successfully preserves the fertility without compromising treatment and survival.

The stage-wise best management practices followed in India are presented in Table 3.

The targeted therapies, like bevacizumab, which have demonstrated clinical benefits to these patients (in clinical studies as well as clinical experience of some of the Indian experts) need to be widely utilized in India, as per this expert group's opinion.

Conclusion

The treatment of cervical cancer is stage-specific and necessitates cognizance of patient's age, desire to preserve fertility, overall health, clinician's expertise, and accessibility to healthcare infrastructure. The panel concluded that a uniform, multi-disciplinary treatment approach across patient care centers using advanced therapeutics

Table 2 Availability of Resources for Management of Cervical Cancer in India

Resources	Availability in India
Loop Electrocautery Excision Procedure	It is a safer procedure as compared to cold knife conization, but is not very common in India as it requires expensive machines [62].
Radical trachelectomy	It is an expensive surgical option, thus unaffordable by women in poor-resource setting who are known to be more commonly diagnosed with cervical cancer.
Surgical expertise	As per the ASCO resource-stratified clinical practice guideline, fertility sparing treatment requires surgical expertise which may not be easily available in the basic or limited settings [63].
Radiotherapy	There is a one radiotherapy machine per 2-5 million cancer patients which highlights the lack of accessibility to radiotherapy. The use of brachytherapy in India is limited due to following reasons. • Lack of radiation oncologists and radiotherapy technologists. • Private hospitals favour other techniques including IMRT and IGRT over brachytherapy. • Implementation of latest advancements in brachytherapy is limited to a few premier hospitals [64]. However, despite all these challenges, the use of brachytherapy has shown a surge in India.
Chemotherapy	Chemotherapeutic drugs are available in India, but the associated cost is high. • A recent observational study by Kolasani et al. (2016) assessed the variation in prices of anti-cancer drugs (chemotherapy) in India. Physicians might not prescribe the low-priced drug due to lack of information on quality, conflict of interest, and a belief that new drug is better than the older [65]. • Thus, if awareness is raised among the treating physicians about the quality of the low-priced drugs, it will increase the accessibility and affordability of the treatment to lower and middle-class patients in India. • Pharmaceutical companies and government should also make efforts to reduce the drug prices to lower the economic burden on the patients. [64]
CCRT	Annually, 38,771 patients with cervical cancers in India do not receive CCRT, resulting in poorer survival. [66]
HDR and interstitial brachytherapy	• Ir-192 is commonly used for HDR brachytherapy in state government funded hospital in India, but its replacement with Co-60 will be a cost-effective option in developing countries like India. [64] • Few studies in Indian settings have assessed the applicability of interstitial brachytherapy in patients not suitable to undergo intracavitary brachytherapy. [67–69]
Bevacizumab	• The cost-effectiveness analysis of bevacizumab has been conducted using the Markov decision tree in 240 patients enrolled in the GOG trial. The study concluded that ICER associated with bevacizumab could be reduced by introducing biosimilars, and/or other cheaper and efficacious anti-angiogenesis agents. [70] • Roche is currently running 'The Blue Tree' program for cancer patients in India. This program covers several aspects to help cancer patients ranging from "diagnostics, funding of treatment, information, post-treatment job search, assistance with documentation for reimbursement and free medicines where possible."
Pelvic exenteration procedure	• This procedure requires tremendous economic and psychosocial support which a developing country like India largely lacks. • Poverty and illiteracy further makes optimal rehabilitation of these patients difficult [50]. • There is a need of increase in beds at ICUs in both private and public hospitals with the expected rise in number of cancer patients. The associated high cost of ICUs in private hospitals and lack of its coverage under health insurance, the oncology patients has to borrow or sell assets for admission to ICUs [71].
Palliative Care	• There is a huge lack of manpower in Indian hospitals to provide palliative care to cancer patients [72]. • Thus, it is not possible to provide palliative care to all cancer patients in India.

Abbreviations: *ASCO* American Society of Clinical Oncology, *IMRT* Intensity-modulated radiotherapy, *IGRT* Image-guided radiotherapy, *Ir* Iridium, *CCRT* Concurrent radiotherapy, *Co* Cobalt, *ICER* Incremental cost-effectiveness ratio, *ICU* Intensive care units

Table 3 Summary of Cervical Cancer Management Practices Followed in India

Cone biopsy and radical trachelectomy with pelvic lymph node dissection are the best treatment option for fertility preservation in early stage (IA1, IA2, IB1 and IB2) cervical cancer patients.

Patients not interested to maintain fertility can undergo radical hysterectomy with PLND and tailored adjuvant radiotherapy/chemoradiation and/or brachytherapy.

Stage IA2-IB1 cervical cancer patients are typically treated with radical hysterectomy with PLND with or without para-aortic lymph node sampling. They are further managed with adjuvant CCRT depending on the surgico-pathologic findings. Radiation therapy includes both EBRT and brachytherapy.

In a developing country like India, radiotherapeutic facilities are limited and generally patients have a lengthy waiting period, hence, neo-adjuvant chemotherapy with cisplatin and paclitaxel is the preferred alternative for early stage cervical cancer patients. The high cost of chemotherapeutic agents increases the economic burden on the patients.

For stage IB2-IVA, primary CCRT plus brachytherapy with or without adjuvant cisplatin or carboplatin based chemotherapy is an effective management option

Cervical cancer stage IVB is incurable and the main treatment option is palliation. Incorporation of bevacizumab with chemotherapy doublets may improve survival by a median 3.7 months.

Pelvic exenteration may be curative for a patient with a central, isolated recurrence but if the patient is not an exenteration candidate (eg., non-central recurrence or metastatic disease or refuses exenteration).

Legend: *PLND* Pelvic lymph node dissection, *CCRT* Concurrent chemoradiation therapy, *EBRT* External beam radiation therapy

should be widely utilized in India. The panel acknowledges that prevention represents the most feasible and effective path forward but that requires commitment to develop a VIA screening infrastructure and national endoresment of a HPV vaccination program.

Abbreviations
AAIR: Age-Adjusted Incidence Rate; AAMR: Age-Adjusted Mortality Rate; ASCO: American Society of Clinical Oncology; CCRT: Concomitant Chemo-Radiation Therapy; CI: Confidence Interval; CT: Computed Tomography; EBRT: External Beam Radiation Therapy; FIGO: International Federation of Gynecology and Obstetrics; HDR: High Dose Rate; HPV: Human Papilloma Virus; HR: Hazard Ratio; ICRU: International Commission on Radiation Units and Measurements; IMRT: Intensity-Modulated Radiation Therapy; LDR: Low dose rate; LVSI: Lymphovascular Space Invasion; MRI: Magnetic Resonance Imaging; NCCN: National Comprehensive Cancer Network; ORR: Overall Response Rate; OS: Overall Survival; PALN: Para-Aortic Lymph Node; PET: Positron Emission Tomography; PLND: Pelvic Lymph Node Dissection; RR: Rate Ratios; VIA: Visual Inspection with Acetic Acid; VIAM: Visual Inspection with Acetic Acid Magnified; WHO: World Health Organization

Acknowledgements
Medical writing and editing support was provided by Ritika P of Turacoz and Priyanka Bhattacharya of Roche Products (India) Pvt. Ltd.

Funding
Roche Products (India) Pvt. Ltd. provided financial support for this scientific/educational project at no detriment to the freedom to prescribe and to choose treatment. Roche does not recommend or endorse any use, preparation or administration of the products, which is outside of their Prescribing Information.

Authors' contributions
KST conceived and led the expert opinion meeting and critically reviewed all three drafts of the meeting report and developed the final version through substantial writing contributions. BU, SJ, BS helped conduct the meeting and draft the meeting report. AA, AP, AR, BP, MS, GS, SV, NH, SG, SN, SG, SR, SSA,VG, and AK contributed towards the discussion at the meeting and critically reviewed the meeting report. All authors read and approved the final expert opinion meeting report.

Competing interests
The authors declare that they have no competing interests except for Dr. Balaji Ugile, Dr. Suyog Jain, Dr. Binay Swarup and Dr. Anil Kukreja who are full time employees of Roche Products (India) Pvt. Ltd.

Author details
[1]Division of Gynecologic Oncology, Department of Obstetrics & Gynecology, University of California, Irvine, The City Tower, 333 City Blvd, West - Suite 1400, Orange, CA, USA. [2]Medical Oncology, Dr. B.L. Kapur Memorial Hospital, New Delhi, India. [3]Cancer Care Hospital, Nagpur, Maharashtra, India. [4]Apollo Speciality Hospital, Chennai, Tamil Nadu, India. [5]Bombay Hospital, Mumbai, Maharashtra, India. [6]Indraprastha Apollo Hospitals, New Delhi, India. [7]Max Super Speciality Hospital, Vaishali, India. [8]KIMS Hospital, Hyderabad, Telangana, India. [9]Nanavati Hospital, Mumbai, Maharashtra, India. [10]Nizams Institute Medical Sciences, Hyderabad, Telangana, India. [11]Medanta Hospital, Gurgaon, Haryana, India. [12]Indraprastha Apollo Hospital, Delhi, India. [13]Dharamshila Hospital, New Delhi, India. [14]Apollo Hospitals, Ahmedabad, Gujarat, India. [15]Fortis Hospital, Noida, Uttar Pradesh, India. [16]Roche Products (India) Pvt. Ltd., Mumbai, Maharastra, India.

References
1. GLOBOCAN. Cervical Cancer Estimated Incidence, Mortality and Prevalence Worldwide in 2012. Available at: http://globocan.iarc.fr/old/FactSheets/cancers/cervix-new.asp. Accessed 11 July 2018.
2. NICPR. Cancer Statistics. Available at: http://cancerindia.org.in/statistics/ Accessed 11 July 2018.
3. Chatterjee S, Chattopadhyay A, Samanta L, et al. HPV and Cervical Cancer Epidemiology - Current Status of HPV Vaccination in India. *Asian Pac J Cancer Prev.* 2016;17:3663–73.
4. Sreedevi A, Javed R, Dinesh A. Epidemiology of cervical cancer with special focus on India. *International Journal of Women's Health.* 2015;7:405–14.
5. Ernst & Young. Call for Action: Expanding cancer care in India. Available at: https://www.ey.com/Publication/vwLUAssets/EY-Call-for-action-expanding-cancer-care-in-india/$FILE/EY-Call-for-action-expanding-cancer-care-in-india.pdf Accessed 11 July 2018.
6. Mohanty G, Ghosh SN. Risk factors for cancer of cervix, status of screening and methods for its detection. *Arch Gynecol Obstet.* 2015;291:247–9.
7. HPV information center. Summary report. Available at: http://hpvcentre.net/statistics/reports/IND_FS.pdf. Accessed 11 July 2018.
8. Khan SH. Cancer and positron emission tomography imaging in India: Vision 2025. *Indian J Nucl Med.* 2016;31:251–4.
9. Tests for Cervical Cancer. Available at: https://www.cancer.org/cancer/cervical-cancer/detection-diagnosis-staging/how-diagnosed.html. Accessed 11 July 2018.
10. Bobdey S, Sathwara J, Jain A, et al. Burden of cervical cancer and role of screening in India. *Indian Journal of Medical and Paediatric Oncology.* 2016;37:278–85.
11. National Programme for Prevention and Control of Diabetes, Cardiovascular Disease and Stroke. Available at: http://www.searo.who.int/india/topics/cardiovascular_diseases/NCD_Resources_COMBINED_MANUAL_for_medical_officer.pdf. Accessed 11 July 2018.

12. Sankaranarayanan R, Nene BM, Shastri SS, et al. HPV screening for cervical cancer in rural India. *N Engl J Med*. 2009;360:1385–94.

13. Shastri SS, Mittra I, Mishra GA, et al. Effect of VIA screening by primary health workers: randomized controlled study in Mumbai, India. *J Natl Cancer Inst* 2014;106:dju009.

14. HPV Vaccination information for clinicians. Available at: https://www.cdc.gov/hpv/hcp/need-to-know.pdf. Accessed 11 July 2018.

15. Punjab launches HPV vaccine with WHO support. Available at: http://www.searo.who.int/india/mediacentre/events/2016/Punjab_HPV_vaccine/en/. Accessed 11 July 2018.

16. American cancer society. Treatment options for cervical cancer by stage. Available at: https://www.cancer.org/cancer/cervical-cancer/treating/by-stage.html Accessed 11 July 2018.

17. Pesee M, Kirdpon W, Puapairoj A, et al. Palliative treatment of advanced cervical cancer with radiotherapy and thai herbal medicine as supportive remedy - analysis of survival. *Asian Pac J Cancer Prev*. 2013;14:1593–6.

18. K I, Saba I H, Gopi A, et al. Awareness of health insurance in a rural population of Bangalore, India. *Int J Med Sci Public Health*. 2016;5:2162–7.

19. Indian Insurance Industry Overview & Market Development Analysis. Available at: https://www.ibef.org/industry/insurance-sector-india.aspx. Accessed 29 Aug 2017.

20. NCCN. Cervical cancer. Available at: https://www.nccn.org/professionals/physician_gls/pdf/cervical.pdf Accessed 11 July 2018

21. Chuang LT, Feldman S, Nakisige C, et al. Management and Care of Women With Invasive Cervical Cancer: ASCO Resource-Stratified Clinical Practice Guideline. *J Clin Oncol*. 2016;34:3354–5.

22. Wright JD, NathavithArana R, Lewin SN, et al. Fertility-conserving surgery for young women with stage IA1 cervical cancer: safety and access. *Obstet Gynecol*. 2010;115:585–90.

23. Bratila E, Bratila CP, Coroleuca CB. Radical Vaginal Trachelectomy with Laparoscopic Pelvic Lymphadenectomy for Fertility Preservation in Young Women with Early-Stage Cervical Cancer. *Indian J Surg*. 2016;78:265–70.

24. Johansen G, Lönnerfors C, Falconer H, et al. Reproductive and oncologic outcome following robot-assisted laparoscopic radical trachelectomy for early stage cervical cancer. *Gynecol Oncol*. 2016;141:160–5.

25. Shepherd JH, Spencer C, Herod J, et al. Authors response to: Regarding radical vaginal trachelectomy as a fertility-sparing procedure in women with early-stage cervical cancer-cumulative pregnancy rate in a series of 123 women. *BJOG*. 2007;114:116.

26. Kasuga Y, Nishio H, Miyakoshi K, et al. Pregnancy outcomes after abdominal radical trachelectomy for early-stage cervical cancer: a 13-year experience in a single tertiary-care center. *Int J Gynecol Cancer*. 2016;26:163–8.

27. Candelaria M, Garcia-Arias A, Cetina L, et al. Radiosensitizers in cervical cancer. Cisplatin and beyond. *Radiat Oncol*. 2006;1:15.

28. Sedlis A, Bundy BN, Rotman MZ, et al. A randomized trial of pelvic radiation therapy versus no further therapy in selected patients with stage IB carcinoma of the cervix after radical hysterectomy and pelvic lymphadenectomy: A Gynecologic Oncology Group Study. *Gynecol Oncol*. 1999;73:177–83.

29. Peters WA 3rd, Liu PY, Barrett RJ 2nd, et al. Concurrent chemotherapy and pelvic radiation therapy compared with pelvic radiation therapy alone as adjuvant therapy after radical surgery in high-risk early-stage cancer of the cervix. *J Clin Oncol*. 2000;18:1606–13.

30. Loiselle C, Koh WJ. The emerging use of IMRT for treatment of cervical cancer. *J Natl Compr Canc Netw*. 2010;8:1425–34.

31. Morris M, Eifel PJ, Lu J, et al. Pelvic radiation with concurrent chemotherapy compared with pelvic and para-aortic radiation for high-risk cervical cancer. *N Engl J Med*. 1999;340:1137–43.

32. Kang YJ, O'Connell DL, Lotocki R, et al. Effect of changes in treatment practice on survival for cervical cancer: results from a population-based study in Manitoba, Canada. *BMC Cancer*. 2015;15:642.

33. Au-Yeung G, Mileshkin L, Bernshaw DM, Kondalsamy-Chennakesavan S, Rischin D, Narayan K. Radiation with cisplatin or carboplatin for locally advanced cervix cancer: the experience of a tertiary cancer centre. *J Med Imaging Radiat Oncol*. 2013;57:97–104.

34. Sebastião AM, da Silva Rocha LS, Gimenez RD, et al. Carboplatin-based chemoradiotherapy in advanced cervical cancer: an alternative to cisplatin-based regimen? *Eur J Obstet Gynecol Reprod Biol*. 2016;201:161–5.

35. Hashemi FA, Akbari EH, Kalaghchi B, et al. Concurrent chemoradiation with weekly gemcitabine and cisplatin for locally advanced cervical cancer. *Asian Pac J Cancer Prev*. 2013;14:5385–9.

36. Narayan S, Sharma N, Kapoor A, et al. Pros and Cons of Adding of Neoadjuvant Chemotherapy to Standard Concurrent Chemoradiotherapy in Cervical Cancer: A Regional Cancer Center Experience. *J Obstet Gynaecol India*. 2016;66:385–90.

37. Gill BS, Kim H, Houser CJ, et al. MRI-guided high-dose-rate intracavitary brachytherapy for treatment of cervical cancer: The University of Pittsburgh experience. *Int J Radiat Oncol Biol Phys*. 2015;91:540–7.

38. Li XY, Liu L, Xie XM, et al. The role of raltitrexed/cisplatin with concurrent radiation therapy in treating advanced cervical cancer. *Age*. 2014;40:40.

39. Asiri MA, Tunio MA, Mohamed R, et al. Is extended-field concurrent chemoradiation an option for radiologic negative paraaortic lymph node, locally advanced cervical cancer? *Cancer Manag Res*. 2014;6:339–48.

40. Atahan IL, Onal C, Ozyar E, et al. Long-term outcome and prognostic factors in patients with cervical carcinoma: a retrospective study. *Int J Gynecol Cancer*. 2007;17:833–42.

41. Perez CA, Kavanagh BD. Uterine cervix. In: Halperin ECPC, Brady LW, editors. 5th ed. Philadelphia: Lippincott William & Wilkins; 2008. p. 1532–609.

42. Nagase S, Inoue Y, Umesaki N, et al. Evidence-based guidelines for treatment of cervical cancer in Japan: Japan Society of Gynecologic Oncology (JSGO) 2007 edition. *Int J Clin Oncol*. 2010;15:117–24.

43. International Commission on Radiation Units and measurement. Report 38 Dose and volume specification for intracavitary, Inc 1985. USA: Bethesda; 1985. Available at: http://www.icru.org. Accessed Feburary 3, 2017.

44. Castelnau-Marchand P, Chargari C, Maroun P, et al. Clinical outcomes of definitive chemoradiation followed by intracavitary pulsed-dose rate image-guided adaptive brachytherapy in locally advanced cervical cancer. *Gynecol Oncol*. 2015;139:288–94.

45. Haie-Meder C, Gerbaulet A, Potter R. Interstitial Brachytherapy in Gynaecological Cancer, Avaialble at: https://www.estro.org/binaries/content/assets/estro/about/gec-estro/handbook-of-brachytherapy/id-17-30072002-interstitial-gyn-print_proc.pdf. Accessed 6 Nov 2017.

46. Banerjee S, Mahantshetty U, Shrivastava S. Brachytherapy in India - a long road ahead. *J Contemp Brachytherapy*. 2014;6:331–5.

47. Winarto H, Febia E, Purwoto G, et al. The need for laparoscopic ovarian transposition In young patients with cervical cancer undergoing radiotherapy. *Int J Reprod Med*. 2013;2013:173568.

48. Gadducci A, Tana R, Cosio S, et al. Treatment options in recurrent cervical cancer (Review). *Oncol Lett*. 2010;1:3–11.

49. Yoo HJ, Lim MC, Seo SS, et al. Pelvic exenteration for recurrent cervical cancer: ten-year experience at National Cancer Center in Korea. *J Gynecol Oncol*. 2012;23:242–50.

50. Pandey D, Zaidi S, Mahajan V, et al. Pelvic exenteration: a perspective from a regional cancer center in India. *Indian J Cancer*. 2004;41:109–14.

51. Pálfalvi L. Ungár L. Pelvic Exenteration. Available from: http://eacademy.esgo.org/esgo/2013/ebook.textbook/document?c_id=42825&type=pdf_book. Accessed 10 Oct 2017

52. Cibula D, Babjuk M, Freitag P, et al. Reconstruction procedures following pelvic exenterations. *Ceska Gynekol*. 2005;70:205–10.

53. Angioli R, Panici PB, Mirhashemi R, et al. Continent urinary diversion and low colorectal anastomosis after pelvic exenteration. Quality of life and complication risk. *Crit Rev Oncol Hematol*. 2003;48:281–5.

54. Zbar A. Reconstructive surgery of the rectum, anus and perineum: Springer; 2013.

55. Moore DH, Blessing JA, McQuellon RP, et al. Phase III study of cisplatin with or without paclitaxel in stage IVB, recurrent, or persistent squamous cell carcinoma of the cervix: a gynecologic oncology group study. *J Clin Oncol*. 2004;22:3113–9.

56. Thigpen T, Shingleton H, Homesley H, et al. Cis-platinum in treatment of advanced or recurrent squamous cell carcinoma of the cervix: a phase II study of the Gynecologic Oncology Group. *Cancer*. 1981;48:899–903.

57. Long HJ 3rd, Bundy BN, Grendys EC Jr, et al. Randomized phase III trial of cisplatin with or without topotecan in carcinoma of the uterine cervix: a Gynecologic Oncology Group Study. *J Clin Oncol*. 2005;23:4626–33.

58. Pfaendler K, Tewari K. Changing paradigms in the systemic treatment of advanced cervical cancer. *Am J Obstet Gynecol*. 2016;214:22–30.

59. Smith SC, Koh WJ. Palliative radiation therapy for gynaecological malignancies. *Best Pract Res Clin Obstet Gynaecol*. 2001;15:265–78.

60. Friedlander M, Grogan M, Force USPST. Guidelines for the treatment of recurrent and metastatic cervical cancer. *Oncologist*. 2002;7:342–7.

61. Kamura T, Ushijima K. Chemotherapy for advanced or recurrent cervical cancer. *Taiwan J Obstet Gynecol*. 2013;52:161–4.

62. Rema P, Ahmed I. Conservative Surgery for Early Cervical Cancer. Indian J Surg Oncol. 2016;7:336–40.

63. Chuang LT, Feldman S, Nakisige C, Temin S, Berek JS. Management and Care of Women With Invasive Cervical Cancer: ASCO Resource-Stratified Clinical Practice Guideline. J Clin Oncol. 2016;34:3354–5.

64. Nikam DSJA, Vinothraj R. Resolving the brachytherapy challenges with government funded hospital. Indian journal of cancer. 2016;53:132.

65. Kolasani BP, Malathi DC, Ponnaluri RR. Variation of Cost among Anti-cancer Drugs Available in Indian Market. J Clin Diagn Res. 2016;10:FC17–20.

66. Nandakumar AKRG, Chandra Kataki A, Poonamalle Bapsy P, Gupta PC, Gangadharan P, Mahajan RC, Nath Bandyopadhyay M, Kumaraswamy VE, Visweswara RN. Concurrent Chemoradiation for Cancer of the Cervix: Results of a Multi-Institutional Study From the Setting of a Developing Country (India). Journal of Global Oncology. 2015;1:11–22.

67. Sharma DN, Gandhi AK, Sharma S, Rath GK, Jagadesan P. Julka PK. Interstitial brachytherapy vs. intensity-modulated radiation therapy for patients with cervical carcinoma not suitable for intracavitary radiation therapy. Brachytherapy. 2013;12:311–6.

68. Murakami N, Kobayashi K, Kato T, Nakamura S, Wakita A, Okamoto H, et al. The role of interstitial brachytherapy in the management of primary radiation therapy for uterine cervical cancer. J Contemp Brachytherapy. 2016;8:391–8.

69. Mahantshetty U, Shrivastava S, Kalyani N, Banerjee S, Engineer R, Chopra S. Template-based high-dose-rate interstitial brachytherapy in gynecologic cancers: a single institutional experience. Brachytherapy. 2014;13:337–42.

70. Tewari KS, Sill MW, Long HJ 3rd, Penson RT, Huang H, Ramondetta LM, et al. Improved survival with bevacizumab in advanced cervical cancer. N Engl J Med. 2014;370:734–43.

71. Suhag V, Sunita BS, A. S. Intensive Care For Cancer Patients: An Overview. Asian Austral J Anim. 2014;13:193–201.

72. Nair M, Varghese C. Cancer: Current scenario, intervention strategies and projections. Available at: http://www.searo.who.int/india/topics/cancer/Cancer_resource_Commision_on_Macroeconomic_and_Health_Bg_P2_Cancers_current_scenario.pdf?ua=1. Accessed 11 July 2018.

24

New therapies for advanced, recurrent, and metastatic endometrial cancers

Vicky Makker[1*], Angela K. Green[1], Robert M. Wenham[2], David Mutch[3], Brittany Davidson[4] and David Scott Miller[5]

Abstract

Endometrial cancer is the most common gynecologic malignancy in the United States, accounting for 6% of cancers in women. In 2017, an estimated 61,380 women were diagnosed with endometrial cancer, and approximately 11,000 died from this disease. From 1987 to 2008, there was a 50% increase in the incidence of endometrial cancer, with an approximate 300% increase in the number of associated deaths. Although there are many chemotherapeutic and targeted therapy agents approved for ovarian, fallopian tube and primary peritoneal cancers, since the 1971 approval of megestrol acetate for the palliative treatment of advanced endometrial cancer, only pembrolizumab has been Food and Drug Administration (FDA)-approved for high microsatellite instability (MSI-H) or mismatch repair deficient (dMMR) endometrial cancer; this highlights the need for new therapies to treat advanced, recurrent, metastatic endometrial cancer. In this review, we discuss current and emerging treatment options for endometrial cancer, including chemotherapy, targeted therapy, and immunotherapy. The National Cancer Institute (NCI) and others are now focusing their efforts on the design of scientifically rational targeted therapy and immunotherapy trials for specific molecular phenotypes of endometrial cancer. This is essential for the advancement of cancer care for women, which is threatened by a severe enrollment decline of approximately 80% for gynecologic oncology clinical trials.

Keywords: Endometrial cancer, Targeted therapy, Chemotherapy, Immunotherapy

Introduction

Endometrial cancer (EC) is the most common gynecologic malignancy in the United States, with an estimated 61,380 new cases and 11,000 deaths in 2017 [1]. The incidence of EC is increasing annually by an estimated 1–2%. The number of deaths attributed to EC are also increasing, while the mortality rate for ovarian cancer is declining [2, 3]. Obesity is a strong risk factor for the development of EC, accounting for approximately 50% of cases in Europe and the United States; it also has been associated with a relative increased risk of death of up to 6.25 [4].

Reduced birth rates, improvements in health and nutrition, and changes in the social structure of developed countries have led to an increasing elderly population, at a rate of 2.4% per year [5]. With the aging population, health promotion and disease prevention initiatives are warranted for individuals older than 50 years of age [6]. Of note, most EC diagnoses are made in women aged 45 to 74 years [3].

From 1987 to 2008, there was a 50% increase in the incidence of EC, with an approximate 300% increase in the number of associated deaths; however, no new agents were approved for treating EC. Although there are many drugs approved for the treatment of ovarian, fallopian tube, and primary peritoneal cancers, to date, there are only two FDA-approved drugs for EC, highlighting the need for new therapies to treat advanced, recurrent, metastatic EC [7].

Review

Types of endometrial cancer

Endometrial adenocarcinomas can be classified into two histologic categories—type 1 or type 2 [8]. Approximately 70–80% of new cases are classified as type 1 endometrial carcinomas, which are of endometrioid histology, lower grade, and often confined to the uterus at diagnosis. These tumors are estrogen-mediated, and often, women diagnosed with type 1 endometrial carcinomas are obese, with excess endogenous estrogen production. Type 1 carcinomas (estrogen dependent) have high rates of *K-ras* and PTEN loss or mutation, as well

* Correspondence: makkerv@mskcc.org
[1]Gynecologic Medical Oncology Service, Department of Surgery, Memorial Sloan Kettering Cancer Center and Weill Cornell Medical College, 1275 York Avenue, New York, TX 10065, USA
Full list of author information is available at the end of the article

as defects in mismatch repair genes, which lead to microsatellite instability (MSI) [9–13]. Type 2 (non-estrogen dependent) carcinomas are higher-grade adenocarcinomas and are of non-endometrioid histology, occurring in older, leaner women, although an association with increasing body mass index (BMI) has been observed. Type 2 cancers have *p53* mutations, may have overexpression of human epidermal growth factor receptor 2 (HER-2/neu), and show aneuploidy [14–20]. It should be noted that there are limitations to this dualistic classification of ECs, as there is heterogeneity and often overlap of the underlying genetics; for example, many high-grade endometrioid cancers can harbor p53 mutations and behave like other type 2 cancers. A recent Gynecologic Oncology Group (GOG) study evaluated the etiologic heterogeneity of ECs and reported that women with type 2 cancers, compared with type 1 cancers, were less likely to be obese but more likely to be older, non-white, multiparous, and current smokers [21]. Women with grade 3 endometrioid carcinomas displayed characteristics that were similar to those of type 2 cancers, but more often had histories of breast cancer without tamoxifen exposure.

Uterine carcinosarcomas, a poorly differentiated subgroup of uterine carcinomas, account for less than 5% of all uterine malignancies and are rare, aggressive biphasic neoplasms that consist of high-grade malignant epithelial and mesenchymal elements [22]. Five-year progression-free survival (PFS) rates for uterine-confined disease range from 40 to 75%, compared with 20–35% for disease with extra-uterine extension [23, 24].

The Cancer Genome Atlas (TCGA) Research Network has performed the most comprehensive molecular study of EC, integrating genomic, transcriptomic, and proteomic characterizations of EC based on array and sequencing technologies in 373 primary EC surgical specimens [25]. These data revealed that EC can be classified into four molecularly phenotypically different groups: 1) DNA polymerase epsilon catalytic subunit (POLE) ultra-mutated (very high mutation rate, hot spot mutations in POLE, endometrioid histology, frequently grade 3 [>50%], associated with a good prognosis, comprises 1% of cases of recurrent disease, and characterized by mutations in PTEN [94%], PIK3CA [71%], PIK3R1 [65%], FBXW7 [82%], ARID1A [76%], KRAS [53%], and ARID5B [47%]); 2) MSI hypermutated (high mutation rate, microsatellite unstable, frequently with MLH-1 promoter hypermethylation, endometrioid histology, comprises approximately 25% of cases of recurrent disease, and characterized by mutations in PTEN [88%], RPL22 [33%], KRAS [35%], PIK3CA [54%], PIK3R1 [40%], and ARID1A [37%]); 3) copy-number low (lower mutation rate, microsatellite stable (MSS), endometrioid histology, grade 1/2 tumors, and characterized by mutations in

PTEN [77%], CTNNB1 [52%], PIK3CA [53%], PIK3R1 [33%], and ARID1A [42%]); and 4) copy-number high serous-like (lowest mutation rate, serous, comprises approximately 25% of grade 3 endometrioid cases, poorest prognosis, and characterized by mutations in TP53 [92%], PPP2R1A [22%], PIK3CA [47%], and chromosomal instability).

The classification of EC by morphologic features is irreproducible and imperfectly reflects tumor biology. A molecular classification system based on the TCGA genomic subgroups, referred to as the Proactive Molecular Risk Classifier for Endometrial Cancer (ProMisE), was developed to confirm the feasibility and prognostic ability in a separate cohort of ECs [26]. ProMisE successfully categorized all cases and improved subgroup discrimination compared with the European Society of Medical Oncology (ESMO) risk classification system.

A TCGA analysis of 57 primary uterine carcinosarcoma tumor samples revealed extensive copy-number alterations and highly recurrent somatic mutations. Similar to endometrioid and serous endometrial carcinomas, mutations in TP53 (91%), PIK3CA (35%), PPP2R1A (28%), FBXW7 (28%), PTEN (19%), FBXW7, and KRAS (12%) were identified. A strong epithelial-to-mesenchymal transition (EMT) gene signature was observed in a subset of analyzed cases; the range of EMT scores was the largest among all tumors studied thus far by TCGA. Multiple somatic mutations and copy-number alterations in genes that are therapeutic targets were identified; 62% of tumors had one or more potentially clinically relevant mutations in the PI3K/AKT/mTOR pathway, and approximately 23% of cases had alterations in cell-cycle genes [27].

Risk factors

Risk factors for EC include endometrial hyperplasia, unopposed estrogen therapy, tamoxifen use, obesity, reproductive factors (early menarche/late menopause, nulliparity, or polycystic ovarian syndrome), family history/genetic predisposition, and hyperinsulinemia [28–34]. Lynch syndrome, an autosomal dominant inherited cancer susceptibility syndrome, is caused by a germline mutation in mismatch repair (MMR) genes (MLH1, MSH2, MSH6, and PMS2) and accounts for 2–5% of endometrial carcinomas [35–37]. Women with Lynch syndrome have an approximate 70% lifetime risk of developing EC [38, 39]. MMR is a single-strand DNA repair mechanism critical to maintaining genomic stability. MMR genes can be lost via mutation or methylation, with MMR deficiency associated with up to 30% of all ECs [25].

Type I EC oncogenesis is primarily estrogen dependent, having a positive correlation with high circulating estrogen levels [40, 41]. Prolonged exposure to estrogens through early menarche, late menopause, or the use of hormone replacement therapy are known risk factors [42]. Furthermore, sex hormone production from adipose tissue leads to estrogen stimulation of the endometrial lining [43].

Emerging data identify hyperinsulinemia, hyperglycemia, and chronic inflammation as potentially modifiable risk factors for the development and progression of multiple malignancies, including EC. Numerous etiologies lead to the development of the metabolic syndrome; however, obesity is dominant and has rising prevalence [44].

Based on National Health and Nutrition Examination Survey (NHANES) data, since 1960, the percentages of adults classified as overweight, obese, or extremely obese have continued to increase [45]. Obese women (BMI >30 kg/m^2), compared with normal-weight women, are at an increased risk of developing EC, with each 5 kg/m^2 increase in BMI conferring additional risk [46, 47]. A recent meta-analysis reported that, compared with normal-weight women, the risk of developing EC was 1.34 times higher in overweight women and 2.54 times higher in obese women [48]. Outcomes for EC also are affected by obesity. A retrospective study of patients with EC managed with surgery demonstrated that obese women had significantly more perioperative complications [49]. In obese women, death rates from EC are much higher compared with death rates in obese patients with other malignancies, suggesting the importance of the angiogenic tumor microenvironment related to adiposity [46–48]. Currently, there are a myriad of studies evaluating the impact of calorie restriction and exercise in promoting weight loss in obese patients with EC (NCT02665962, NCT02665962), as well as the impact of ketogenic diet in overweight or obese patients with newly diagnosed EC (NCT03285152).

Signaling pathways in endometrial cancer

One of the hallmarks of cancer is metabolic "addiction" to glucose, which is partially due to alterations in mitochondrial structure and function that result from genetic, epigenetic, and enzymatic alterations within cancer cells [50–53]. Current research suggests that this preferential metabolism of glucose through glycolysis may arise as a selective advantage in the hypoxic conditions experienced during early tumor development [54]. This cellular reprogramming of glucose metabolism to fuel tumor cell growth is largely thought to be driven by the AKTphosphoinositide 3-kinase (PI3K)/mammalian target of rapamycin (mTOR) pathway, which is commonly activated in endometrial carcinomas.

In fact, EC demonstrates the highest rate of PI3K pathway alterations of all solid tumors. The PI3K pathway also regulates cell growth, survival and motility, all key aspects of cancer cell biology. There are three classes of PI3K enzymes, which are grouped according to structure and function. Class IA PI3Ks are most associated with promoting carcinogenesis. Pathway activation begins with membrane-associated receptor tyrosine kinases (RTKs), such as the insulin-like growth factor receptor (IGFR), which has more than five-fold increased expression in endometrial adenocarcinoma compared with normal endometrium [55]. Upon stimulation of RTKs, PI3K phosphorylates the lipid phosphatidylinositol 4,5- biphosphate (PIP2), creating phosphatidylinositol 3,4,5- triphosphate (PIP3). PIP3 recruits protein kinase AKT to the membrane, where it is phosphorylated and activated by mTOR complex 2 (mTORC2) and 3-phosphoinositide-dependent protein kinase 1 (PDK1). Among its targets, AKT phosphorylates and inhibits tuberous sclerosis complex 2 (TSC2) within the TSC complex, which indirectly inhibits mTOR complex 1 (mTORC1). PI3K-AKT signaling activates mTORC1 [56], a key regulator of metabolism and biosynthetic processes, including activation of hypoxia-inducible factor 1 (HIF1) and other transcription factors. HIF1 stimulates glucose transporter expression on the cell surface, thereby increasing cellular glucose influx, and shifts metabolic pathways towards glycolysis through inhibitory mitochondrial pyruvate dehydrogenase kinase activation [49, 57].

Obesity, due to physical inactivity and excess caloric intake, leads to high glucose, insulin, and insulin-like growth factor 1 (IGF-1) levels. Increased signaling via the insulin/IGF-1 pathway culminates in activation of the mTOR pathway, resulting in increased cell proliferation and cancer development. Elevated glucose levels reduce 5′ adenosine monophosphate-activated protein kinase (AMPK) levels, which in turn increase mTOR stimulation and cell proliferation. Components of the mTOR pathway are often mutated, amplified, or aberrantly expressed in ECs, further supporting the link between obesity and this disease [49].

Metastatic disease

Most women with EC are diagnosed at an early stage. The 5-year survival rate for those diagnosed with localized disease is 95%; however, women diagnosed with advanced or recurrent disease have a poor prognosis, with a 5-year survival rate of 17% [3, 58]. In a study of four GOG trials evaluating the relationship between histology and outcomes of women with advanced, recurrent EC, the median overall survival (OS) was less than 12 months, with PFS ranging from 3 to 6 months based on histology [59]. Unfortunately, most current chemotherapeutic options for advanced EC are associated with significant toxicity and limited efficacy, highlighting the need to continue with efforts to exploit the molecular underpinnings and biology of this disease for target-specific and immunotherapeutic approaches.

Novel approaches for treating endometrial cancer
Adjuvant chemotherapy

Based on the findings of several GOG trials, platinum doublet chemotherapy remains the mainstay for first-line systemic therapy in patients with advanced EC. A phase 3 study of cisplatin plus doxorubicin demonstrated improved response rates and PFS (5.7 vs 3.8 months) compared with doxorubicin alone, but the regimen was not associated with increased OS (9.0 vs 9.2 months) [60]. Following this trial, the GOG-122 study accrued 396 patients with stage III or IV EC and a maximum of 2 cm of postoperative residual disease and randomized them to treatment with whole-abdominal irradiation or doxorubicin-cisplatin chemotherapy [61]. With a median 74 months of follow-up, patients in the chemotherapy arm, compared with those in the radiation arm, had a significantly improved 5-year survival rate (55% vs. 42%, respectively); however, the chemotherapy arm was also associated with greater toxicity. This pivotal study led to a paradigm shift in the management of advanced-stage EC.

To further improve efficacy, the GOG-177 study was designed to compare doxorubicin, cisplatin, paclitaxel and filgrastim support (TAP) with doxorubicin and cisplatin. Findings from the study demonstrated a significantly improved response rate (57% vs 34%, respectively), PFS (8.3 vs 5.3 months, respectively), and OS (15.3 vs 12.3 months, respectively; $p = 0.037$) with the former regimen, albeit with significantly higher patient-reported neurotoxicity [62]. In an effort to develop a less toxic regimen, GOG-209 was designed to compare carboplatin and paclitaxel (CT) to the triplet TAP regimen. This study demonstrated that CT was not inferior to TAP in terms of PFS (14 months in both arms) and OS (32 vs 38 months, respectively; HR 1.01) [63]. The toxicity profile for CT was significantly more favorable, and this regimen serves as the acceptable backbone for chemotherapy trials.

A myriad of ongoing studies using CT as the chemotherapy backbone include a phase 1 study of the selective inhibitor of nuclear export selinexor in combination with CT in patients with advanced ovarian or endometrial cancers (NCT02269293), a phase 2 study of the androgen-receptor inhibitor enzalutamide in combination with CT in advanced endometrioid EC (NCT02684227), a randomized phase 2 trial of CT compared to CT plus bevacizumab in advanced-stage or recurrent EC (NCT01770171), a phase 2 study of pembrolizumab in combination with CT in advanced EC (NCT02549209), and a randomized phase 2/3 study of CT plus metformin (NSC#91485) versus CT plus placebo as initial therapy in advanced-stage or recurrent EC (NCT02065687).

Chemotherapy for uterine carcinosarcomas

In the GOG-108 study, patients with advanced or recurrent carcinosarcoma treated with the combination of ifosfamide and cisplatin exhibited increased response rates and longer PFS compared with patients who received ifosfamide alone; no significant difference in survival was reported [64]. Results from a follow-up trial (GOG-161) demonstrated an increased response rate (29 vs 45%), median PFS (3.6 vs 5.8 months), and OS (8.4 vs 13.5 months) in patients receiving a 3-day regimen of ifosfamide plus paclitaxel versus paclitaxel alone [65]. As with ixabepilone for EC treatment, a nearly identical and modest response rate (12%), median PFS 1.7 months), and OS (7.7 months) were seen in 34 patients with uterine carcinosarcoma in the GOG-130F study [66]. Furthermore, as with treatment of other ECs, the use of CT in uterine carcinosarcoma is an appropriate option based on apparent equivalent efficacy and better tolerability [67].

A phase 2 trial using CT as the chemotherapy backbone and BSI-201 in advanced uterine carcinosarcomas was recently completed (NCT00687687). BSI-201, by activating gamma-H2AX, induces cell cycle arrest in the G2/M phase in tumor cell lines, and potentiates the cell cycle effects of DNA damaging modalities in tumor cell lines. Other ongoing studies include a feasibility trial of CT and galunisertib (inhibitor of the kinase domain of Type 1 TGF-B receptor) in patients with newly diagnosed or recurrent carcinosarcoma of the uterus or ovary (NCT03206177) and the phase 1 study of selinexor in combination with CT in patients with advanced ovarian or endometrial cancers (NCT02269293).

Advanced-disease treatments

Recent chemotherapy trials in the advanced/recurrent disease setting have not shown significant outcome improvements over prior single-agent chemotherapy studies. For example, a phase 3 randomized trial of second-line ixabepilone, an anti-tubulin epothilone, versus paclitaxel or doxorubicin in women with advanced EC failed to meet its primary objective of improving OS in the ixabepilone arm compared with the control chemotherapy arm. At interim analysis, the study of futility for OS favored the control chemotherapy arm (HR = 1.3; 95% CI: 1.0–1.7; stratified log-rank test $P = 0.0397$), and the study was discontinued based on the interim OS results [68].

Hormonal strategies and antibody drug conjugates

Given the endocrine sex hormone relationship with most ECs, agents that target these receptors and pathways have been evaluated and are in clinical use for EC of low-grade endometrioid histology; however, they are associated with limited efficacy. Megestrol acetate, a progestin, was approved more than 40 years ago for the palliative treatment of recurrent, metastatic breast and endometrial cancers. More recently, the GOG-153 study evaluated the combined hormonal strategy of alternating tamoxifen and megestrol acetate based on the hypothesis that tamoxifen increases the expression of progesterone receptors and thereby increases the efficacy of megestrol acetate. Megestrol acetate at 80 mg twice daily every 3 weeks, alternating with tamoxifen 20 mg twice daily every 3 weeks, was associated with an overall response rate of 27% [69]. Responses were attenuated by grade, which is correlated with hormone receptor status, with rates of 38%, 24%, and 22% for grade 1, 2, and 3 disease, respectively. Estrogen reduction by aromatase inhibitors, specifically anastrozole and letrozole, has shown little activity in EC in two prior studies [64, 65].

Elevated cyclin-dependant kinase 4 (CDK4) expression is observed in 34% to 77% of endometrioid endometrial cancers (EECs) and is considered to be an early event of neoplastic transformation in EEC [70]. CDK4/6 mediate the transition from G1 to S phase by associating with D-type cyclins and regulating the phosphorylation state of retinoblastoma. CDK4/6SA is significantly higher ($P = 0.002$) in pathologically low-risk patients (not receiving adjuvant chemotherapy, $n = 74$) than in intermediate- or high-risk patients (receiving adjuvant chemotherapy, $n = 35$). Patients with high CDK4/6SA (>3.0) have significantly ($P = 0.024$) shorter PFS than those with low CDK4/6SA (<3.0) [71]. CDK4/6 inhibitors restore cell-cycle control and halt tumor growth. In an effort to improve the efficacy of treatment in this setting, a randomized phase 2 trial of palbociclib (CDK4/6 inhibitor) in combination with letrozole versus placebo in combination with letrozole for patients with estrogen receptor (ER)-positive advanced or recurrent EC (NCT02730429) and a phase 2 trial of ribociclib (cyclin D1 and CDK4/6 inhibitor) and letrozole in ER-positive advanced ovarian, fallopian tube, primary peritoneal carcinomas and EC (NCT02657928) are currently recruiting patients.

Luteinizing hormone-releasing hormone receptors (LHRH-Rs) mediate antiproliferative activity in endometrial cell lines, and approximately 80% of ECs express LHRH-Rs, offering a potentially useful target in these tumors [66, 67]. Zoptarelin doxorubicin is an [D-Lys6]LHRH linked to doxorubicin, with activity in LHRH-R-positive cancer cell lines [72, 73]. Zoptarelin doxorubicin is internalized via LHRH-R and induces apoptosis without activating the MDR-1 efflux pump system, and it is less toxic than doxorubicin [73–76]. In an initial study of 17 women with ovarian, endometrial, or breast cancer who received various doses of zoptarelin doxorubicin, 3 patients who received 160 mg/m^2 and 3 patients who received 267 mg/m^2 (maximally tolerated dose) responded [77]. In a phase 2 study of 43 patients with LHRH-R-positive advanced EC, 2 patients achieved complete remission and 8 achieved partial remission following zoptarelin doxorubicin administration [78]. The overall objective response and stable disease rates were 23% and 47%, respectively. The ZoptEC phase 3 trial

compared the efficacy and safety of zoptarelin doxorubicin to doxorubicin alone. Patients were centrally randomized in a 1:1 ratio and received either zoptarelin doxorubicin (267 mg/m^2) or doxorubicin (60 mg/m^2) intravenously every 3 weeks for up to 9 cycles. The median OS period for patients treated with zoptarelin doxorubicin was 10.9 months compared with 10.8 months for patients treated with doxorubicin. This was not a statistically significant, clinically meaningful increase in OS, and thus the ZoptEC phase 3 clinical study did not meet its primary endpoint (unpublished data).

Folate receptor alpha (FRα) expression is associated with high-grade, advanced-stage EC and a poor prognosis, particularly in serous-type tumors, [79, 80], thus providing an attractive candidate for novel, targeted therapeutic strategies in advanced EC. Mirvetuximab soravtansine is an antibody-drug conjugate (ADC) comprised of an FRα-binding antibody, cleavable linker, and the maytansinoid DM4, a potent tubulin-targeting agent. A phase 1 expansion study of mirvetuximab soravtansine in patients with EC is currently ongoing (NCT02606305).

Other targeted therapies
Antiangiogenic therapies
Vascular endothelial growth factor (VEGF) is expressed in most ECs and is associated with higher histologic grade, lymphovascular space invasion, lymph node metastasis, and deep myometrial invasion [81–86]. In the GOG-229E study, bevacizumab therapy led to an overall response rate of 14% in 52 women with persistent or recurrent EC treated with one or two prior cytotoxic regimens [87]. Multiple phase 2 trials have demonstrated improved PFS with bevacizumab monotherapy or in combination with an mTOR inhibitor [88, 89]. The ongoing GOG-86P trial of bevacizumab with cytotoxic agents has demonstrated a potential survival benefit [90], and final results are anticipated in the near future.

Other anti-angiogenic agents have been investigated but have shown limited activity; these agents include thalidomide, aflibercept, sorafenib, and the small-molecule tyrosine kinase inhibitors (TKIs) dovitinib, nintedanib, brivanib, and sunitinib [91–94]. The GOG-229F trial of aflibercept (VEGF ligand binding fusion) in 44 patients with advanced EC met its study endpoint of PFS at 6 months but was associated with significant toxicities at the studied dose and schedule [95]. Cediranib, a multi-target TKI, targets VEGF 1–3 and platelet-derived growth factor β (PDGFβ) receptors, as well as c-Kit. The recent GOG-229 J study of cediranib in advanced EC demonstrated its sufficient activity and tolerability as monotherapy treatment (Table 1) [87, 92, 95–101].

Lenvatinib, an oral receptor TKI, targets VEGF receptors 1–3, fibroblast growth factor receptos1–4, RET, KIT, and PDGFβ. Confirmed complete responses and

Table 1 Anti-angiogenic Therapies

Study Drug	Target	Prior Lines of Therapy	Patients	ORR	mTTP/PFS (months)	mOS (months)
Dalantercept [98]	BMP9/10	1–2	28	0%	2.1	14.5
Trebananib [99]	Tie2 Receptor	1–2	32	3.1%	2	6.6
Cediranib [96]	VEGF/c-kit	1–2	48	12.5%	3.7	12.5
Sunitinib [91]	VEGF/KIT/PDGFR	≤ 1	33	18.2%	3.0	19.4
Nintedanib [92]	VEGF/FGFR/PDGFR	1–2	32	9.4%	3.1	10.1
Lenvatinib [97]	VEGFR/FGFR/RET/KIT/PDGFRβ	1–2	133	14.3%	5.6	10.6
Aflibercept [95]	VEGFR	1–2	44	7%	2.9	14.6
Bevacizumab [87]	VEGFR	1–2	52	13.5%	4.2	10.6
Sorafenib [100]	VEGF/Raf/Ras	≤ 1	39	5%	3.2	11.4
Thalidomide [101]	VEGFR/bFGF	1–2	21	12.5%	1.7	6.3

ORR objective response rate, mTTP median time to progression, PFS progression-free survival, mOS median overall survival

partial responses were observed in 19 patients (14%) and 29 patients (22%) treated with lenvatinib by independent review and investigator assessment, respectively [97]. The median PFS was 5.4 months, and the median OS was 10.6 months. Lenvatinib is being developed further in combination with immunotherapy.

EGFR pathway inhibitors

In EC, epidermal growth factor receptor (EGFR) overexpression is common, and is associated with deep myometrial invasion, tumor grade, and a poor prognosis [102–104]. Low response rates have been reported for the oral EGFR inhibitors gefitinib and erlotinib in phase 2 trials [105, 106].

HER2/neu is a member of the human epidermal growth factor receptor (HER/EGFR/ERBB) family. HER2/neu overexpression leads to alterations in cell proliferation, migration, differentiation, and survival, as well as the upregulation of the Ras/Raf/MAPK and PI3K/AKT/mTOR pathways [107]. HER2/neu overexpression is seen in advanced type 2 cancers and is associated with a poor prognosis [108, 109]. ERBB2/HER2 is an RTK that mediates signaling via the PI3K and mitogen-activated protein kinase (MAPK) pathways. Importantly, ERBB2 was focally amplified with protein overexpression in 25% of the serous or serous-like tumors based on TCGA data [25]. A phase 2 trial of the HER2/EGFR inhibitor lapatinib in molecularly unselected advanced EC revealed limited activity, with an ORR of 3.3% and median PFS of 1.8 months [110]. A randomized phase 2 trial (NCT01367002) evaluating CT in combination with trastuzumab, which as a single agent showed limited activity in a previous phase 2 trial (ORR, 0%; median PFS, 1.8 months) [111], closed due to poor accrual. Ongoing trials of ado-trastuzumab emtansine and afatinib (irreversible EGFR, HER2, and HER4 inhibitor)

for patients with EC and HER2-amplified or mutant cancers are accruing (NCT02675829, NCT02491099).

Inhibitors of the PI3K/Akt/mTOR pathway

Since the initial studies of nearly 20 years ago, a myriad of approaches to target this pathway have been explored. The initial studies of rapamycin analogs (rapalogs) that bind directly to and allosterically inhibit mTOR1 revealed modest but reproducible antitumor activity across the serous, endometrioid and clear cell histologic subtypes, with some patients experiencing prolonged stable disease. Several phase 2 trials have investigated the use of mTOR inhibitors as single agents in advanced EC. The objective response rates (ORRs) in those studies ranged form 0% to 24%, and responses were higher in chemotherapy-naïve patients (Table 2) [112–117].

The modest activity shown in these studies could be secondary to the existence of intra- or inter-pathway feedback loops (e.g., MAPK pathway) and from the incomplete blockage of the pathway provided by the rapalogs. Correlative analyses of archival biospecimens have failed to identify a predictive biomarker in EC, and these initial studies also did not enrich for patients with abnormalities in the PI3K/Akt/mTOR pathway. These studies may have been strengthened by limiting eligibility to patients with alterations in this pathway, although it is also possible that a single or multiple target biomarkers may be insufficient to predict for response due to the inherent complexity of this pathway.

Rapalogs have also been evaluated in combination trials. A phase 2 study of everolimus plus letrozole reported a response rate of 32% and a clinical benefit rate (CBR) of 40% [118]. Interim results of an ongoing phase 2 trial of everolimus, letrozole and metformin showed a partial response rate of 29%, and 38% of patients achieved stable disease [119]. The GOG-248 study of temsirolimus with or without megestrol acetate in 71 patients revealed that adding the combination of megestrol

Table 2 Single-Agent mTOR Inhibitor Studies in Endometrial Cancer

Agent	Patients	Prior Chemotherapy Regimens	Molecular Selection of Patients	Objective Response Rate	Other Activity
Temsirolimus [112]	29	None	No	24%	SD ≥ 8 weeks: 69%
	25	1–2	No	4%	SD ≥ 8 weeks: 46%
Everolimus [113]	28	1–2	No	0%	SD: 43%
Everolimus [114]	44	1–2	No	9%	SD: 27%
Ridaforolimus IV [115]	45	1–2	No	11%	CBR: 29%
Ridaforolimus PO [116]	30	Adjuvant only	No	9%	SD: 52.9%
Ridaforolimus PO [117]	64	1–2	No	0%	SD: 35%

IV intravenous, *PO* oral, *SD* stable disease, *CBR* clinical benefit rate

acetate and tamoxifen to temsirolimus did not enhance activity. The study was closed early due to an excess of venous thrombosis in the combination arm [120].

Due to the incomplete inhibition of mTORC1 targets by rapalogs, and the feedback loops that exist, activation of upstream PI3K signals [54, 55] can result. It has been hypothesized that newer PI3K pathway agents, which target further upstream in the pathway, will be more clinically effective. Numerous phase 1b/2 clinical trials evaluating catalytic mTOR, AKT, pan-PI3K, and dual PI3K/mTOR inhibitors are underway.

mTOR inhibitors have also been combined with chemotherapy. Two phase 1 trials in solid tumors using CT with either ridaforolimus [121] or temsirolimus [122] showed response rates of 25% and 82%, respectively, in EC populations. However, a randomized phase 2 trial (GOG-86P) comparing CT with either temsirolimus or bevacizumab or carboplatin plus ixabepilone and bevacizumab to CT showed improved OS when bevacizumab, but not temsirolimus, was added to CT [90].

Non-rapalog PI3K/AKT/mTOR inhibitors

There are multiple completed or ongoing single-agent phase 2 clinical trials examining non-rapalog PI3K/mTOR agents in EC. A phase 2, two-stage, two-arm PIK3CA mutation stratified trial of MK-2206, an allosteric inhibitor of AKT, of previously treated endometrial cancer also revealed limited single-agent activity in both mutant (1 partial response) and wild-type (1 partial response) EC populations, although activity was detected in serous histology tumors with exploratory analysis, revealing that all patients with a 6-month PFS had serous EC. This study may have suffered from small patient numbers in the mutant group, as well as poor drug tolerance [123]. A phase 2 trial of the pan class I PI3K inhibitor pilaralisib demonstrated minimal activity, with an ORR of 6%, as did the phase 2 MAGGIE study of GDC-0980, a dual PI3K/mTOR inhibitor, which also demonstrated an ORR of 6% and limited antitumor activity [124, 125]. Both studies were limited in that they did not require an alteration in the PI3K/Akt/mTOR

axis. Similarly, a phase 2 double-strata (low grade vs high grade) trial of BKM120, a pure PI3K inhibitor, in previously treated EC demonstrated an ORR of 0%, and was discontinued early due to excessive toxicity [126]. A phase 2 trial of LY3023414, a PI3K/mTOR inhibitor (NCT02549989), in EC with PI3K pathway activation without concurrent resistance mutations is ongoing. HER2/neu gene amplification and PIK3CA driver mutations are common in uterine serous carcinoma. Preclinical studies have shown that HER2-amplified serous cell lines were more sensitive to growth inhibition by PI3K inhibitors than HER2 non-amplified serous EC cell lines, a potential future direction [127]. Of additional interest is the combination with poly (ADP-ribose) polymerase (PARP) inhibitors, as drugs targeting the PIK3/AKT/mTOR pathway may interfere with DNA repair mechanisms, as described below.

Metformin

Metformin is an oral biguanide agent that is known to inhibit cellular proliferation and induce apoptosis, potentially through inhibition of Mitochondrial complex 1 and AMPK activation and mTOR inhibition [128–131]. An association between metformin use and improved outcomes in patients on prior single-agent mTOR inhibitors, as well as in the everolimus and letrozole combination, has been shown [118, 132]. Currently, there are numerous metformin chemoprevention studies, as well as studies of metformin combinations with standard chemotherapy (NCT02065687) and with hormonal and mTOR agents (NCT01797523).

PARP inhibitors

Preclinical studies have shown that inhibition of the PI3K/akt/mTOR pathway may sensitize EC cell lines to PARP inhibitors, and that loss of PTEN function may predict sensitivity to PARP due to a synthetic lethality process. This appears to be particularly true in a low-estrogenic setting [123, 133]. A phase 2 study of the PARP inhibitor niraparib in recurrent EC (NCT03016338) is active but not yet recruiting.

In addition, a phase I study is exploring the role of the PARP inhibitor olaparib in combination with the mTORC1/2 inhibitor AZD2014 or the AKT inhibitor AZD5363 for gynecological cancers, including advanced ECs (NCT02208375).

Immunotherapy

Immune checkpoint inhibitors in the treatment of EC, although potentially promising, have had until recently limited reportable data. Programmed cell death-1 (PD-1) and its ligand PD-L1 are expressed on the tumor-infiltrating immune cells of 61% to 80% of primary ECs [134, 135] and in 100% of metastatic ECs [134, 135]. Presence of tumor-infiltrating lymphocytes is also an independent prognostic factor in type I and II ECs [136]. The high mutation load in the POLE-mutated and MSI-H EC subgroups is correlated with PD-1 expression [133]. Approximately 26% of recurrent ECs harbor mismatch repair deficiency (MMD-D) or POLE-E exomuclease domain mutations (POLE EDM) in the recurrent disease setting, and may be excellent candidates for PD-1 targeting immunotherapies [137]. The vast majority of recurrent ECs are the copy-number low endometrioid and copy-number high serous-like ECs, which may warrant more tailored immunotherapy and combination treatment approaches.

A phase 2 study evaluating the clinical activity of the PD-1 inhibitor pembrolizumab in patients with colorectal cancer demonstrated an immune-related PFS rates of 78% in patients with MMR-deficient cancer and 11% in patients with MMR-proficient cancer, demonstrating that MMR status predicts the clinical benefit of pembrolizumab [138]. In preliminary results from the phase 1b KEYNOTE-028 study, there was a partial response of 13% among 24 pretreated patients with advanced EC and PD-L1 expression ≥1% [139].

Pembrolizumab recently was granted FDA accelerated approval for tissue or site agnostic use in the treatment of patients with unresectable or metastatic solid tumors, including EC, associated with MSI-H or MMR-deficient disease. This was the FDA's first tissue or site agnostic approval, which was based on data from five single-arm, multi-cohort, multi-center, clinical trials of 149 patients with MSI-H or MMR-deficient disease. The overall ORR based on independent review was 39.6%, with 11 complete responses and 48 partial responses. Responses lasted 6 months or longer in 78% of patients who responded.

Observations in several mouse models have shown that the oral TKI lenvatinib appears to significantly decrease the tumor-associated macrophage population, leading to increased antitumor activity and upregulation of PD-1 signal inhibitors [140, 141]. A phase 1b/2 trial of lenvatinib plus pembrolizumab in patients with selected solid tumors, including EC, is ongoing (NCT02501096). Interim

results in 23 patients with advanced EC revealed an ORR of 52% by independent review. Importantly, responses were seen in both MSI-high and MSS patients [142].

Multiple monotherapy trials (NCT02628067, NCT 02912572, NCT02899793, NCT02630823), combination immunotherapy trials (NCT03015129 NCT02982486), and immunotherapy trials in combination with paclitaxel and carboplatin (NCT02549209) are planned or ongoing.

Conclusions

Based on the increasing incidence and mortality associated with EC, and with only one recently approved therapy for a subset of patients with advanced EC, the NCI has published priorities for research on treating EC, with a goal to integrate molecular and/or histologic stratification into EC management. A recent international survey reported that 94% of participants supported the concept of treating patients in appropriate clinical trials. Since 2011, there has been a severe enrollment decline of 80% for gynecologic oncology clinical trials due to decreased federal funding and the consolidation of cooperative groups within the NCI. A focus on designing clinical trials to study new rationally combined therapeutic agents, including molecularly targeted agents and immunotherapy, in patients with EC is essential to the advancement of cancer care and the improvement of outcomes among women with advanced EC.

Acknowledgements
Not applicable.

Funding
Drs. Makker and Green are supported in part by the MSK Cancer Center Support Grant P30 CA008748.

Authors' contributions
DSM conceived the project, performed the literature review, and contributed to the composition and editing of this manuscript. DM, BD, AG and VM performed the literature review, and contributed to the composition and editing of this manuscript. All authors read and approved the final manuscript.

Competing interests
Dr. Robert M. Wenham has received study grant support from Merck and honoraria from Tesaro, Genentech, Clovis, and Jansen. Dr. Vicky Makker has received an honorarium from Eisai, as well as study support from Lilly, AstraZeneca, and Kryopharm. Dr. David Mutch has served as speaker for Clovis. Dr. David Miller has received grant funding from Tracon, Arno, Tesaro, Aprea, AstraZeneca, Janssen, Aeterna Zentaris, and Millenium; honorariums from Clovis, Eisai, Tesaro, AstraZeneca, Gaurdant, Genentech, and Alexion; and speaks for Genentech and Clovis. The other authors declare that they have no competing interests.

Author details

[1]Gynecologic Medical Oncology Service, Department of Surgery, Memorial Sloan Kettering Cancer Center and Weill Cornell Medical College, 1275 York Avenue, New York, TX 10065, USA. [2]Department of Gynecologic Oncology, H. Lee Moffitt Cancer Center, Tampa, FL, USA. [3]Division of Gynecologic Oncology, Washington University School of Medicine, St Louis, MO, USA. [4]Division of Gynecologic Oncology, Duke University Medical Center, Duke Cancer Institute, Durham, NC, USA. [5]Division of Gynecologic Oncology, University of Texas Southwestern Medical Center, Dallas, USA.

References

1. American Cancer Society. Cancer Facts and Figures, 2017. https://www.cancer.org/content/dam/cancer-org/research/cancer-facts-and-statistics/annual-cancer-facts-and-figures/2017/cancer-facts-and-figures-2017.pdf. Accessed 11 July 2017.

2. American Cancer Society. Cancer Facts and Figures, 2016. https://www.cancer.org/content/dam/cancer-org/research/cancer-facts-and-statistics/annual-cancer-facts-and-figures/2016/cancer-facts-and-figures-2016.pdf. Accessed 11 July 2017.

3. INational Cancer Institute Surveillance, Epidemiology, and end results program. Cancer Stat Facts: Endometrial Cancer. https://seer.cancer.gov/statfacts/html/corp.html. Accessed 11 July 2017.

4. Calle EE, Rodriguez C, Walker-Thurmond K, Thun MJ. Overweight, obesity, and mortality from cancer in a prospectively studied cohort of U.S. adults. N Engl J Med. 2003;348:1625–38.

5. Kinsella K, Suzman R, Robine JM. Demography of older populations in developed countries. J Family Issues. 2000;21:541–58.

6. The Second Fifty Years. Promoting health and preventing disability. Report of a study undertaken by the committee on health promotion and disease prevention for the second fifty. Washington, DC: Institute of Medicine; 1990.

7. National Cancer Institute. Drugs Approved for Endometrial Cancer. https://www.cancer.gov/about-cancer/treatment/drugs/endometrial. Accessed 11 July 2017.

8. Bokhman JV. Two pathogenetic types of endometrial carcinoma. Gynecol Oncol. 1983;15:10–7.

9. Maxwell GL, Risinger JI, Gumbs C, Shaw H, Bentley RC, Barrett JC, et al. Mutation of the PTEN tumor suppressor gene in endometrial hyperplasias. Cancer Res. 1998;58:2500–3.

10. Basil JB, Goodfellow PJ, Rader JS, Mutch DG, Herzog TJ. Clinical significance of microsatellite instability in endometrial carcinoma. Cancer. 2000;89:1758–64.

11. Mutter GL, Lin MC, Fitzgerald JT, Kum JB, Baak JP, Lees JA, et al. Altered PTEN expression as a diagnostic marker for the earliest endometrial precancers. J Natl Cancer Inst. 2000;92:924–30.

12. Bilbao C, Rodriguez G, Ramirez R, Falcon O, Leon L, Chirino R, et al. The relationship between microsatellite instability and PTEN gene mutations in endometrial cancer. Int J Cancer. 2006;119:563–70.

13. Hecht JL, Mutter GL. Molecular and pathologic aspects of endometrial carcinogenesis. J Clin Oncol. 2006;24:4783–91.

14. Zheng W, Cao P, Zheng M, Kramer EE, Godwin TA. p53 overexpression and bcl-2 persistence in endometrial carcinoma: comparison of papillary serous and endometrioid subtypes. Gynecol Oncol. 1996;61:167–74.

15. Lax SF, Kendall B, Tashiro H, Slebos RJ, Hedrick L. The frequency of p53, K-ras mutations, and microsatellite instability differs in uterine endometrioid and serous carcinoma: evidence of distinct molecular genetic pathways. Cancer. 2000;88:814–24.

16. Santin AD, Bellone S, Gokden M, Palmieri M, Dunn D, Agha J, et al. Overexpression of HER-2/neu in uterine serous papillary cancer. Clin Cancer Res. 2002;8:1271–9.

17. Risinger JI, Maxwell GL, Chandramouli GV, Jazaeri A, Aprelikova O, Patterson T, et al. Microarray analysis reveals distinct gene expression profiles among different histologic types of endometrial cancer. Cancer Res. 2003;63:6–11.

18. Slomovitz BM, Broaddus RR, Burke TW, Sneige N, Soliman PT, Wu W, et al. Her-2/neu overexpression and amplification in uterine papillary serous carcinoma. J Clin Oncol. 2004;22:3126–32.

19. Zorn KK, Bonome T, Gangi L, Chandramouli GV, Awtrey CS, Gardner GJ, et al. Gene expression profiles of serous, endometrioid, and clear cell subtypes of ovarian and endometrial cancer. Clin Cancer Res. 2005;11:6422–30.

20. Doll A, Abal M, Rigau M, Monge M, Gonzalez M, Demajo S, et al. Novel molecular profiles of endometrial cancer-new light through old windows. J Steroid Biochem Mol Biol. 2008;108:221–9.

21. Brinton LA, Felix AS, McMeekin DS, Creasman WT, Sherman ME, Mutch D, et al. Etiologic heterogeneity in endometrial cancer: evidence from a gynecologic oncology group trial. Gynecol Oncol. 2013;129:277–84.

22. Kurman RJ, International Agency for Research on Cancer, World Health Organization. WHO classification of Tumours of female reproductive organs, fourth edition. International Agency for Research on Cancer: Lyon; 2014.

23. Ferguson SE, Tornos C, Hummer A, Barakat RR, Soslow RA. Prognostic features of surgical stage I uterine carcinosarcoma. Am J Surg Pathol. 2007;31:1653–61.

24. Yamada SD, Burger RA, Brewster WR, Anton D, Kohler MF, Monk BJ. Pathologic variables and adjuvant therapy as predictors of recurrence and survival for patients with surgically evaluated carcinosarcoma of the uterus. Cancer. 2000;15(88):2782–6.

25. Cancer Genome Atlas Research Network, Kandoth C, Schultz N, Cherniack AD, Akbani R, Liu Y, et al. Integrated genomic characterization of endometrial carcinoma. Nature. 2013;497:67–73.

26. Talhouk A, McConechy MK, Leung S, Yang W, Lum A, Senz J, et al. Confirmation of ProMisE: a simple, genomics-based clinical classifier for endometrial cancer. Cancer. 2017;123:802–13.

27. Cherniack AD, Shen H, Walter V, Stewart C, Murray BA, Bowlby R, et al. Integrated molecular characterization of uterine Carcinosarcoma. Cancer Cell. 2017;31:411–23.

28. Ziel HK, Finkle WD. Increased risk of endometrial carcinoma among users of conjugated estrogens. N Engl J Med. 1975;293:1167–70.

29. Jick SS, Walker AM, Jick H. Estrogens, progesterone, and endometrial cancer. Epidemiology. 1993;4:20–4.

30. van Leeuwen FE, Benraadt J, Coebergh JW, Kiemeney LA, Gimbrere CH, Otter R, et al. Risk of endometrial cancer after tamoxifen treatment of breast cancer. Lancet. 1994;343:448–52.

31. Fisher B, Costantino JP, Redmond CK, Fisher ER, Wickerham DL, Cronin WM. Endometrial cancer in tamoxifen-treated breast cancer patients: findings from the National Surgical Adjuvant Breast and bowel project (NSABP) B-14. J Natl Cancer Inst. 1994;86:527–37.

32. Lu KH, Schorge JO, Rodabaugh KJ, Daniels MS, Sun CC, Soliman PT, et al. Prospective determination of prevalence of lynch syndrome in young women with endometrial cancer. J Clin Oncol. 2007;25:5158–64.

33. Lynch HT, Lynch J, Conway T, Watson P, Coleman RL. Familial aggregation of carcinoma of the endometrium. Am J Obstet Gynecol. 1994;171:24–7.

34. Nead KT, Sharp SJ, Thompson DJ, Painter JN, Savage DB, Semple RK, et al. Evidence of a Causal Association Between Insulinemia and Endometrial Cancer: A Mendelian Randomization Analysis. J Natl Cancer Inst 2015;107:1–7.

35. Lancaster JM, Powell CB, Chen LM, Richardson DL, SGO Clinical Practice Committee. Society of Gynecologic Oncology statement on risk assessment for inherited gynecologic cancer predispositions. Gynecol Oncol. 2015;136:3–7.

36. Kwon JS, Scott JL, Gilks CB, Daniels MS, Sun CC, Lu KH. Testing women with endometrial cancer to detect lynch syndrome. J Clin Oncol. 2011;29:2247–52.

37. Guillotin D, Martin SA. Exploiting DNA mismatch repair deficiency as a therapeutic strategy. Exp Cell Res. 2014;329:110–5.

38. Barrow E, Robinson L, Alduaij W, Shenton A, Clancy T, Lalloo F, et al. Cumulative lifetime incidence of extracolonic cancers in lynch syndrome: a report of 121 families with proven mutations. Clin Genet. 2009;75:141–9.

39. Koornstra JJ, Mourits MJ, Sijmons RH, Leliveld AM, Hollema H, Kleibeuker JH. Management of extracolonic tumours in patients with lynch syndrome. Lancet Oncol. 2009;10:400–8.

40. Cavalieri E, Chakravarti D, Guttenplan J, Hart E, Ingle J, Jankowiak R, et al. Catechol estrogen quinones as initiators of breast and other human cancers: implications for biomarkers of susceptibility and cancer prevention. Biochim Biophys Acta. 1766;2006:63–78.

41. Allen NE, Key TJ, Dossus L, Rinaldi S, Cust A, Lukanova A, et al. Endogenous sex hormones and endometrial cancer risk in women in the European prospective investigation into cancer and nutrition (EPIC). Endocr Relat Cancer. 2008;15:485–97.

42. Rutkowska AZ, Szybiak A, Serkies K, Rachon D. Endocrine disrupting chemicals as potential risk factor for estrogen-dependent cancers. Pol Arch Med Wewn. 2016;126:562–70.

43. Richardson LC, Thomas C, Bowman BA. Obesity and endometrial cancer: challenges for public health action. Womens Health (Lond). 2009;5:595–7.

44. Gunter MJ, Hoover DR, Yu H, Wassertheil-Smoller S, Rohan TE, Manson JE, et al. Insulin, insulin-like growth factor-I, and risk of breast cancer in postmenopausal women. J Natl Cancer Inst. 2009;101:48–60.

45. Fryar CD, Carroll MD, Ogden CL. Prevalence of overweight, obesity, and extreme obesity among adults: United States, trends 1960–1962 through 2009–2010. https://www.cdc.gov/nchs/data/hestat/obesity_adult_09_10/obesity_adult_09_10.pdf. Accessed 11 July 2017.

46. Reeves GK, Pirie K, Beral V, Green J, Spencer E, Bull D, et al. Cancer incidence and mortality in relation to body mass index in the million women study: cohort study. BMJ. 2007;335(7630):1134. doi:10.1136/bmj.39367.495995.AE.

47. Renehan AG, Tyson M, Egger M, Heller RF, Zwahlen M. Body-mass index and incidence of cancer: a systematic review and meta-analysis of prospective observational studies. Lancet. 2008;371:569–78.

48. Jenabi E, Poorolajal J. The effect of body mass index on endometrial cancer: a meta-analysis. Public Health. 2015;129(7):872–80. doi:10.1016/j.puhe.2015.04.017.

49. Bouwman F, Smits A, Lopes A, Das N, Pollard A, Massuger L, et al. The impact of BMI on surgical complications and outcomes in endometrial cancer surgery–an institutional study and systematic review of the literature. Gynecol Oncol. 2015;139:369–76.

50. Arismendi-Morillo GJ, Castellano-Ramirez AV. Ultrastructural mitochondrial pathology in human astrocytic tumors: potentials implications pro-therapeutics strategies. J Electron Microsc. 2008;57:33–9.

51. Seyfried TN, Shelton LM. Cancer as a metabolic disease. Nutr Metab (Lond). 2010;7:7.

52. Zhou Y, Zhou Y, Shingu T, Feng L, Chen Z, Ogasawara M, et al. Metabolic alterations in highly tumorigenic glioblastoma cells: preference for hypoxia and high dependency on glycolysis. J Biol Chem. 2011;286:32843–53.

53. Westhoff MA, Karpel-Massler G, Bruhl O, Enzenmuller S, La Ferla-Bruhl K, Siegelin MD, et al. A critical evaluation of PI3K inhibition in Glioblastoma and Neuroblastoma therapy. Mol Cell Ther. 2014;2:32.

54. Whiteman EL, Cho H, Birnbaum MJ. Role of Akt/protein kinase B in metabolism. Trends Endocrinol Metab. 2002;13:444–51.

55. Elstrom RL, Bauer DE, Buzzai M, Karnauskas R, Harris MH, Plas DR, et al. Akt stimulates aerobic glycolysis in cancer cells. Cancer Res. 2004;64:3892–9.

56. Eritja N, Yeramian A, Chen BJ, Llobet-Navas D, Ortega E, Colas E, et al. Endometrial carcinoma: specific targeted pathways. Adv Exp Med Biol. 2017;943:149–207.

57. Garg SK, Maurer H, Reed K, Selagamsetty R. Diabetes and cancer: two diseases with obesity as a common risk factor. Diabetes Obes Metab. 2014;16:97–110.

58. Siegel RL, Miller KD, Jemal A. Cancer statistics, 2016. CA Cancer J Clin. 2016;66:7–30.

59. McMeekin DS, Filiaci VL, Thigpen JT, Gallion HH, Fleming GF, Rodgers WH, et al. The relationship between histology and outcome in advanced and recurrent endometrial cancer patients participating in first-line chemotherapy trials: a gynecologic oncology group study. Gynecol Oncol. 2007;106:16–22.

60. Thigpen JT, Brady MF, Homesley HD, Malfetano J, DuBeshter B, Burger RA, et al. Phase III trial of doxorubicin with or without cisplatin in advanced endometrial carcinoma: a gynecologic oncology group study. J Clin Oncol. 2004;22:3902–8.

61. Randall ME, Filiaci VL, Muss H, Spirtos NM, Mannel RS, Fowler J, et al. Randomized phase III trial of whole-abdominal irradiation versus doxorubicin and cisplatin chemotherapy in advanced endometrial carcinoma: a gynecologic oncology group study. J Clin Oncol. 2006;24:36–44.

62. Fleming GF, Brunetto VL, Cella D, Look KY, Reid GC, Munkarah AR, et al. Phase III trial of doxorubicin plus cisplatin with or without paclitaxel plus filgrastim in advanced endometrial carcinoma: a gynecologic oncology group study. J Clin Oncol. 2004;22:2159–66.

63. Miller DFV, Fleming G, Mannel R, Cohn D, Matsumoto T, Tewari K, DiSilvestro P, Pearl M, Zaino R. Randomized phase III noninferiority trial of first line chemotherapy for metastatic or recurrent endometrial carcinoma: a gynecologic oncology group study. Gynecol Oncol. 2012;125:771–3.

64. Sutton G, Brunetto VL, Kilgore L, Soper JT, McGehee R, Olt G, et al. A phase III trial of ifosfamide with or without cisplatin in carcinosarcoma of the uterus: a gynecologic oncology group study. Gynecol Oncol. 2000;79:147–53.

65. Homesley HD, Filiaci V, Markman M, Bitterman P, Eaton L, Kilgore LC, et al. Phase III trial of ifosfamide with or without paclitaxel in advanced uterine carcinosarcoma: a gynecologic oncology group study. J Clin Oncol. 2007;25:526–31.

66. McCourt CK, Deng W, Dizon DS, Lankes HA, Birrer MJ, Lomme MM, et al. A phase II evaluation of ixabepilone in the treatment of recurrent/persistent carcinosarcoma of the uterus, an NRG oncology/gynecologic oncology group study. Gynecol Oncol. 2017;144:101–6.

67. Lorusso D, Martinelli F, Mancini M, Sarno I, Ditto A, Raspagliesi F. Carboplatin-Paclitaxel versus Cisplatin-Ifosfamide in the treatment of uterine carcinosarcoma: a retrospective cohort study. Int J Gynecol Cancer. 2014;24:1256–61.

68. McMeekin S, Dizon D, Barter J, Scambia G, Manzyuk L, Lisyanskaya A, et al. Phase III randomized trial of second-line ixabepilone versus paclitaxel or doxorubicin in women with advanced endometrial cancer. Gynecol Oncol. 2015;138:18–23.

69. Fiorica JV, Brunetto VL, Hanjani P, Lentz SS, Mannel R, Andersen W, et al. Phase II trial of alternating courses of megestrol acetate and tamoxifen in advanced endometrial carcinoma: a gynecologic oncology group study. Gynecol Oncol. 2004;92:10–4.

70. Tsuda H, Yamamoto K, Inoue T, Uchiyama I, Umesaki N. The role of p16-cyclin d/CDK-pRb pathway in the tumorigenesis of endometrioid-type endometrial carcinoma. Br J Cancer. 2000;82(3):675–82.

71. Ikeda Y, Oda K, Ishihara H, Wada-Hiraike O, Miyasaka A, Kashiyama T, et al. Prognostic importance of CDK4/6-specific activity as a predictive marker for recurrence in patients with endometrial cancer, with or without adjuvant chemotherapy. Br J Cancer. 2015;113:1477–83.

72. Volker P, Grundker C, Schmidt O, Schulz KD, Emons G. Expression of receptors for luteinizing hormone-releasing hormone in human ovarian and endometrial cancers: frequency, autoregulation, and correlation with direct antiproliferative activity of luteinizing hormone-releasing hormone analogues. Am J Obstet Gynecol. 2002;186:171–9.

73. Westphalen S, Kotulla G, Kaiser F, Krauss W, Werning G, Elsasser HP, et al. Receptor mediated antiproliferative effects of the cytotoxic LHRH agonist AN-152 in human ovarian and endometrial cancer cell lines. Int J Oncol. 2000;17:1063–9.

74. Nagy A, Schally AV. Targeting of cytotoxic luteinizing hormone-releasing hormone analogs to breast, ovarian, endometrial, and prostate cancers. Biol Reprod. 2005;73:851–9.

75. Gunthert AR, Grundker C, Bongertz T, Schlott T, Nagy A, Schally AV, et al. Internalization of cytotoxic analog AN-152 of luteinizing hormone-releasing hormone induces apoptosis in human endometrial and ovarian cancer cell lines independent of multidrug resistance-1 (MDR-1) system. Am J Obstet Gynecol. 2004;191:1164–72.

76. Grundker C, Volker P, Griesinger F, Ramaswamy A, Nagy A, Schally AV, et al. Antitumor effects of the cytotoxic luteinizing hormone-releasing hormone analog AN-152 on human endometrial and ovarian cancers xenografted into nude mice. Am J Obstet Gynecol. 2002;187:528–37.

77. Emons G, Kaufmann M, Gorchev G, Tsekova V, Grundker C, Gunthert AR, et al. Dose escalation and pharmacokinetic study of AEZS-108 (AN-152), an LHRH agonist linked to doxorubicin, in women with LHRH receptor-positive tumors. Gynecol Oncol. 2010;119:457–61.

78. Emons G, Gorchev G, Harter P, Wimberger P, Stahle A, Hanker L, et al. Efficacy and safety of AEZS-108 (LHRH agonist linked to doxorubicin) in women with advanced or recurrent endometrial cancer expressing LHRH receptors: a multicenter phase 2 trial (AGO-GYN5). Int J Gynecol Cancer. 2014;24:260–5.

79. Brown Jones M, Neuper C, Clayton A, Mariani A, Konecny G, Thomas MB, et al. Rationale for folate receptor alpha targeted therapy in "high risk" endometrial carcinomas. Int J Cancer. 2008;123:1699–703.

80. Senol S, Ceyran AB, Aydin A, Zemheri E, Ozkanli S, Kösemetin D, et al. Folate receptor a expression and significance in endometrioid endometrium carcinoma and endometrial hyperplasia. Int J Clin Exp Pathol. 2015;8:5633–41.

81. Papa A, Zaccarelli E, Caruso D, Vici P, Benedetti Panici P, Tomao F. Targeting angiogenesis in endometrial cancer - new agents for tailored treatments. Expert Opin Investig Drugs. 2016;25:31–49.

82. Mazurek A, Telego M, Pierzynski P, Lapuc G, Niklinska W, Juczewska M, et al. Angiogenesis in endometrial cancer. Neoplasma. 1998;45:360–4.

83. Lee CN, Cheng WF, Chen CA, Chu JS, Hsieh CY, Hsieh FJ. Angiogenesis of endometrial carcinomas assessed by measurement of intratumoral blood flow, microvessel density, and vascular endothelial growth factor levels. Obstet Gynecol. 2000;96:615–21.

84. Hirai M, Nakagawara A, Oosaki T, Hayashi Y, Hirono M, Yoshihara T. Expression of vascular endothelial growth factors (VEGF-A/VEGF-1 and

VEGF-C/VEGF-2) in postmenopausal uterine endometrial carcinoma. Gynecol Oncol. 2001;80:181–8.

85. Holland CM, Day K, Evans A, Smith SK. Expression of the VEGF and angiopoietin genes in endometrial atypical hyperplasia and endometrial cancer. Br J Cancer. 2003;89:891–8.

86. Kamat AA, Merritt WM, Coffey D, Lin YG, Patel PR, Broaddus R, et al. Clinical and biological significance of vascular endothelial growth factor in endometrial cancer. Clin Cancer Res. 2007;13:7487–95.

87. Aghajanian C, Sill MW, Darcy KM, Greer B, McMeekin DS, Rose PG, et al. Phase II trial of bevacizumab in recurrent or persistent endometrial cancer: a gynecologic oncology group study. J Clin Oncol. 2011;29:2259–65.

88. Alvarez EA, Brady WE, Walker JL, Rotmensch J, Zhou XC, Kendrick JE, et al. Phase II trial of combination bevacizumab and temsirolimus in the treatment of recurrent or persistent endometrial carcinoma: a gynecologic oncology group study. Gynecol Oncol. 2013;129:22–7.

89. Simpkins F, Drake R, Escobar PF, Nutter B, Rasool N, Rose PG. A phase II trial of paclitaxel, carboplatin, and bevacizumab in advanced and recurrent endometrial carcinoma (EMCA). Gynecol Oncol. 2015;136:240–5.

90. Aghajanian C, Filiaci V, Dizon DS. A randomized phase II study of paclitaxel/carboplatin/bevacizumab, paclitaxel/carboplatin/temsirolimus and ixabepilone/carboplatin/bevacizumab as initial therapy for measurable stage III or IVA, stage IVB or recurrent endometrial cancer, GOG-86P. J Clin Oncol. 2015;(suppl):abstr 5500.

91. Castonguay V, Lheureux S, Welch S, Mackay HJ, Hirte H, Fleming G, et al. A phase II trial of sunitinib in women with metastatic or recurrent endometrial carcinoma: a study of the Princess Margaret, Chicago and California consortia. Gynecol Oncol. 2014;134:274–80.

92. Dizon DS, Sill MW, Schilder JM, McGonigle KF, Rahman Z, Miller DS, et al. A phase II evaluation of nintedanib (BIBF-1120) in the treatment of recurrent or persistent endometrial cancer: an NRG oncology/gynecologic oncology group study. Gynecol Oncol. 2014;135:441–5.

93. Konecny GE, Finkler N, Garcia AA, Lorusso D, Lee PS, Rocconi RP, et al. Second-line dovitinib (TKI258) in patients with FGFR2-mutated or FGFR2-non-mutated advanced or metastatic endometrial cancer: a non-randomised, open-label, two-group, two-stage, phase 2 study. Lancet Oncol. 2015;16:686–94.

94. Powell MA, Sill MW, Goodfellow PJ, Benbrook DM, Lankes HA, Leslie KK, et al. A phase II trial of brivanib in recurrent or persistent endometrial cancer: an NRG oncology/gynecologic oncology group study. Gynecol Oncol. 2014; 135:38–43.

95. Coleman RL, Sill MW, Lankes HA, Fader AN, Finkler NJ, Hoffman JS, et al. A phase II evaluation of aflibercept in the treatment of recurrent or persistent endometrial cancer: a gynecologic oncology group study. Gynecol Oncol. 2012;127:538–43.

96. Bender D, Sill MW, Lankes HA, Reyes HD, Darus CJ, Delmore JE, et al. A phase II evaluation of cediranib in the treatment of recurrent or persistent endometrial cancer: an NRG oncology/gynecologic oncology group study. Gynecol Oncol. 2015;138:507–12.

97. Vergote I, Teneriello M, Powell MA, Miller DS, Garcia AA, Mikheeva ON, et al. A phase II trial of lenvatinib in patients with advanced or recurrent endometrial cancer: angiopoietin-2 as a predictive marker for clinical outcomes. J Clin Oncol. 2013;31(suppl):abstract 5520.

98. Makker V, Filiaci V, Chen LM, Darus CJ, Kendrick JE, Sutton G, et al. Phase II evaluation of dalantercept, a soluble recombinant activin receptor-like kinase 1 (ALK1) receptor fusion protein, for the treatment of recurrent or persistent endometrial cancer: an NRG oncology/gynecologic oncology group study 0229N. Gynecol Oncol. 2015;138:24–9.

99. Moore KN, Sill MW, Tenney ME, Darus CJ, Griffin D, Werner TL, et al. A phase II trial of trebananib (AMG 386; IND#111071), a selective angiopoietin 1/2 neutralizing peptibody, in patients with persistent/recurrent carcinoma of the endometrium: an NRG/gynecologic oncology group trial. Gynecol Oncol. 2015;138:513–8.

100. Nimeiri HS, Oza AM, Morgan RJ, Huo D, Elit L, Knost JA, et al. A phase II study of sorafenib in advanced uterine carcinoma/carcinosarcoma: a trial of the Chicago, PMH, and California phase II consortia. Gynecol Oncol. 2010;117:37–40.

101. McMeekin DS, Sill MW, Benbrook D, Darcy KM, Stearns-Kurosawa DJ, Eaton L, et al. A phase II trial of thalidomide in patients with refractory endometrial cancer and correlation with angiogenesis biomarkers: a gynecologic oncology group study. Gynecol Oncol. 2007;105:508–16.

102. Niikura H, Sasano H, Kaga K, Sato S, Yajima A. Expression of epidermal growth factor family proteins and epidermal growth factor receptor in human endometrium. Hum Pathol. 1996;27:282–9.

103. Brys M, Semczuk A, Rechberger T, Krajewska WM. Expression of erbB-1 and erbB-2 genes in normal and pathological human endometrium. Oncol Rep. 2007;18:261–5.

104. De Luca A, Carotenuto A, Rachiglio A, Gallo M, Maiello MR, Aldinucci D, et al. The role of the EGFR signaling in tumor microenvironment. J Cell Physiol. 2008;214:559–67.

105. Oza AM, Eisenhauer EA, Elit L, Cutz JC, Sakurada A, Tsao MS, et al. Phase II study of erlotinib in recurrent or metastatic endometrial cancer: NCIC IND-148. J Clin Oncol. 2008;26:4319–25.

106. Leslie KK, Sill MW, Fischer E, Darcy KM, Mannel RS, Tewari KS, et al. A phase II evaluation of gefitinib in the treatment of persistent or recurrent endometrial cancer: a gynecologic oncology group study. Gynecol Oncol. 2013;129:486–94.

107. Graus-Porta D, Beerli RR, Daly JM, Hynes NE. ErbB-2, the preferred heterodimerization partner of all ErbB receptors, is a mediator of lateral signaling. EMBO J. 1997;16:1647–55.

108. Bansal N, Yendluri V, Wenham RM. The molecular biology of endometrial cancers and the implications for pathogenesis, classification, and targeted therapies. Cancer Control. 2009;16:8–13.

109. Black JD, English DP, Roque DM, Santin AD. Targeted therapy in uterine serous carcinoma: an aggressive variant of endometrial cancer. Womens Health (Lond). 2014;10:45–57.

110. Leslie KK, Sill MW, Lankes HA, Fischer EG, Godwin AK, Gray H, et al. Lapatinib and potential prognostic value of EGFR mutations in a gynecologic oncology group phase II trial of persistent or recurrent endometrial cancer. Gynecol Oncol. 2012;127:345–50.

111. Fleming GF, Sill MW, Darcy KM, McMeekin DS, Thigpen JT, Adler LM, et al. Phase II trial of trastuzumab in women with advanced or recurrent, HER2-positive endometrial carcinoma: a gynecologic oncology group study. Gynecol Oncol. 2010;116:15–20.

112. Oza AM, Elit L, Tsao MS, Kamel-Reid S, Biagi J, Provencher DM, et al. Phase II study of temsirolimus in women with recurrent or metastatic endometrial cancer: a trial of the NCIC clinical trials group. J Clin Oncol. 2011;29:3278–85.

113. Slomovitz BM, Lu KH, Johnston T, Coleman RL, Munsell M, Broaddus RR, et al. A phase 2 study of the oral mammalian target of rapamycin inhibitor, everolimus, in patients with recurrent endometrial carcinoma. Cancer. 2010;116:5415–9.

114. Ray-Coquard I, Favier L, Weber B, Roemer-Becuwe C, Bougnoux P, Fabbro M, et al. Everolimus as second- or third-line treatment of advanced endometrial cancer: ENDORAD, a phase II trial of GINECO. Br J Cancer. 2013;108:1771–7.

115. Colombo N, McMeekin DS, Schwartz PE, Sessa C, Gehrig PA, Holloway R, et al. Ridaforolimus as a single agent in advanced endometrial cancer: results of a single-arm, phase 2 trial. Br J Cancer. 2013;108:1021–6.

116. Tsoref D, Welch S, Lau S, Biagi J, Tonkin K, Martin LA, et al. Phase II study of oral ridaforolimus in women with recurrent or metastatic endometrial cancer. Gynecol Oncol. 2014;135:184–9.

117. Oza AM, Pignata S, Poveda A, McCormack M, Clamp A, Schwartz B, et al. Randomized phase II trial of Ridaforolimus in advanced endometrial carcinoma. J Clin Oncol. 2015;33:3576–82.

118. Slomovitz BM, Jiang Y, Yates MS, Soliman PT, Johnston T, Nowakowski M, et al. Phase II study of everolimus and letrozole in patients with recurrent endometrial carcinoma. J Clin Oncol. 2015;33:930–6.

119. Soliman PT, Westin SN, Iglesias DA, Munsell MF, Slomovitz BM, Lu KH, et al. Phase II study of everolimus, letrozole, and metformin in women with advanced/recurrent endometrial cancer. J Clin Oncol. 2016; 34(suppl):abstr 5506.

120. Fleming GF, Filiaci VL, Marzullo B, Zaino RJ, Davidson SA, Pearl M, et al. Temsirolimus with or without megestrol acetate and tamoxifen for endometrial cancer: a gynecologic oncology group study. Gynecol Oncol. 2014;132:585–92.

121. Chon HS, Kang S, Lee JK, Apte SM, Shahzad MM, Williams-Elson I, Wenham RM. Phase I study of oral ridaforolimus in combination with paclitaxel and carboplatin in patients with solid tumor cancers. BMC Cancer. 2017;17:407.

122. Kollmannsberger C, Hirte H, Siu LL, Mazurka J, Chi K, Elit L, et al. Temsirolimus in combination with carboplatin and paclitaxel in patients with advanced solid tumors: a NCIC-CTG, phase I, open-label dose-escalation study (IND 179). Ann Oncol. 2012;23:238–44.

123. Janzen DM, Paik DY, Rosales MA, Yep B, Cheng D, Witte ON, et al. Low levels of circulating estrogen sensitize PTEN-null endometrial tumors to PARP inhibition in vivo. Mol Cancer Ther. 2013;12:2917–28.

124. Makker V, Recio FO, Ma L, Matulonis UA, Lauchle JO, Parmar H, et al. A multicenter, single-arm, open-label, phase 2 study of apitolisib (GDC-0980) for the treatment of recurrent or persistent endometrial carcinoma (MAGGIE study). Cancer 2016 doi:10.1002/cncr.30286.

125. Matulonis U, Vergote I, Backes F, Martin LP, McMeekin S, Birrer M, et al. Phase II study of the PI3K inhibitor pilaralisib (SAR245408; XL147) in patients with advanced or recurrent endometrial carcinoma. Gynecol Oncol. 2015; 136:246–53.

126. Heudel PE, Fabbro M, Roemer-Becuwe C, Treilleux I, Kaminsky MC, Arnaud A, et al. J Clin Oncol. 2015;33(15_suppl):5588.

127. Lopez S, Cocco E, Black J, Bellone S, Bonazzoli E, Predolini F, et al. Dual HER2/PIK3CA targeting overcomes single-agent acquired resistance in HER-2 amplified uterine serous carcinoma cell lines in vitro and in vivo. Mol Cancer Ther. 2015;14:2519–26.

128. Viollet B, Guigas B, Sanz Garcia N, Leclerc J, Foretz M, Andreelli F. Cellular and molecular mechanisms of metformin: an overview. Clin Sci (Lond). 2012;122:253–70.

129. Cantrell LA, Zhou C, Mendivil A, Malloy KM, Gehrig PA, Bae-Jump VL. Metformin is a potent inhibitor of endometrial cancer cell proliferation–implications for a novel treatment strategy. Gynecol Oncol. 2010;116:92–8.

130. Xie Y, Wang YL, Yu L, Hu Q, Ji L, Zhang Y, et al. Metformin promotes progesterone receptor expression via inhibition of mammalian target of rapamycin (mTOR) in endometrial cancer cells. J Steroid Biochem Mol Biol. 2011;126:113–20.

131. Ko EM, Walter P, Jackson A, Clark L, Franasiak J, Bolac C, et al. Metformin is associated with improved survival in endometrial cancer. Gynecol Oncol. 2014;132:438–42.

132. Mackay HJ, Eisenhauer EA, Kamel-Reid S, Tsao M, Clarke B, Karakasis K, et al. Molecular determinants of outcome with mammalian target of rapamycin inhibition in endometrial cancer. Cancer. 2014;120:603–10.

133. Koppensteiner R, Samartzis EP, Noske A, Koppensteiner R, Samartzis EP, Noske A, et al. Effect of MRE11 loss on PARP-inhibitor sensitivity in endometrial cancer in vitro. PLoS One. 2014;9(6):e100041.

134. Mo Z, Liu J, Zhang Q, Chen Z, Mei J, Liu L, et al. Expression of PD-1, PD-L1 and PD-L2 is associated with differentiation status and histological type of endometrial cancer. Oncol Lett. 2016;12:944–50.

135. Gatalica Z, Snyder C, Maney T, Ghazalpour A, Holterman DA, Xiao N. Programmed cell death 1 (PD-1) and its ligand (PDI1) in common cancers and their correlaio ith moleculat cancer type. Cancer Epidemiol Biomark Prev. 2014;23:2965–70.

136. de Jong RA, Leffers N, Boezen HM, ten Hoor KA, van der Zee AG, Hollema H, et al. Presence of tumor-infiltrating lymphocytes is an independent prognostic factor in type I and type II endometrial cancer. Gynecol Oncol. 2009;114:105–10.

137. Ott PA, Elez E, Hiret S, Kim DW, Morosky A, Saraf S, et al. Pembrolizumab in Patients with Extensive-Stage Small-Cell Lung Cancer: Results From the Phase Ib KEYNOTE-028 Study. J Clin Oncol 2017 16: [Epub ahead of print].

138. Le DT, Uram JN, Wang H, Bartlett BR, Kemberling H, Eyring AD, et al. PD-1 blockade in tumors with mismatch-repair deficiency. N Engl J Med. 2015;372:2509–20.

139. Ott PA, Bang Y, Berton-Rigaud D, Elez E, Pishvanian MJ, Rugo HA, et al. Pembrolizumab in advanced endometrial cancer: preliminary results from the phase Ib KEYNOTE-028 study. J Clin Oncol. 2016;34(suppl):Abstract 5581.

140. Kato Y, Bao X, Macgrath S, Tabata K, Hori Y, Tachino M, et al. Lenvatinib mesilate (LEN) enhanced antitumor activity of a PD-1 blockade agent by potentiating Th1 immune response. Ann Oncol. 2016;27:1–14. Abstract 2008

141. Kato Y, Tabata K, Hori Y, Tachino KS, Okamoto K, Matsui J. Effects of lenvatinib on tumor-associated macrophages enhance antitumor activity of PD-1 signal inhibitors. AACR. 2015;14(suppl. 2):Abstract A92.

142. Makker V, Rasco D, Dutcus C, Stephen DE, Li D, Schmidt E, et al. A phase Ib/2 trial of Lenvatinib plus Pembrolizumab in patients with endometrial carcinoma. ASCO 2017. J Clin Oncol. 2017;35(suppl):abstract 5598.

25

The utility of patient reported data in a gynecologic oncology clinic

D. Barnes[1]* ⓘ, R. Rivera[1], S. Gibson[2], C. Craig[1], J. Cragun[2], B. Monk[1] and D. Chase[1]

Abstract

Background: Measuring QoL is essential to the field of gynecologic oncology but there seems to be limited standardized data regarding collecting QoL assessments throughout a patient's cancer treatment especially in non-clinical trial patients. The aim of this study is to explore patient characteristics that may be associated with poor quality of life (QoL) in women with gynecologic cancers at two University of Arizona Cancer Center (UACC) sites.

Methods: A cross-sectional survey was conducted among English speaking women with gynecologic malignancies at the University of Arizona Cancer Centers in Phoenix and Tucson from April 2012 to July 2015. The survey was a paper packet of questions that was distributed to cancer patients at the time of their clinic visit. The packet contained questions on demographic information, treatment, lifestyle characteristics, pelvic pain and Health-related quality of life (HRQoL). Measures included the generic and cancer-specific scores on the Functional Assessment of Cancer Therapy–General (FACT-G) and the Female Genitourinary Pain Index (GUPI). The total scores and subdomains were compared with descriptive variables (age, body mass index (BMI), diet, exercise, disease status, treatment and support group attendance) using Cronbach alpha (α), Spearman rank correlations (ρ), and Holm's Bonferroni method.

Results: One–hundred and forty-nine women completed the survey; 55% ($N = 81$) were older than 60 years, 38% ($N = 45$) were obese (BMI > 30), 46% ($N = 66$) exercised daily, and 84% ($N = 111$) ate one or more daily serving of fruit and vegetables. Women in remission, those who exercised daily and ate fruits/vegetables were less likely to have their symptoms impact their QoL. Younger women were more likely to report genitourinary issues ($p = -0.22$) and overall problems with QoL ($p = -0.29$) than older women. Among FACT-G support group responses, we found those that did not attend support groups had a significantly higher emotional wellbeing ($p = 0.05$).

Conclusions: This study identified potential areas of clinical focus, which aid in understanding our approach to caring for gynecologic cancer patients and improvement of their HRQoL. We identified that age, pelvic pain, and lifestyle characteristics have indicators to poor QoL in women with gynecologic cancers. In this population, younger women and those with pelvic pain complaints, poor diet and exercise habits should be targeted early for supportive care interventions to improve QoL throughout both treatment and survivorship.

Background

The impact of illness and treatment on quality of life (QoL) has received increasing recognition in recent years with the both the National Cancer Institute and the Food and Drug Administration who have mandated that the goals of cancer research should be to improve both survival and QoL [1]. Measuring QoL is essential to the field of gynecologic oncology but there seems to be limited standardized data regarding collecting QoL

assessments throughout a patient's cancer treatment especially in non-clinical trial patients [2, 3]. Prior studies have demonstrated that a patient's QoL changes over the course of treatment; however this is unknown in non-clinical trial patients [4, 5].

QoL is defined as the level of satisfaction a person has with their physical (PWB), emotional (EWB), and social wellbeing (SWB) [6]. The diagnosis of cancer in a woman encompasses not only the physical effects of the disease but also the short and long-term side effects of treatment, its cost, potential economic loss, and the reaction of family and friends, each of which influence QoL [6–12]. Since QoL is a multidimensional concept it

* Correspondence: Nikky.barnes@gmail.com
[1]Department of Gynecologic Oncology, Creighton University School of Medicine at St. Joseph's Hospital and Medical Center, Phoenix, AZ, USA
Full list of author information is available at the end of the article

is important to assess how it affects various communities and populations so that interventions can be designed to help improve overall wellbeing in patients. Numerous instruments have been created and aim to measure patients' QoL [13]. One of these measures is the Health Related Quality of Life (HRQoL), which allows patients to self-report symptoms using patient-reported outcome (PRO) measures [4, 14]. The use of PRO, especially in oncology, has been shown to help with detection of problematic symptoms, symptom monitoring, satisfaction with patient care, and communication between clinicians and patients [15–17].

The aim of this study is to examine HRQoL in a community oncology setting. The goal of this research is to ultimately identify and then address areas to target QoL interventions in a non-clinical trial population.

Methods
Study design
Following Institutional Review Board approval, we performed a cross-sectional HRQoL survey among women aged 21–89 years with gynecologic malignancies (cervical, ovarian, and/or uterine) seen at the University of Arizona Cancer Center locations in Phoenix and Tucson from April 2012 to July 2015.

Patient selection
Participants were comprised of women who had survived cancer and were undergoing care at our two sites. Eligibility criteria included: 1) age ≥ 21 years, 2) current gynecologic malignancy 3) current history of gynecologic malignancy 4) ability to read, write, and understand English (as a primary or secondary language). Women were excluded if they did not complete at least 50% of the questionnaire.

QoL assessments and instruments
We used a questionnaire packet that included the Functional Assessment of Cancer Therapy Female Genitourinary Pain Index, and self-reported demographic information. The QoL questionnaires were scored separately.

Functional Assessment of Cancer Therapy – General (FACT-G), is a 27-item QoL instrument that consisted of four well-being subscales: physical, functional, social, and emotional [18, 19]. Within each subdomain, questions are answered on a 5-point Likert scale, ranging from 1 (not at all) to 4 (very much). The items are summed to give a score for each subdomain. The subdomain scores are then summed to give a total FACT score; higher subscale and total scores indicate better QoL [20].

The Genitourinary Pain Index (GUPI) is a 15-item instrument intended to measure, within the past week, the intensity of three constructs: (a) pelvic pain or discomfort, (b) urinary symptoms, and (c) quality of life [21]. Lower subscale and total scores indicate better QoL.

Construct A: Pelvic pain or discomfort was measured by ten items: eight of these items, which consisted of binary response options (0 = no, 1 = yes), were indicative of pain/discomfort stemming both from the pelvic area (e.g., urethra, vagina) and activities involving the pelvic area (e.g., sexual intercourse, urinating). The ninth item measured pelvic pain frequency with six-point response options ranging from 0 (never) to 5 (always), and the tenth item used an 11-point average pain scale ranging from 0 to 10. The scores were summed to create a total score that could range from 0 to 23.

Construct B: Urinary symptoms (e.g., urinating frequency) were measured with two GUPI items with response options that ranged from 0 (not at all) to 5 (almost always). The mean of the two items were computed creating a score ranging from 0 to 5 with higher scores being indicative of higher urinary symptoms.

Construct C: GUPI- QoL consisted of three items that measured the impact of the symptoms on decreasing respondent's QoL. The first two items have response options ranging from 0 (none) to 3 (a lot). The third item, which had response scale ranging from 1 (pleased) to 6 (terrible), measured how respondents felt about symptoms if they had them for the rest of their life. The three items were summed to create a total score, which could range from 1 to 12, with higher values being indicative of worse impact on QoL.

Self-reported demographic information such as age, weight, height, BMI, disease status (current disease verses cancer remission), cancer stage, past medical history, past surgical history, previous cancer treatment, and current chemotherapy treatment cycle was collected via self-reported questionnaire. The survey also included questions on exercise frequency (defined as ≥30 min of moderate activity), amount of daily consumption of fruits of vegetables, and support group attendance.

Data collection
Potential study participants were approached after registering for their appointment at a clinic visit, and the objective of the study was explained. If they choose to participate, they were given the questionnaire, and patients self-reported their answers. Informed consent was obtained and presumed when patients proceeded with the questionnaire. The self-administered survey took approximately 15–20 min to complete.

Study measures
Socio-demographic
Descriptive statistics were calculated for demographic and clinical characteristics. Differences in demographic, clinical, and symptoms characteristics, as well as QoL outcomes, were evaluated using Cronbach alpha (α),

Spearman rank correlations (ρ), and Holm's Bonferroni method were used to correct for type-I error rates.

Statistical analysis

For each lifestyle behavior a one-way analysis of covariance was used to examine the association with HRQoL. Descriptive statistics and frequency distributions were performed while controlling for potential demographic and medical confounders for each lifestyle behavior. Logistic regression was then used for analysis with significance set at $p < 0.05$.

Results

A total of 149 women participated in the study. Of the completed questionnaires 100% of patients completed the questions for age, 80% completed BMI and disease status, 88% completed diet questions, 97% completed questions for exercise, history of surgery, and support group attendance, 44% completed treatment questions, and 77% completed questions on their disease status.

Baseline self-reported demographics for the final analytic cohort are reported in Table 1. A little over half (55.4%, $N = 81$) of the women were older than 60 years, and over two-thirds (68.6%, N = 81) self-reported they were overweight or obese. About 46% reported exercising daily ($N = 66$) and 31% ($N = 45$) exercised weekly.

Roughly 84% ($N = 111$) had more than one daily serving of fruit and vegetables. Only 13% ($N = 19$) of the women attended a support group.

Treatment, cancer stage, and disease status of the final analytic cohort are presented in Table 2. Prior treatment was defined as chemotherapy and/or surgery, and there were no documented treatments available for 23 individuals. Of the participants with documented treatment, 61 (48%) had a history of receiving chemotherapy, while another 61 (48%) were currently receiving chemotherapy. Only five (4%) were re-initiating chemotherapy. Among the 61 women who had a previous chemotherapy, 56% had their last treatment less than a year prior to study participation. Of the 61 patients who were currently receiving chemotherapy, 82% were in the middle (cycles 2–5) of their treatment cycle. The majority (83%, $N = 120$) of participants had either a recent or a historical report of surgery. Disease status was obtained from the questionnaires for 119 women and a little more than a quarter (27%, $N = 32$) had received their first chemotherapy dose, almost a third (33%, $N = 39$) had a recurrence of cancer, and 40% ($N = 48$) were in remission. Among participants with a documented cancer stage ($N = 114$), 60% had stage III or IV disease.

Table 3 summarizes the Spearman's rho rank-order correlations (ρ) of three GUPI subscales, as well as four

Table 1 Demographic Characteristics of Participant from April 2012 to July 2015 ($N = 149$)

		F	%
Age (years)	21–40	15	10.07
	41–50	19	12.75
	51–60	34	22.82
	61–70	50	33.56
	> 70	31	20.81
	Total	149	100
BMI Categories (kg/m²)	Underweight (< 18.5)	0	0.00
	Healthy (18.5–24.99)	37	31.36
	Overweight (25–29.99)	36	30.51
	Obese (30+)	45	38.14
	Total	118	100
Exercise	Never	34	23.45
	Weekly	45	31.03
	Daily	66	45.52
	Total	145	100
Daily Amount of Fruit/ Vegetables (servings)	< 1	21	16.03
	1–2	68	51.91
	≥3	42	32.06
	Total	131	100
Attends Support Group	Yes	19	13.10
	No	126	86.90
	Total	145	100

Table 2 Frequency and Percent Distribution of Historical/Current Treatment and Disease Progression from April 2012 to July 2015

			F	%
Last Previous Treatment	< 1 month		13	19.70
	2–6 month		11	16.67
	6–12		13	19.70
	13–24		7	10.61
	> 2 years		22	33.33
		Total[a]	66	100
Chemotherapy Cycle of Current Treatment	First		3	4.55
	Middle		54	81.82
	Last		9	13.64
		Total[a]	66	100
History / Recent Surgery	Yes		120	83.33
	No		24	16.67
		Total	144	100
Disease Status	1st Chemotherapy Treatment		32	26.89
	Recurrent		39	32.77
	Remission		48	40.34
		Total	119	100
Cancer Stage	I		25	21.93
	II		20	17.54
	III		43	37.72
	IV		26	22.81
		Total	114	100

[a]127 participants had a record either of only a previous treatment (*n* = 66), only a current chemotherapy treatment (*n* = 66), and for 23 cases the treatment status was not known

FACT-G dimensions, with age, BMI, healthy behaviors, surgery, and disease status. Pelvic pain or discomfort was not correlated to patient's age, BMI, healthy behaviors (exercise engagement, daily consumption of vegetables/fruit, and group therapy attendance), or disease status (1st chemo-therapy, cancer recurrence and remission). Urinary symptoms were inversely related with age ($\rho = -.22$, $p < .05$) with younger patients being more likely to report urinating more frequently than older patients. BMI, exercise, history of or recent surgery, and remission had clinically significant pain severity ($p < .05$). Although the results suggest that urinary symptoms may correlate with cancer recurrence ($\rho = .22$, ns), the correlation was not significant.

Table 3 shows that poorer QoL scores correlated with having both surgery ($\rho = 0.25$, $p < 0.05$) and first chemotherapy treatment ($\rho = 0.22$, $p < 0.05$). Women who were older were less likely to have symptoms negatively impact their QoL than younger women ($\rho = -0.29$, $p < 0.05$). The more servings of fruits/vegetables ($\rho = -0.23$, $p < 0.05$), a woman consumed each day or the more frequently she engaged in exercise ($\rho = -0.20$, $p < 0.05$), the less likely she reported symptoms that negatively impacted

her QoL. Those who were in remission were less likely to have their symptoms that affected their QoL ($\rho = -0.35$, $p < 0.05$).

Participants were more likely to have higher PWB scores and fewer complaints about fatigue if they were older ($\rho = 0.31$, $p < 0.05$), engaged in exercise ($\rho = 0.22$, $p < 0.05$), had daily intake of fruits/vegetables ($\rho = 0.22$, $p < 0.05$), or were in remission ($\rho = 0.46$, $p < 0.05$). Having surgery ($\rho = -0.24$, $p < 0.05$), first chemotherapy ($\rho = -0.27$, $p < 0.05$), or recurrent cancer ($\rho = -0.23$, $p < .05$) resulted in lower PWB. Support from friends and family as well as SWB score were positively correlated with age ($\rho = 0.23$). Older patients were more likely to have an increased sense of friends or family support than those who were younger. FWB had a positive association with age ($\rho = 0.23$, $p < 0.05$), exercise ($\rho = 0.23$, $p < 0.05$), and being in remission ($\rho = 0.38$, $p < 0.05$). FWB was negatively correlated with cancer recurrence and positively correlated with exercise. Older patients had higher FWB scores than younger patients, and those who were in remission or did not have recurrence of cancer were more functional than their counterparts.

Table 3 Spearman's Rho (ρ) Rank Correlations between Patient characteristics and pain, quality of life, social support and Wellbeing from April 2012 to July 2015

Patient Characteristics		GUPI Symptoms			FACT-G Well-Being			
		Pelvic Pain	Urinary symptoms	Impact on QoL	Physical Well-Being	Social Well-Being	Emotional Well-Being	Functional Well-Being
Age	P	0.09	−.22[a]	−.29[a]	.31[a]	.23[a]	0.09	.23[a]
	N	135	131	134	146	145	142	141
BMI	P	0.04	−0.13	0.03	0.04	0.04	−0.04	0.09
	N	120	116	119	121	121	118	117
Exercise	P	0.05	−0.03	−.20a	.22[a]	0.15	0.02	.23[a]
	N	130	127	129	141	140	137	136
Daily Fruit/ Vegetables	P	0.09	0.04	−.23[c]	.22[a]	0.02	0.06	0.17
	N	127	123	126	127	127	124	124
Support Group	P	0.08	−0.08	−0.01	−0.04	−0.16	−0.18	−0.03
	N	134	130	133	145	144	141	140
History/Recent Surgery	P	0.05	0.10	.25[a]	−.24[a]	−0.03	0.04	−0.17
	N	133	129	132	144	143	140	139
1st Chemo	P	0.13	−0.05	.22a	−.27[a]	−0.02	0.05	−0.17
	N	108	106	107	119	118	116	115
Recurrent Cancer	P	0.08	0.22	0.16	−.23[a]	−0.09	−0.19	−.24[a]
	N	108	106	107	119	118	116	115
Remission	P	0.04	−0.16	−.35[a]	.46[a]	0.10	0.14	.38[a]
	N	108	106	107	119	118	116	115
	N	135	131	134	146	145	142	141
	M	8.54	1.46	4.39	20.88	22.84	18.51	19.69
	SD	4.85	1.38	3.44	6.29	5.70	4.35	6.22
	Mdn	9.00	1.00	4.00	23.00	24.50	19.00	20.00

[a]Significant at.05 level after correcting for type I error rate with Holm–Bonferroni method

Discussion

Based on the survey results, we identified that age, pelvic pain, and lifestyle characteristics are indicators to poor HRQoL in women with gynecologic cancers. Previous studies have shown promise when investigating the influence of lifestyle on QoL in gynecologic cancers [22–25]. Lifestyle modifications have been shown to relieve fatigue, improve treatment induced anemia, maintain a healthy BMI, and enhance quality of sleep [26–28]. Our findings support this and indicate that weekly exercise (≥30 min of moderate activity) and a diet rich in fruits/vegetables (≥3 servings per day) positively impacted HRQoL. Almost a quarter of our population did not partake in any physical activity. This is drastically different from previous research in breast and prostate cancer survivors who reported at least > 50% of physical activity [22, 29–32]. Inferences may be that our population and the studies characteristics were different. In those studies some patients were from higher socio-economic and education backgrounds, which may be different from our patient cohort, and it would be prudent to investigate these barriers in future studies.

Alarming, however, is the finding that 44% of our younger patients ≤60 years of age reported having more issues with QoL. This is consistent with previous research among breast cancer and chronic disease patients. Younger patients have more issues adapting to their condition and have significant impairments in QoL, wellbeing, and recovery [13, 33–39]. Our data reinforces what other studies have found in chronic disease (Alzheimer's, Multiple Sclerosis, Bone, Breast, and Non-Small Cell Lung Cancer) and in gynecologic cancers such as Ovarian Cancer; that all patients especially those younger need to be targeted and counseled early in their care about the potential side effects in their disease and treatment [36, 40–47]. This has been shown to help patients have a more realistic expectation for their outcome, decrease patient anxiety, depression, and anticipate challenges that may lie ahead during and after their treatment. Multiple studies have shown that counseling patients on chemotherapy improved QoL and physiological and physical health scores when performed by a physician [17, 48].

Another principal finding was more then half of our sample reported clinically significant pelvic pain. BMI, exercise, history of or recent surgery, and remission had clinically significant pain. Pelvic pain is a distressing symptom and a common QoL concerns for women with gynecologic cancer, and may be an influential variable of QoL in Gynecologic malignancies [47, 48]. Our data supports that pelvic pain is a direct correlate of HRQoL.

This study is not without limitations. We conducted a cross-sectional convenience sample; therefore, our results may not be generalizable, especially since only two institutions were involved within this study. By limiting our respondents to women who only spoke English as a primary or secondary language, we may have excluded a portion of our population where cultural or language factors could have influenced our results. Although we sampled patients with different disease severity (first treatment, recurrent, or remission), selection bias is still possible, but given the nature of QoL concerns, radical difference across populations seems unlikely. We did not correlate symptoms based on specific gynecologic cancers and age, and no associations were made to see how the quality or location of pelvic pain varied within the study cohort. Finally, we have not yet investigated the responsiveness of this packet and its ability to detect baseline or important changes over time, even if that change is small.

Conclusions

This study identified potential areas of clinical focus, which aid in understanding our approach to caring for gynecologic cancer patients and improvement of their HRQoL. We identified that age, pelvic pain, and lifestyle characteristics have indicators to poor QoL in women with gynecologic cancers. In this population, younger women and those with pelvic pain complaints, poor diet and exercise habits should be targeted early for supportive care interventions to improve QoL throughout both treatment and survivorship.

Highlights

- Lifestyle interventions may be targeted towards specific populations to improve QoL in women with gynecologic cancers
- Further studies are needed to evaluate these effects on Health Related Quality of Life (HRQoL) in non-clinical trial patient population

Abbreviations
EMB: Emotional Wellbeing; FACT-G: Functional Assessment of Cancer Therapy–General; FWB: Functional Wellbeing; GUPI: Female Genitourinary Pain Index; HRQoL: Health-related quality of life; PRO: Patient Reported Outcome; PWB: Physical Wellbeing; QoL: Quality of Life; SWB: Social Wellbeing

Acknowledgements
Dr. Heather Dalton and Dr. Ekwutosi Okoroh for revising manuscript critically for important intellectual content and drafting the manuscript.

Authors' contributions
DC and BM were involved in the conception and the design of the study. CC and SG took part in data collection. RR, DB, DC were responsible for data analysis and interpretation. DB, RR, SG were involved with drafting the manuscript or revisions for manuscript submission. DC and BM conceived the study design and participated in coordination and helped with the manuscript. All authors read and approved the final manuscript.

Competing interests
The authors declare that they have no competing interests.

Author details
[1]Department of Gynecologic Oncology, Creighton University School of Medicine at St. Joseph's Hospital and Medical Center, Phoenix, AZ, USA. [2]University of Arizona Cancer Center, Tucson, AZ, USA.

References
1. Arriba LN, Fader AN, Frasure HE, von Gruenigen VE. A review of issues surrounding quality of life among women with ovarian cancer. Gynecol Oncol. 2010;119:390–6. https://doi.org/10.1016/j.ygyno.2010.05.014.
2. Pignata S, Ballatori E, Favalli G, Scambia G. Quality of life: Gynaecological cancers. Ann Oncol. 2001;12:37–42. https://www.researchgate.net/publication/11555496_Quality_of_life_Gynaecological_cancers (Accessed 19 Jan 2018).
3. Pearman T. Quality of life and psychosocial adjustment in gynecologic cancer survivors. Health Qual Life Outcomes. 2003;1:33. https://doi.org/10.1186/1477-7525-1-33.
4. Doll KM, Barber EL, Bensen JT, Snavely AC, Gehrig PA. The health-related quality of life journey of gynecologic oncology surgical patients: implications for the incorporation of patient-reported outcomes into surgical quality metrics ☆. Gynecol Oncol. 2016;141:329–35. https://doi.org/10.1016/j.ygyno.2016.03.003.
5. Moss HA, Havrilesky LJ. The use of patient-reported outcome tools in gynecologic oncology research, clinical practice, and value-based care, 2017. https://doi.org/10.1016/j.ygyno.2017.11.011.
6. Goker FKA, Guvenal T, Yanikkerem E. Turham, quality of life in women with gynecologic cancer in Turkey, Asian Pacific. J Cancer Prev. 2011;12:3121–8. https://www.researchgate.net/profile/Tevfik_Guvenal/publication/221680950_Quality_of_life_in_women_with_gynecologic_cancer_in_Turkey/links/00b4953b6cbc00ed37000000.pdf (Accessed 10 Apr 2017
7. Guidozzi F. Living with ovarian Cancer. Gynecol Oncol. 1993;50:202–7. https://doi.org/10.1006/gyno.1993.1193.
8. Rannestad T, Skjeldestad FE, Platou TF, Hagen B. Quality of life among long-term gynaecological cancer survivors. Scand J Caring Sci. 2008;22:472–7. https://doi.org/10.1111/j.1471-6712.2007.00557.x.
9. Reis N, Beji NK, Coskun A. Quality of life and sexual functioning in gynecological cancer patients: results from quantitative and qualitative data. Eur J Oncol Nurs. 2010;14:137–46. https://doi.org/10.1016/j.ejon.2009.09.004.
10. Özaras G, Özyurda F. Quality of Life and Influencing Factors in Patients with a Gynaecologic Cancer Diagnosis at Gazi University, Turkey. Asian Pacific J Cancer Prev. 2010;11(5):1403–8. Article 45.
11. Wilailak S, Lertkhachonsuk A, Lohacharoenvanich N, Luengsukcharoen SC, Jirajaras M, Likitanasombat P, Sirilerttrakul S. Quality of life in gynecologic cancer survivors compared to healthy check-up women. J Gynecol Oncol. 2011;22:103. https://doi.org/10.3802/jgo.2011.22.2.103.

12. Ersek M, Ferrell BR, Dow KH, Melancon CH. Quality of life in women with ovarian Cancer. West J Nurs Res. 1997;19:334–50. https://doi.org/10.1177/019394599701900305.

13. Burckhardt CS, Anderson KL. The quality of life scale (QOLS): reliability, validity, and utilization. Health Qual Life Outcomes. 2003;1:60. https://doi.org/10.1186/1477-7525-1-60.

14. Stover AM, Basch EM. Using patient-reported outcome measures as quality indicators in routine cancer care. Cancer. 2016;122:355–7. https://doi.org/10.1002/cncr.29768.

15. Basch E, Deal AM, Kris MG, Scher HI, Hudis CA, Sabbatini P, Rogak L, Bennett AV, Dueck AC, Atkinson TM, Chou JF, Dulko D, Sit L, Barz A, Novotny P, Fruscione M, Sloan JA, Schrag D. Symptom monitoring with patient-reported outcomes during routine Cancer treatment: a randomized controlled trial. J Clin Oncol. 2016;34:557–65. https://doi.org/10.1200/JCO.2015.63.0830.

16. Velikova G, Booth L, Smith AB, Brown PM, Lynch P, Brown JM, Selby PJ. Measuring quality of life in routine oncology practice improves communication and patient well-being: a randomized controlled trial. J Clin Oncol. 2004;22:714–24. https://doi.org/10.1200/JCO.2004.06.078.

17. Detmar SB, Muller MJ, Schornagel JH, Wever LDV, Aaronson NK. Health-related quality-of-life assessments and patient-physician communication. JAMA. 2002;288:3027. https://doi.org/10.1001/jama.288.23.3027.

18. Cella DF, Tulsky DS, Gray G, Sarafian B, Linn E, Bonomi A, Silberman M, Yellen SB, Winicour P, Brannon J. The Functional Assessment of Cancer Therapy scale: development and validation of the general measure. J Clin Oncol. 1993;11:570–9. http://www.ncbi.nlm.nih.gov/pubmed/8445433 (Accessed 18 July 2016)

19. von Gruenigen VE, Huang HQ, Gil KM, Frasure HE, Armstrong DK, Wenzel LB. The association between quality of life domains and overall survival in ovarian cancer patients during adjuvant chemotherapy: a gynecologic oncology group study. Gynecol Oncol. 2012;124:379–82. https://doi.org/10.1016/j.ygyno.2011.11.032.

20. Yost KJ, Thompson CA, Eton DT, Allmer C, Ehlers SL, Habermann TM, Shanafelt TD, Maurer MJ, Slager SL, Link BK, Cerhan JR. The Functional Assessment of Cancer Therapy - General (FACT-G) is valid for monitoring quality of life in patients with non-Hodgkin lymphoma. Leuk Lymphoma. 2013;54:290–7. https://doi.org/10.3109/10428194.2012.711830.

21. Clemens JQ, Calhoun EA, Litwin MS, McNaughton-Collins M, Kusek JW, Crowley EM, Landis JR. Urologic Pelvic Pain Collaborative Research Network, Validation of a modified National Institutes of Health chronic prostatitis symptom index to assess genitourinary pain in both men and women. Urology. 2009;74:983–7. https://doi.org/10.1016/j.urology.2009.06.078. NaN-3

22. Blanchard CM, Stein KD, Baker F, Dent MF, Denniston MM, Courneya KS, Nehl E. Association between current lifestyle behaviors and health-related quality of life in breast, colorectal, and prostate cancer survivors. Psychol Health. 2004;19:1–13. https://doi.org/10.1080/08870440310001606507.

23. Knols R, Aaronson NK, Uebelhart D, Fransen J, Aufdemkampe G. Physical exercise in Cancer patients during and after medical treatment: a systematic review of randomized and controlled clinical trials. J Clin Oncol. 2005;23:3830–42. https://doi.org/10.1200/JCO.2005.02.148.

24. Courneya KS. Exercise in cancer survivors: an overview of research. Med Sci Sports Exerc. 2003;35:1846–52. https://doi.org/10.1249/01.MSS.0000093622.41587.B6.

25. Bellizzi KM, Rowland JH, Jeffery DD, McNeel T. Health behaviors of cancer survivors: examining opportunities for cancer control intervention. J Clin Oncol. 2005;23:8884–93. https://doi.org/10.1200/JCO.2005.02.2343.

26. Ghavami H, Akyolcu N. The impact of lifestyle interventions in breast Cancer women after completion of primary therapy: a randomized study. J Breast Heal. 2017;13:94-9.

27. Mosher CE, Sloane R, Morey MC, Snyder DC, Cohen HJ, Miller PE, Demark-Wahnefried W. Associations between lifestyle factors and quality of life among older long-term breast, prostate, and colorectal cancer survivors. Cancer. 2009;115:4001–9. https://doi.org/10.1002/cncr.24436.

28. Ravasco P, Monteiro-Grillo I, Marques Vidal P, Camilo ME. Impact of nutrition on outcome: a prospective randomized controlled trial in patients with head and neck cancer undergoing radiotherapy. Head Neck. 2005;27:659–68. https://doi.org/10.1002/hed.20221.

29. Blanchard CM, Courneya KS, Stein K. American Cancer Society's SCS-II, Cancer survivors' adherence to lifestyle behavior recommendations and associations with health-related quality of life: results from the American Cancer Society's SCS-II. J Clin Oncol. 2008;26:2198–204. https://doi.org/10.1200/JCO.2007.14.6217.

30. Maunsell E, Drolet M, Brisson J, Robert J, Deschênes L. Dietary change after breast cancer: extent, predictors, and relation with psychological distress. J Clin Oncol. 2002;20:1017–25. https://doi.org/10.1200/JCO.2002.20.4.1017.

31. Meyerhardt JA, Heseltine D, Niedzwiecki D, Hollis D, Saltz LB, Mayer RJ, Thomas J, Nelson H, Whittom R, Hantel A, Schilsky RL, Fuchs CS. Impact of physical activity on cancer recurrence and survival in patients with stage III colon cancer: findings from CALGB 89803. J Clin Oncol. 2006;24:3535–41. https://doi.org/10.1200/JCO.2006.06.0863.

32. Doyle C, Kushi LH, Byers T, Courneya KS, Demark-Wahnefried W, Grant B, McTiernan A, Rock CL, Thompson C, Gansler T, Andrews KS. 2006 nutrition, physical activity and Cancer survivorship advisory committee, American Cancer Society, nutrition and physical activity during and after cancer treatment: an American Cancer Society guide for informed choices. CA Cancer J Clin. n.d.;56:323–53. http://www.ncbi.nlm.nih.gov/pubmed/17135691 (Accessed 20 Jan 2018)

33. Avis NE, Crawford S, Manuel J. Quality of life among younger women with breast cancer. J Clin Oncol. 2005;23:3322–30. https://doi.org/10.1200/JCO.2005.05.130.

34. Wenzel LB, Fairclough DL, Brady MJ, Cella D, Garrett KM, Kluhsman BC, Crane LA, Marcus AC. Age-related differences in the quality of life of breast carcinoma patients after treatment. Cancer. 1999;86:1768–74. http://www.ncbi.nlm.nih.gov/pubmed/10547550 (accessed January 20, 2018)

35. Canuet L, Ishii R, Iwase M, Ikezawa K, Kurimoto R, Azechi M, Takahashi H, Nakahachi T, Teshima Y, Takeda M. Factors associated with impaired quality of life in younger and older adults with epilepsy. Epilepsy Res. 2009;83:58–65. https://doi.org/10.1016/J.EPLEPSYRES.2008.09.001.

36. Brod M. Pilot study - quality of life issues in patients with diabetes and lower extremity ulcers: patients and care givers. Qual Life Res. 1998;7:365–72. https://doi.org/10.1023/A:1024994232353.

37. Bifulco G, De Rosa N, Tornesello ML, Piccoli R, Bertrando A, Lavitola G, Morra I, Di A, Sardo S, Buonaguro FM, Nappi C. Quality of life, lifestyle behavior and employment experience: a comparison between young and midlife survivors of gynecology early stage cancers. Gynecol Oncol. 2012;124:444–51. https://doi.org/10.1016/j.ygyno.2011.11.033.

38. Paraskevi T. Quality of life outcomes in patients with breast cancer. Oncol Rev. 2012;6:e2. https://doi.org/10.4081/oncol.2012.e2.

39. Wenzel L, Vergote I, Cella D, Quality of Life in Patients Receiving Treatment for Gynecologic Malignancies: Special considerations for patient care, (n.d.). http://www.unipd.it/esterni/wwwginec/Assistenza-Documenti/Unita'%20operative/Ginecologia%20Oncologica/B5%20-%20QUALITY%20OF%20LIFE.pdf (Accessed 6 May 2018).

40. Howell D, Fitch MI, Deane KA. MN Institution: From the Psychosocial and Behavioral Research Unit, Toronto Sunnybrook Regional Cancer Centre, Toronto Ontario. Impact of Ovarian Cancer Perceived by Women. Cancer Nurs. 2003;26(1):1-9.

41. Armstrong DK. Disease Relapsed Ovarian Cancer: Challenges and Management Strategies for a Chronic Relapsed Ovarian Cancer: Challenges and Management Strategies for a Chronic Disease, 2002. doi:https://doi.org/10.1634/theoncologist.7-suppl_5-20.

42. Sørensen LV, Waldorff FB, Waldemar G. Early counselling and support for patients with mild Alzheimer's disease and their caregivers: a qualitative study on outcome. Aging Ment Health. 2008;12:444–50. https://doi.org/10.1080/13607860802224342.

43. Fawzy FI, Fawzy NW, Hyun CS, Elashoff R, Guthrie D, Fahey JL, Morton DL. Malignant Melanoma. Arch Gen Psychiatry. 1993;50:681. https://doi.org/10.1001/archpsyc.1993.01820210015002.

44. Temel JS, Greer JA, Muzikansky A, Gallagher ER, Admane S, Jackson VA, Dahlin CM, Blinderman CD, Jacobsen J, Pirl WF, Billings JA, Lynch TJ. Early palliative Care for Patients with metastatic non–small-cell lung Cancer. N Engl J Med. 2010;363:733–42. https://doi.org/10.1056/NEJMoa1000678.

45. Felder-Puig R, Formann AK, Mildner A, Bretschneider W, Bucher B, Windhager R, Zoubek A, Puig S, Topf R. Quality of life and psychosocial adjustment of young patients after treatment of bone cancer. Cancer. 1998;83:69–75. https://doi.org/10.1002/(SICI)1097-0142(19980701)83:1<69::AID-CNCR10>3.0.CO;2-A.

46. Periasamy U, Mohd Sidik S, Rampal L, Fadhilah SI, Akhtari-Zavare M, Mahmud R. Effect of chemotherapy counseling by pharmacists on quality of life and psychological outcomes of oncology patients in Malaysia: a randomized control trial. Health Qual Life Outcomes. 2017;15:104. https://doi.org/10.1186/s12955-017-0680-2.

26

A retrospective evaluation of activity of gemcitabine/platinum regimens in the treatment of recurrent ovarian cancer

Tran N. Le[1], Rachel E. Harvey[2], Christine K. Kim[3], Jubilee Brown[4], Robert L. Coleman[3] and Judith A. Smith[1,5*]

Abstract

Background: While many of these agents have been compared in prospective clinical trials, the gemcitabine/platinumbased regimens have not been compared in a prospective, randomized clinical trial. While bothgemcitabine/carboplatin and gemcitabine/cisplatin have a similar ORR in separate clinical trials, the tworegimens have never been directly been compared. With overlapping dose-limiting toxicity of thrombocytopenia, the gemcitabine/carboplatin regimen has been challenging to employ in the clinical setting in previously treated ovarian cancer patients and is often associated with treatment delays and/or dose reductions. Gemcitabine/cisplatin can also be a challenge due to its dose limiting neuropathy and renal toxicity, especially in previously treated patients. In the absence of any prospective, head to head comparison this retrospective study was embarked upon to compare the response rate and toxicity profiles of gemcitabine/cisplatin verses gemcitabine/carboplatin for the treatment of platinum-sensitive verses platinum-resistant recurrent ovarian cancer.

Methods: This was a retrospective chart review study that identified patients that had received either gemcitabine/cisplatin or gemcitabine/carboplatin for treatment of recurrent ovarian cancer and compared documented hematological and non-hematological toxicity and response based on RECIST (v1.1). Data was evaluated based upon platinum sensitivity/resistance as well.

Results: A total of 93 patients were identified that had received a gemcitabine/platinum regimen with 48 with recurrent ovarian cancer that were included in the study. There were 21 patients in the gemcitabine/cisplatin arm and 27 patients identified in the gemcitabine/carboplatin arm. Objective response rate (ORR) was greater in platinum-sensitive patients that received gemcitabine/carboplatin compared to gemcitabine/cisplatin (8 (67%) vs 2 (25%), $p < 0.05$). Conversely, ORR was greater in platinum-resistant patients treated with gemcitabine/cisplatin (4 (57%) vs 1 (25%), NS). Mean time to progression was greater in gemcitabine/cisplatin patients (7.2 vs 5.1 months, $p < 0.03$). Patients treated with gemcitabine/carboplatin discontinued due to toxicity at a greater rate (8 (33%) vs 5 (24%)). Specifically gemcitabine/carboplatin had a greater incidence (85%) of grade 2 or greater leukopenia, thrombocytopenia, and neutropenia compared to gemcitabine/cisplatin (19%) However, there was no significant difference in dose reductions, treatment delays, or granulocyte-colony stimulating factor (G-CSF) administration between regimens.

(Continued on next page)

* Correspondence: Judith.Ann.Smith@uth.tmc.edu
[1]Department of Obstetrics, Gynecology, and Reproductive Sciences,
UTHealth McGovern Medical School, 6431 Fannin Street, Rm. 3.152, Houston,
TX 77030, USA
[5]UTHealth-Memorial Hermann Cancer Center-TMC, Houston, TX, USA
Full list of author information is available at the end of the article

(Continued from previous page)

Conclusions: Gemcitabine/cisplatin appears to have greater efficacy in platinum-resistant patients, while gemcitabine/carboplatin seems to have greater efficacy in platinum-sensitive patients. Overall, gemcitabine/carboplatin was associated with a greater incidence of myelosuppression and discontinuation due to toxicity. Similar to findings in endometrial cancer, gemcitabine/cisplatin may have benefit specifically in platinum-resistant ovarian cancer.

Keywords: Gemcitabine, Cisplatin, Carboplatin, Recurrent ovarian cancer, Efficacy, Toxicity

Background

Ovarian cancer is one of the most common cancers of, and the leading cause of death from gynecologic cancers [1]. This cancer is often undiagnosed until its progression to stage III/IV, at which point the 5-year survival rate is less than 50% [2]. Most patients with advanced ovarian cancer develop recurrent disease which is usually resistant to many chemotherapeutic agents [2]. There is no official standard second-line treatment of recurrent ovarian cancer. The selection of chemotherapy for recurrent disease include is often based upon platinum-sensitivity, residual toxicity, and patient/physician preferences. It may include a combination regimen or single-agent regimen with various agents showing some benefit for treatment of recurrent ovarian cancer including: carboplatin, cisplatin, paclitaxel, pegylated liposomal doxorubicin, gemcitabine, topotecan, bevacizumab, or more recently one of the new PARP inhibitors.

While many of these agents have been compared in prospective clinical trials, the gemcitabine/platinum-based regimens have not been compared in a prospective, randomized clinical trial. Gemcitabine is a nucleoside analog which exerts its chemotherapeutic activity by incorporation into DNA causing apoptosis [3]. Gemcitabine possesses activity in ovarian cancer resistant to treatment with paclitaxel/carboplatin combination regimen, demonstrating synergy with cisplatin and a mild toxicity profile [3]. Neutropenia was the most commonly reported toxicity with gemcitabine [3]. Other reported toxicities include hematologic toxicity, flu-like symptoms, nausea, vomiting, and appetite suppression [3]. Cisplatin and carboplatin are platinum-based antineoplastic agents which bind to and cross-link DNA [4]. Both are used in combination with gemcitabine as treatment for recurrent ovarian cancer. Cisplatin-based chemotherapy has a high toxicity potential, most commonly causing nausea, vomiting, and other GI symptoms. [4] The primary dose-limiting toxicity of cisplatin is nephrotoxicity resulting in reduced renal perfusion and concentrating defect [5]. Carboplatin has lower reactivity and slower DNA binding kinetics in comparison to cisplatin [6]. Nausea and vomiting are less severe and easier to control in carboplatin compared to cisplatin [6]. Primary toxicities associated with carboplatin are myelosuppression and neutropenia [6].

Based on a previous randomized study by Pfisterer and colleagues, carboplatin in combination with gemcitabine demonstrates greater efficacy through improved overall response rate (ORR) and median progression free survival in comparison to carboplatin alone [7]. Gemcitabine/carboplatin also results in increased myelosuppression requiring increased supplementation with G-CSF, but sequelae such as febrile neutropenia and infections were uncommon. [7] While both gemcitabine/carboplatin and gemcitabine/cisplatin have a similar ORR in separate clinical trials [8, 9], the two regimens have never been directly been compared. With overlapping dose-limiting toxicity of thrombocytopenia, the gemcitabine/carboplatin regimen has been challenging to employ in the clinical setting in previously treated ovarian cancer patients and is often associated with treatment delays and/or dose reductions. Gemcitabine/cisplatin can also be a challenge due to its dose limiting neuropathy and renal toxicity, especially in previously treated patients. In the absence of any prospective, head to head comparison this retrospective study was embarked upon to compare the response rate and toxicity profiles of gemcitabine/cisplatin verses gemcitabine/carboplatin for the treatment of platinum-sensitive verses platinum-resistant recurrent ovarian cancer.

Methods

Patients

This retrospective review of medical records was performed on patients with recurrent ovarian cancer who completed treatment with either gemcitabine 1000 mg/m^2 and cisplatin 40 mg/m^2 biweekly regimen or gemcitabine 800 mg/m^2 and carboplatin AUC 5 given once every 21 days at the University of Texas M.D. Anderson Cancer Center (UTMDACC) Gynecologic Oncology Center between 1 January 2002 to 30 September 2012. The protocol was reviewed and approved by the UTMDACC Institutional Review Board and granted a waiver of consent. Inclusion criteria included medical records of patients with recurrent ovarian cancer that received at least one cycle of gemcitabine/platinum based regimen. Medical records were excluded if patients were on concomitant biotherapy and/or other chemotherapy agents with gemcitabine/platinum regimen and patients with incomplete or restricted medical records.

Data collection

Patient data extracted from medical records included: patient demographics, body mass index (BMI) at start of therapy, documented comorbidities, stage at diagnosis, tumor histology, tumor debulking history, chemotherapy history, baseline complete metabolic panel and complete blood count prior to each cycle of chemotherapy, number of dose reductions during treatment, number of treatment delays, complications of chemotherapy (use of rescue antiemetics, electrolyte replacement, IV hydration), and reason for discontinuation of regimen. Criteria established by Gordon and colleagues [10] were used to determine platinum-sensitive and –resistant disease. When patients stopped their respective regimen, response to treatment was evaluated by modified RECIST (version 1.1) based on measurable tumor progression [11].

Statistical and data analysis

Within each gemcitabine/platinum group data were further sorted into platinum-sensitive and –resistant groups. The student t-test analysis was used to evaluate for statistically significant differences ($p \leq 0.05$) between treatment groups in age, BMI, number of prior chemotherapy regimens, and number of cycles of gemcitabine/platinum completed. Time to progression was calculated as the interval between the start of the first gemcitabine/platinum cycle and the end of the last gemcitabine/platinum cycle; the end of the gemcitabine/cisplatin regimen was determined as 28 days after the last cycle start date, while the end of the gemcitabine/carboplatin regimen was determined as 21 days after the last cycle start date. The student t-test analysis was performed to evaluate for differences in time to progression, differences in dose reductions, treatment delays, and G-CSF administration between each treatment group with p values less than or equal to 0.05 considered significant. ORR was calculated on patients who completed treatment with the following responses considered an objective response: partial response to treatment, complete response, and stable disease. The chi-square test was performed to evaluate for differences in ORR. The incidence of grade 2 or greater leukopenia, thrombocytopenia, and neutropenia was measured and defined, respectively, as: white blood count < 3000/µL, platelet count < 75,000/µL, absolute neutrophil count < 1500/µL.

Results

Patient characteristics

A total of 93 charts were identified of patients that had received a gemcitabine/platinum regimen with 48 charts included from patients that had received gemcitabine/platinum for recurrent ovarian cancer from January 1st, 2002 to September 30th, 2012. Other than number of prior treatments, there were no statistical differences between patient demographics/characteristics as summarized in Table 1 by treatment group and by platinum sensitivity. Briefly there were 21 charts from patients that had received gemcitabine/cisplatin which included ten platinum-sensitive

patients, ten platinum-resistant patients, and one patient whose platinum-sensitivity was unknown. There were 27 charts from patients that had received gemcitabine/carboplatin which included 18 platinum-sensitive patients, eight platinum-resistant patients, and one patient whose platinum-sensitivity was unknown. The majority of patients in both groups had serous tumors that were stage IIIC or IV whose tumor had been optimally debulked (<1 cm) prior to treatment. The gemcitabine/carboplatin group had a higher percentage of platinum-sensitive patients (66% vs 48%). There was no statistically significant difference between age or BMI in treatment groups. The mean number of prior chemotherapy regimens was significantly greater in the gemcitabine/cisplatin group, 3.5 ± 1.7 regimens (1–6, $p = 0.003$) compared to the gemcitabine/carboplatin group 2 ± 1.5 (0–6). When comparing treatment groups by platinum sensitivity, the gemcitabine/cisplatin platinum-sensitive subgroup had a greater number of mean prior chemotherapy regimens 3.2 ± 1.5 (1–5, $p = 0.025$) compared to the gemcitabine/carboplatin platinum-sensitive subgroup 1.8 ± 1.5 (0–6). There was no statistically significant difference in mean number of cycles of gemcitabine/platinum between groups.

Efficacy

Table 2 summarizes response rates in each treatment group overall and by platinum-sensitivity. ORR was greater in the overall gemcitabine/carboplatin group (56% vs 38%). When comparing platinum-sensitive patients alone, the gemcitabine/carboplatin group again had a greater ORR (67% vs 25%, $p < 0.05$). However, when comparing platinum-resistant patients alone, the gemcitabine/cisplatin group had a greater ORR (57% vs 25%). Mean time to progression was significantly greater in the overall gemcitabine/cisplatin group 7.2 ± 2(3.2–9.7, $p = 0.03$) compared to the overall gemcitabine/carboplatin group 5.1 ± 1.7 (2.3–7.2). There was a higher percentage of patients who discontinued treatment due to toxicity in the overall gemcitabine/carboplatin group (33% vs 24%), in the platinum-sensitive gemcitabine/carboplatin subgroup (29% vs 20%), and in the platinum-resistant gemcitabine/carboplatin subgroup (75% vs 30%).

Toxicities

Table 3 summarizes toxicity profiles of each treatment group. Use of rescue antiemetics was greater in the gemcitabine/cisplatin group compared to the gemcitabine/carboplatin group (29% vs 4%). Use of electrolyte replacement was greater in the gemcitabine/carboplatin group (33% vs 24%). Change in renal function from baseline occurred more often in the gemcitabine/cisplatin group (19% vs 4%). Change in liver function from baseline occurred more often in the overall gemcitabine/carboplatin group (22% vs 10%).

Table 1 Summary of patient characteristics

Patient Demographics	Gem/Cis Overall	Gem/Carbo Overall	Gem-]/Cis Plt Sensitive	Gem/Carbo Plt Sensitive	Gem/Cis Plt Resistant	Gem/Carbo Plt Resistant
	N = 21	N = 27	N = 10	N = 18	N = 10	N = 8
Mean Age [# ± SD (Range)]	61.4 [±10.2(42–84)]	62.0 [+9.1(43–79)]	60.8 [+9.4(49–81)]	60.8 [+8.3(47–79)]	61.6 [+11.9(42–84)]	65.8 [+10.7(43–78)]
Race						
-White	16	20	7	14	8	5
-Hispanic	3	4	2	3	1	1
-African American	0	1	0	0	0	1
-Asian	0	1	0	1	0	0
-Unreported race	2	0	1	0	1	1
Mean # of Comorbidities	1.48	1.48	0.70	1.11	2.30	2.50
Tumor Histology						
-Serous	15	17	8	11	6	6
-Clear Cell	0	1	0	1	0	0
-Adenocarcinoma	2	2	2	0	0	1
-Mixed	1	3	0	3	1	1
-Unreported histology	3	3	0	3	3	0
Tumor Stage						
-I	0	1	0	0	0	1
-II	2	1	2	0	0	0
-III	12	17	5	11	6	5
-IV	3	3	2	3	1	0
-Unreported stage	4	6	1	4	3	2
Tumor Debulking						
-Optimal (<1 cm)	10	16	5	11	5	4
-Suboptimal	5	7	2	6	2	1
-Not a surgical candidate	0	1	0	0	0	1
-Unreported tumor debulking	6	3	3	1	3	2
Plt sens/resis/unkn	10/10/1	18/8/1	NA	NA	NA	NA
Mean # of prior regimens [# ± SD (Range)]	3.5 [+1.7(1–6)] P < 0.003	2 [+1.5(0–6)]	3.2 [+1.5(1–5)] P < 0.025	1.8 [+1.5(0–6)]	4 [+1.9(1–6)]	2.5 [+1.4(1–5)]
Mean # of cycles Gem/Plt [# ± SD (Range)]	6.2 [+3.5(1–12)]	5.44 [+2.5(2–12)]	6.7 [+3.5(2–12)]	5.3 [+2.2(2–9)]	5.2 [+3.0(1–9)]	6.3 [+3.0(3–12)]

Abbreviations: *Gem-Cis* Gemcitabine-cisplatin, *Gem-Carbo* Gemcitabine-carboplatin, *Plt* Platinum, *SD* Standard deviation, sens = sensitive; resis = resistant, unkn = unknown

There was no statistically significant difference in dose reductions or treatment delays in either treatment group. Mean rate of G-CSF administration per patient was greater in the gemcitabine/carboplatin group 4.2 ± 3.2 (0–9) compared to the gemcitabine/cisplatin group 2.9 ± 3.3 (0–9), however the difference was not statistically significant. In the gemcitabine/carboplatin group there was a greater rate of grade 2 or higher leukopenia (37% vs 0%), thrombocytopenia (7% vs 0%), and neutropenia (41% vs 19%). Of the 13 patients that discontinued due to toxicity, eight patients were from the gemcitabine/carboplatin group; five of these eight patients also had grade 2 or greater or myelosuppression.

Discussion

The results of this study comparing gemcitabine/carboplatin and gemcitabine/cisplatin regimens show that gemcitabine/carboplatin has greater efficacy in platinum-sensitive patients, but gemcitabine/cisplatin demonstrates greater efficacy in platinum-resistant patients. Toxicity profiles demonstrate decreased use of rescue antiemetics but greater myelosuppression with gemcitabine/carboplatin.

Table 2 Summary of response rates

Response Rates	Gemcitabine +Cisplatin	Gemcitabine + Carboplatin
Overall	N = 21	N = 24
Progression #(%)	10 (63)	7(44)
Complete response #(%)	2(13)	3(19)
Partial response #(%)	2(13)	3(19)
Stable disease #(%)	2(13)	3(19)
Discontinued due to toxicity #(%)	5(24)	8(33)
Objective response rate (PR + CR + SD) #(%)	6(38)	9(56)
Mean time to progression (months) [# ± SD (Range)] p = 0.03	7.2 [±2(3.2–9.7)]	5.1 [±1.7(2.3–7.2)]
Response Rates	Gemcitabine +Cisplatin	Gemcitabine + Carboplatin
Platinum Sensitive	N = 10	N = 17
Progression #(%)	6(75)	4(33)
Complete response #(%)	1(13)	3(25)
Partial response #(%)	0(0)	3(25)
Stable disease #(%)	1(13)	2(17)
Discontinued due to toxicity #(%)	2(20)	5(29)
Objective response rate (PR + CR + SD) #(%) p = 0.05	2(25)	8(67)
Mean time to progression (months) [# ± SD (Range)]	7.2 [±2.5(3.2–9.5)]	5.1 [±1.8(2.3–7.2)]
Response Rates	Gemcitabine +Cisplatin	Gemcitabine + Carboplatin
Platinum Resistant	N = 10	N = 7
Progression #(%)	3(43)	3(75)
Complete response #(%)	1(14)	0(0)
Partial response #(%)	2(29)	0(0)
Stable disease #(%)	1(14)	1(25)
Discontinued due to toxicity #(%)	3(30)	3(75)
Objective response rate (PR + CR + SD) #(%)	4(57)	1(25)
Mean time to progression (months) [# ± SD (Range)]	7.2 [±1.6(5.7–9.7)]	5.1 [±1.8(2.5–6.8)]

Abbreviations: SD Standard deviation, PR Partial response, CR Complete response, SD Stable disease

Table 3 Summary of toxicity profiles

Toxicity Profiles	Gemcitabine +Cisplatin	Gemcitabine + Carboplatin
Overall	N = 21	N = 27
Use of rescue antiemetics #(%)	6(29)	1(4)
Use of electrolyte replacement #(%)	5(24)	9(33)
Use of additional IV hydration	7(33)	8(30)
Change in renal function from baseline #(%)	4(19)	1(4)
Change in liver function from baseline #(%)	2(10)	6(22)
Mean dose reductions per patient [# + SD (Range)]	1.9 [+0.7(1–3)]	1.9 [+0.7(1–3)]
Mean treatment delays per patient[# + SD (Range)]	0.8 [+0.9(0–3)]	0.7 [+1(0–4)]
Mean rate of G-CSF administration per patient [# + SD (Range)]	2.9 [+3.3(0–9)]	4.2 [+3.2(0–9)]
Leukopenia, Grade 2 or greater #(%)	0	10(37)
Thrombocytopenia, Grade 2 or greater #(%)	0	2(7)
Neutropenia, Grade 2 or greater #(%)	4(19)	11(41)

Abbreviation: SD Standard deviation

No previous studies have compared gemcitabine/cisplatin and gemcitabine/carboplatin in the treatment of recurrent ovarian cancer. However, the controversy of which platinum to used in combination with paclitaxel three randomized studies have compared efficacy and toxicity of paclitaxel/carboplatin with paclitaxel/cisplatin in the first-line treatment of advanced ovarian cancer. In a phase III study, Nejit and colleagues randomized 208 patients with advanced ovarian cancer to paclitaxel/cisplatin or paclitaxel/carboplatin to compare toxicity profiles [11]. Overall, paclitaxel/carboplatin was less toxic with fewer patients discontinuing due to toxicity, less nausea and vomiting, and less peripheral neurotoxicity. However, paclitaxel/carboplatin resulted in a greater incidence of granulocytopenia and thrombocytopenia. In another phase III trial, Ozols and colleagues randomized 792 patients with optimally resected stage III ovarian cancer to receive paclitaxel/cisplatin or paclitaxel/carboplatin [12]. Again, paclitaxel/cisplatin demonstrated increased gastrointestinal, renal, and metabolic toxicity while paclitaxel/carboplatin had a greater incidence of grade 2 or greater thrombocytopenia. No significant difference was observed in the regimens' efficacy measured by median progression-free survival, overall survival, relative risk of progression, and relative risk of death. Similarly, Du Bois and colleagues also concluded paclitaxel/carboplatin and paclitaxel/cisplatin are comparable in terms of efficacy, but paclitaxel/carboplatin led to a higher frequency of hematologic toxicity [13].

Similar to the three randomized studies comparing paclitaxel/cisplatin with paclitaxel/carboplatin, this study indicates gemcitabine/carboplatin results in greater myelosuppression than gemcitabine/cisplatin. Grade 2 or greater leukopenia, thrombocytopenia, and neutropenia occurred at a markedly greater rate in the gemcitabine/carboplatin group compared to the gemcitabine/cisplatin group. Although there was no significant difference in dose reductions, treatment delays, or rate of G-CSF administration per patient, the gemcitabine/carboplatin displayed a greater rate of discontinuation due to toxicity. Due to the retrospective nature of this study, the reason for discontinuation due to toxicity was not specified for all patients. However, most of the gemcitabine/carboplatin patients who discontinued due to toxicity also demonstrated grade 2 or greater leukopenia, neutropenia or thrombocytopenia. This is in agreement with studies showing greater myelosuppression with gemcitabine/carboplatin than carboplatin alone, as well as with paclitaxel/carboplatin compared to paclitaxel/cisplatin [7, 11–13]. To further emphasize this observation of greater myelosuppression in the gemcitabine/carboplatin group, it is important to note that the gemcitabine/cisplatin group actually had a significantly greater mean number of prior chemotherapy regimens that would increase the likelihood of being more susceptible to the development of myelosuppression.

Other aspects of the toxicity profile of gemcitabine/carboplatin compared to gemcitabine/cisplatin in this study are similar to previous studies [11, 12]. In particular, a greater rate of use of rescue antiemetics and incidence of change in renal function was observed more often in the gemcitabine/cisplatin group. The greater incidence of change in renal function in the gemcitabine/cisplatin patients was expected since carboplatin dosing is based on individualized renal function and *cisplatin* is not.

In contrast to prior studies on paclitaxel/cisplatin and paclitaxel/carboplatin that found no difference in efficacy between regimens [12, 13], this retrospective study observed a greater ORR in the gemcitabine/carboplatin group overall. When the response rates were evaluated based on platinum sensitivity, gemcitabine/carboplatin had a greater ORR in platinum-sensitive patients compared to gemcitabine/cisplatin. However, this study observed that gemcitabine/cisplatin had a greater ORR in platinum-resistant patients than those that received gemcitabine/carboplatin. Previous studies have demonstrated gemcitabine/cisplatin activity in platinum-resistant patients [14] and clinically it is predominantly administered to patients with platinum-resistant disease [15, 16]. A larger is study is needed to ascertain whether gemcitabine/cisplatin is more effective in platinum-resistant patients compared to gemcitabine/carboplatin.

Furthermore, the mean time to progression was statistically significantly greater in gemcitabine/cisplatin patients regardless of platinum -sensitivity even though tumor stage, histology, and rate of optimal debulking were similar between the treatment groups. Interestingly, gemcitabine/cisplatin patients had a statistically significantly greater mean number of prior regimens, which would theoretically cause greater rates of drug resistance and decrease mean time to progression. However, Smith and colleagues have previously demonstrated in-vitro the increase cytotoxicity observed with gemcitabine/cisplatin was attributed to gemcitabine modulation of cisplatin-resistance in a panel of human endometrial cancer cell lines [17, 18]. These findings translated to clinical practice as demonstrated in follow up phase II clinical study by Brown and colleagues that observed an significantly improved PFS and objective response in platinum-resistant endometrial carcinoma [19]. In addition, Smith and colleagues went onto confirm combination as well as sequential treatment with gemcitabine with cisplatin demonstrated a greater improvement in growth inhibitory activity in both the chemosensitive and chemoresistant ovarian cancer cell lines which was attributed to modulation of the steroid xenobiotic receptor/multi-drug resistance (SXR/MDR) pathway [20]. In this study gemcitabine/cisplatin was found to be more active than gemcitabine/carboplatin in the platinum-resistant patients perhaps this is because gemcitabine and cisplatin are given on the same day twice a cycle which allows for optimal time for the gemcitabine modulation of the platinum-resistance pathways leading to improved sensitivity to the cisplatin activity. In the gemcitabine/carboplatin regimen both drugs are given on day one only then day 8 is the gemcitabine alone which has less cytotoxicity activity by itself in recurrent, platinum-resistant ovarian cancer. A definitive reason is currently unknown.

Since this was a retrospective study design, the study does have limitations that could not be controlled. First, the overall small sample size for the study. There are multiple options for chemotherapy treatment options for recurrent ovarian cancer, hence this limited sample size. Patients that did not have confirmed diagnosis of ovarian cancer were excluded to attempt to limit sources of variability in response rates. The patients on the gemcitabine/cisplatin arm did have slightly higher number of prior treatments overall as well as when evaluated by platinum-sensitivity too. It likely contributed to the lower overall response rate and lower response in the "platinum-sensitive" patients too. Conversely, despite having a higher number of prior treatments, the gemcitabine/cisplatin regimen had better response in those patients with documented platinum-resistance. This observation supports the hypothesis that gemcitabine modulated multi-drug resistance pathways. In the absence of confirmatory data, selection of which gemcitabine/platinum regimen should be based on the common principles of selection of chemotherapy for recurrent ovarian cancer including patient convenience and residual toxicity. In those patients with known platinum resistance, the current pre-clinical and clinical data suggests gemcitabine/cisplatin appears to have more likelihood of achieving a response.

Conclusion

This study is the first study to directly compare gemcitabine/carboplatin to gemcitabine/cisplatin in patients with recurrent ovarian cancer. Overall the incidence of toxicity was similar between the two regimens and consistent with previous studies of carboplatin, gemcitabine/carboplatin leads to greater myelosuppression than gemcitabine/cisplatin. It appears that efficacy of gemcitabine/carboplatin seems to have greater efficacy in platinum-sensitive patients. Similar to findings in platinum-resistant endometrial cancer and well as recent clinical trials in platinum-resistant ovarian cancer, gemcitabine/cisplatin appears to have greater efficacy in platinum-resistant patients [14, 15, 18]. Preliminary in vitro data suggests gemcitabine may have a role in modulation of the SXR/MDR which would improve sensitivity of multiple chemotherapy agents in used for the treatment recurrent drug resistant tumors [19]. Based on this current study, additional research efforts should focus on way optimize the role of gemcitabine/cisplatin for treatment of platinum-resistant ovarian cancer.

Abbreviations

BMI: Body Mass Index; G-CSF: Granulocyte-colony stimulating factor; NS: Not significant; ORR: Objective response rate; SXR/MDR: Steroid xenobiotic receptor/multi-drug resistance; UTMDACC: University of Texas M.D. Anderson Cancer Center

Acknowledgements

Not applicable.

Funding

No funding was received related to this submission.

Authors' contributions

TL - data analysis, manuscript preparation. RH- protocol development, data collection. CKK- protocol development, data collection. JB- protocol collaborator, data interpretation, manuscript preparation. RC- protocol collaborator, data interpretation, manuscript preparation. JAS- research concept, principal investigator, data collection oversight, data analysis & interpretation, manuscript preparation. All authors read and approved the final manuscript.

Competing interest

The authors declare that they have no competing interests.

Author details

[1]Department of Obstetrics, Gynecology, and Reproductive Sciences, UTHealth McGovern Medical School, 6431 Fannin Street, Rm. 3.152, Houston, TX 77030, USA. [2]MBS Pharmacy, Round Rock, TX, USA. [3]University of Texas M.D. Anderson Cancer Center, Houston, TX, USA. [4]Levine Cancer Institute, Carolinas HealthCare System, Charlotte, NC, USA. [5]UTHealth-Memorial Hermann Cancer Center-TMC, Houston, TX, USA.

References

1. Ozols RF. Advanced ovarian cancer: a clinical update on first-line treatment, recurrent disease, and new agents. J Natl Compr Cancer Netw. 2004;2:S60–73.
2. Heintz AP, Odcino F, Maisonneuve P, et al. Carcinoma of the ovary. FIGO 26th annual report on the results of treatment in gynecological cancer. Int J Gynaecol Obstet. 2006;1:S161–92.
3. Thigpen T. The role of gemcitabine in first-line treatment of advanced ovarian carcinoma. Semin Oncol. 2006;33:S26–32.
4. Surendiran A, Balamurugan N, Gunaseelan K, et al. Adverse drug reaction profile of cisplatin-based chemotherapy in a tertiary care hospital in India: an evaluative study. Indian J Pharmacol. 2010;42:40–3.
5. Arany I, Safirstein RL. Cisplatin nephrotoxicity. Semin Nephrol. 2003;23:460–4.
6. Pecorelli S, Pasinetti B, Tisi G, et al. Optimizing gemcitabine regimens in ovarian cancer. Semin Oncol. 2006;33:S17–25.
7. Pfisterer J, Plante M, Vergote I, et al. Gemcitabine plus carboplatin compared with carboplatin in patients with platinum-sensitive recurrent ovarian cancer: an intergroup trial of the AGO-OVAR, the NCIC CTG, and the EORTC GCG. J Clin Oncol. 2006;24:4699–707.
8. Lorusso D, Di Stefano A, Fanfani F, et al. Role of gemcitabine in ovarian cancer treatment. Ann Oncol. 2006;17:v1188–94.
9. Fruscella E, Gallo D, Ferrandina G, et al. Gemcitabine: current role and future options in the treatment of ovarian cancer. Crit Rev Oncol Hematol. 2003;48:81–8.
10. Gordon AN, Fleagle JT, Gutherie D, et al. Recurrent epithelial ovarian carcinoma: a randomized phase III trial of pegylated liposomal doxorubicin versus topotecan. J Clin Oncol. 2001;15:3312–22.
11. Eisenhauer EA, Therasse P, Bogaerts J, et al. New response evaluation criteria in solid tumours: revised RECIST guideline (version 1.1). Eur J Cancer. 2009;45:228–47.

12. Nejit JP, Engelholm SA, Tuxen MK, et al. Exploratory phase III study of paclitaxel and cisplatin versus paclitaxel and carboplatin in advanced ovarian cancer. J Clin Oncol. 2000;18:3084–92.

13. Ozols RF, Bundy BN, Greer BE, et al. Phase III trial of carboplatin and paclitaxel compared with cisplatin and paclitaxel in patients with optimally resected stage III ovarian cancer: a gynecologic oncology group study. J Clin Oncol. 2003;21:3194–200.

14. du Bois A, Luck HJ, Meier W, et al. A randomized clinical trial of cisplatin/paclitaxel versus carboplatin/paclitaxel as first-line treatment of ovarian cancer. J Natl Cancer Inst. 2003;95:1320–9.

15. Rose PG, Mossbruger K, Fusco N, et al. Gemcitabine reverses cisplatin resistance: demonstration of activity in platinum-and multidrug-resistant ovarian and peritoneal carcinoma. Gynecol Oncol. 2003;88:17–21.

16. Bozas G, Bamias A, Koutsoukou V, et al. Biweekly gemcitabine and cisplatin in platinum-resistant/refractory, paclitaxel-pretreated, ovarian and peritoneal carcinoma. Gynecol Oncol. 2007;104:580–5.

17. Smith JA, Brown J, Martin MC, Ramondetta LM, Wolf JK. An in vitro study of the inhibitory activity of gemcitabine and platinum agents in human endometrial carcinoma cell lines. Gynecol Oncol. 2004;92(1):314–9.

18. Smith JA, Gaikwad A, Ramondetta LM, Wolf JK, Brown J. Determination of the mechanism of gemcitabine modulation of cisplatin drug resistance in panel of human endometrial cancer cell lines. Gynecol Oncol. 103(2):518–22. 11/2006. e-Pub 5/2006

19. Brown J, Smith JA, Ramondetta LM, Sood AK, Ramirez PT, Coleman RL, Levenback CF, Munsell MF, Jung M, Wolf JK. Combination gemcitabine and cisplatin is highly active in endometrial carcinoma: results of a prospective phase II trial. Cancer. 2010;116(21):4973–9.

20. Smith JA, Gaikwad A, Hanks A, Coleman R. Evaluation of gemcitabine modulation of multidrug resistance in a cisplatin-resistant human ovarian cancer cell lines. Pharmacotherapy. 2011;31(10):362e (#187).

27

Options in human papillomavirus (HPV) detection for cervical cancer screening: comparison between full genotyping and a rapid qualitative HPV-DNA assay in Ghana

Dorcas Obiri-Yeboah[1*], Yaw Adu-Sarkodie[2], Florencia Djigma[3], Kafui Akakpo[4], Ebenezer Aniakwa-Bonsu[1], Daniel Amoako-Sakyi[1], Jacques Simpore[3] and Philippe Mayaud[5]

Abstract

Background: Modern cervical cancer screening increasingly relies on the use of molecular techniques detecting high-risk oncogenic human papillomavirus (hr-HPV). A major challenge for developing countries like Ghana has been the unavailability and costs of HPV DNA-based testing. This study compares the performance of *care*HPV, a semi-rapid and affordable qualitative detection assay for 14 hr-HPV genotypes, with HPV genotyping, for the detection of cytological cervical squamous intraepithelial lesions (SIL).

Methods: A study comparing between frequency matched HIV-1 seropositive and HIV-seronegative women was conducted in the Cape Coast Teaching Hospital, Ghana. A systematic sampling method was used to select women attending clinics in the hospital. Cervical samples were tested for HPV by *care*HPV and Anyplex-II HPV28 genotyping assay, and by conventional cytology.

Results: A total of 175 paired results (94 from HIV-1 seropositive and 81 from HIV-seronegative women) were analyzed based on the ability of both tests to detect the 14 hr-HPV types included in the *care*HPV assay. The inter-assay concordance was 94.3% (95%CI: 89.7–97.2%, kappa = 0.88), similar by HIV serostatus. The *care*HPV assay was equally sensitive among HIV-1 seropositive and seronegative women (97.3% vs. 95.7%, $p = 0.50$) and slightly more specific among HIV-seronegative women (85.0% vs. 93.1%, $p = 0.10$). *care*HPV had good sensitivity (87.5%) but low specificity (52.1%) for the detection of low SIL or greater lesions, but its performance was superior to genotyping (87.5 and 38.8%, respectively). Reproducibility of *care*HPV, tested on 97 samples by the same individual was 82.5% (95%CI: 73.4–89.4%).

Conclusions: The performance characteristics of *care*HPV compared to genotyping suggest that this simpler and cheaper HPV detection assay could offer a suitable alternative for HPV screening in Ghana.

Keywords: Human papillomavirus (HPV), *care*HPV, Genotyping, Cervical cancer, Screening, HIV, Ghana

* Correspondence: d.obiri-yeboah@uccsms.edu.gh; castella.oy@gmail.com
[1]Department of Microbiology and Immunology, School of Medical Sciences, University of Cape Coast, Cape Coast, Ghana
Full list of author information is available at the end of the article

Background

Persistent infection with high-risk oncogenic human papillomavirus (hr-HPV) genotypes is aetiologically linked with cervical cancer and its precursor histological cervical intraepithelial neoplasia (CIN) or cytological squamous intraepithelial lesions (SIL) [1, 2]. Modern cervical cancer screening increasingly relies on the use of HPV testing in developed countries because of its high sensitivity to detect CIN/SIL [3, 4]. Resource intensive molecular methods, such as genotyping using polymerase chain reaction (PCR) are able to detect and type HPV but are mostly unavailable in developing countries like Ghana. However, simplified molecular assays are becoming available which will enable HPV molecular diagnosis in resource-constrained settings. The careHPV assay (Qiagen, Gaithersburg, MD), a simplified version of the better known Digene Hybrid Capture 2 (HC2), has shown promise with high sensitivity and specificity against histological end points when tested in diverse setting and heterogeneou populations as Africa and China [5–7]. A study conducted among 149 women living with HIV in Burkina Faso and South Africa was the first head to head evaluation of careHPV versus HC2 among African women and reported an excellent agreement between the two tests (94.6%, 95% confidence interval [CI]: 89.7 to 97.7%, Kappa value = 0.88) and concluded that careHPV assay could be as suitable as HC2 for cervical cancer screening among HIV-infected African women [6].

In Ghana, HPV testing has remained confined to research laboratories where genotyping is used. One such genotyping assay is the recently developed Anyplex™ II HPV28 (Seegene, Seoul, Korea). The assay detects 28 HPV genotypes including 19 hr-HPV types of which 13 are considered carcinogenic (HPV16, 18, 31, 33, 35, 39, 45, 51, 52, 56, 58, 59 and 68), six possible carcinogenic (HPV26, 53, 66, 69, 73 and 82), and nine low-risk HPV types (HPV6, 11, 40, 42, 43, 44, 54, 61 and 70), according to the Interagency for Research on Cancer (IARC) classification [8]. The addition of a high performing, semi-rapid and affordable test such as careHPV would considerably enhance access to HPV-based cervical cancer screening in the country. In particular, since HPV molecular assays have very high negative predictive value for the detection of cervical cancer lesions, they could become very useful as a primary screening test or as triage in combination with cytology. However, because they cannot distinguish between transient and persistent infections, their specificity is low. They are thus recommended for use among women aged 30 years and older when most HPV infections should have cleared. Molecular tests can also indicate complete viral eradication if the result is negative 12 months following cervical lesions treatment, hence they can be useful for patients' follow-up. Studies have compared various strategies including those which combine HPV genotyping with concurrent cytology and those which offer HPV screening without concurrent cytology. The results of the ATHENA trial conducted among 42,209 women in the United States of America comparing various single or combination screening strategies suggest that both strategies are feasible and have equivalent performance depending on factors like age of the woman [9]. Other important factors in selecting a particular screening strategy include its ability to restrict the number of unnecessary colposcopies while maintaining a high negative predictive value [7, 10].

The present study aimed at comparing careHPV with HPV genotyping for the molecular diagnosis of HPV and at evaluating the performance of both assays against cytology among HIV-1 seropositive and HIV-seronegative women in Ghana. This is an essential step as the country is looking to inform the development of its cervical cancer screening algorithms.

Methods

Study design and subjects

Participants were recruited as part of a larger HPV/cervical cancer epidemiological study (comparing HIV-1 seropositive to HIV-seronegative women) conducted in the Cape Coast Teaching Hospital (CCTH) in Ghana. Briefly, a comparative frequency-matched study was conducted in a systematic (1 in 5) sample of women attending the HIV and the general outpatient clinics at CCTH. Every fifth woman aged ≥18 years was systematically selected from the list of attendants, starting by a randomly selected attendance number for the first woman. If a woman was deemed not eligible (i.e. who had previous total abdominal hysterectomy, was menstruating that day, or was pregnant), the next available patient was offered her place, and every fifth woman whence, to a maximum of 10 women per clinic day. Participants who met the inclusion criteria (i.e. aged ≥18 years and willing to be tested for HIV) were given an explanation of the protocol after which written informed consent was obtained. This method was used to recruit the women for the parent study and then a sub set target of about 50% of participants (every other recruited woman) were asked to be part of the careHPV evaluation study.

Clinical sample collection

Gynaecological examination with speculum was performed, during which cervical swabs were collected from the ecto and endocervix targeting the squamo-columnar junction using a DNA PAP™ Cervical Sampler™ and transported in Swab Specimen Collection Kit (Qiagen, Gaithersburg, MD) for genotyping by Anyplex II HPV 28. For careHPV testing, the careHPV specific brush and transport medium were used (Qiagen, Gaithersburg,

MD). Cervical smears were taken for cytology with a cervical brush and immediately alcohol-fixed at the clinic.

HPV DNA detection

The Anyplex II HPV 28 test was performed from its specific transport medium as per manufacturer's protocol previously described [11]. The isolation of nucleic acid was by QIAamp DNA Mini kit (Qiagen, USA) as per established protocol by the manufacturer using 500 µl of the sample. The process from DNA extraction to the RT-PCR for a full panel of 96 plate takes at least 6 h to complete. The careHPV test was performed on the samples collected into the careHPV transport medium. This test is a semi-rapid test designed based on simplification of the Digene HC2 test technology to be used for the detection of the DNA for 14 hr-HPV types (HPV16, 18, 31, 33, 35, 39, 45, 52, 56, 58, 59, 66 and 68; HPV66 being the addition). This test takes 2.5 to 3 h to perform for a 96 well and involves 6 easy-to-follow steps of denaturation, hybridization and capturing, conjugation, washing, additions of substrate and detection with the illuminometer. The results obtained are qualitative for hr-HPV without indicating the specific genotype [7, 12, 13]. In order to verify testing reproducibility, a random 50% of samples were retested without knowledge of prior result.

Cervical cytology

Cervical smears were prepared in the laboratory following a standardized protocol for Papanicolaou (Pap) staining. Slides were read by a consultant cytopathologist at CCTH using the Bethesda 2001 guidelines for SIL classification [14].

Statistical analysis

Analysis of careHPV performance compared with genotyping was done for 14 hr-HPV genotypes detectable by both tests (HPV16, 18, 31, 33, 35, 39, 45, 51, 52, 56, 58, 59, 66 and 68). Sensitivity, specificity, positive and negative predictive values (PPV and NPV), and Cohen's Kappa values for agreement between the two tests were calculated with their 95%CI. These were calculated for the total results and then also done separately for HIV-1 seropositive and HIV-seronegative women separately. Data analyses were performed using Stata version 13 software (Stata Corp, Texas USA).

Ethics

Ethical approval for this study was obtained from the Committee on Human Research Publications and Ethics (CHRPE) of the School of Medical Sciences (SMS), Kwame Nkrumah University of Science and Technology (KNUST) before the study commenced. Study participants were recruited only after obtaining signed written informed consent.

Results

Overall, 333 eligible women were included in the parent study, 163 HIV-1 seropositive women (mean age 43.8 years, standard deviation [SD] ±9.4) and 170 HIV-seronegative women (mean age 44.3 years, SD ±12.8). A total of 197 paired careHPV and genotyping samples from the subsample of women (100 HIV-1 seropositive (mean age 44.7 years, SD ±9.7) and 97 HIV-seronegative (mean age 43.7 years, SD ±12.8) randomly selected into the careHPV validation study were tested, and 175 results (89%) were available for analysis based on the ability of both tests to detect the 14 hr-HPV types. For 21 careHPV results (6 from HIV-1 seropositive and 15 from HIV-seronegative women), Anyplex II HPV 28 detected genotypes which are undetectable by careHPV (i.e., low-risk types, as well as HPV26, 53, 69, 73 and 82). In addition, one careHPV sample (from an HIV-seronegative woman) gave an invalid result despite repeat testing. These 22 samples (11.1%) were not included in the analysis of careHPV performance.

The hr-HPV prevalence by careHPV was 55% (95%CI: 48.0–62.9) overall, 79% (95%CI: 69.0–86.5) among HIV-1 seropositive women and 28.0% (95%CI: 19.0–39.5) among HIV-seronegative women (p ≤ 0.0001) (Table 1). Similarly, the hr-HPV prevalence by genotyping was 57% (95%CI: 49.0–64.0), 79% (95%CI: 69.0–86.5) among HIV-1 seropositive women and 31% (95%CI: 12.0–42.1) among HIV-seronegative women (p ≤ 0.0001).

There was excellent agreement (94.3%, 95%CI: 89.7–97.2%) between careHPV and genotyping overall (kappa = 0.88, 95%CI: 0.81–0.95, p < 0.0001), and the agreement was similar among HIV-1 seropositive (94.7%, 95%CI: 88.0–98.3%) and seronegative (93.8%, 95%CI: 86.2–98.0%) women (Kappa of 0.84 and 0.85, respectively) (Table 1). The careHPV assay was equally sensitive among HIV-1 seropositive and HIV-seronegative women (97.3% vs. 95.7%, p = 0.50) and slightly more specific among HIV-seronegative women (85.0% vs. 93.1%, p = 0.10), but these differences were not statistically significant (Table 1).

For 9 of the hr-HPV types (HPV18, 31, 33, 35, 39, 45, 51, 52 and 68), the concordance between careHPV and Anyplex II HPV 28 was 100%. For 4 genotypes careHPV missed one positive sample, and for HPV58 it missed 2 samples (Table 2).

careHPV prevalence increased according to severity of cytological lesions, from 47.8% among women with normal cytology to 100% among women with high-grade lesions (HSIL/ASC-H) (p-trend = 0.08). Similarly, hr-HPV prevalence by genotyping increased by cytological grade severity (p-trend = 0.07) (Fig. 1). careHPV and genotyping had the same sensitivity for detection of lesions low SIL and above of 87.5% (95%CI: 43.3–99.7%) but careHPV had statistically significantly higher specificity (52.1% vs.

Table 1 Performance characteristics of *care*HPV assay for the detection of 14 high-risk (hr) HPV genotypes compared with HPV genotyping among 175 women in Cape Coast, Ghana

	All women (N = 175) % (95% CI)	HIV-1 seropositive women (N = 94) % (95% CI)	HIV seronegative women (N = 81) % (95% CI)	*P-value
hr-HPV prevalence	55.0 (48.0–62.9)	79.0 (69.0–86.5)	28.0 (19.0–39.5)	0.0001
Sensitivity	96.9 (91.2–99.4)	97.3 (90.6–99.7)	95.7 (78.1–99.9)	0.50
Specificity	91.0 (82.4–96.3)	85.0 (62.1–96.8)	93.1 (83.3–98.1)	0.10
PPV	93.1 (86.2–97.2)	96.0 (88.8–99.2)	84.6 (65.1–95.6)	0.01
NPV	95.9 (88.8–99.2)	89.5 (66.9–98.7)	98.2 (90.3–100.0)	0.02
Agreement	94.3 (89.7–97.2)	94.7 (88.0–98.3)	93.8 (86.2–98.0)	0.77
Kappa value (95%CI)	0.88 (0.81–0.95)	0.84 (0.70–0.98)	0.85 (0.73–0.98)	0.86
P-value for Kappa	<0.0001	<0.0001	<0.0001	

PPV positive predictive valuem, NPV negative predictive value
* comparing HIV-1 seropositive and HIV-seronegative women

38.8%, 95%CI: 31.8–46.2%, p < 0.0001), PPV and NPV than genotyping (Table 3).

A random sample of approximately 50% of all *care*HPV samples was tested twice by the same individual with *care*HPV to check the reproducibility of results. Of these, 80/97 produced the same results giving a reproducibility rate of 82.5% (95%CI: 73.4–89.4%). In 5/97 initially negative *care*HPV results the second result was positive, 2/97 became invalid and in 8/97 positive *care*HPV result, the second result was negative, and 2 became invalid.

Discussion

Given the high cost and resource intensive nature of genotyping for HPV screening, both in terms of skills and materials, it is essential that developing countries find acceptable alternatives to move into the modern

Table 2 Agreement between results of *care*HPV and genotyping with Anyplex II HPV28 for the detection of 14 high-risk HPV genotypes, among 175 women in Cape Coast, Ghana

HPV genotypes	Anyplex II HPV28 No. Positive (%)	*care*HPV No. Positive (%)	Agreement %
16	15 (8.6)	14 (8.0)	93.3
18	15 (8.6)	15 (8.6)	100.0
31	13 (7.4)	13 (7.4)	100.0
33	12 (6.9)	12 (6.9)	100.0
35	17 (9.7)	17 (9.7)	100.0
39	8 (4.6)	8 (4.6)	100.0
45	8 (4.6)	8 (4.6)	100.0
51	1 (0.6)	1 (0.6)	100.0
52	16 (9.1)	16 (9.1)	100.0
56	12 (6.9)	11 (6.3)	91.7
58	20 (11.4)	18 (10.3)	90.0
59	6 (3.4)	5 (2.9)	83.3
66	7 (4.0)	6 (3.4)	85.7
68	12 (6.9)	12 (6.9)	100.0

cervical cancer screening era. The advantage of full genotyping is its higher analytical sensitivity and ability to specifically identify the genotypes present in a population. While this is essential for research or epidemiological monitoring purposes, it is not absolutely necessary for clinical care. The role of HPV screening for clinical practice is to help establish a protocol of screening which is cost effective and helps identify women having hr-HPV infection so they can have further evaluation [7], whilst helping reduce the number of unnecessary colposcopies and histology. Since molecular testing of HPV does not necessarily require representative samples from the cervix to be taken, an additional potential benefit is the possible use of self-collected vaginal samples. This might increase testing by women especially in settings where self-collection might be preferred either due to cultural reasons or the convenience of not necessarily having to visit a health facility to provide samples [15–17]. Full genotyping requires DNA extraction (an additional cost) and molecular testing. Samples for DNA extraction for PCR have strict temperature control: they must be immediately extracted or kept in a fridge, and once extracted the DNA must be stored at 20 °C until used. Both DNA extraction and PCR testing require extensive technical training and appropriate setup. There is also the need to ensure continuous supply of electrical power throughout the processing until results are generated. All of these factors pose a tremendous challenge for resource-constrained countries like Ghana.

*care*HPV represents an alternative HPV screening assay that has been specifically developed for resource-constrained settings. This assay requires just bench top and 3 portable equipment which has a backup battery to store power enough to run a full set of 96 samples without the need for an external supply of electricity. The samples for *care*HPV can also be stored at room temperature for up to 4 weeks, do not require DNA

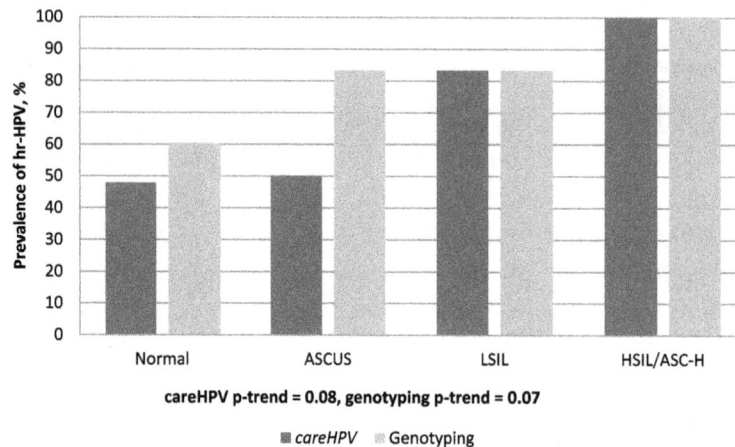

Fig. 1 14 hr-HPV prevalence by *care*HPV and genotyping according to cytological findings among women, Cape Coast, Ghana. Cytology readings: Normal = no abnormal findings found; ASCUS = atypical squamous cells of undetermined significance; LSIL = low grade squamous intraepithelial lesions; HSIL = high grade squamous intraepithelial lesions; ASC-H = Atypical squamous cells cannot rule out HSIL. Hr-HPV = high risk HPV types

extraction and require very limited technical knowledge to be performed. While *care*HPV has been evaluated in some settings, this research presents the first such evaluation done among women including HIV seropositive and seronegative women in Ghana. The simplicity of the assay and its relative robustness in the context of a resource-constrained laboratory setting was confirmed in this study. Various studies have been conducted using this assay including in Uganda [12], rural China [18], rural Thailand [19] with good outcomes.

This study found an excellent agreement (94.3%, $k = 0.88$) between *care*HPV and full HPV genotyping for the detection of 14 hr-HPV genotypes, and the result was similar among HIV-1 seropositive and HIV-seronegative women. The *care*HPV assay was slightly more sensitive among HIV-1 seropositive women but more specific among HIV-seronegative women. Investigators in Burkina Faso and South Africa found very similar excellent agreement (94.6%) for *care*HPV compared to HC2 [6], a well-validated HPV qualitative assay used in many settings, and when compared to genotyping using the InnoLiPA assay [20]. The clinical performance though not extensively investigated in this study was good as *care*HPV detected 83.3% of all cases with LSIL and all cases (100%) of HSIL/ASC-H.

Other studies have demonstrated good clinical performance of *care*HPV in HIV-seronegative African women [21] and in African women living with HIV-1. Segondy et al. [20] found the sensitivity and specificity of *care*HPV for the diagnosis of HSIL among 929 HIV-1 seropositive women in Burkina Faso and South Africa to be 88.8 and 61.8% respectively. The negative predictive value of *care*HPV for detection of cytological lesions was 99.0% in this study. This is very important because it implies that it could serve as an essential screening tool. Given its good sensitivity but low specificity, *care*HPV testing might be best performed as triage test with cytology or visual inspection (VIA) to reduce unnecessary referrals for colposcopy. It will be useful to study the cost effectiveness of such strategies in the Ghanaian socio-economic context.

To check reproducibility and hence reliability of results, 97 samples were tested in duplicate in this study by the same individual. Reproducibility was found to be 82.5%. This is good but still implies that all of the 6 processing steps be completed without fault by a meticulous lab technician to reduce the risk of having variable results, and that quality control should be routinely implemented. The positive and negative controls included for each plate serve to ensure that only valid

Table 3 Performance of *care*HPV and genotyping to detect cases of cytological abnormalities (LSIL and greater, $n = 8$) among 197 study participants in Cape Coast, Ghana

Performance Indicators	*care*HPV % (95%CI)	Anyplex II HPV 28 % (95%CI)
Number of LSIL+ cases detected by assay	7	7
Sensitivity	87.5 (47.3–99.7)	87.5 (47.3–99.7)
Specificity	52.1 (44.7–59.5)	38.8 (31.8–46.2)
Positive predictive value (PPV)	7.2 (3.0–14.3)	5.7 (2.3–11.5)
Negative predictive value (NPV)	99.0 (94.5–100.0)	98.6 (92.7–100.0)

results are read, and only a small proportion of retests we found invalid (4%). To assess the reliability of results in a study evaluating *care*HPV assay in Nigeria, researchers checked intra-rater (reproducibility of results by the same local technician) and inter-rater (reproducibility of results between 2 different local technicians) agreements. Intra-rater agreement was 98.8% ($k = 0.97$) and 98.9% ($k = 0.97$) for Technicians 1 and 2, respectively, and the inter-rater agreement was 96.3% ($k = 0.90$), suggesting that *care*HPV results were reliable [5], which is very encouraging for countries in the region. However, the higher agreement values found in the Nigerian study suggest that this can also be very dependent on locale/staff.

The present study had some limitations. The number of samples tested by *care*HPV was relatively low, owing to financial constraints and dependence on donated *care*HPV kits; and for the same reasons a more extensive repeat testing could not be organized. Furthermore, a full economic evaluation of cervical cancer screening was beyond the scope of this study. However, based on market prices and personal communication with relevant people, the cost of genotyping (including reagents and technician time) would come to approximately US$ 100.00 per sample, whereas *care*HPV cost could be about US$ 15–20.00 per sample. Other forms of cervical screening include cytology (Pap smears) being offered at a minimum of US$ 15.00 in Ghana (personal communication from facilities offering these tests), whereas visual inspection using VIA could cost as little as US$ 5.00 (up to US$ 15) [22]. As indicated by the study by Quentin et al., the feasibility of increasing uptake to achieve economies of scale in Ghana is essential for choosing a screening method [22]. The fact that HPV-based screening protocols can increase screening intervals [23, 24] and allow for possible patient self-collection [25] are important advantages that could reduce costs and increase access for both health services and Ghanaian women.

Conclusion

This study has demonstrated that *care*HPV has very good concordance with, and good performance characteristics compared to, HPV genotyping for the detection of cervical squamous intraepithelial lesions, and whilst reproducibility could be improved, the findings support the possibility of setting up HPV screening without the need for resource-intensive genotyping as a suitable alternative for cervical cancer screening in countries like Ghana.

Abbreviations

ASCUS: Atypical squamous cells of undetermined significance; CCTH: Cape Coast Teaching Hospital; CD4+: Activated T-lymphocytes CD4; CI: Confidence interval; CIN: Cervical intraepithelial neoplasia; HIV: Human Immunodeficiency Virus; HPV: Human Papilloma Virus; hr-HPV: High-Risk Human Papilloma Virus; H-SIL: High grade squamous intraepithelial lesions; KNUST: Kwame Nkrumah University of Science and Technology; LSIL: Low grade squamous

intraepithelial lesions; PLHIV: People Living with HIV; SIL: Squamous intraepithelial lesions; SSA: Sub Saharan Africa; VIA: Visual Inspection with Acetic acid

Acknowledgements
We wish to thank the staff at CCTH who helped with recruitment and follow-up management of the women, Mr Latif Abdul and Miss Anna Hayfron-Benjamin. The Commonwealth Secretariat Commission, UK, provided support to Dr. Dorcas Obiri-Yeboah to study at Kwame Nkrumah University of Science and Technology, Kumasi, Ghana and at the London School of Hygiene & Tropical Medicine, UK. Qiagen Company donated the *care*HPV brushes and the reagents for this study. Also the CERBA/LABIOGEN and Kumasi Center Collaborative Research (KCCR) laboratory staff for allowing and supporting testing in their facilities.

Funding
Funding for this research was mainly obtained from the University of Cape Coast, Ghana.

Authors' contributions
DOY study concept and design, participants' recruitment and sample collection, laboratory testing (HPV genotyping), data entry and analysis, first manuscript writing. YAS study concept and design, data review/interpretation of research findings, first manuscript writing. FD laboratory method (careHPV) and testing. KA proposal development, laboratory method (cytology). EAB data entry and analysis. DAS proposal development, data entry and analysis. JS oversight laboratory (careHPV). PM study concept and design, data review/interpretation of research findings, first manuscript writing. All authors reviewed/contributed to the manuscript and accepted final version for submission.

Competing interests
The authors declare that they have no competing interests.

Author details
[1]Department of Microbiology and Immunology, School of Medical Sciences, University of Cape Coast, Cape Coast, Ghana. [2]Department of Clinical Microbiology, School of Medical Sciences, Kwame Nkrumah University of Science and Technology, Kumasi, Ghana. [3]Laboratory of Molecular Biology and Genetics (LABIOGENE), University of Ouagadougou, Ouagadougou, Burkina Faso. [4]Department of Pathology, School of Medical Sciences, University of Cape Coast, Cape Coast, Ghana. [5]Department of Clinical Research, Faculty of Infectious and Tropical Diseases, London School of Hygiene and Tropical Medicine, London, UK.

References
1. Denny L, et al. Human papillomavirus prevalence and type distribution in invasive cervical cancer in sub-Saharan Africa. Int J Cancer. 2014; 134(6):1389–98.
2. Clifford GM, et al. Comparison of HPV type distribution in high-grade cervical lesions and cervical cancer: a meta-analysis. Br J Cancer. 2003;89(1):101–5.
3. Cuzick J, et al. New technologies and procedures for cervical cancer screening. Vaccine. 2012;30 Suppl 5:F107–16.
4. Roberts CC, et al. Comparison of real-time multiplex human papillomavirus (HPV) PCR assays with the linear array HPV genotyping PCR assay and influence of DNA extraction method on HPV detection. J Clin Microbiol. 2011;49(5):1899–906.

5. Gage JC, et al. Effectiveness of a simple rapid human papillomavirus DNA test in rural Nigeria. Int J Cancer. 2012;131(12):2903–9.

6. Ngou J, et al. Comparison of careHPV and hybrid capture 2 assays for detection of high-risk human Papillomavirus DNA in cervical samples from HIV-1-infected African women. J Clin Microbiol. 2013;51(12):4240–2.

7. Qiao YL, et al. Lower cost strategies for triage of human papillomavirus DNA-positive women. Int J Cancer. 2013;134(12):2891–901.

8. Bouvard V, et al. A review of human carcinogens; Part B: biological agents. Lancet Oncol. 2009;10(4):321–2.

9. Wright TC, et al. Primary cervical cancer screening with human papillomavirus: end of study results from the ATHENA study using HPV as the first-line screening test. Gynecol Oncol. 2015;136(2):189–97.

10. Luttmer R, et al. Comparing triage algorithms using HPV DNA genotyping, HPV E7 mRNA detection and cytology in high-risk HPV DNA-positive women. J Clin Virol. 2015;67:59–66.

11. Kwon MJ, et al. Comparison of the Anyplex II HPV28 assay with the Hybrid Capture 2 assay for the detection of HPV infection. J Clin Virol. 2014;59(4):246–9.

12. Mitchell SM, et al. Factors associated with high-risk HPV positivity in a low-resource setting in sub-Saharan Africa. Am J Obstet Gynecol. 2014;210(1):81.e1–7.

13. Qiao Y-l, et al. A new HPV-DNA test for cervical-cancer screening in developing regions: a cross-sectional study of clinical accuracy in rural China. Lancet Oncol. 2008;9(10):929–36.

14. Solomon D, et al. The 2001 Bethesda System: terminology for reporting results of cervical cytology. JAMA. 2002;287(16):2114–9.

15. Vanderpool RC, et al. Self-collecting a cervico-vaginal specimen for cervical cancer screening: An exploratory study of acceptability among medically underserved women in rural Appalachia. Gynecol Oncol. 2013;132(01):S21–25.

16. Darlin L, et al. Comparison of use of vaginal HPV self-sampling and offering flexible appointments as strategies to reach long-term non-attending women in organized cervical screening. J Clin Virol. 2013;58(1):155–60.

17. Sancho-Garnier H, et al. HPV self-sampling or the Pap-smear: a randomized study among cervical screening nonattenders from lower socioeconomic groups in France. Int J Cancer. 2013;133(11):2681–7.

18. Zhao FH, et al. An evaluation of novel, lower-cost molecular screening tests for human papillomavirus in rural China. Cancer Prev Res (Phila). 2013;6(9):938–48.

19. Trope LA, Chumworathayi B, Blumenthal PD. Feasibility of community-based careHPV for cervical cancer prevention in rural Thailand. J Low Genit Tract Dis. 2013;17(3):315–9.

20. Segondy M, et al. Performance of careHPV for detecting high-grade cervical intraepithelial neoplasia among women living with HIV-1 in Burkina Faso and South Africa: HARP study. Br J Cancer. 2016;115(4):425–30.

21. Jeronimo J, et al. A Multicountry Evaluation of careHPV Testing, Visual Inspection With Acetic Acid, and Papanicolaou Testing for the Detection of Cervical Cancer. Int J Gynecol Cancer. 2014;24(3):576–85.

22. Quentin W, et al. Costs of cervical cancer screening and treatment using visual inspection with acetic acid (VIA) and cryotherapy in Ghana: the importance of scale. Trop Med Int Health. 2011;16(3):379–89.

23. Kitchener HC, et al. The clinical effectiveness and cost-effectiveness of primary human papillomavirus cervical screening in England: extended follow-up of the ARTISTIC randomised trial cohort through three screening rounds. Health Technol Assess. 2014;18(23):1–196.

24. Lew JB, et al. Effectiveness Modelling and Economic Evaluation of Primary HPV Screening for Cervical Cancer Prevention in New Zealand. PLoS One. 2016;11(5):e0151619.

25. Jentschke M, Soergel P, Hillemanns P. Evaluation of a multiplex real time PCR assay for the detection of human papillomavirus infections on self-collected cervicovaginal lavage samples. J Virol Methods. 2013;193(1):131–4.

Permissions

All chapters in this book were first published in GORP, by BioMed Central; hereby published with permission under the Creative Commons Attribution License or equivalent. Every chapter published in this book has been scrutinized by our experts. Their significance has been extensively debated. The topics covered herein carry significant findings which will fuel the growth of the discipline. They may even be implemented as practical applications or may be referred to as a beginning point for another development.

The contributors of this book come from diverse backgrounds, making this book a truly international effort. This book will bring forth new frontiers with its revolutionizing research information and detailed analysis of the nascent developments around the world.

We would like to thank all the contributing authors for lending their expertise to make the book truly unique. They have played a crucial role in the development of this book. Without their invaluable contributions this book wouldn't have been possible. They have made vital efforts to compile up to date information on the varied aspects of this subject to make this book a valuable addition to the collection of many professionals and students.

This book was conceptualized with the vision of imparting up-to-date information and advanced data in this field. To ensure the same, a matchless editorial board was set up. Every individual on the board went through rigorous rounds of assessment to prove their worth. After which they invested a large part of their time researching and compiling the most relevant data for our readers.

The editorial board has been involved in producing this book since its inception. They have spent rigorous hours researching and exploring the diverse topics which have resulted in the successful publishing of this book. They have passed on their knowledge of decades through this book. To expedite this challenging task, the publisher supported the team at every step. A small team of assistant editors was also appointed to further simplify the editing procedure and attain best results for the readers.

Apart from the editorial board, the designing team has also invested a significant amount of their time in understanding the subject and creating the most relevant covers. They scrutinized every image to scout for the most suitable representation of the subject and create an appropriate cover for the book.

The publishing team has been an ardent support to the editorial, designing and production team. Their endless efforts to recruit the best for this project, has resulted in the accomplishment of this book. They are a veteran in the field of academics and their pool of knowledge is as vast as their experience in printing. Their expertise and guidance has proved useful at every step. Their uncompromising quality standards have made this book an exceptional effort. Their encouragement from time to time has been an inspiration for everyone.

The publisher and the editorial board hope that this book will prove to be a valuable piece of knowledge for researchers, students, practitioners and scholars across the globe.

List of Contributors

Lisa Grace, Regina Whitaker and Angeles Alvarez Secord
Division of Gynecologic Oncology, Duke Cancer Institute, Durham, NC 27710, USA

Micael Lopez-Acevedo
Division of Gynecologic Oncology, Duke Cancer Institute, Durham, NC 27710, USA
DUMC 3079, Gynecologic Oncology, Duke University Medical Center, Durham, NC 27710, USA

Deanna Teoh
Division of Gynecologic Oncology, University of Minnesota, Minneapolis, MN 55455, USA

David J Adams and Andrew B Nixon
Department of Medicine, Duke University Medical Center, Durham, NC 27710, USA

Jingquan Jia
East Carolina University School of Medicine, Greenville, NC 27834, USA

Krishnansu S. Tewari
The Division of Gynecologic Oncology, University of California, Irvine Medical Center, The City Tower, 333 City Blvd W., Orange, CA 92868, USA

Netsanet Belete
Ethiopian Public Health Institute, Health System Research Directorate, Addis Ababa, Ethiopian

Yosief Tsige
Addis Ababa University, Allied School of Health Science, Addis Ababa, Ethiopian

Habtamu Mellie
Debre Markos University, College of Medicine and Health Science, Department of Public Health, Debre Markos, Ethiopia

Andreas Obermair
Queensland Centre for Gynaecological Cancer, The University of Queensland, Brisbane, QLD, Australia.
2Greenslopes Private Hospital, Brisbane, QLD, Australia
Queensland Centre for Gynaecological Cancer, c/o Royal Brisbane and Women's Hospital, Butterfield Street, Herston, Brisbane, QLD 4029, Australia

Donal J. Brennan
Rotunda Hospital, Dublin, Ireland

Eva Baxter
QIMR Berghofer Medical Research Institute, Brisbane, QLD, Australia.

Jane E. Armes
Anatomical Pathology Mater Health Services, Mater Adult Hospital, and Mater Research Institute-University of Queensland, Brisbane, QLD, Australia

Val Gebski
University of Sydney NHMRC Clinical Trials Centre, Sydney, NSW, Australia

Monika Janda
School of Public Health, Institute for Health and Biomedical Innovation, Queensland University of Technology, Brisbane, QLD, Australia

Neville F. Hacker and Archana Rao
Gynaecological Cancer Centre, Royal Hospital for Women, Randwick, NSW 2031, Australia
School of Women's and Children's Health, University of New South Wales, Kensington, NSW 2052, Australia

John H Farley
Division of Gynecologic Oncology, Department of Obstetrics and Gynecology, University of Arizona Cancer Center, 500 W. Thomas Road, Suite 600, Phoenix, AZ 85013, USA

Cassandra D Foss, Bradley J Monk and Dana M Chase
Division of Gynecologic Oncology, Department of Obstetrics and Gynecology, University of Arizona Cancer Center, 500 W. Thomas Road, Suite 600, Phoenix, AZ 85013, USA
Creighton University School of Medicine at Dignity Health St. Joseph's Hospital and Medical Center, 500 W. Thomas Road, Suite 600, Phoenix, AZ 85013, USA

Heather J Dalton
Department of Gynecologic Oncology and Reproductive Medicine, The University of Texas MD Anderson Cancer Center, Houston, TX, USA

Jonathan R. Foote, Stephanie Gaillard, Brittany Davidson, Angeles Alvarez Secord, Monica B. Jones and Laura J. Havrilesky
Division of Gynecologic Oncology, Duke University Medical Center, 2301 Erwin Rd, Durham, NC 27710, USA

Gloria Broadwater
Biostatistics, Duke Cancer Institute, Duke University, 2301 Erwin Rd, Durham, NC 27710, USA

Mohamed A. Adam
Department of Surgery, Duke University Medical Center, 2301 Erwin Rd, Durham, NC 27710, USA

Julie A. Sosa
Department of Surgery, Duke University Medical Center, 2301 Erwin Rd, Durham, NC 27710, USA
Duke Clinical Research Institute, Durham, USA

Junzo Chino
Division of Radiation Oncology, Duke University Medical Center, 2301 Erwin Rd, Durham, NC 27710, USA

Robert S. Meehan and Alice P. Chen
Early Clinical Trials Development Program Division of Cancer Treatment and Diagnosis (DCTD), National Institutes of Health (NIH) National Cancer Institute (NCI), 10 Center Drive, Bldg 31, 3A44, Bethesda MD 20892, USA

Sarah E. Paraghamian, Teresa C. Longoria and Ramez N. Eskander
Department of Obstetrics and Gynecology, Division of Gynecologic Oncology, University of California Irvine Medical Center, 33 City Blvd. West #1400, Orange, CA 92868, USA

Gillian E. Hanley, Jessica N. McAlpine and Janice S. Kwon
Department of Gynaecology and Obstetrics, Division of Gynaecologic Oncology, University of British Columbia, Vancouver, BC, Canada

Gillian Mitchell
Hereditary Cancer Program, BC Cancer Agency, Vancouver, BC, Canada
Department of Medicine, University of British Columbia, Vancouver, BC, Canada

Steven J Gibson, Bradley J Monk and Dana M Chase
The Division of Gynecologic Oncology, University of Arizona Cancer Center, 500 West Thomas Road, Suite 600, Phoenix, AZ 85013, USA

Creighton University School of Medicine, St. Joseph's Hospital and Medical Center, A Dignity Health Member, 500 West Thomas Road, Suite 600, Phoenix, AZ 85013, USA

Krishnansu S Tewari
The Division of Gynecologic Oncology, Department of Obstetrics and Gynecology, The Chao Family Comprehensive Cancer Center, University of California, Irvine Medical Center, 101 The City Drive South, Building 56, Room 275, Orange, CA 92868, USA.

Melissa K. Frey
Division of Gynecologic Oncology, Weill Cornell Medicine, 525 East 68th Street, Suite J-130, New York, NY 10065, USA

Bhavana Pothuri
Division of Gynecologic Oncology, New York University Langone Medical Center, 240 E. 38th St, 19th floor, New York, NY 10016, USA

Nimisha Agrawal and Hanoon P. Pokharel
Department of Obstetrics and Gynaecology, B.P. Koirala Institute of Health Sciences, Dharan, Nepal

Reshu Agrawal Sagtani and Shyam Sundar Budhathoki
School of Public Health and Community Medicine, B.P. Koirala Institute of Health Sciences, Dharan, Nepal.

Heather J Dalton
The University of Texas MD Anderson Cancer Center, Houston, TX, USA

James Fiorica
Sarasota Memorial Hospital, Sarasota, FL, USA

Candace K McClure
Precision Therapeutics, Inc, Pittsburgh, PA, USA

Rodney P Rocconi
University of South Alabama Mitchell Cancer Institute, Mobile, AL, USA

Fernando O Recio
South Florida Center for Gynecologic Oncology, Boca Raton, FL, USA

John L Levocchio
North Shore LIJ Health System/Biomedical Research Alliance of New York, Manhassett, NY, USA

Matthew O Burrell
Georgia Gynecologic Oncology, Atlanta, GA, USA

Bradley J Monk
University of Arizona Cancer Center, Creighton University School of Medicine at Dignity Health St. Joseph's Hospital and Medical Center, 500 W. Thomas Road, Suite 600, Phoenix, AZ 85013, USA

Karla Willows and Genevieve Lennox1
Division of Gynecologic Oncology, Department of Obstetrics and Gynecology, University of Toronto, M700-610 University Avenue, Toronto M5G 2 M9, ON, Canada

Allan Covens
Division of Gynecologic Oncology, Department of Obstetrics and Gynecology, University of Toronto, M700-610 University Avenue, Toronto M5G 2 M9, ON, Canada
Division of Gynecologic Oncology, T2051 Odette Cancer Centre, University of Toronto, 2075 Bayview Avenue, Toronto M4N 3 M5, ON, Canada

Hassan Errihani
Department of Oncology, National Institute of Oncology, Avenue Allal El Fassi, BP 6542, Rabat 10100, Maroc

Ablavi Adani-Ifè
Department of Oncology, National Institute of Oncology, Avenue Allal El Fassi, BP 6542, Rabat 10100, Maroc
Department of Oncology, Paul Brousse University Hospital AP-HP, 12-14 Avenue Paul Vaillant Couturier, 94800 Villejuif, France

Emma Goldschmidt, Pasquale Innominato, Ayhan Ulusakarya and Jean François Morère
Department of Oncology, Paul Brousse University Hospital AP-HP, 12-14 Avenue Paul Vaillant Couturier, 94800 Villejuif, France

Philippe Bertheau
Laboratory of Cytopathology, Saint Louis Hospital AP-HP, Avenue Claude Vellefaux, 75010 Paris, France

Radoslav Chekerov Yoana Nedkova and Isil Yalcinkaya
Department of Gynaecology, European Competence Centre for Ovarian Cancer, Charité Universitätsmedizin, Berlin, Germany

Jalid Sehouli
Department of Gynaecology, European Competence Centre for Ovarian Cancer, Charité Universitätsmedizin, Berlin, Germany
North-Eastern German Society for Gynaecologic Oncology, Ovarian Cancer Study Group, Berlin, Germany

Philipp Harter
Department of Gynaecology and Gynaecologic Oncology, Kliniken Essen Mitte, Essen, Germany

Stefan Fuxius
Onkologische Schwerpunktpraxis Heidelberg, Heidelberg, Germany

Lars Christian Hanker
Department of Gynaecology and Obstetrics, Gynaecological Cancer Center of the University Schleswig-Holstein, Campus Lübeck, Lübeck, Germany

Linn Woelber
Department of Gynaecology and Gynaecologic Oncology, University Medical Center Hamburg-Eppendorf, Hamburg, Germany

Lothar Müller
Onkologische Schwerpunktpraxis Leer, Leer, Germany

Peter Klare
Praxisklinik Krebsheilkunde für Frauen, Berlin, Germany

Gülten Oskay-Oezcelik
Praxisklinik Krebsheilkunde für Frauen, Berlin, Germany
North-Eastern German Society for Gynaecologic Oncology, Ovarian Cancer Study Group, Berlin, Germany

Wolfgang Abenhardt
Onkologische Schwerpunktpraxis im Elisenhof, Munich, Germany

Georg Heinrich
Gynäkologisch-onkologische Schwerpunktpraxis, Fürstenwalde, Germany

Harald Sommer and Sven Mahner
Department of Gynaecology and Obstetrics and Comprehensive Cancer Center, University of Munich, Munich, Germany

Pauline Wimberger
Department of Gynecology and Obstetrics, Technische Universität Dresden, Dresden, Germany

Dominique Koensgen-Mustea
Department of Gynaecology and Obstetrics, University Medicine Greifswald, Greifswald, Germany

Rolf Richter
North-Eastern German Society for Gynaecologic Oncology, Ovarian Cancer Study Group, Berlin, Germany

Nancy Innocentia Ebu
Department of Public Health, School of Nursing and Midwifery, University of Cape Coast, Cape Coast, Ghana

Brett Miles
Department of Otolaryngology, Icahn School of Medicine at Mount Sinai, New York, NY, USA

Howard P. Safran
Brown University Oncology Research Group, Providence, RI, USA

Bradley J. Monk
Division of Gynecologic Oncology, Arizona Oncology (US Oncology Network), University of Arizona College of Medicine, Creighton University School of Medicine at St. Joseph's Hospital, 2222 E. Highland Ave, Suite 400, Phoenix, AZ 85016, USA

Amsalu Degu and Peter Karimi
Department of Pharmaceutics and Pharmacy Practice, University of Nairobi, College of Health Sciences, School of Pharmacy, Nairobi, Kenya

Peter Njogu
Department of Pharmaceutical Chemistry, University of Nairobi, College of Health Sciences, School of Pharmacy, Nairobi 19676-00202, Kenya

Irene Weru
Kenyatta National Hospital, Division of Pharmacy, Nairobi 20723-00202, Kenya

Neville F. Hacker
Gynaecologic Cancer Centre, Royal Hospital for Women, Sydney, Australia
School of Women's and Children's Health, University of New South Wales, Sydney, Australia

Hanoon P. Pokharel
Gynaecologic Cancer Centre, Royal Hospital for Women, Sydney, Australia
School of Women's and Children's Health, University of New South Wales, Sydney, Australia
Department of Obstetrics and Gynaecology, B P Koirala Institute of Health Sciences, Dharan, Nepal

Lesley Andrews
Hereditary Cancer Clinic, Prince of Wales Hospital, Sydney, Australia
School of Medicine, University of New South Wales, Sydney, Australia

Brett A. Miles
Division of Head and Neck Cancer Surgery, Department of Otolaryngology, Icahn School of Medicine at Mount Sinai, One Gustave L. Levy Place, New York, NY 10029, USA

Bradley J. Monk
Division of Gynecologic Oncology, University of Arizona College of Medicine, Creighton University School of Medicine at Dignity Health St. Joseph's Hospital and Medical Center, Phoenix, AZ, USA.

Howard P. Safran
Brown University Oncology Research Group, Providence, RI, USA

K. S. Tewari
Division of Gynecologic Oncology, Department of Obstetrics and Gynecology, University of California, Irvine, The City Tower, 333 City Blvd, West – Suite 1400, Orange, CA, USA

A. Agarwal
Medical Oncology, Dr. B.L. Kapur Memorial Hospital, New Delhi, India

A. Pathak
Cancer Care Hospital, Nagpur, Maharashtra, India

A. Ramesh
Apollo Speciality Hospital, Chennai, Tamil Nadu, India

B. Parikh
Bombay Hospital, Mumbai, Maharashtra, India

M. Singhal
Indraprastha Apollo Hospitals, New Delhi, India

G. Saini
Max Super Speciality Hospital, Vaishali, India

P. V. Sushma
KIMS Hospital, Hyderabad, Telangana, India

N. Huilgol
Nanavati Hospital, Mumbai, Maharashtra, India

S. Gundeti
Nizams Institute Medical Sciences, Hyderabad, Telangana, India

S. Gupta
Medanta Hospital, Gurgaon, Haryana, India

S. Nangia
Indraprastha Apollo Hospital, Delhi, India

S. Rawat
Dharamshila Hospital, New Delhi, India

S. Alurkar
Apollo Hospitals, Ahmedabad, Gujarat, India

V. Goswami
Fortis Hospital, Noida, Uttar Pradesh, India

B. Swarup, B. Ugile, S. Jain and A. Kukreja
Roche Products (India) Pvt. Ltd., Mumbai, Maharastra, India

Vicky Makker and Angela K. Green
Gynecologic Medical Oncology Service, Department of Surgery, Memorial Sloan Kettering Cancer Center and Weill Cornell Medical College, 1275 York Avenue, New York, TX 10065, USA

Robert M. Wenham
Department of Gynecologic Oncology, H. Lee Moffitt Cancer Center, Tampa, FL, USA

David Mutch
Division of Gynecologic Oncology, Washington University School of Medicine, St Louis, MO, USA

Brittany Davidson
Division of Gynecologic Oncology, Duke University Medical Center, Duke Cancer Institute, Durham, NC, USA

David Scott Miller
Division of Gynecologic Oncology, University of Texas Southwestern Medical Center, Dallas, USA

D. Barnes, R. Rivera, C. Craig, B. Monk and D. Chase
Department of Gynecologic Oncology, Creighton University School of Medicine at St. Joseph's Hospital and Medical Center, Phoenix, AZ, USA

S. Gibson and J. Cragun
University of Arizona Cancer Center, Tucson, AZ, USA

Tran N. Le
Department of Obstetrics, Gynecology, and Reproductive Sciences, UTHealth McGovern Medical School, 6431 Fannin Street, Rm. 3.152, Houston, TX 77030, USA

Judith A. Smith
Department of Obstetrics, Gynecology, and Reproductive Sciences, UTHealth McGovern Medical School, 6431 Fannin Street, Rm. 3.152, Houston, TX 77030, USA
UTHealth-Memorial Hermann Cancer Center-TMC, Houston, TX, USA

Rachel E. Harvey
MBS Pharmacy, Round Rock, TX, USA

Christine K. Kim and Robert L. Coleman
University of Texas M.D. Anderson Cancer Center, Houston, TX, USA

Jubilee Brown
Levine Cancer Institute, Carolinas HealthCare System, Charlotte, NC, USA

Dorcas Obiri-Yeboah, Ebenezer Aniakwa-Bonsu and Daniel Amoako-Sakyi
Department of Microbiology and Immunology, School of Medical Sciences, University of Cape Coast, Cape Coast, Ghana

Yaw Adu-Sarkodie
Department of Clinical Microbiology, School of Medical Sciences, Kwame Nkrumah University of Science and Technology, Kumasi, Ghana

Florencia Djigma and Jacques Simpore
Laboratory of Molecular Biology and Genetics (LABIOGENE), University of Ouagadougou, Ouagadougou, Burkina Faso

Kafui Akakpo
Department of Pathology, School of Medical Sciences, University of Cape Coast, Cape Coast, Ghana

Philippe Mayaud
Department of Clinical Research, Faculty of Infectious and Tropical Diseases, London School of Hygiene and Tropical Medicine, London, UK

Index

www.ingramcontent.com/pod-product-compliance
Lightning Source LLC
Chambersburg PA
CBHW080505200326
41458CB00012B/4090